ATLAS OF
PEDIATRIC PHYSICAL DIAGNOSIS

A **Slide Atlas of Pediatric Physical Diagnosis**, based on the material presented in this book, is also available. The Slide Atlas is organized into 20 topic-based volumes, each of which corresponds to a chapter in the book. Each volume consists of superbly illustrated text, with 35mm color slides corresponding to the photographs in the text. In this unique format, all of the slides are labeled, numbered, and indexed for easy reference. In addition, each unit is presented in a durable vinyl binder, and the complete collection comes in an attractive and sturdy presentation slip case. In its entirety, the **Slide Atlas of Pediatric Physical Diagnosis** comprises over 1000 slides and 400 pages of text.

The **Slide Atlas of Pediatric Physical Diagnosis** may be purchased as a complete set of 20 volumes or in individual volumes.

Volume 1 Genetics: Common Chromosomal Disorders	25 slides
Volume 2 Neonatology	46 slides
Volume 3 Developmental Pediatrics	48 slides
Volume 4 Pediatric Allergy and Immunology	58 slides
Volume 5 Pediatric Cardiology	35 slides
Volume 6 Child Abuse and Neglect	25 slides
Volume 7 Pediatric Rheumatology	37 slides
Volume 8 Pediatric Dermatology	100 slides
Volume 9 Pediatric Endocrinology	25 slides
Volume 10 Pediatric Nutrition and Gastroenterology	37 slides
Volume 11 Pediatric Hematology	67 slides
Volume 12 Pediatric Infectious Disease	67 slides
Volume 13 Renal and Genitourinary Disorders	40 slides
Volume 14 Pediatric Neurology	40 slides
Volume 15 Pediatric Surgery	92 slides
Volume 16 Pediatric and Adolescent Gynecology	40 slides
Volume 17 Pediatric Ophthalmology	80 slides
Volume 18 Oral Disorders	52 slides
Volume 19 Pediatric Orthopedics	84 slides
Volume 20 Pediatric Otolaryngology	78 slides

For further information, please contact:
Gower Medical Publishing
101 Fifth Avenue
New York, NY 10003

ATLAS OF
PEDIATRIC PHYSICAL DIAGNOSIS

Edited by

Basil J. Zitelli, M.D.
Associate Professor of Pediatrics
University of Pittsburgh
School of Medicine
Staff Pediatrician
Children's Hospital of Pittsburgh

Holly W. Davis, M.D.
Assistant Professor of Pediatrics
University of Pittsburgh
School of Medicine
Medical Director
Emergency Department
Children's Hospital of Pittsburgh

Foreword by
Frank A. Oski, M.D.
Given Professor of Pediatrics
The Johns Hopkins University
School of Medicine
Baltimore

The C.V. Mosby Company
St. Louis • Toronto

Gower Medical Publishing
New York • London

Distributed in all countries except USA, Canada and
Japan by:

Edward Arnold
A Division of Hodder and Stoughton
LONDON   MELBOURNE   AUCKLAND

Distributed in the USA by:

C.V. Mosby Company
11830 Westline Industrial Drive
St Louis
Missouri 63146
USA

Distributed in Canada by:

C.V. Mosby Limited
5240 Finch Avenue East
Scarborough
Ontario M1S 4P2
Canada

Library of Congress Cataloging in Publication Data

   Atlas of pediatric physical diagnosis.

      Includes bibliographies and index.
      1. Children – Diseases – Diagnosis.   2. Physical
diagnosis.   I. Zitelli, Basil J. (Basil John),
1946-   . II. Davis, Holly W., 1945-
[DNLM: 1. Diagnosis – in infancy & childhood –
atlases.   2. Physical Examination – in infancy &
childhood – atlases.   WS 17 A881]
RJ50.A86   1987   618.92'00754   86-19492
   ISBN 0 912143 053 (Gower)
        0 7131 45390 (Edward Arnold)
        0-8016-5728-8 (C.V. Mosby)

Project Editors
   Abe Krieger
   Joy Noel Travalino
Book Design
   Lisa Altomare
   Rebecca Brackett
   Carol Drozdyk
Illustration
   Alan Landau
   Laura Pardi

Reprinted in Singapore in 1989 by Imago Productions FE (PTE) Ltd.

Print number 7 6 5 4 3 2 1

FOREWORD

There are four basic methods by which a physician makes a diagnosis. The four methods are: instant recognition, hypothesis generation and testing, the use of algorithm, and sampling of the universe in apparently random fashion.

When instant recognition is possible, the other means of making a diagnosis, more time consuming and more expensive, become unnecessary. Instant recognition is usually based on experience—"I've seen that before"—the older clinician will more often remark.

The more you know the more you will see, and conversely, the more you see the more you will know. Although there may not be any true substitute for experience, the superb collection of photographs assembled by Doctors Basil Zitelli and Holly Davis in this **Atlas of Pediatric Physical Diagnosis** comes as close to being there as any I have ever seen.

All diseases and syndromes have their characteristic signs and symptoms, but a sign is not a sign when it cannot be read. Hours spent with these nearly 1200 photographs will lead to improved sign-reading and a heightened capacity for diagnosis by instant recognition.

Frank A. Oski, M.D.
Given Professor of Pediatrics
The Johns Hopkins University
School of Medicine

To our parents, who were our first teachers

Hannah L. Zitelli and Patsy A. Zitelli
Ruth Holmes Davis and William S. Davis

To those exceptional teachers we have had,
whose dedication, enthusiasm and creativity
helped make the acquisition, application and
sharing of knowledge more fun than hard
work, and who inspired us not only to perform
to the best of our ability, but also to become
teachers as well as physicians

John Altrocchi, Ph.D., Morton Bogdanoff, M.D.,
Arthur Ferguson, Ph.D., Henry Furrie, Paul C. Gaffney, M.D.,
Arthur Glaeser, Robert Kudra, Hans Lowenbach, M.D.,
Lois A. Pounds, M.D., Francis G. Reilly, M.D., Elizabeth Robenheimer,
Elizabeth Seipel, Estelle Tankard, Catherine M. Wilfert, M.D.,
William H. Zinkham, M.D., J.R. Zuberbueller, M.D.

To our residents and students, whose eagerness
to learn and to put their knowledge to use
keeps us learning actively and makes teaching
so rewarding

PREFACE

For many disorders, visual recognition is a major factor in making the correct diagnosis, hence, the advantage of the experienced clinician who has seen so much and the spectra of so many disorders. This book was developed for students, residents, practitioners and nurses who care for children, to aid them in diagnosing pediatric disorders through inspection of the patient or review of simple laboratory tests. Our goal is to broaden the visual experience of the clinician. This Atlas is by no means encyclopedic but rather presents an overview of problems that lend themselves to visual diagnosis. The accompanying text deliberately emphasizes pertinent historical factors, visual findings and techniques of examination and diagnostic methods, rather than therapy. We have also attempted to select disorders that are common and/or important, and where relevant, to describe the spectrum of clinical findings. It is our hope that this Atlas will serve as a useful and practical reference whether in an office, a clinic, or an emergency department.

Basil J. Zitelli, M.D.
Holly W. Davis, M.D.

ACKNOWLEDGMENTS

The seed for this Atlas was planted by Dr. Sylvan Stool, a pediatric otolaryngologist with an intense interest in visual diagnosis and teaching. The staff at Gower Medical Publishing helped us to get the project off the ground and have nurtured it from inception to fruition. This effort could not have succeeded without the organizational skills and initiative of Sandra Arjona, our editorial consultant. Photographs were gathered by the authors largely from their patient populations and clinical material at Children's Hospital of Pittsburgh. Most of these were taken by our Department of Photography. Norman Rabinowitz, Douglas Sellars, William Winstein, Jr., and Kathleen Muffie deserve special credit for being at our beck and call for months on end. Bernadette Marshalek merits high praise for scouring the radiology teaching files for many of the radiographs that appear in the book.

Dr. Ellen Wald, Dr. Kenneth Schuit, and Mrs. Sue Evans Hughes also have been exceptionally helpful in reviewing chapters. Darleen Chiponis, PNP, and Joy Harris, RN, devoted a great deal of time to proofreading, and Mrs. Helen Schorner worked tirelessly typing and retyping many of the manuscripts. We would also like to acknowledge the assistance of all the other secretaries who helped in manuscript preparation.

Special acknowledgment must go to the contributing authors who unselfishly devoted their valuable time, effort, and case material. Indeed, their work supports the old maxim, "The whole art of medicine is in observation."

CONTENTS

CONTRIBUTORS

Ellis D. Avner, M.D.
Associate Professor of Pediatrics and Nephrology
University of Pittsburgh School of Medicine
Staff Nephrologist, Children's Hospital of Pittsburgh

Roberta E. Bauer, M.D.
Clinical Instructor of Pediatrics
University of Pittsburgh School of Medicine
Medical Director, Infant and Family Development
  Program, D.T. Watson Rehabilitation Hospital
  for Children and Adults, Pittsburgh

Julie Blatt, M.D.
Assistant Professor of Pediatrics
University of Pittsburgh School of Medicine
Director of Research, Hematology/Oncology, Children's
  Hospital of Pittsburgh

A'Delbert Bowen, M.D.
Associate Professor of Radiology
University of Pittsburgh School of Medicine
Staff Radiologist, Children's Hospital of Pittsburgh

Holly W. Davis, M.D.
Assistant Professor of Pediatrics
University of Pittsburgh School of Medicine
Medical Director, Emergency Department, Children's
  Hospital of Pittsburgh

Rodrigo Dominguez, M.D.
Associate Professor of Radiology
The University of Texas Medical School at Houston
Staff Radiologist, The University Children's Hospital
Houston, Texas

Demetrius Ellis, M.D.
Associate Professor of Pediatrics and Nephrology
University of Pittsburgh School of Medicine
Director, Nephrology, Children's Hospital of Pittsburgh

David N. Finegold, M.D.
Assistant Professor of Pediatrics and Medicine
University of Pittsburgh School of Medicine
Staff Endocrinologist, Children's Hospital of Pittsburgh

Philip Fireman, M.D.
Professor of Pediatrics
University of Pittsburgh School of Medicine
Director, Allergy and Immunology, Children's Hospital of
  Pittsburgh

Roger A. Friedman, M.D.
Assistant Clinical Professor of Allergy
Ohio State University School of Medicine
Assistant Clinical Professor of Pediatrics,
  Columbus Children's Hospital
Columbus, Ohio

J. Carlton Gartner, Jr., M.D.
Associate Professor of Pediatrics
University of Pittsburgh School of Medicine
Director, Diagnostic Referral Service, Children's Hospital
  of Pittsburgh

Melissa Hamp, M.D.
Assistant Professor of Pediatrics
University of Pittsburgh School of Medicine
Director of Adolescent Medicine, Ambulatory Care
  Center, Children's Hospital of Pittsburgh

Edward N. Hanley, Jr., M.D.
Assistant Professor of Orthopedic Surgery
University of Pittsburgh School of Medicine
Staff Orthopedic Surgeon, Presbyterian-University
  Hospital and Children's Hospital of Pittsburgh

David A. Hiles, M.D.
Clinical Professor of Ophthalmology
University of Pittsburgh School of Medicine
Chief of Ophthalmology, Children's Hospital of
  Pittsburgh

Ian R. Holzman, M.D.
Associate Professor of Pediatrics, Obstetrics and
  Gynecology
University of Pittsburgh School of Medicine
Staff Neonatologist, Magee-Women's Hospital
Pittsburgh

Jocyline Ledesma-Medina, M.D.
Professor of Radiology
University of Pittsburgh School of Medicine
Staff Radiologist, Children's Hospital of Pittsburgh

Cora C. Lenox, M.D.
Professor Emeritus of Pediatrics
University of Pittsburgh School of Medicine
Emeritus Staff, Children's Hospital of Pittsburgh

David A. Lloyd, M.D.
Associate Professor of Pediatric Surgery

University of Pittsburgh School of Medicine
Staff Pediatrician, Children's Hospital of Pittsburgh

J. Jeffrey Malatack, M.D.
Associate Professor of Pediatrics
University of Pittsburgh School of Medicine
Staff Pediatrician, Children's Hospital of Pittsburgh

Susan Bayliss Mallory, M.D.
Assistant Professor of Dermatology and Pediatrics
University of Arkansas for Medical Sciences
Staff Dermatologist, University Hospital
Little Rock, Arkansas

Mamoun M. Nazif, D.D.S.
Clinical Professor
University of Pittsburgh School of Dental Medicine
Chief, Dental Services, Children's Hospital of Pittsburgh

Lila Penchansky, M.D.
Associate Professor of Pathology
University of Pittsburgh School of Medicine
Director of Hematology, Children's Hospital of Pittsburgh

Mary Ann Ready, D.M.D.
Assistant Professor of Pediatric Dentistry
Medical College of Georgia
Staff, Eugene Talmadge Memorial Hospital
Augusta, Georgia

James S. Reilly, M.D.
Associate Professor, Department of Surgery, Division of
  Otorhinolaryngology
University of Alabama at Birmingham
Otorhinolaryngologist in Chief, Children's Hospital of
  Alabama

David P. Skoner, M.D.
Assistant Professor of Pediatrics
University of Pittsburgh School of Medicine
Director, Asthma Clinic; Clinical Associate Physician of
  the Clinical Research Center, Children's Hospital of
  Pittsburgh

Mark W. Steele, M.D.
Associate Professor of Pediatrics
University of Pittsburgh School of Medicine
Director, Division of Medical Genetics, Children's
  Hospital of Pittsburgh

Paul K. Stillwagon, M.D.
Allergy/Immunology Fellow
Children's Hospital of Pittsburgh

Andrew H. Urbach, M.D.
Assistant Professor of Pediatrics
University of Pittsburgh School of Medicine
Staff Pediatrician, Children's Hospital of Pittsburgh

W. Timothy Ward, M.D.
Assistant Professor of Orthopedic Surgery
University of Pittsburgh School of Medicine
Staff Physician, Pediatric Orthopedics, Children's
  Hospital of Pittsburgh

Henry B. Wessel, M.D.
Assistant Professor of Pediatrics and Neurology
University of Pittsburgh School of Medicine
Staff, Division of Child Neurology, Children's Hospital of
  Pittsburgh

Lionel W. Young, M.D.
Professor of Radiology and Pediatrics
University of Pittsburgh School of Medicine
Director of Radiology, Children's Hospital of Pittsburgh

Basil J. Zitelli, M.D.
Associate Professor of Pediatrics
University of Pittsburgh School of Medicine
Staff Pediatrician, Children's Hospital of Pittsburgh

John A. Zitelli, M.D.
Associate Professor of Dermatology
University of Pittsburgh School of Medicine
Chief, Cutaneous Surgery, Dermatology Department,
  Falk Clinic
Pittsburgh

GENETICS: COMMON CHROMOSOMAL DISORDERS

Mark W. Steele, M.D.

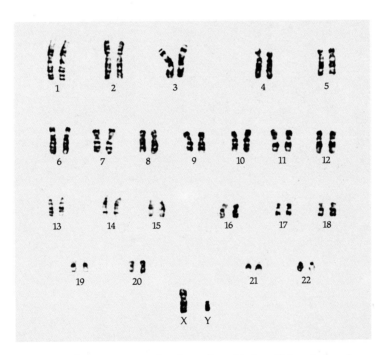

FIG. 1.1 *Photomicrographs show that this is a G-banded male karyotype (a female would have two X chromosomes and no Y chromosome). The horizontal banding produced by the Giemsa staining technique allows for precise identification of homologous chromosomes.*

GENERAL PRINCIPLES

The Nature of Chromosomes

The human hereditary factors are located in the genes (the genome): 5 percent (about 50,000) structural genes that code for proteins (such as enzymes), and the other 95 percent whose function is not clear. The genes are composed of deoxyribonucleic acid (DNA) and are stored in intranuclear cell organelles called chromosomes. Each chromosome contains one linear DNA molecule folded over onto itself several times, as well as ribonucleic acid (RNA) and proteins. Since all genes exist in pairs, all chromosomes must likewise exist in pairs. The members of each pair of genes are called alleles; and of each pair of chromosomes, homologues. The conventional depiction of the constitution of homologues in the nucleus is called the cell's karotype (Fig. 1.1). If at any gene locus the alleles are identical, that gene locus is said to be homozygous. If the alleles are not identical, the gene locus is heterozygous.

Except for gametes, normal human cells contain 23 pairs of chromosomes, 46 in all. One of these pairs is concerned, in part, with inducing the primary sex of the embryonic gonads. These sex chromosomes are called the X and Y chromosomes, and are not genetically homologous except in a few areas. Females have two X chromosomes while males have an X and a Y chromosome. The remaining 22 pairs are called autosomes and determine non-sex-related (somatic) characteristics.

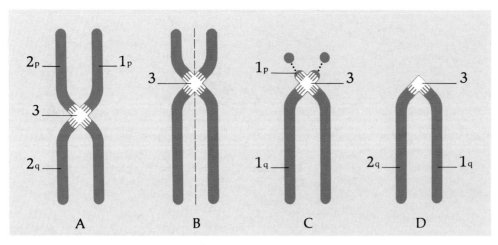

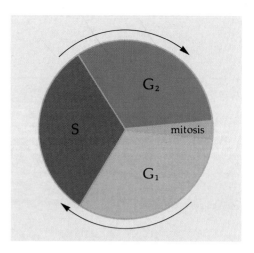

FIG. 1.2 The morphology of a chromosome during metaphase. **A** Metacentric chromosome with centromere (3) in middle; **B** submetacentric chromosome with centromere off center; **C** acrocentric chromosome with centromere near one end; **D** telocentric chromosome (not found in humans) with centromere at one end. The DNA of the chromosome has replicated to form two chromatids: lp and lq represent one complete chromatid, 2p and 2q the other complete chromatid. The chromosome will then divide longitudinally as shown in **B**.

FIG. 1.3 The in vitro life cycle of a somatic cell. Interphase lasts 21 hours and can be divided into three stages:
G_1 (7 hours)—cell performs its tasks;
S (7 hours)—DNA replicates;
G_2 (7 hours)—cell prepares to divide (mitosis).

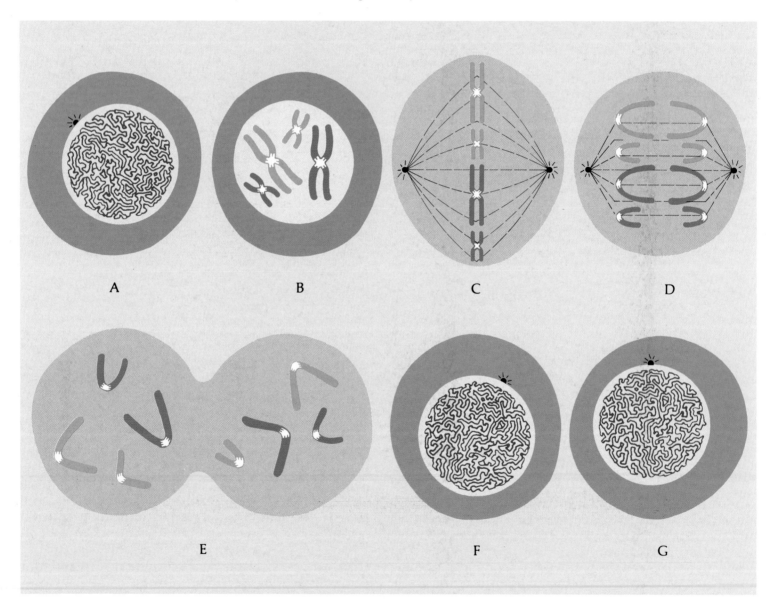

FIG. 1.4 Mitosis lasts about 1 hour, during which time the cell divides. **A** Interphase cell at end of G_2. **B** Prophase—replicated DNA condenses and is visible. **C** Metaphase—46 duplicated chromosomes align randomly on spindle and can be photographed for karyotyping. **D** Anaphase—chromosomes divide longitudinally, and half of each one moves to the opposite poles of the cell. **E** Telophase—cell wall divides. **F** and **G** Interphase at G_1—two daughter cells each with 46 chromosomes.

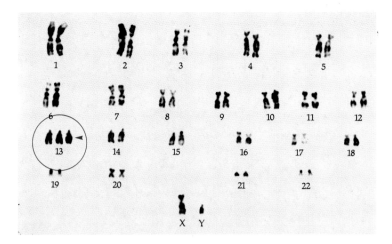

FIG. 1.5 *Karyotype of a patient with trisomy 13 demonstrates aneuploidy. Note the extra chromosome 13, causing the cell to have 47 instead of 46 chromosomes.*

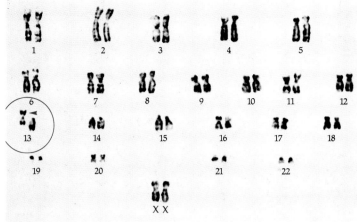

FIG. 1.6 *Pericentric inversion* (arrow) *of chromosome 13.*

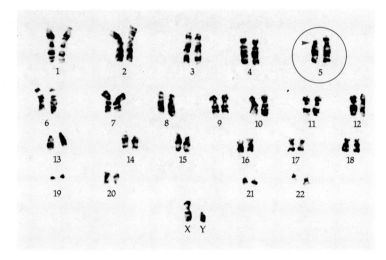

FIG. 1.7 *Deletion* (arrow) *of the p arm of chromosome 5 (cri-du-chat syndrome).*

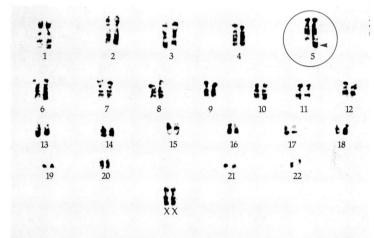

FIG. 1.8 *Unbalanced translocation. The additional DNA was translocated onto the q arm of chromosome 5. The abnormality was inherited from a normal carrier father (Fig. 1.9) with a balanced reciprocal translocation between the q arms of chromosome 3 and chromosome 5. The patient died of multiple birth defects, and in essence had a partial trisomy of the distal portion of the q arm of chromosome 3.*

During most of a cell's life cycle, chromosomes are diffusely spread throughout the nucleus and cannot be morphologically identified. Only when the cell divides does chromosome morphology become apparent (Fig. 1.2). The in vitro life cycle and the cellular division, or mitosis, of a somatic cell are illustrated in Figures 1.3 and 1.4, respectively. The life cycle and divisions, or meiosis, of a germ cell are much more complex and are not suitable for ordinary clinical evaluation.

Any somatic cell which can divide in tissue culture can be used for chromosomal (cytogenetic) analyses. The most convenient tissue source is peripheral blood from which lymphocytes can be stimulated to divide during 2 or 3 days' incubation in tissue culture media. After death, lung tissue is best to culture for chromosomal analyses, although the process requires a 4- to 6-week incubation period. When a treatment decision requires urgency, preliminary chromosomal evaluation can be made within 24 to 36 hours using uncultured bone marrow aspirate.

An abnormality in chromosome number less than an even multiple of 23 (the haploid number) is called aneuploidy (Fig. 1.5). Usually, aneuploidy is 45 or 47 chromosomes; rarely, multiples of the X or Y chromosome will result in individuals with 48 or 49 chromosomes. If aneuploidy occurs in a gamete as a result of a chromosomal division error (nondysjunction

or anaphase lag) during meiosis, all cells will be affected in the fertilized embryo. Subsequently, the parents' recurrent risk for another affected offspring is increased, but is still less than 2 percent.

If the one-celled embryo (zygote) is chromosomally normal and aneuploidy occurs after fertilization in an embryonic somatic cell because of a division error during mitosis, only one or two lines of embryonic cells will be affected. The remaining embryonic cells will be chromosomally normal. This mixed chromosomal state is called mosaicism, and cannot have been inherited since it occurred after conception. However, with a mosaic child, the parent's recurrent risk may still be significantly increased over that of the general population since the zygote may have been aneuploid to start with. In the latter case, the chromosomally normal cell line resulted from a division error during somatic cell mitosis.

Chromosomes can be normal in number (diploid), but still be abnormal in structure. Inversions (Fig. 1.6), deletions (Fig. 1.7), and translocations (Fig. 1.8) are examples of structural chromosomal abnormalities. These abnormalities can arise as

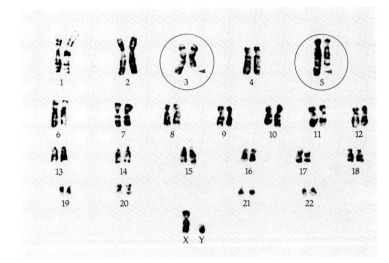

FIG. 1.9 A "balanced" reciprocal translocation of chromosomes 3 and 5 in a normal male (the father of the defective newborn in Fig. 1.8).

INCIDENCE OF CHROMOSOMAL ABNORMALITIES*

Among Spontaneous Abortuses	%
1st trimester	62
After 1st trimester	5
Type of Abnormality	
Trisomy 16	8
Other trisomies	18
Triploidy	8
45XO	9
Miscellaneous	7
Overall incidence	50

Among Liveborns	per 1000
Abnormality of autosomes	4.0
Trisomies	1.4
Balanced rearrangements	2.0
Unbalanced rearrangements	0.6
Abnormality of sex chromosomes	2.2
In males (XXY, XYY, mosaics)	3.0
In females	1.4
45XO	0.1
XXX, mosaics	1.3
Overall incidence	6.2

*About one-quarter of all conceptuses are chromosomally abnormal. About 50 in 1000 stillborns have a chromosomal abnormality.

FIG. 1.10 Incidence of chromosomal abnormalities.

new (sporadic) mutations in the egg or sperm from which the embryo was formed, in which case the parents' recurrent risk for another affected offspring is 1 percent or less. However, the abnormality may also be inherited from a phenotypically normal carrier parent (Fig. 1.9).

About 1 in 350 normal individuals carry a balanced, structurally abnormal set of chromosomes. "Balanced" here means that the structural abnormality does not appear on cytogenetic analysis to have resulted in any net loss or gain of genetic material. If the balanced chromosomal abnormality runs in the family (i.e., is inherited from a parent), the carrier is usually phenotypically normal. However, if the carrier state resulted from a new mutation, there is a sixfold increased risk that the carrier will have some degree of mental retardation (albeit, most such carriers are still phenotypically normal).

Incidence of Chromosomal Abnormalities

At least 25 percent and perhaps as high as 40 percent of all pregnancies terminate in spontaneous abortion. Most such abortions are so early in gestation that pregnancy is not recognized. The earlier the abortion, the more probable that the fetus had a chromosomal abnormality. Of first trimester abortuses, 62 percent are chromosomally abnormal, compared to 5 percent of later abortuses. On the average, 50 percent of all spontaneous abortuses are chromosomally abnormal, with triploidy (69 chromosomes), trisomy 16, and 45XO being by far the most common findings (Fig. 1.10). While the former two are not found among liveborns, 45XO is relatively common and results in Turner syndrome. Nevertheless, 98 percent of embryos with Turner syndrome abort. Since most chromosomally abnormal embryos abort spontaneously, it is not surprising that the incidence of chromosomal abnormalities among liveborns in general is only about 6 in 1000 (see Fig. 1.10), or that it is about 50 in 1000 among stillborns and other perinatal deaths.

When to Suspect a Chromosomal Abnormality

Chromosomal abnormalities, either in number or structure, are likely to have a detrimental effect on the phenotype.

Aneuploidy of an autosome is either lethal or interferes significantly with physical and mental development. However, aneuploidy of an X or Y chromosome may have little effect on the phenotype. Aneuploidy is not entirely a random event, and familial clustering is well known. Consequently, if a normal couple has an aneuploid offspring, their recurrent risk is 1 to 2 percent, which is significantly greater than that of the general population. The reason for this increase is still obscure, but such couples should have prenatal diagnostic counseling.

Carriers of an inherited, reciprocal translocation are usually genetically balanced and are subsequently normal. Carriers of a de novo reciprocal translocation, however, may not be entirely genetically balanced since the incidence of mental retardation in such individuals is about six times greater than that in the general population. In either case, conceptions are likely to be genetically unbalanced, and may abort spontaneously or be born with major congenital anomalies. A history of unexplained infertility, multiple spontaneous abortions (three or more), and particularly the prior birth of a defective baby to the couple or to a close relative should make one suspect that one of the parents carries a balanced chromosome translocation. A chromosome study on the couple is thus indicated, and if translocation is found, they should have prenatal diagnostic counseling.

Physical anomalies at birth are categorized as minor or major types (Figs. 1.11, 1.12, and 1.13). Minor anomalies, such as epicanthal folds (in Caucasians), simian creases, and raised hemangiomas, are of little physiologic significance,

EXAMPLES OF CONGENITAL ANOMALIES*

Category	Minor	Major
Craniofacial	Bony occipital spur Flat occiput Slight micrognathia (3)	Choanal atresia Severe scaphocephaly Cleft lip and/or palate (1.5)
Eye	Inner epicanthal folds (4) Short palpebral fissures	Coloboma of iris Cataract
Auricle	Sinus Skin tags (2)	Severely malformed Rudimentary
Skin	Raised hemangioma Cafe au lait spots	Multiple hemangiomas Posterior webbed neck
Hand	Simian crease (20) Duplication of thumbnail Rudimentary polydactyly Clinodactyly of the fifth digit (10)	Polydactyly Absence of thumbs Complete cutaneous syndactyly Absence of all metacarpals
Foot	Partial syndactyly of second and third toes (2) Recessed fifth toes	Absence of nails Equinovarus
Other skeletal regions	Shieldlike chest Cubitus valgus	Short thoracic cage Absence of radius
Miscellaneous	Diastasis recti (>3 cm) Ectopic femoral testes	Neural tube defects Severe hypospadias

Except as noted in parentheses, the incidence of each is < 1 in 1000 liveborns.

FIG. 1.11 Examples of congenital anomalies.

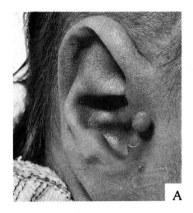 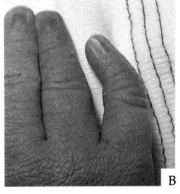 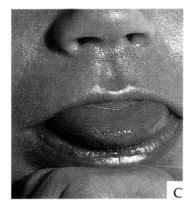 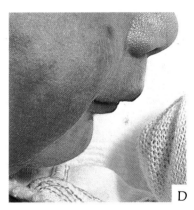

FIG. 1.12 Clinical photographs show several minor anomalies seen at birth. **A** Preauricular skin tag; **B** clinodactyly of the fifth finger; **C** macroglossia; **D** micrognathia. (Courtesy of Dr. Christine L. Williams, Scarsdale, New York)

and each one occurs in less than 4 percent of the population. In contrast, major anomalies, such as coloboma of the iris, polydactyly, and multiple hemangiomas, have a greater adverse effect on the individual.

Among 7000 newborn infants surveyed, 45 percent had one or more minor anomalies; 9 percent had three or more. Many of these minor anomalies represent the effects of multifactorial inheritance, i.e., they are simply familial. About 1.5 percent of newborns have at least one major anomaly, and this incidence is severalfold greater among prematures. Infants with a single major anomaly (e.g., congenital heart disease, polydactyly, cleft lip) do not present an increased incidence of minor anomalies and usually represent multifactorial or simple mendelian inheritance. In contrast, infants with two or more major anomalies usually show an increased incidence of minor anomalies and often represent a specific syndrome of congenital anomalies. Most such syndromes, particularly when there are two or more primary defects in morphogenesis, represent the effects of simple mendelian inheritance; a few represent the effect of environmental teratogens on the fetus in utero (e.g., rubella, maternal alcohol ingestion, antiepileptic medication). About 10 percent of these syndromes represent the effect of unique or known chromosome abnormalities, with translocations illustrating the former and aneuploidies such as trisomy 21 (Down syndrome) or 45XO (Turner syndrome) characteristic of the latter.

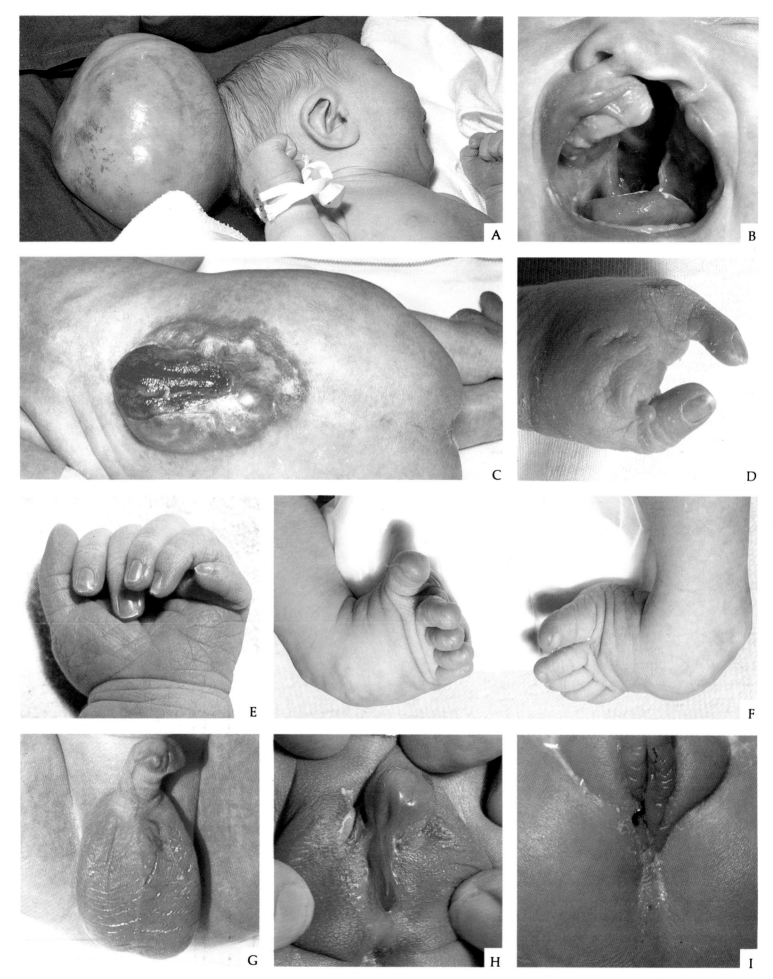

FIG. 1.13 *Clinical photographs show several major anomalies seen at birth.* **A** *Encephalocele;* **B** *cleft lip and palate;* **C** *men-ingomyelocele;* **D** *lobster-claw hand;* **E** *polydactyly (postaxial);* **F** *bilateral clubfoot;* **G** *hypospadias;* **H** *fused labia with enlarged clitoris;* **I** *imperforate anus. (Courtesy of Dr. Christine L. Williams, Scarsdale, New York)*

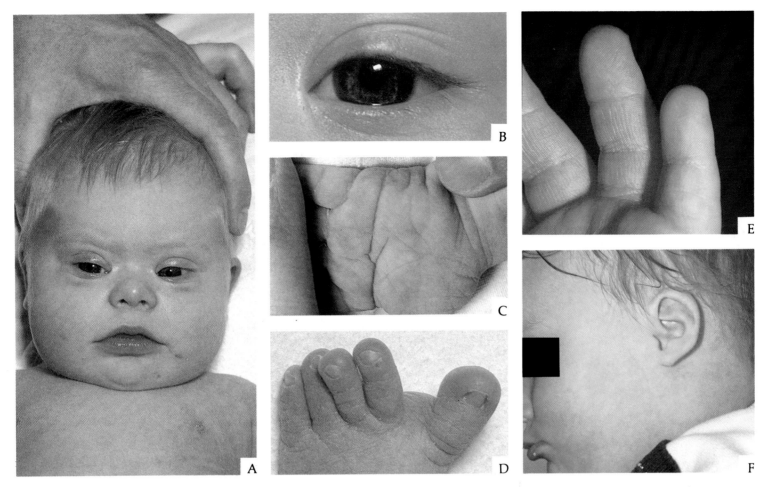

FIG. 1.14 Clinical photographs show several minor anomalies associated with Down syndrome. **A** Typical facies (note epican-thal folds); **B** Brushfield spots; **C** simian crease; **D** wide space between first and second toes; **E** short fifth finger; **F** small ears.

ABNORMALITIES OF AUTOSOMES

Down Syndrome

The worldwide incidence of Down syndrome among liveborns is 1 in 700, with 45 percent of affected individuals being born to women over 35 years of age. In the United States the incidence is somewhat lower: about 1 in 1100 liveborns and only 28 percent born to women over age 35. This difference represents the effect of elective infertility among older U.S. women, and, to a lesser extent, the impact of prenatal diagnosis leading to selective abortion of Down syndrome fetuses. The incidence of Down syndrome among conceptuses is three times greater than among liveborns, but about two-thirds of Down syndrome fetuses spontaneously abort.

There is no single physical stigma of Down syndrome; rather, the clinical diagnosis rests on a gestalt of many minor and a few major anomalies. Although any one of the minor anomalies may be found in a normal person, it is the constellation of several anomalies in one individual which characterizes Down syndrome (Fig. 1.14). These minor anomalies include brachycephaly, inner epicanthal folds, upward slanting eyes, Brushfield spots, small ears, a small upturned nose with saddle bridge, a small mouth with protruding tongue which fissures with age, a short neck with redundant skinfolds, simian crease(s), clinodactyly of the fifth finger(s) with single digital crease due to hypoplasia of the middle phalanx, and a wide space between first and second toes. The number of these minor anomalies present in any particular case is variable.

Other features of Down syndrome are infection-prone dry skin; relatively short stature; rapid aging with premature graying of hair; hypotonia during infancy; wide, flat iliac wings; and a narrow acetabular angle on radiographs. Adult males have reduced libido and are usually impotent (or perhaps sterile). Adult females may have normal libido and are fertile; about one-third of their liveborns may have Down syndrome, the rest should be normal. In both sexes, puberty is delayed.

Several major anomalies are commonly associated with Down syndrome. Congenital heart disease is found in 45 percent of cases, particularly atrioventricular communis and ventricular septal defects. About 7 percent have a gastrointestinal anomaly, most often duodenal atresia. There is also an increased incidence of thyroid disorders (particularly of the autoimmune type) in Down syndrome individuals, their mothers, and their close relatives. Acute and neonatal leukemia occur 20 times more frequently than in the general population. Quantitative abnormalities are found in many enzyme systems. However, the most consistent major anomaly is mental retardation.

With rare exceptions, Down syndrome individuals are

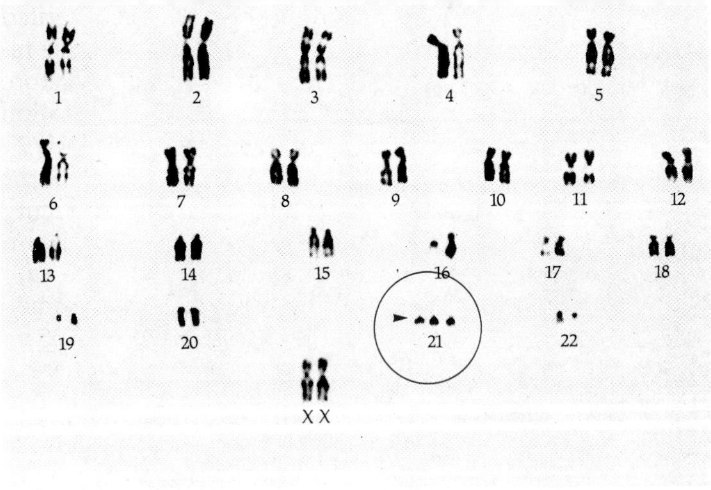

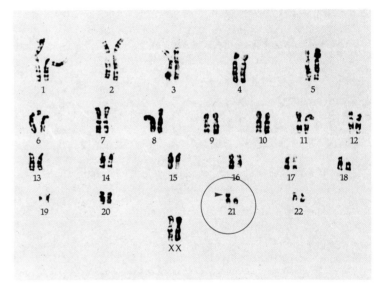

Age (years)	Risk Factor
<25	1 in 1600
25–29	1 in 1100
30–34	1 in 700
35–39	1 in 250
40–42	1 in 80
>42	1 in 40

Note: Risk for any chromosomal abnormality in liveborns: maternal age <35 years—1 in 200; 35 to 40 years—1 in 100; >40 years—1 in 50.

FIG. 1.15 Karyotype of a Down syndrome patient indicates trisomy 21.

FIG. 1.16 Risk of Down syndrome in liveborns, by maternal age.

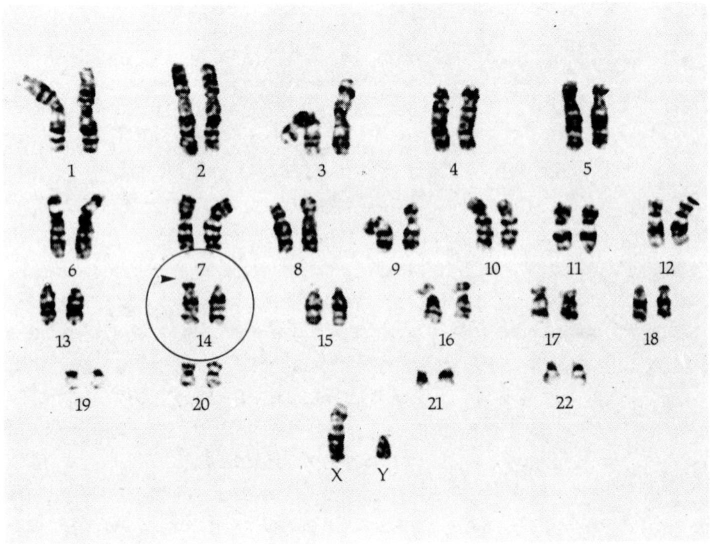

FIG. 1.17 Karyotype of a Down syndrome patient shows 14/21 centric fusion translocation.

FIG. 1.18 Karyotype of a Down syndrome patient shows 21/21 centric fusion translocation.

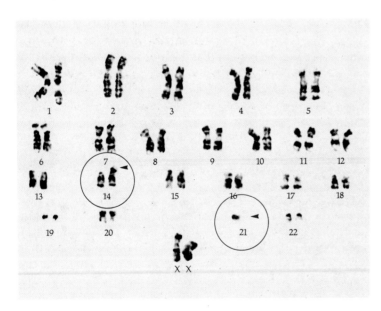

FIG. 1.19 Karyotype of a normal female 14/21 centric fusion translocation carrier (the mother of the Down syndrome patient in Fig. 1.17).

mentally retarded. The degree of retardation varies, with intelligence quotients (IQs) ranging from 20 to 80, and is significantly related to the environment in which the Down syndrome child is raised. A warm, accepting, stimulating home upbringing with early special education maximizes the child's intellectual potential. With such an upbringing, over 95 percent are highly trainable to educable retardates who, as adults, should be capable of a semi-independent existence within the parents' home or in a sheltered workshop. This is helped by the fact that their social quotients (SQs) are relatively higher than their IQs. Additionally, mosaic Down syndrome individuals tend to be somewhat brighter than their nonmosaic counterparts, given a comparable positive rearing. There may even be a slight positive correlation between parental IQ and that of their Down syndrome child, but whether this reflects genetic or environmental influences is not known. With rare exceptions, institutionalization is contraindicated since it has been found to have an extremely negative effect on the patients' mental development.

The apparent decline in both IQ and SQ with age in Down syndrome individuals is an artifact of testing. Most Down

PHYSICAL ABNORMALITIES IN TRISOMY 13 AND 18 SYNDROMES*

Abnormality	Trisomy 13	Trisomy 18
Severe developmental retardation	††††	††††
>90% dead within 1st year	††††	††††
Cryptorchidism in males	††††	††††
Low-set, malformed ears	††††	††††
Multiple major congenital anomalies	††††	††††
Prominent occiput	†	††††
Cleft lip and/or palate	†††	†
Micrognathia	††	†††
Microphthalmos	†††	††
Coloboma of iris	†††	†
Short sternum	†	†††
Rocker-bottom feet	††	†††
Congenital heart disease	††	††††
Scalp defects (of skin)	†††	†
Flexion deformities of fingers	††	††††
Polydactyly	†††	†
Hypoplasia of nails	††	†††
Hypertonia in infancy	†	†††
Apneic spells in infancy	†††	†
Midline brain defects	†††	†
Persistance of Hgb F	††††	†
Horseshoe kidney	†	†††

*Relative frequency: ††††, usual; † rare.

FIG. 1.20 Physical abnormalities in trisomy 13 and 18 syndromes.

syndrome children should be tested between the ags of 6 and 8 years for the best estimate of their intellectual potential. Given proper rearing, most Down syndrome children will have an IQ between 45 and 55, though rare cases are known with IQ scores between 60 and 85.

The etiology of Down syndrome is trisomy 21 (Fig. 1.15). In 94 percent of cases, this is a consequence of meiotic nondysjunction. The extra chromosome 21 is maternally derived in two-thirds of instances, paternally derived in one-third. Meiotic nondysjunction increases with maternal but not paternal age. Consequently, a couple's risk of having a liveborn child with Down syndrome is directly correlated with maternal age (Fig. 1.16). However, once a couple has had a trisomy 21 child, their recurrent risk is 1 to 2 percent at any maternal age.

About 2 percent of Down syndrome cases are chromosomal mosaics with a mixture of normal and trisomy 21 cells. Although mosaicism represents a chromosomal division error occurring after conception, recurrent risk for the couple may still be appreciably increased.

About 4 percent of Down syndrome cases represent a centric fusion translocation between the long arm of a chromosome 21 and those of either a D (Fig. 1.17) or G (Fig. 1.18) group chromosome. Of these, about one-third are inherited from a clinically normal, balanced carrier (Fig. 1.19); the remainder are sporadic. Chromosome studies should therefore be performed on the parents and siblings of a translocation Down syndrome individual. If a parent carries a 21/21 translocation, all liveborns will have Down syndrome; for the remaining 21/D or G group translocations, the empiric recurrent risk for a Down syndrome liveborn is 2 percent if the father is the carrier and 5 to 10 percent if the mother is the carrier. Amniocentesis for prenatal diagnosis of fetal chromosomes is therefore recommended for gravid women age 35 or older, couples with a Down syndrome child, and where a parent carries a centric fusion translocation. (The various chromosomal types of Down syndrome cannot be distinguished clinically.)

About 40 percent of Down syndrome individuals die prior to age 5, most often because of congenital heart disease or respiratory and other infections. The mean survival after 5 years is to age 45, and 25 percent may even survive both parents.

Trisomy 13 and 18

Trisomy 13 and 18 are relatively rare chromosomal abnormalities, the incidence of each being about 1 in 8000 liveborns. About 95 percent of trisomy 18 fetuses abort early, while trisomy 13 fetuses rarely abort spontaneously. The major physical features of each abnormality are listed in Figure 1.20, and illustrated in Figures 1.21 and 1.22. There is often much overlap in physical findings between the two syndromes, making it occasionally difficult to distinguish one from the other solely on the basis of clinical evaluation. Both syndromes result in profound mental retardation and usually lead to death within 1 year. Therefore, heroic attempts at medical intervention should be discouraged.

As in Down syndrome, meiotic nondysjunction is the mechanism for the chromosome error in most cases of trisomy 13 and 18, with risk increasing with maternal age. Occasionally, cases result from centric fusion translocations (spontaneous or inherited) or postconception mosaicism. The latter may have a slightly better prognosis, at least for survival. The recurrence risk is 1 to 2 percent at any maternal age (but higher when resulting from an inherited translocation), and amniocentesis for prenatal diagnosis of fetal chromosome abnormalities is recommended with subsequent pregnancies.

About 20 percent of liveborns with the physical features of trisomy 13 are chromosomally normal, probably resulting from single-gene-dominant mutations, or, less often, recessive inheritance. Less common are chromosomally normal liveborns with the physical features of trisomy 18. Such instances may indicate Smith-Lemli-Opitz syndrome (autosomal-recessive trait) or the effects of maternal ingestion of methotrexate early in pregnancy. The occasional infant who has survived methotrexate embryopathy has had normal intelligence. However, the prognosis for these other chromosomally normal mimics of trisomy 13 or 18 is little better than that for the other two. Unfortunately, the negative prognosis is often resisted by parents, physicians, and other health care providers, resulting in fruitless medical-surgical interventions with subsequent frustration and bitterness by all involved. Early frank discussions of the realities may be painful, but in the long run may be better for all concerned.

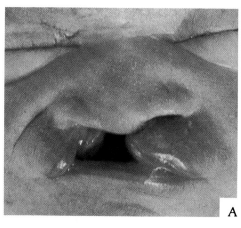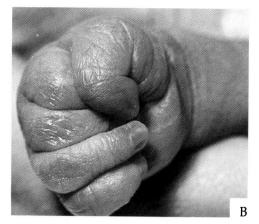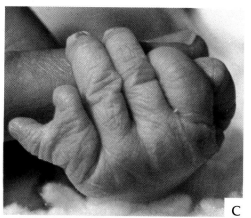

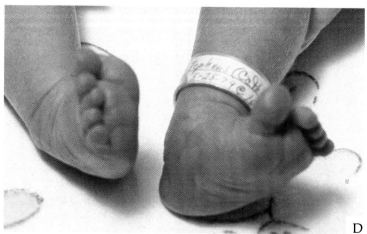

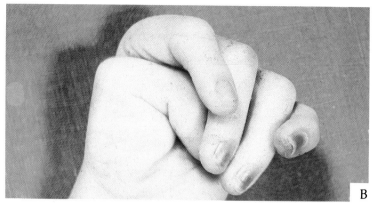

FIG. 1.21 Clinical photographs show several physical manifestations of trisomy 13. **A** Facies showing midline defect; **B** clenched hand with overlapping fingers; **C** preaxial polydactyly; **D** equino-varus deformity; **E** typical punched-out posterior scalp lesions.

(**A** courtesy of Dr. T. Kelly, University of Virginia Medical Center, Charlottesville; **B–E** courtesy of Dr. Kenneth Garver, Magee-Women's Hospital, Pittsburgh)

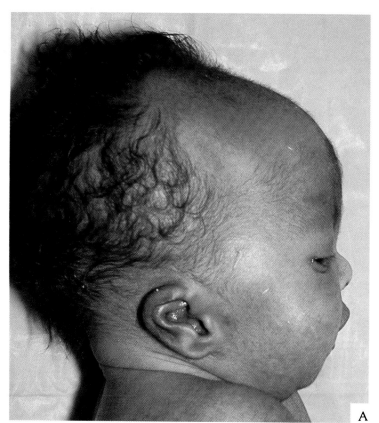

FIG. 1.22 Clinical photographs show several physical manifestations of trisomy 18. **A** Typical profile showing prominent occiput and low-set, malformed auricles; **B** clenched hand showing typical pattern of overlapping fingers; **C** rocker-bottom feet. (**A** courtesy of Dr. Kenneth Garver, Magee-Women's Hospital, Pittsburgh)

GENETICS: COMMON CHROMOSOMAL DISORDERS

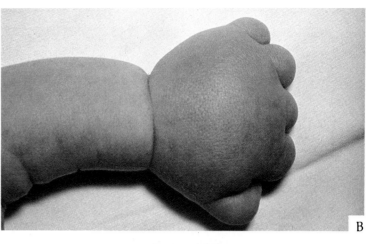

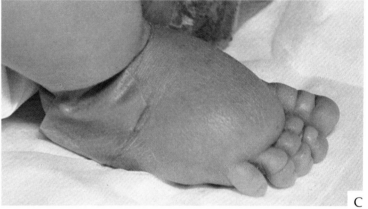

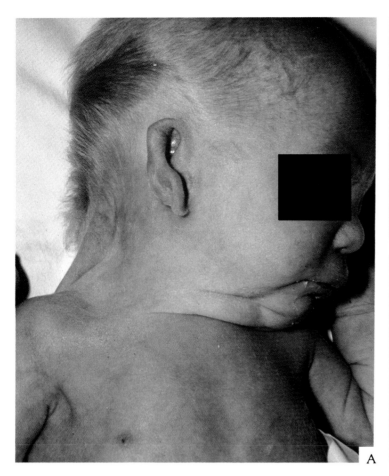

FIG. 1.23 Clinical photographs show several physical manifest-ations associated with Turner syndrome. **A** Web neck, widespread nipples, abnormal ears, and micrognathia; lymphedema of hands (**B**) and feet (**C**).

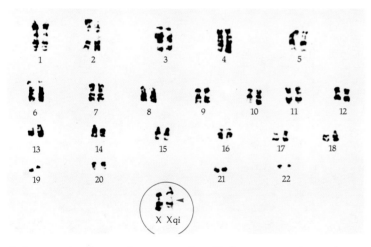

FIG. 1.24 Isochrome long arm of an X chromosome (arrow) in a female with Turner syndrome. Essentially this child has lost the short arms of one X chromosome.

ABNORMALITIES OF SEX CHROMOSOMES

Turner Syndrome

This is one of the three most common chromosomal abnor-malities found in early spontaneous abortions; in fact, only 2 percent of affected fetuses are ever born. The phenotype is female. Primary amenorrhea, sterility, sparse pubic-axillary hair, underdeveloped breasts, and short stature (4½ to 5 feet) are the usual manifestations. These women have an infantile uterus, and their ovaries are only strands of fibrous connec-tive tissue. Other physical features may include webbing of the neck, cubitus valgus, a low hairline, shield chest, and coarctation of the aorta (in 20 percent of cases) (Fig. 1.23). Newborns often have lymphedema of the feet and/or hands which can reappear briefly during adolescence. Mental devel-opment is usually normal.

The chromosome error in 60 percent of individuals with Turner syndrome is 45XO. Most often the missing sex chromosome is paternally derived, so the risk of Turner syn-drome does not increase with parental age. Another 15 per-cent of individuals with Turner syndrome are mosaics (XO/XX, XO/XX/XXX, or XO/XY). The physical stigma may be less marked in mosaics, and fertility is rarely reported. If an XY cell line is present, the intra-abdominal gonads should be removed since they are prone to malignant change. The remaining cases of Turner syndrome have 46 chromo-somes, including one normal plus one structurally abnormal X. The latter may have a deletion or may be an isochrome (Fig. 1.24); usually it is paternally derived.

While loss of the short arm of an X chromosome results in full-blown Turner syndrome, deletion of the long arm usually produces only streak (fibrous) gonads with consequent sterili-ty, amenorrhea, and infantile secondary sex characteristics. A buccal smear for sex chromatin is a poor diagnostic test for Turner syndrome since mosaics, partial deletions, and isochromes can be sex chromatin positive. If the diagnosis is clinically suspected, a G-banded chromosome study should be ordered. Should the affected child be 45XO or a mosaic, the parental recurrent risk is not greatly increased, though it may be increased if a parent carries a structurally abnormal X chromosome.

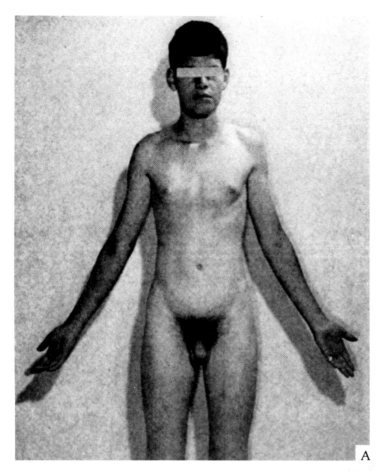

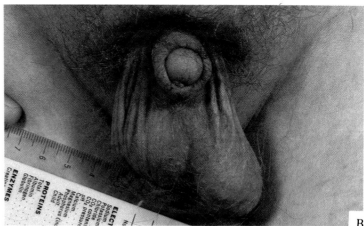

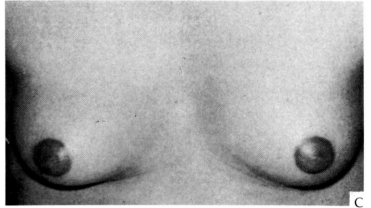

FIG. 1.25 Clinical photographs show several physical manifestations of Klinefelter syndrome. **A** Eunuchoid body habitus, relatively narrow shoulders, increased carrying angle of arms, female distribution of pubic hair, normal penis, small scrotum due to small size of testes; **B** small testes and penis; **C** gynecomastia. (**B** courtesy of Dr. Peter Lee, University of Pittsburgh School of Medicine)

Prenatal diagnosis of affected fetuses should be discussed with the parents, and the *relatively* good prognosis for Turner syndrome liveborns should not be overlooked. Girls with Turner syndrome should receive appropriate hormone therapy during adolescence to develop their secondary sex characteristics and simulate menses. Although hormonal efforts to promote growth have not yet been very successful, newer therapeutic approaches hold promise for the future.

A chromosomally normal phenotypic mimic of Turner syndrome is Noonan syndrome. This autosomal-dominant trait occurs in 1 to 1000 liveborns and affects both sexes. Microcephaly, pulmonary stenosis, and normal stature are more common than in Turner syndrome; unfortunately, about half of affected individuals are mildly to moderately mentally retarded. Noonan females menstruate and are fertile, but males are usually sterile. Most cases represent fresh mutations, and the empiric recurrent risk without a family history is 10 percent.

Klinefelter Syndrome

About 20 percent of aspermic adult males have Klinefelter syndrome, as do 1 in 250 males over 6 feet tall. The physical stigmata usually are not obvious until puberty, at which time the normal onset of spermatogenesis is blocked by the presence of two X chromosomes. Consequently, the germ cells die, the seminiferous tubules become hyalinized and scarred,

and the testes become small. Testosterone levels are below the normal male adult level, though the level varies from case to case (the average is about half normal). This then leads to a wide range of virilization in these cases. At one extreme is the eunuchoid male with a small penis and gynecomastia (Fig. 1.25); at the opposite extreme is the virile mesomorph with a normal penis. Scoliosis may develop during adolescence, and behavioral problems may become significant during school years. The average IQ in Klinefelter syndrome is about 87, and perhaps 10 percent are mentally retarded. Libido may be reduced in adult males, virtually all of whom are sterile.

Testosterone treatment should begin at about 11 or 12 years of age if in vivo levels do not result in virilization. Such treatment will also prevent gynecomastia, which occurs in 40 percent of cases. Once gynecomastia occurs, it can only be corrected by surgery. Testosterone treatment may also improve libido in some patients, but whether this reflects a pharmacotherapeutic or a psychological effect remains unclear. Although men with Klinefelter syndrome can be homosexual, there is little evidence to suggest a predisposition in that direction.

The karyotype in Klinefelter syndrome is XXY in 80 percent of cases and mosaic (XY/XXY) in the other 20 percent. The latter rarely may be fertile. About 60 percent of cases reflect a chromosome error in oogenesis, 40 percent an error in spermatogenesis. Risk of having an affected child increases with maternal age. Males with more than two X chromosomes (XXXY, XXXXY) are usually mentally retarded and are more likely to have skeletal and other major congenital anomalies.

XXX and XYY Syndromes

Triple X females have no characteristic physical stigmata. However, average intelligence is reduced, and about one-fourth are mildly retarded. The parental risk for an XXX daughter increases with maternal age. XXX females are fertile, and the offspring are usually chromosomally normal.

About 1 in 350 males over 6 feet tall are XYY. Such males have no pathognomonic physical stigmata, but average IQ is about 87. The prevalence of XYY males in a prison population is manyfold greater than their proportion of the general population. This has led to the erroneous conclusion that XYY males must be overly aggressive and antisocial, presumably due to the extra Y chromosome. In fact, XYY males are typically neither. Their disproportion in prisons—usually for nonaggressive crimes—reflects their diminished average intelligence; that is, they are more likely to get caught when breaking the law. Since XYY males reflect a chromosomal error in their father's spermatogenesis, the recurrent risk does not increase with parental age. XYY males are fertile, and the offspring are usually chromosomally normal.

Sex and Gender

Sex is determined by chromosomes, but gender is a psychosocial definition. It is the latter which should be the prime consideration to the medical practitioner. When sex and gender are not compatible, anatomic, physiologic, and psychosocial considerations should determine the final gender assignment of the individual. Finally, although XO, XXY, XYY, and XXX fetuses can be detected in utero by amniocentesis and in newborns by routine chromosome screening, the relatively benign clinical course of these conditions should be an important factor in deciding to pursue such genetic diagnostic approaches.

BIBLIOGRAPHY

Bergsma D (ed.): Birth Defects Compendium, 2nd ed. Alan Liss, New York, 1979.

Milunsky A: Genetic Disorders and the Fetus. Plenum, New York, 1979.

Smith DW: Recognizable Patterns of Human Malformations. Saunders, Philadelphia, 1982.

Steele MW, Golden WL: Syndromes of congenital anomalies. In Kelley VC (ed.) Practice of Pediatrics. Lippincott, Philadelphia, 1984.

NEONATOLOGY

Ian R. Holzman, M.D.

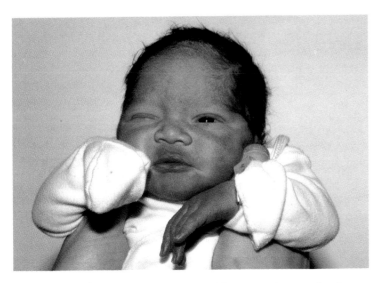

Fig. 2.1 Examination techniques. Holding an infant under the arms and gently rocking him calms the infant and reflexively induces eye opening.

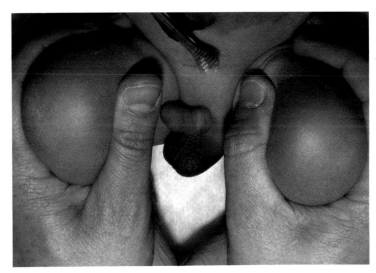

Fig. 2.2 Ortolani's maneuver. The proper hand positioning for this maneuver is demonstrated. Abducting the femur produces a palpable "clunk" in the infant with congenital hip dislocation.

GENERAL PHYSICAL EXAMINATION TECHNIQUES

Examination of the newborn requires specialized techniques because of lack of cooperation on the part of the patient, the infant's small size, and developmental immaturity. As much observation as is feasible must be accomplished before disturbing a quiet infant. By visual inspection one can readily assess skin and facies; general tonus and symmetry of movement; respiratory rate, retractions, and color; and abdominal contour. Auscultation of the heart and lungs should be done before more stressful portions of the examination, which are likely to make the infant fussy. Allowing the baby to suck on a pacifier or clean finger can be helpful in quieting him. The latter also allows for an assessment of strength of suck as well as of integrity of the palate. Lifting the infant under the arms (Fig. 2.1) and gently rocking him (such that the head swings toward and away from the examiner) is usually calming. This maneuver induces a reflex opening of the eyes, which facili-

tates the ophthalmologic examination. Sucking also induces eye opening and can be useful.

When examining the abdomen it is often helpful to gently flex the hip on the side being examined, since this relaxes the abdominal muscles. Most structures in the abdomen are smaller (pyloric olive), softer (liver), more superficial (spleen tip), or deeper (kidneys) than expected. The use of any part of the hand other than the fingertips is to be discouraged, since maximal sensitivity is essential.

Careful evaluation of the hip joints is a crucial part of every newborn examination because identification and early treatment of congenital dislocation can prevent later disability. While visual inspection for asymmetry of buttocks and skin creases or of femoral length can be a clue to dislocation, the performance of at least one of a number of active motion tests is essential. Ortolani's maneuver involves placing the third or fourth finger over the greater trochanter, and the thumb on the medial aspect of the thighs (Fig. 2.2). The thighs are adducted and then abducted with the fingers pushing toward the

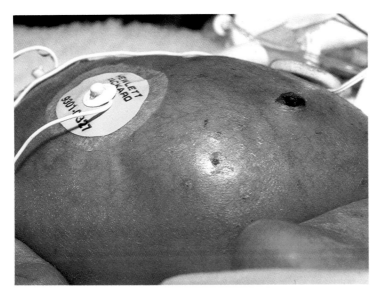

Fig. 2.3 Premature skin. This premature infant demonstrates translucent, paper-thin skin with a prominent venous pattern.

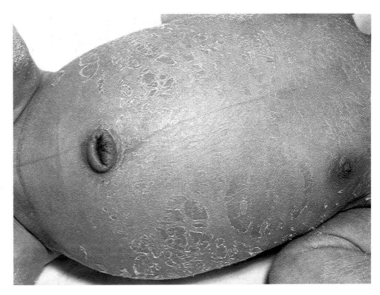

Fig. 2.4 Postterm skin. Peeling and cracking of the skin are characteristic of the infant delivered after 42 weeks gestation.

midline and the thumbs away. A definite clunk can be felt and often heard if the femoral head is dislocating. Often, higher pitched clicks and snaps can be heard and felt which do not represent anything more than tendons passing over bone or cartilage.

Assessment of Gestational Age

One of the unique considerations in the examination of the newborn is an assessment of the infant's gestational age. Accurate determination should actually be the first part of any newborn examination since this provides the context for the remainder of the evaluation. No differential diagnosis of newborn disease can be made without knowing whether the infant is premature or full-term, and whether the infant is small, large, or appropriate for gestational age. While an accurate menstrual and pregnancy history usually provides firm evidence of gestational age, there are many instances when data such as the date of the last menses or the date of the onset of fetal movement are either unavailable or unreliable.

A number of different investigators (see Bibliography) have developed examination criteria, both morphologic and neurologic, for the assessment of gestational age. While these criteria are generally useful because of the ordered patterns of fetal development, no single item or even small group of items can be relied upon to develop at the same rate in all infants. In fact, assessment of paired structures, such as ears, may reveal slightly different degrees of maturation from one side to the other. Thus, all of the available methods involve *numerous* physical and neurologic items, and at best have a 2-week range of error.

While morphologic criteria tend to be uninfluenced by events occurring around the time of delivery, neurologic findings may be unreliable in the presence of a number of conditions, including depression secondary to medication, asphyxia, seizures, metabolic diseases, infections, and severe respiratory distress. Even morphologic criteria may be inaccurate if the infant is born with severe edema, growth retardation, or suffers effects from maternal drug use. Such factors must be considered in estimating gestational age.

MORPHOLOGIC CRITERIA

As it is not possible to illustrate all of the physical signs that are helpful in determining gestational age, this section will emphasize some of the more easily observed and generally agreed upon findings.

Among the most striking differences among infants of various gestational ages is the quality of the skin. As intrauterine development proceeds, the chemical nature of skin changes. There is a gradual decrease in water content and a thickening of the keratin layer. The most premature infants (24 to 28 weeks) exhibit nearly translucent, paper-thin skin (Fig. 2.3) which is easily abraded. A diffuse red hue and a prominent venous pattern are characteristic. At term, the skin no longer appears thin and the general color is a pale pink. Some superficial peeling and cracking around the ankles and wrists may be visible. Postterm infants (42 to 44 weeks) often have more diffuse peeling and cracking of the skin as the outermost layers are sloughed (Fig. 2.4).

The general quality of scalp hair changes during development from rather fine, thin hair (24 to 28 weeks) to coarser and thicker hair at term. There are, of course, racial differences in hair quality which can make this change difficult to assess. A second type of hair, known as lanugo, appears and disappears during development. Lanugo is very fine body hair which resembles "peach fuzz." It is absent prior to approximately 20 to 22 weeks, becomes diffuse until 30 to 32 weeks, and then begins to thin. Assessment of presence and extent of lanugo hair is best accomplished by observing the back tangentially (Fig. 2.5).

Transverse creases begin to appear on the anterior portion of the soles of the feet at approximately 32 weeks (Fig. 2.6). By 36 weeks of gestation, the anterior two-thirds of the sole is covered with creases. To adequately assess this feature, it is necessary to stretch the skin over the sole gently so as to distinguish wrinkling from true creases. Infants with congenital neurologic dysfunction involving the lower extremities may lack normal creases, as might infants born with severe pedal edema. It is sometimes possible to learn something about gestational age long after birth by reviewing the sole prints made for identification in many hospitals.

Cartilaginous development proceeds in an orderly manner

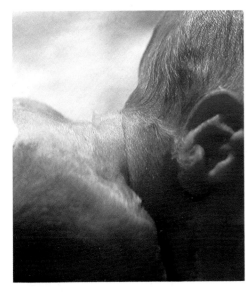

Fig. 2.5 Lanugo. This fine body hair resembling "peach fuzz" is present on infants of 24 to 32 weeks gestation.

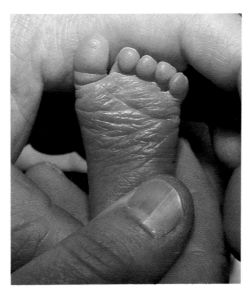

Fig. 2.6 Sole creases. Transverse sole creases cover approximately one-half the sole in this infant, indicating approximately 34 weeks gestational age.

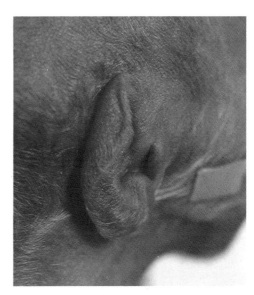

Fig. 2.7 Ear cartilage. The lack of cartilage and easy foldability (lack of recoil) of the premature ear at 26 weeks is evident.

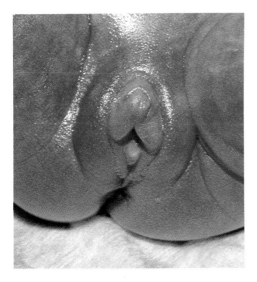

Fig. 2.8 Premature female genitalia. Prominence of the labia minora in a premature female infant at 28 weeks.

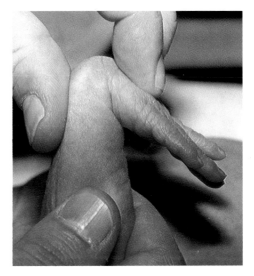

Fig. 2.9 Square-window test. The position for assessing the square window is shown. The 45° angle seen between palm and forearm is consistent with an infant of 30 to 32 weeks gestation.

during gestation and can be assessed by examination of the external ear. While the normal incurving of the upper pinnae begins at 33 to 34 weeks and is complete at term, it is more reliable to assess the extent of cartilage in the pinnae by feeling its edge and folding the ear (Fig. 2.7). Until approximately 32 weeks, there is only minimal recoil of a folded ear, but by term there is instant recoil.

The appearance of genitalia can be used to assess gestational age. In the male, the testes descend into the scrotum during the last month of gestation but are often palpable in the inguinal canal by 28 to 30 weeks. The appearance of rugae on the scrotum parallels testicular migration. Absence of testicular descent will alter the appearance of the scrotum at term. Clearly, congenital cryptorchidism complicates this evaluation. In the female, the labia majora tend to be overshadowed by the clitoris and labia minora until 34 to 36 weeks (Fig. 2.8). In cases of fetal malnutrition, lack of subcutaneous fat which should normally be present in the latter part of gestation can interfere with assessment of the female genitalia.

NEUROLOGIC CRITERIA

There are numerous neurologic tests and observations which can be used in attempting to assess gestational age. Many tend to be redundant and most examiners use those that seem to best cover the various facets of neurologic function, including range of motion, tone, reflexes, and posture. None are particularly reliable in the face of illness, and the entire neurologic examination is best done between 12 and 24 hours after birth to allow recovery from the stress of delivery.

Tests for flexion angles, including those of the ankle, wrist, and knee, assess a combination of muscle tone, ligament and tendon laxity, and flexion-extension development. The inexperienced examiner usually assumes that the most premature will be the most flexible, but observation of flexion angles demonstrates this to be false. The square-window test of the wrist (Fig. 2.9) is performed by gently flexing the hand upon the wrist and assessing the resultant angle. Infants less than approximately 32 weeks can be flexed only to 45°–90°, while term infants undergo full flexion. Sometime between birth and adulthood this flexion ability is lost. It is essential to emphasize gentleness in these evaluations, since any result can be achieved if undue force is used.

Resting tone can be assessed in a number of ways, one of which is the heel-to-ear maneuver. With the infant on its back, a foot is moved as near to the ipsilateral ear as possible without exerting undue force. The pelvis must be kept flat

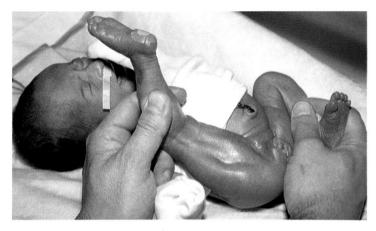

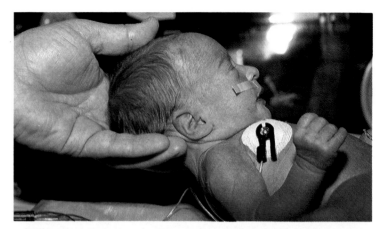

Fig. 2.10 Heel-to-ear maneuver. The position for assessing heel-to-ear maneuver is demonstrated. The degree of extension seen is consistent with a 28- to 30-week infant.

during the evaluation. The most premature infants can easily touch their heel to their ear (Fig. 2.10), while this becomes somewhat more difficult after 30 weeks and impossible by approximately 34 weeks of gestational age.

A large number of primitive reflexes can be elicited in the normal newborn. Usually a selection of these, including sucking and rooting reflexes, tonic neck reflex, and the Moro reflex suffice for evaluation. Certain other reflexes may take on importance in individual cases. The Moro reflex evaluates both vestibular maturation and the relationship between flexor and extensor tone. It, like all other reflexes in the newborn, is affected by the overall status of the infant. A marked asymmetry in the response can be used as a clue to physical and neurologic problems, such as a brachial plexus injury or a fracture. Elicitation of the reflex involves a short (10 cm) sudden drop of the head when the infant is supine. The full response involves extension and then flexion of the arms, ending in a cry (Fig. 2.11). A similar response is seen with "startling" but is not the true vestibular reflex. An incomplete but identifiable reflex becomes apparent at approximately 32 weeks of gestation, and by 38 weeks is essentially complete. The more immature infants demonstrate extension of the arms and fingers, but no true flexion or sustained cry.

Abnormalities of Growth

One of the important advances in newborn medicine has been the realization that the size of an infant at birth does not necessarily reflect gestational age (Fig. 2.12). The parameter most commonly affected is weight, especially in infants who are small for gestational age. A number of terms have been applied to small infants, including small for gestational age (SGA), intrauterine growth retardation (IUGR), and fetal malnutrition (FM). The last is probably most descriptive of those infants whose weight is inappropriately low in relation to length and head circumference. These infants, who appear long and thin, often have an obvious loss of subcutaneous tissue which is best seen over the buttocks and within the folds of the neck.

The relationship among weight, length, and head circumference can be useful in understanding the etiology of the small size. Conditions that affect growth during the third trimester of pregnancy, such as preeclampsia, tend to interfere with the normal acquisition of fatty tissue while sparing brain growth (and thus head circumference) and linear growth.

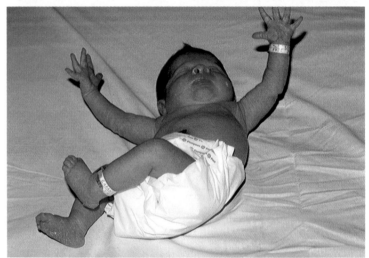

Fig. 2.11 The Moro reflex. (Top) To elicit the reflex, the head is supported and allowed to drop to the level of the bed. (Bottom) This is the initial extension response to vestibular stimulation. The complete response includes secondary flexion and cry.

These infants have an asymmetrical form of growth retardation. In more severe cases, the onset of protein catabolism will affect muscle mass. By comparing length or head circumference percentiles to the weight percentile at any given gestational age, one can detect growth retardation even if the actual weight still falls within two standard deviations of normal. Often infants who are postmature (> 42 weeks) have some decrease in weight compared to length or head circumference. Problems beginning earlier than the third trimester tend to produce more generalized growth retardation (Fig. 2.13). In the more premature infants, such global decreases in growth often complicate assessment of gestational age since the tools are rather limited in infants of 24 to 28 weeks gestational age. Two of the most important causes of generalized growth retardation are chromosomal syndromes and congenital infections. A thorough investigation for such problems should be undertaken in any unexplained instance of generalized growth retardation.

Multiple gestation pregnancies often produce infants who are both premature and symmetrically small. Size discordancy (> 10 percent difference in weight) between identical twins is fairly common, as their placentas can share vascular connections, resulting in overperfusion of one twin and underperfusion of the other. This leads to a marked difference in size, with the underperfused twin being symmetrically growth retarded. Discordancy may also occur in dizygotic twins (Fig. 2.14) if one of the pair has inadequate placentation.

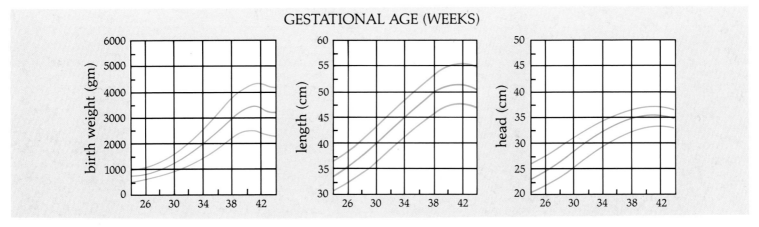

GESTATIONAL AGE (WEEKS)

Fig. 2.12 The mean (± 2 standard deviations) weight, length, and head circumference for infants born at various gestational ages. Infants above or below the curves are considered too large or too small for gestational age. (From Usher R, McLean F: J Pediatr 74:901, 1969, with permission)

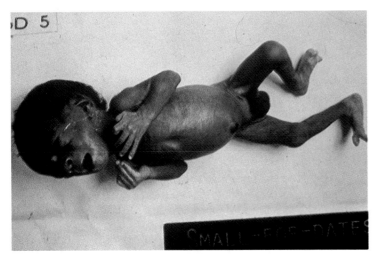

Fig. 2.13 Intrauterine growth retardation. This term baby weighed only 1.7 kg. The head appears disproportionately large for the thin, wasted body. This results from placental insufficiency late in pregnancy. Hypoglycemia may be a complication. (Courtesy of TALC, Institute of Child Health)

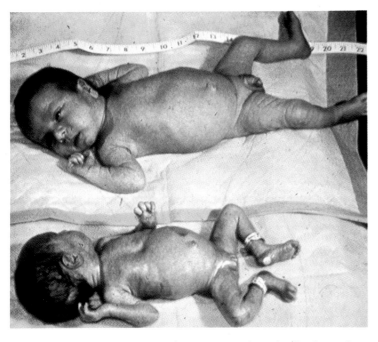

Fig. 2.14 Discordant twins. This is a pair of markedly discordant dizygotic twins. Disturbed placentation accounted for the marked reduction in size of the smaller twin.

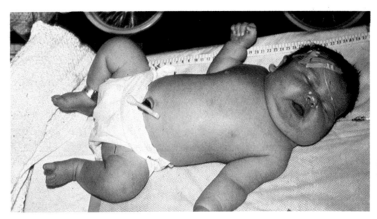

Fig. 2.15 Large-for-gestational age infant. This infant of a diabetic mother weighed 5.0 kg at birth and exhibits the typical rounded facies.

Rarely, one of a pair of twins may be afflicted with a chromosomal abnormality or a congenital infection, while the other is normal.

Infants who are too large for gestational age (LGA) often are the products of pregnancies in diabetic or prediabetic mothers. The effect is usually noted during the third trimester, with infants at term weighing greater than 8 pounds. Weight is the most affected parameter but length and head circumference are often increased as well. Infants of diabetic mothers often are identifiable by their macrosomia, round facies (Fig. 2.15), and sometimes by plethora and hirsutism (especially of the pinnae). They may also demonstrate visceromegaly, with enlargement particularly of the liver and heart.

While infants greater than 8 pounds are more likely to be from diabetic pregnancies, a significant number of large term infants are the products of normal pregnancies. Nevertheless, all LGA infants should be routinely screened for hypoglycemia, and their mothers investigated for the possibility of undiagnosed diabetes mellitus. Two fairly unusual syndromes can also serve as the cause for excessive newborn size: (1) cerebral gigantism, or Soto syndrome, in which infants have macrosomia, macrocephaly, large hands and feet, and ultimately poor coordination and variable mental deficiency; and (2) Beckwith-Wiedemann syndrome, whose prominent features include macrosomia, macroglossia, omphalocele, linear ear fissures, and neonatal hypoglycemia (see Chapter 9).

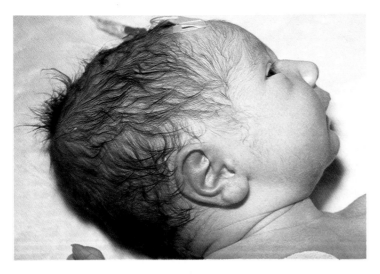

Fig. 2.16 *Caput succedaneum. This infant has significant scalp edema as a result of compression during transit through the birth canal. The edema crosses suture lines.*

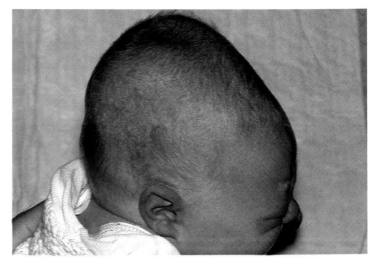

Fig. 2.17 *Cephalohematoma. In this infant with bilateral cephalohematomas, the midline sagittal suture remained palpable, confirming the subperiosteal location of the hematomas.*

BIRTH TRAUMA

In the vast majority of cases, a newborn infant is left relatively unscathed by the birth process. However, there are times when both transient and permanent stigmata of birth trauma are evident. Prompt identification of such injuries is not only important for good management, but also can prevent inappropriate speculation, diagnostic tests, and treatment. This section will review some of the more common birth-related physical signs and appropriate therapy.

Caput Succedaneum

Normal transit of the fetal head through the birth canal induces both molding of the skull and scalp edema, especially if labor is prolonged. The edema, which can be massive, is known as a caput succedaneum (Fig. 2.16). Much of this edema is present at birth and tends to overlie both the occipital bones and portions of the parietal bones bilaterally. In some cases, bruising of the scalp may also be present (especially if a vacuum extractor was employed). The presence of a caput requires no therapy, and spontaneous resolution in a few days is the rule. At times it can be difficult to distinguish a caput from a rare but serious subgaleal (subaponeurotic) hematoma, which is a collection of blood within scalp tissues extending under the epicranial aponeurosis. Such infants, however, will show signs of progressive hypovolemia; while the exact source and location of bleeding may be unclear initially, awareness of the possibility of massive blood loss extending under a large portion of the scalp and prompt replacement can be lifesaving.

Cephalohematoma

Often, confusion arises between the diagnosis of a caput and that of a cephalohematoma. The latter is a localized collection of blood beneath the periosteum of one of the calvarial bones. It is distinguished from a caput by the fact that its borders are limited by suture lines, usually those surrounding the parietal bones. However, diagnosis can be difficult in the immediate newborn period when there may be overlying scalp edema. Cephalohematoma can be bilateral (Fig. 2.17), but is more often unilateral. On palpation, the border feels elevated and the center depressed. Most patients have an uncomplicated course of slow resolution over 1 or more months, with possible calcification. Occasionally complications are seen, the most common being jaundice, resulting from breakdown and resorption of a large hematoma. Secondary anemia should also be considered when the hematoma is large. Underlying hairline skull fractures occur with some regularity, but are rarely of clinical significance. The exception is the uncommon development of a leptomeningeal cyst. Radiologic investigation for an underlying depressed fracture is indicated in those infants whose history suggests significant trauma, and those having a depressed level of consciousness and/or neurologic abnormalities on examination. Another potentially serious, though rare, complication is infection. This is more likely to occur when the integrity of the overlying skin is broken. Needle aspiration of a cephalohematoma is contraindicated because of the risk of introducing microorganisms.

Meconium Staining

Meconium is noted in the amniotic fluid in as many as 10 percent of deliveries. The meconium may have been recently expelled or many have been present in the amniotic fluid for hours or days. Since the timing of the passage of meconium may have significance for the diagnosis of asphyxia, it is useful to examine infants for the presence of meconium staining. It apparently takes at least 4 to 6 hours of contact before staining of the umbilicus, skin, and nails occurs (Fig. 2.18). Often, the meconium-stained infant is postmature and has diffuse peeling of the skin as well as a shriveled, stained umbilical cord.

Bruises and Petechiae

Superficial bruising can occur whenever delivery is difficult. This is relatively common with breech presentations (Fig. 2.19), and can include swelling and discoloration of the labia and of the scrotum (to be distinguished from an incarcerated inguinal hernia). When bruises are extensive, significant secondary jaundice may develop as the extravasated blood is broken down and resorbed. In those infants in whom a nuchal

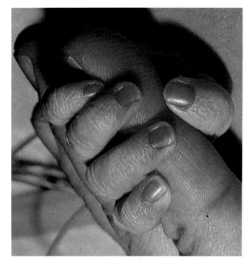

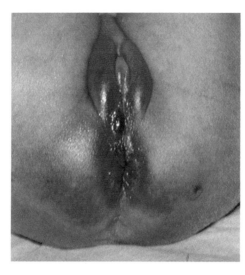

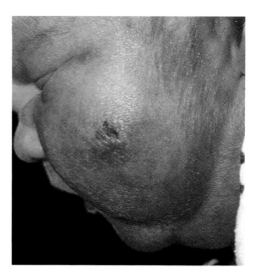

Fig. 2.18 Meconium staining. The marked discoloration of this infant's fingernails resulted from longstanding meconium staining of the amniotic fluid prior to delivery.

Fig. 2.19 Bruising. This severe bruising of the perineum was the result of a difficult breech labor and delivery.

Fig. 2.20 Fat necrosis. This discolored nodular lesion on the cheek is characteristic of subcutaneous necrosis of fat secondary to forceps trauma.

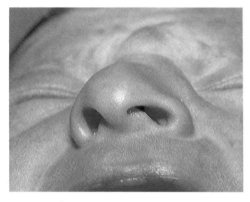

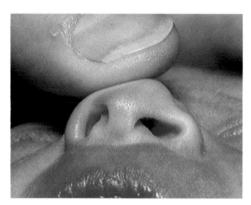

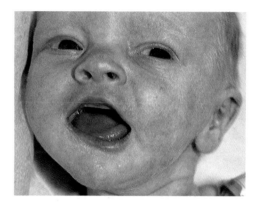

Fig. 2.21 Nasal deformity. This infant has incurred dislocation of the triangular cartilage of the nasal septum during delivery. (Left) Inspection of the nose reveals deviation of the septum to the right and asym-

metry of the nares. (Right) When the septum is manually moved toward the midline, the asymmetry persists, confirming the dislocation.

Fig. 2.22 Facial nerve palsy. This infant incurred injury to the right facial nerve, resulting in loss of the nasolabial fold on the affected side and asymmetrical movement of the mouth. The side of the mouth which appears to droop is the normal side.

cord is found at delivery, the presence of diffuse petechiae around the head and neck is a common occurrence and does not warrant further investigation. The appearance of new bruises or petechiae after delivery should alert the physician and nurse to the possibility of a bleeding disorder.

Fat Necrosis

Many infants delivered with the aid of forceps show forceps marks after delivery, which tend to fade over 24 to 48 hours. Occasionally, a well-circumscribed, firm nodule with purplish discoloration may appear at the site of a forceps mark. This is felt to represent fat necrosis (Fig. 2.20), and resolves spontaneously over weeks to months. The phenomenon may occur at other sites of trauma as well.

Nasal Deformities

Abnormalities of the nose are commonly seen after delivery, the majority consisting of transient flattening or twisting of the nose induced during transit through the birth canal. Less than 1 percent of nasal deformities are due to actual disloca-

tions of the triangular cartilage of the nasal septum. These can be differentiated from positional deformities by manually moving the septum to the midline and observing the resultant shape of the nares. In a true dislocation, marked asymmetry of the nares persists (Fig. 2.21). Returning the septum to its proper position can be accomplished in the nursery with the guidance of an otolaryngologist. Failure to recognize and treat dislocation may lead to permanent deformity.

Peripheral Nerve Damage

Injury to the peripheral nervous system, especially the facial and brachial nerves, is one of the more common serious occurrences related to birth. Unilateral facial nerve palsy is the most common peripheral nerve injury, with an incidence as high as 1.4 per 1000 live births. Injury can be the result of direct trauma from forceps or of compression of the nerve against the sacral promontory while the head is in the birth canal. With pronounced nerve injury there is decreased facial movement and forehead wrinkling on the side of the palsy, eyelid elevation, and flattening of the nasolabial folds and corner of the mouth (Fig. 2.22). Crying accentuates the find-

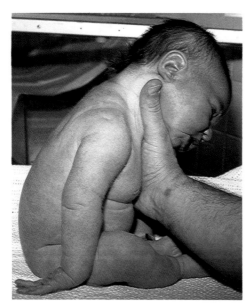

Fig. 2.23 Brachial plexus injury. Traction injury to C5, C6, and C7 (Erb) spinal cord segments produces this palsy. The infant shown demonstrates the characteristic posture of the limply adducted and internally rotated arm.

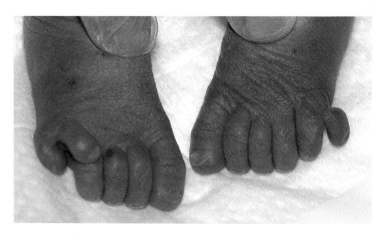

Fig. 2.25 Polydactyly. True bilateral polydactyly of the fifth toe is seen in this infant.

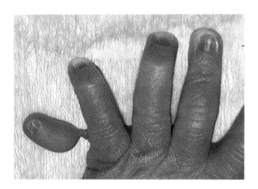

Fig. 2.24 Supernumerary digit. This is the common position for a sixth digit. The thin pedicle distinguishes this anomaly from true polydactyly.

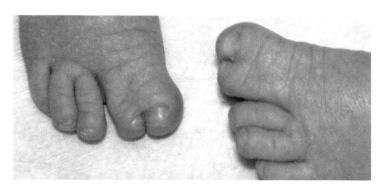

Fig. 2.26 Syndactyly. This child demonstrates bilateral fusion of the soft tissue between the first and second toes.

ings, with the most obvious sign being asymmetrical movement of the mouth. The side which appears to droop when crying is the normal side. The differential diagnosis includes Möbius syndrome (usually bilateral) and absence of the depressor anguli oris muscle. The latter condition is distinguishable from facial nerve palsy by the absence of any involvement of the forehead, eyelid, or nasolabial area. The prognosis for facial nerve palsies is excellent, and recovery usually occurs within the first month. In the meantime, prevention of corneal drying is essential. Surgery is reserved for cases where clear-cut severing of the facial nerve has occurred.

The incidence of brachial plexus trauma with current obstetric management is approximately 0.7 per 1000 live births. The mechanism of injury in most instances is traction on the plexus during delivery. Although lesions have classically been divided into those affecting upper spinal segments (Erb palsy) and those affecting lower segments (Klumpke palsy), the distinction may not be clear-cut in some cases. Injury to the C5 and C6 fibers is probably most often identified with the child's arm hanging limply adducted and internally rotated at the shoulder and extended and pronated at the elbow (Fig. 2.23). Appropriate deep-tendon reflexes are absent. It may be difficult to confirm sensory deficit, and autonomic fibers are often intact. Diagnosis is made clinically, but electromyography may be indicated to assess severity of injury and to determine prognosis in patients not showing improvement after 6 to 8 weeks. Treatment should be deferred for at least 7 to 10 days; then, specific physical therapy and splinting should be undertaken. Most infants with brachial plexus palsies demonstrate complete recovery in the first few months of life. The earlier recovery begins, the better the long-term prognosis.

CONGENITAL ANOMALIES

There are innumerable congenital anomalies, many of a minor nature, which can be noted at birth. While any single minor malformation may be of little medical consequence, the identification of three or more in a single infant may be a clue to more serious errors of morphogenesis. A careful family history, including examination of the parents and siblings, can often place these malformations in proper perspective.

Digits

The majority of minor external anomalies involve the hands, feet, and head. One of the more common abnormalities of digitation, especially in black infants, is the presence of a supernumerary digit (Fig. 2.24). These are most often located lateral to the fifth digit, either on the hand or foot. They are distinguishable from true polydactyly because of the small pedicle which attaches them to the fifth digit. The supernumerary digit may have a fingernail, but often lacks bones. While usually of no consequence, they have on occasion been associated with major CNS malformations. Removal may be accomplished by applying a ligature around the pedicle (assuming it is thin and lacks palpable bony tissue) as close as possible to the surface of the fifth digit and allowing for the digit to fall off naturally. This usually takes approximately 1 week. Care should be taken to observe for infection. True polydactyly (duplication of digits) may also be seen (Fig. 2.25) and is most common on the feet, but can also occur on the hands. There may be a family history of this anomaly or it may occur in association with other more serious patterns of

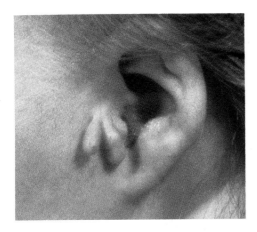

Fig. 2.27 Ear tags. Multiple preauricular skin tags were seen as an isolated finding in this patient.

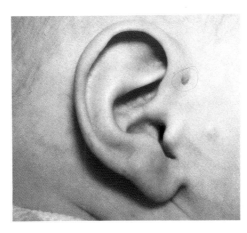

Fig. 2.28 Aural fistula. A pronounced congenital ear pit is seen anterior to the tragus. Its only significance is that it may become infected.

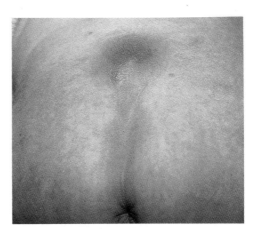

Fig. 2.29 Pilonidal sinus. This midline sinus overlying the sacrum did not extend to the spinal cord.

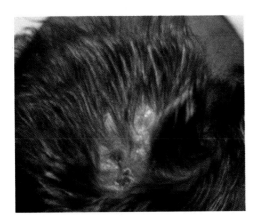

Fig. 2.30 Localized ectodermal dysplasia. An extensive punched-out area lacking all normal dermal elements is seen in the midline of the scalp of this child with trisomy 13.

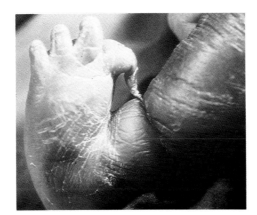

Fig. 2.31 Amniotic bands. A lower extremity amniotic band caused amputation of the toes and constriction around the lower leg.

malformation. While removal is not required, it may be indicated cosmetically. Syndactyly, fusion of the soft tissues between digits, is relatively common (Fig. 2.26). Once again, a family history can be helpful.

External Ear

Careful morphologic examination of the external ear may reveal a number of minor anomalies. One of the more common is the presence of preauricular skin tags located anterior to the tragus (Fig. 2.27). They may be unilateral or bilateral, and represent remnants of the first branchial arch. Although often of little consequence, they may be seen in more serious malformations of branchial arch development involving multiple structures of the head and neck. Surgical removal may be indicated for cosmetic purposes.

A second, often overlooked malformation is the presence of ear pits or congenital aural fistulas located anterior to the tragus (Fig. 2.28). These may be familial, are twice as common in females, and are more common in blacks. They are of little consequence beyond the fact that they may become infected.

Midline Defects

While major malformations of the spinal column such as myelomeningocele are readily identifiable (see Chapter 1), diagnostic differentiation between two other midline defects —pilonidal sinuses and congenital dermal sinuses of the lumbar and sacral spine—can be difficult. A pilonidal sinus tends

to be located over the sacrum (Fig. 2.29). The surface opening is usually larger than that of a dermal sinus, but the tract rarely extends into the spinal canal. Therefore, while infection can occur, CNS extension is unlikely. A congenital dermal sinus is usually located over the lower lumbar region, with a sinus tract that can extend farther down the spinal column. The external orifice may be a small dimple or an easily visible opening surrounded by hair. A hemangioma or a lipoma may lie along the tract. Recognition is important, as there may be an underlying spinal dysraphism, and infection of the tract can extend to the CNS. Both types of sinuses may coexist in the same infant. If diagnostic differentiation is difficult, radiographic and neurosurgical evaluations may be indicated.

Another form of midline defect may occur over the posterior parietal scalp and consists of a localized area of ectodermal dysplasia (Fig. 2.30). This lesion appears "punched out" and lacks all normal dermal elements. It may be associated with chromosomal anomalies, especially trisomy 13, but may be present in otherwise normal infants. Similar-appearing lesions, often located on the extremities, are to be distinguished from those on the scalp, since they often represent a dermatologic defect known as cutis aplasia.

Amniotic Bands

A number of serious structural deformations can result from early in utero amniotic rupture and subsequent bandline compression or amputation. The band-induced abnormalities generally affect the limbs, digits, and craniofacial structures (Fig. 2.31). This phenomenon is usually sporadic.

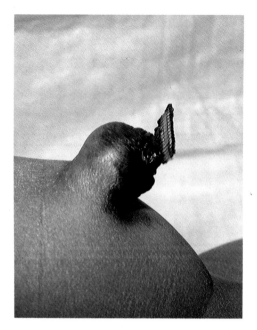

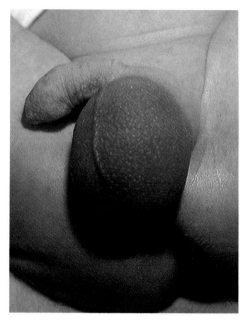

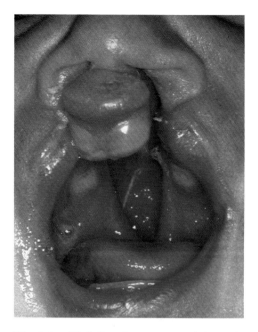

Fig. 2.32 Umbilical hernia. This prominent umbilical hernia was noted at birth
in an otherwise normal black infant.

Fig. 2.33 Scrotal swelling. This infant
demonstrates a unilateral hydrocele which
was noted at birth. Transillumination was
consistent with the diagnosis.

Fig. 2.34 Cleft lip. A prominent bilateral
cleft lip coupled with a complete cleft palate is seen in an infant with trisomy 13.
The cleft extends from the soft to the hard
palate, exposing the nasal cavity.

Umbilical Hernia

A common finding, especially in black infants, is the presence
of an umbilical hernia (Fig. 2.32). The incidence of this defect
of the central fascia beneath the umbilicus is also higher in
premature infants and those with congenital thyroid deficiency. It is important to distinguish between this relatively
benign fascial defect and the more serious defects of those
somites which form the peritoneal, muscular, and ectodermal
layers of the abdominal wall underlying the umbilicus, resulting in an omphalocele. In the latter condition, a portion of the
intestine is located outside of the abdominal wall (see Chapter
15). When large, the distinction is obvious, but in its mildest
form it will resemble a fixed hernia of the umbilicus. A true
umbilical hernia requires no therapy, since the majority
resolve spontaneously in the first few years of life. Those that
remain after the age of 3 years can be surgically repaired. Attempts to reduce the hernia with tape or coins are ineffective.
Incarceration is rare.

Scrotal Swelling

Swelling of the scrotum in the neonate is a relatively common
finding, especially in breech deliveries. While the differential
diagnosis includes hematomas, infections, testicular torsion,
and tumors, the great majority of cases are attributable to
hydroceles or fluid accumulation in the tunica vaginalis. Palpation reveals an extremely smooth, firm, egg-shaped mass
which brightly transilluminates (Fig. 2.33). When the hydrocele is noncommunicating, one can often get above the mass
with a palpatory thumb and finger and feel a normal spermatic cord. The testicle may be difficult to palpate, but is usually visible upon transillumination. It should be noted that
with inguinal hernias the prolapsed intestine may transillumi-

nate as well, but usually presents visible septa under high-
intensity light. Furthermore, on palpation there is significant
thickening of the spermatic cord. While a hydrocele may persist for months, the majority spontaneously resolve. There is
a high association with inguinal hernias, especially in those
hydroceles which persist. In such cases, the spermatic cord is
often noticeably thickened. Because of the association with
hernias, the possibility of bowel incarceration should be kept
in mind. Persistence of a hydrocele for more than 6 months or
other findings suggestive of an inguinal hernia is an indication
for surgical repair. See Chapter 15 for a more detailed discussion of inguinal hernias.

Oral Clefts

Cleft lip and/or palate is among the most common facial
anomalies (Fig. 2.34). These defects represent failure of lip
fusion (at 35 days) and, in some cases, subsequent failure of
closure of the palatal shelves (at 8 to 9 weeks). While many
cases occur spontaneously, others appear to be inherited, and
in a minority of instances the defect is one manifestation of a
chromosomal disorder. Adequate assessment necessitates
careful examination of all the structures of the head and neck
and their relationship to each other. For example, cleft palate
may be coupled with mandibular hypoplasia (Pierre Robin
anomaly), resulting in significant respiratory obstruction.
Because of associated eustachian tube dysfunction, otitis
media is an almost invariable complication of cleft palate.
Specialized feeding techniques are often necessary for these
infants. Even in the absence of an overt cleft, palpation and
visualization of the palate and uvula should be routine since
clefts of the soft palate (associated with a bifid uvula and a
midline notch at the posterior border of the hard palate) can
lead to later speech problems.

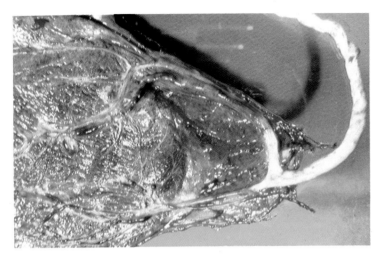

Fig. 2.35 Velamentous cord insertion. The umbilical cord is inserted into the amniotic membranes rather than into the placental disc. This leaves the umbilical vessels relatively unprotected and predisposes them to rupture.

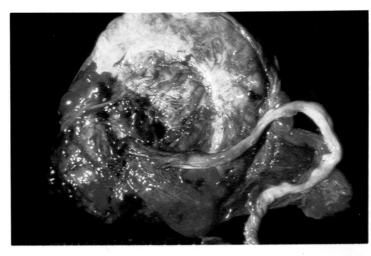

Fig. 2.36 Circumvallate placenta. There is extension of villous tissue beyond the chorionic surface, with a well-defined hyalinized fold at the edge of the chorionic plate.

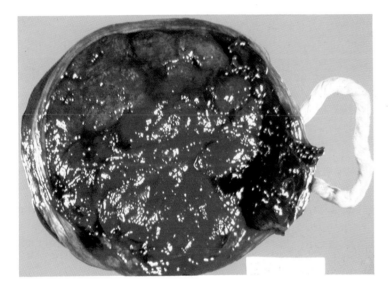

Fig. 2.37 Abruptio placenta. Examination of this placenta reveals a small abruption site, with an adherent blood clot along the margin.

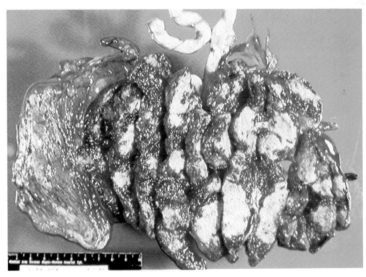

Fig. 2.38 Infarcted placenta. A massive placental infarction comprising the majority of the villous surface is shown. Such an extensive infarction compromises fetal nutrition and oxygenation.

THE PLACENTA

Careful examination of the placenta can prove to be a valuable aid in the diagnosis and treatment of the newborn infant. It is most unfortunate that it has been relegated to an "afterbirth" and is often immediately discarded, without knowing the condition of the offspring. After trimming the membranes and cord, the normal ratio of fetal to placental weight is approximately 4–7 to 1. The configuration, color, condition of the membranes, insertion of the cord, and condition of both the fetal and maternal surfaces are all relevant.

The insertion of the umbilical cord into the placenta, which can be central, eccentric, marginal, or velamentous, can be important in understanding unexplained asphyxia or blood loss. In a velamentous insertion (Fig. 2.35), the cord is inserted into the membranes rather than into the disc, leaving the umbilical vessels unprotected for a variable distance. These vessels are more prone to rupture, with resultant fetal hemorrhage (vasa previa).

At times, placentation itself is abnormal. In a circumvallate placenta (Fig. 2.36), the villous tissue projects beyond the chorionic surface, with a hyalinized fold at the edge of the chorionic plate. This type of placentation has been reported to be a cause of antepartum bleeding, premature labor, and increased perinatal mortality.

Premature placental separation (abruptio placenta) can lead to an accumulation of blood behind the placenta (Fig. 2.37). Although the bleeding is usually of maternal origin, fetal blood loss may also occur. Large abruptions may lead to poor growth, fetal asphyxia, or even death. It is important to distinguish a true abruption, where an adherent clot compresses the maternal surface, from the nonadherent collection of blood which forms upon normal placental separation.

Placental infarctions (Fig. 2.38) are among the more common, easily diagnosed abnormalities. They tend to occur along the margin of the placenta, can vary from red to yellowish-white, and when small are usually of little significance. However, large (> 30 percent of placental volume) central infarcts can be clinically significant by virtue of reducing the placental surface available for fetal oxygenation and nutrition. Infarcts are most common in pregnancies complicated by hypertension.

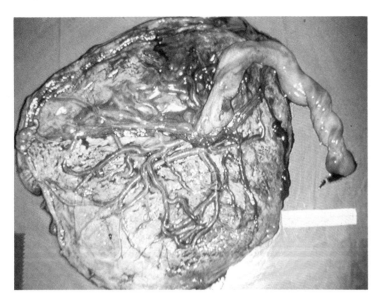

Fig. 2.39 Chorioamnionitis. This is a placental specimen from a pregnancy with documented amniotic fluid infection. The surface of the membranes is opaque and shows yellowish discoloration.

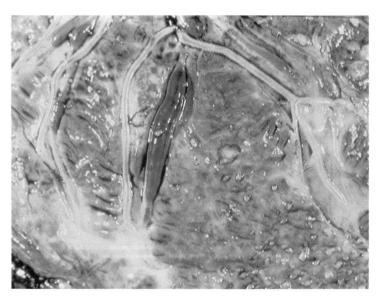

Fig. 2.40 Amnion nodosum. The fetal surface of this placenta from a pregnancy with oligohydramnios demonstrates multiple nodules consistent with amnion nodosum. This finding suggests the strong possibility of renal agenesis or dysgenesis.

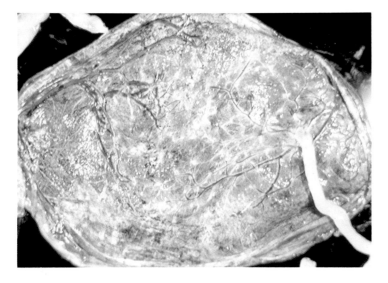

Fig. 2.41 Monochorionic, monoamniotic placenta. Examination of this placenta from monozygotic twins reveals no dividing membranes, thus assuring monozygosity.

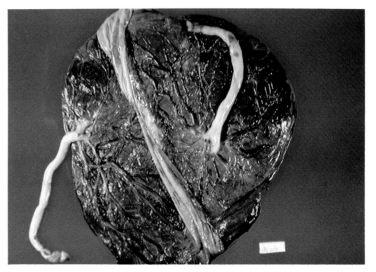

Fig. 2.42 Dichorionic, diamniotic placenta. The presence of two amniotic sacs and separate chorions in this twin placenta precludes determination of zygosity.

Chorioamnionitis (Fig. 2.39), inflammation of the fetal membranes, is an immediate clue to potential neonatal infection. Upon gross examination, the membranes lack their normal sheen and translucency, appearing gray or yellow. Inflammation, confirmable by microscopic examination, can also be found in the fetal vessels of the chorionic plate and the umbilical cord.

In pregnancies in which the quantity of amniotic fluid is decreased (oligohydramnios), examination of the amnion may also reveal shiny, gray, flat nodules known as amnion nodosum (Fig. 2.40). The presence of these nodules can be an immediate clue to the diagnosis of renal dysfunction or agenesis in the newborn. Since such infants may also have hypoplastic lungs and dysmorphic features (such as occurs in Potter syndrome; see Chapter 13 for a full discussion of this syndrome),

this early clue to the diagnosis can be most helpful to the physician and family.

In multiple gestation deliveries, a careful placental evaluation is crucial. The major distinction to be made is whether there is a single chorion or outer layer of the fetal membranes. When twins are present in a single amniotic cavity, and thus a single chorion (Fig. 2.41), monozygosity is assured. For all practical purposes, a single chorion which bridges two amniotic sacs is also evidence for monozygotic twins. In this instance, it is essential to carefully examine the membranes at the site of connection of the two amniotic sacs. When two chorions and two amnions (or a total of four membranes at their interface) are present (Fig. 2.42), twins may be either monozygotic or dizygotic. Approximately 36 percent of monozygotic twins are dichorionic.

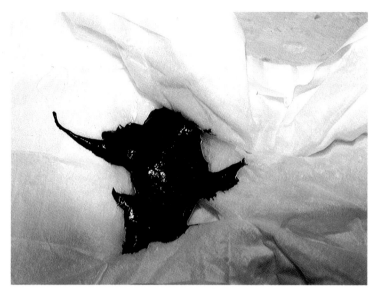

Fig. 2.43 Meconium. A typical, sticky, greenish-black meconium stool is shown. This consists of accumulated intestinal cells, bile, and proteinaceous material formed during intestinal development.

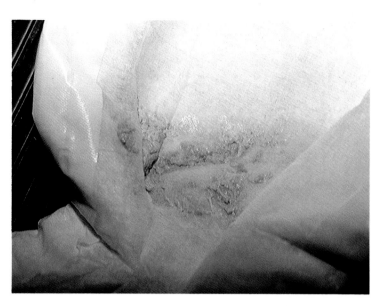

Fig. 2.44 Transitional stool. At 2 to 3 days following delivery, stools become greenish-brown and may contain some milk curds.

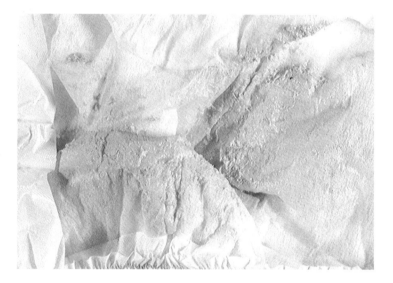

Fig. 2.45 Breast-milk stool. The stools of breast-fed infants are yellow, soft, mild smelling, and typically have the consistency of pea soup.

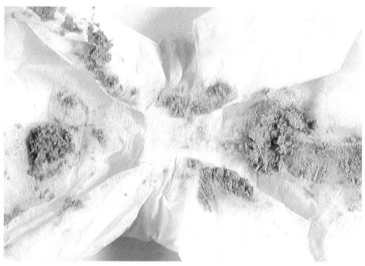

Fig. 2.46 Formula stool. Infants fed commercial formula typically have darker, firmer stools than do breast-fed infants.

NEWBORN STOOLS

An infant's first few bowel movements consist of accumulated intestinal cells, bile, and proteinaceous material formed during intestinal development. The material, termed meconium (Fig. 2.43), is a sticky greenish-black product mirroring the shape of the fetal intestine. When passed prior to delivery into the amniotic fluid, it can, if aspirated into the lung, cause a potentially life-threatening disorder known as meconium aspiration syndrome. Such early passage is generally precipitated by fetal distress or asphyxia. Failure to pass meconium in the first 2 days of life may indicate intestinal obstruction due to stenosis, atresia, or Hirschsprung disease. The possibility of cystic fibrosis with a meconium ileus should also be considered. In premature infants, failure to pass meconium may reflect meconium plug syndrome (small left colon syndrome), which appears to be a disorder of maturation of intestinal motility. In most cases, a Gastrografin enema leads to prompt passage of meconium without recurrence.

By the third day of life, stools change in character and are known as transitional stools (Fig. 2.44). They are greenish-brown to yellowish-brown in color, less sticky than meconium, and may contain some milk curds. In some infants who are fed generous quantities of milk during the first few days, the stool may have an increased liquid component which contains undigested sugar. This diarrheal stool will resolve with moderation in the quantity of feeding, since it is caused by the osmotic effect of undigested lactose.

After the third to fourth day, the quality and frequency of stool are often functions of the type of milk given. Breast-fed infants have stools which are yellow to golden in color, mild smelling, and pasty in consistency, resembling pea soup (Fig. 2.45). Although it is commonly held that the mother's diet directly affects the frequency and consistency of a breast-fed-infant's stool, there is little scientific information on this subject. Infants fed cow-milk–based formula have pale yellow to light brown stools which are firm and somewhat more offensive in odor (Fig. 2.46).

nates. Many infants have a stool after each feeding for the first several weeks, due to an active gastrocolic reflex. Other normal infants may have one stool every few days. In general, infants fed cow milk formula have stools less frequently than those taking breast milk.

A careful history with emphasis on an infant's stool pattern, feeding history, and any parental attempts (laxatives, rectal manipulation) to induce bowel movements can be extremely important. Normal weight gain in the face of true diarrhea is unusual. Difficulty in passing stools (straining, crying, decreased frequency) may reflect local irritation from anal fissure formation, rather than true constipation. The use of a topical lubricant and stool softeners can often overcome constipation. Failure of such measures suggests the possibility of significant pathology (see Chapter 15 for further discussion).

BIBLIOGRAPHY

Avery GB (ed.): Neonatology — Pathophysiology and Management of the Newborn, 2nd ed. Lippincott, Philadelphia, 1981.

Dubowitz LV, Dubowitz C, Goldberger C: Clinical assessment of gestational age in the newborn infant. J Pediatr 77:1–10, 1970.

Fox H: Pathology of the Placenta. In Major Problems in Pathology, vol. 7. Saunders, Philadelphia, 1978.

Painter MJ, Bergman I: Obstetrical trauma to the neonatal central and peripheral nervous system. Semin Perinatol VI (1):89–104, 1982.

Scanlon JW, Nelson T, Grylack LJ, Smith YF: A System of Newborn Physical Examination. University Park Press, Baltimore, 1979.

Smith DW (ed.): Recognizable Patterns of Human Malformation, 3rd ed. In Major Problems in Clinical Pediatrics, vol. 7. Saunders, Philadelphia, 1982.

DEVELOPMENTAL PEDIATRICS

3

Roberta E. Bauer, M.D.

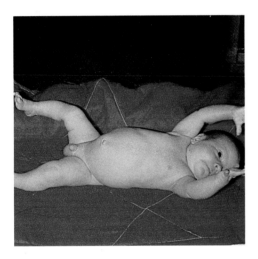

FIG. 3.1 Moro response. Symmetric abduction and extension of the extremities comprises the first phase of the Moro response, following a loud noise or abrupt change in the infant's head position.

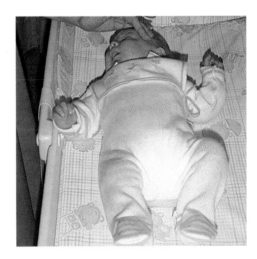

FIG. 3.2 "Fencer" position of the ATNR. Note the elbow and knee flexion on the occipital side, while extension of the extremities dominates on the chin side.

Developmental pediatrics studies the acquisition of functional ability in children as well as the identification of constitutional disorders and/or environmental circumstances that impact upon that acquisition. The development of functional ability extends from birth throughout adulthood and the assessment of development crosses many professional lines, including those of occupational therapy, physical therapy, speech pathology, social work, psychology, teaching, genetics, neurology, and psychiatry. The task of developmental assessment and referral, however, from birth through the preschool years, falls first and often exclusively to the pediatrician.

Although the pediatrician's monitoring of the developmental process continues throughout childhood and adolescence, a pictorial chronicle of developmental assessment at all ages is beyond the scope of this chapter. Because the sensorimotor period of development lends itself best to assessment by physical examination, development will be presented here in terms of the normal milestones that occur during this period as well as their abnormal manifestations. Assessments of development commonly are divided into the following areas: gross motor, cognitive, language, social/emotional, and fine motor and perceptual. This chapter will be divided accordingly.

GROSS MOTOR DEVELOPMENT
Early Reflex Patterns

At birth the infant's random movements consist of alternating flexions and extensions that usually are symmetric and vary in strength with the infant's state of wakefulness. Large muscle groups work together in reflex patterns that appear to be purposeless although they have the effect of exercising and strengthening muscles to be used later for more complex and directed activity.

Perhaps the best known of these patterns is the Moro response (Fig. 3.1), which occurs following a loud noise or an abrupt change in the infant's head position. The first phase of the response consists of symmetric abduction and extension of the arms with extension of the trunk. The second phase is marked by adduction of the upper extremities (as if in an embrace) and is frequently accompanied by crying.

The newborn's limb motions are strongly influenced by head position. In fact, if a neonate's gaze is directed to one side, tone will be increased in the extensor muscles on that side as well as in the flexor muscles on the opposite side. This pattern is termed the asymmetric tonic neck reflex (ATNR) and is seen by 2 weeks of age (Fig. 3.2).

PRIMITIVE REFLEXES AND EQUILIBRIUM RESPONSES

FIG. 3.3 *Primitive Reflexes and Equilibrium Responses.*

Reflex	Appearance	Disappearance
Moro	Birth	4 months
ATNR	2 weeks	6 months
Toe grasp	Birth	8–15 months
Hand grasp	Birth	3 months
Crossed adductor	Birth	7 months
Head righting	4–6 months	Persists voluntarily
Protective equilibrium	4–6 months	Persists voluntarily
Parachute	8–9 months	Persists voluntarily

Different sources may vary on the precise timing of the appearance and disappearance of these primitive reflexes and equilibrium responses.

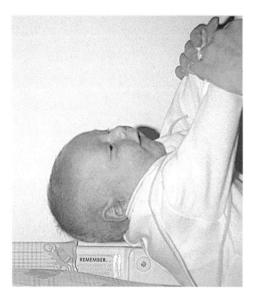 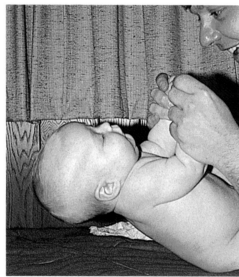 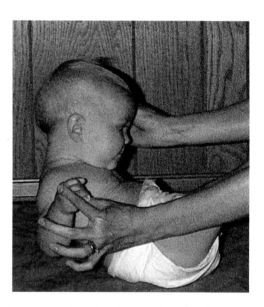

FIG. 3.4 *Children at various levels of ability performing pull to sit maneuver. (Left) At 2 months of age, total head lag is evident. (Center) At 4 months, the head is held nearly even with the body. (Right) At 6 months, the infant's head leads and the body follows.*

With the emergence of voluntary control from higher cortical centers comes the increasing influence of balanced muscular flexion and extension, and of protective equilibrium reactions, to replace the influence of the early primitive reflexes. A timetable listing the expected emergence and disappearance of some of these early reflex patterns is presented in Figure 3.3.

Antigravity Muscular Control

The infant's earliest control task is that of achieving and maintaining stable posture against the influence of gravity. This control develops in a cephalocaudal progression. For example, neck flexors allow head control against gravity in the pull to sit maneuver. The expected developmental progression for this maneuver is demonstrated in Figure 3.4, by children examined at typical checkup intervals.

Next, progressive shoulder and upper trunk control enables the young baby to hold his chest off the surface with his weight supported on the forearms. This so-called puppy position is a favorite of photographers and is expected by 4 months of age (Fig. 3.5).

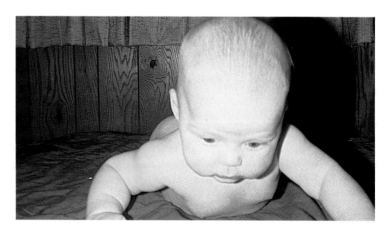

FIG. 3.5 *Puppy position. Increased trunk and shoulder control allows weight bearing on forearms to support chest off the surface. This infant, nearly 6 months old, is beginning to weight shift and lift one arm, as well.*

From the puppy position, the infant can alternate weight bearing on either arm to facilitate the uncontrolled prone to supine roll that normally occurs soon after, at approximately

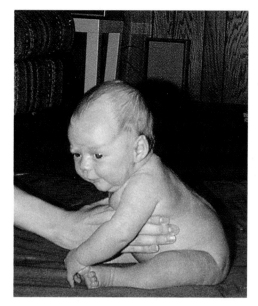 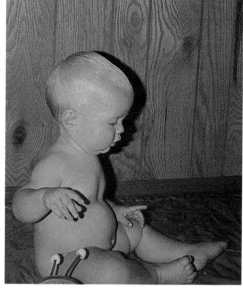 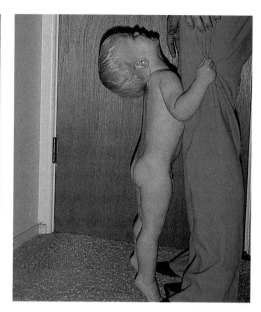

FIG. 3.6 Sitting posture. (Left) At 2 months absent trunk tone prevents the child from sitting independently. Instead he stoops forward with a total C-posture. (Center) By 6 months, the lumbar area is essentially flat with some forward curve remaining. Note how this relatively new sitter keeps hands in guard in case he needs to prop himself up. (Right) By 1 year, the lordotic curve is evident in standing.

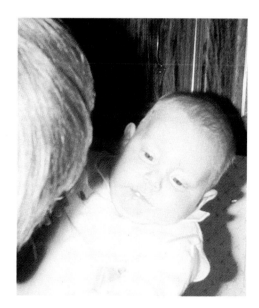 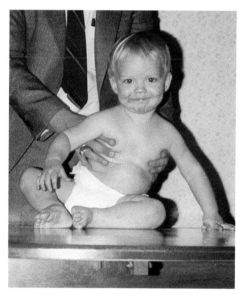 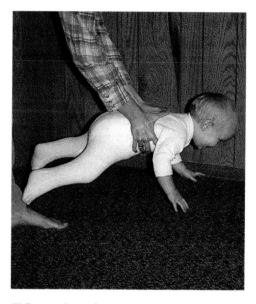

FIG. 3.7 Head righting. The line of vision is maintained parallel to the ground despite a change in the infant's body position.

FIG. 3.8 Protective equilibrium response. As examiner pushes the child laterally, the child flexes his trunk toward the force to regain his center of gravity while one arm extends to protect against falling (lateral propping).

FIG. 3.9 Parachute response. As examiner allows child to freefall in ventral suspension, the child's extremities extend symmetrically to distribute weight over a broader and more stable base upon landing.

4 months of age. Continued evolution of trunk control down the thoracic spine and into the lumbar area results in the lumbar lordotic curve with sitting and standing. This progression is illustrated in Figure 3.6 by a child examined at three typical intervals.

Balance and equilibrium reactions also emerge in sequence. "Head righting" refers to the ability to align the plane of vision parallel to the ground despite the position of one's body (Fig. 3.7). Four-month olds frequently demonstrate this ability when tilted in vertical suspension. Seated protective responses can be elicited by abruptly but gently pushing the child's center of gravity past the midline in one of the horizontal planes in space. This reflex response, which involves increased trunk flexor tone toward the force and an outreached hand and limb away from the force, usually emerges by 6 months of age (Fig. 3.8).

The parachute response, involving outreach of the arms and legs to an abrupt downward motion from suspension in space, must be present by 10 months of age (Fig. 3.9). The absence of equilibrium responses is sometimes taken to be a poor prognostic indicator for unsupported sitting or walking in children with cerebral palsy.

The 6-month-old infant who lacks head control on pull to sit, who cannot clear the table surface with his chest by supporting his weight on his arms in prone, who continues to have a C-posture in sitting, who shows no head righting, or who continues to demonstrate a complete Moro response or ATNR is at significant variance from his peers in gross motor

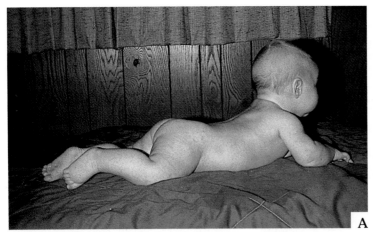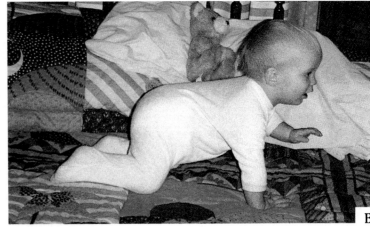

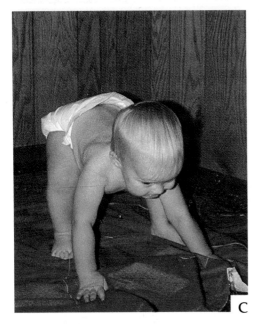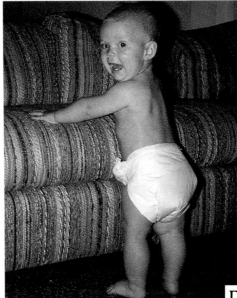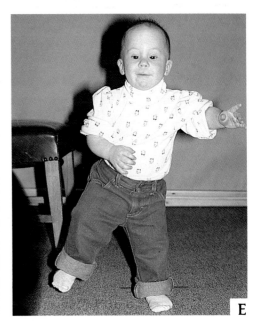

FIG. 3.10 Early forms of locomotion. **A,** Crawling implies that the belly is still on the floor; **B,** creeping refers to hands and knees mobility (quadruped); **C,** bear walking (on hands and feet) is uncommon except in transition from quadruped to free standing; **D,** cruising is supporting weight fully on lower extremities but with two-handed support on stationary objects needed before moving with steps; **E,** early free walking.

development and deserves evaluation for a possible neuromuscular disorder.

Locomotion

Beyond antigravity muscular control, gross motor milestones frequently are described in terms of locomotion. Prone to supine rolling soon is followed by back to front rolling, which usually is present by 5 to 6 months of age. "Commando crawling" often is followed by "creeping" or by "bear walking," which often precedes "cruising." Since these terms though commonly used can be confusing, the forms of locomotion they refer to are depicted in Figure 3.10.

It is important to note that not all children pass through each of these stages in their quest for upright locomotion, and, in fact, there is a wide range for the onset and duration of each stage. Walking three steps alone, for example, occurs at a median age of 11.7 months although the range is from 9 to 17 months of age. Ages at which children are found to be outside of two standard deviations from the group norm may vary relative to the screening test used. The age ranges for early motor development presented in the table in Figure 3.11 were taken from the Bayley sample, a well-known infant testing instrument.

Beyond the attainment of upright mobility, progress in gross motor skills occurs with the child's achieving improved balance and coordination. Typical skills attained include progressive narrowing of the base of the gait (heel to toe walking), balancing on one foot, hopping, and using muscle groups in timed sequences (such as the ability to throw and catch a ball or to pedal a tricycle or bicycle). Typical age ranges for some of these kinds of activities are listed in Figure 3.12.

Evaluating Gross Motor Developmental Delay

Because the achievement of all developmental milestones depends on the successful acquisition of prerequisite abilities, a solid foundation must be established before being built upon,

EARLY GROSS MOTOR MILESTONE NORMALS

Task	Age Range (months)	Median Age
Sits alone momentarily	4.0–8.0	5.3
Rolls back to stomach	4.0–10.0	6.4
Sits steadily	5.0–9.0	6.6
Gets to sitting	6.0–11.0	8.3
Pulls to standing	6.0–12.0	8.6
Stands alone	9.0–16.0	11.0
Walks three steps alone	9.0–17.0	11.7

Wide ranges in the attainment of these gross motor milestones in healthy children are the rule rather than the exception.

FIG. 3.11 Early Gross Motor Milestone Normals. (From Bayley Scales of Infant Development, Psychological Corp., 1969)

HIGHER GROSS MOTOR MILESTONES

Task	Age by Which 75% of Children in Denver Developmental Screening Test Sample Performed Task
Walks well	13½ months
Balances on one foot for 1 second	36 months
Hops on one foot	48 months
Heel to toe walks (75% of time)	4–4¼ years
Throws ball overhand	22½ months
Catches ball bounced (75% of time)	4⅞ years
Pedals tricycle	2¾ years

FIG. 3.12 Higher Gross Motor Milestones. (Selected from Frankenburg WK, Dodds JB: The Denver Developmental Screening Test. J Pediatr 71 [181], 1967)

similar to the construction of a pyramid. Moreover, because these developmental events occur not at a specific time, but rather within a wide age range, the presence or absence of a single skill at a particular age cannot be used as a diagnosis of neurological intactness or dysfunction. Progress in muscular control should be viewed as an ongoing process impacted upon by the child's general health and opportunity for experience, by temperamental characteristics that affect the child's willingness to try new experiences, by genetic endowments for facility of coordination and strength, and by socioeconomic factors that affect child-rearing practices and childhood experiences.

However, when gross motor delays are found to be a part of global delays, when they are related to consistent disuse of one side of the body or of one limb, when they are associated with prolonged or obligatory infantile reflexes or opisthotonic posturing, or when the loss of a previously obtained milestone is historically documented, further diagnostic evaluation is indicated. In such cases, delays in gross motor skills should prompt consideration of a number of possibilities, in-

Global Developmental Delay	Motor Dysfunction	Motor Intact but Otherwise Restricted
Genetic syndromes and chromosomal abnormalities	Central nervous system damage—kernicterus, birth injury, neonatal stroke, trauma, prolonged seizures or metabolic insult, infection	Congenital malformations—bony or soft-tissue defects
Brain morphologic abnormalities		Diminished energy supply—chronic illness, starvation
Endocrine deficiencies—hypothyroidism, prolonged hypoglycemia	Spinal cord damage—Werdnig-Hoffmann disease, myelomeningocele, polio	Environmental deprivation—casted, nonweight-bearing, cultural differences in experience
Neurodegenerative diseases	Peripheral nerve damage—brachial plexus injury, heritable neuropathies	Familial/genetic endowment—slower myelination, racial differences
Congenital infections		Sensory deficits—blindness
Severe mental retardation	Motor end-plate damage—myasthenia gravis	Temperamental effects—low activity level, slow to try new tasks
	Muscular damage—muscular dystrophies	Trauma—child abuse
	Other—benign congenital hypotonia	

FIG. 3.13 Potential Causes of Delayed Gross Motor Development.

cluding those listed in Figure 3.13. A traditional history and physical examination will help to confirm the presence or absence of many of these disorders.

Cerebral Palsy

Cerebral palsy is a static encephalopathy occurring from birth to 2 years of age, resulting from injury to the central motor control areas. It is characterized by abnormal gross motor development, although the child may have normal milestones in other areas as well as a normal examination of the special senses. A diagnosis of cerebral palsy is strongly suggested by findings of four out of six major motor criteria (Fig. 3.14) in a child 1 year of age or older who has no evidence of progressive disease by history.

EARLY PHYSICAL FINDINGS
Hypotonia
Physical findings over the first year of life, in a child with cerebral palsy, will change significantly and may present diversely. Floppy babies—those with diffuse hypotonia but with elicitable reflexes and no evidence of weakness—may well develop increased tone over the first 12 to 18 months and have clearly rigid or spastic hypertonia by the end of the first 2 years. Infants who demonstrate hypotonia in addition to brisk deep tendon reflexes or sustained clonus are at particular risk for the development of cerebral palsy.

Excessive Extensor Posturing
The child who demonstrates increased extensor tone beginning in early infancy also is at risk for cerebral palsy. Under normal circumstances, infants less than 3 months of age, when supported in ventral suspension, will maintain the head in slight flexion with the trunk mildly convex. When ex-

THE LEVINE (POSTER) CRITERIA FOR DIAGNOSIS OF CEREBRAL PALSY

1. Posturing and abnormal movement patterns—extensor thrusts, blocks
2. Oropharyngeal problems—tongue thrusts, grimacing, swallowing difficulties
3. Strabismus
4. Tone—increased or decreased in muscles
5. Evolutional responses—persistent primitive reflexes or failure to develop equilibrium and protective responses
6. Reflexes—deep tendon reflex increased and plantar reflexes up going

FIG. 3.14 The Levine (POSTER) Criteria for Diagnosis of Cerebral Palsy.

aggerated tone is present in the antigravity muscle group, however, the infant may elevate his head above the horizontally level trunk (Fig. 3.15). Similarly, with the child in the prone position on a mat, unknowing parents may be pleased by their child's apparent precocious development of head control or of early belly to back rolling in the first 2 months, when, in fact, both of these findings demonstrate excessive extensor posturing.

Further evidence of abnormally increased tone will be found on the pull to sit maneuver, when the child extends at the hips and knees and comes to standing on pointed toes rather than to the appropriate sitting posture. This child,

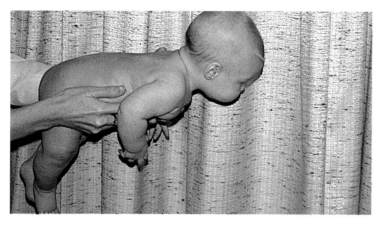

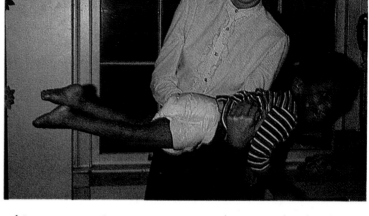

FIG. 3.15 Extensor tone. (Left) Ventral suspension in normal 2-month-old infant shows head held briefly above neutral with lower extremities held below trunk. (Right) Even in this child of 3 years, excessive extensor tone can be seen as head and lower extremities are held above level of trunk.

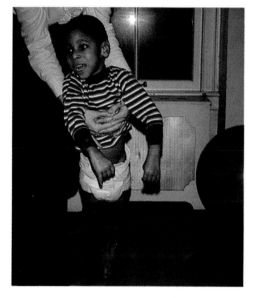

FIG. 3.16 Scissoring. Note how excessive pull of the hip adductors and internal rotators in this child of 3 years results in child's legs crossing in a scissorlike pattern while he is supported in vertical suspension.

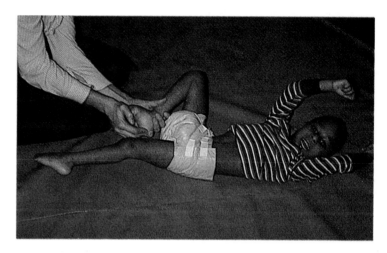

FIG. 3.17 Marie-Foix maneuver. By flexing the child's toes, the therapist can reduce extensor tone enough to obtain abduction of the hip and knee flexion in this child with spastic quadriplegia.

when placed in ventral suspension, will not demonstrate head righting at the expected time and later will scissor the lower extremities as a result of hypertonia of the hip adductors and internal rotators (Fig. 3.16).

Because of the combination of increased trunk extension and scissoring, these infants are predisposed to hip contractures and/or dislocations that deserve careful orthopedic follow-up and intervention. Furthermore, parents will find it difficult to position these infants for activities such as diapering and feeding, and will benefit from knowledge of the Marie-Foix maneuver to break up excessive extension in the lower extremities. Flexing the child's toes will result in flexion of the knee and flexion-abduction of the hip to allow normal perineal hygiene (Fig. 3.17).

Obligatory or Persistent Reflexes

Beyond hypotonia and excessive extensor posturing, the evolutional reflexes are helpful aids in the diagnosis of cerebral palsy. The asymmetric tonic neck reflex, described earlier as a normal primitive reflex in the immature infant's nervous system, is one out of which normal babies can move, with activity. An obligate ATNR, however, will cause the infant to remain in the fencer position until the head position is altered. This finding is not normal in a child of any age and is highly suggestive of the static encephalopathy and motor deficit characterizing cerebral palsy.

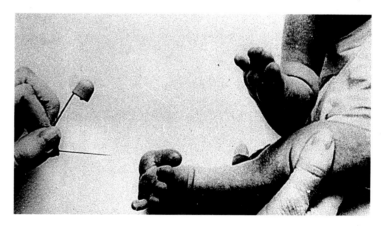

FIG. 3.18 Crossed extensor response in an infant. Stimulation of one foot causes the opposite leg to flex and then abduct and extend.

Also strongly suggestive of cerebral palsy is the non-obligate ATNR that persists beyond 6 months of age. This finding should be considered as abnormal in the baby who *always* prefers to sleep or lie with the head turned in a particular direction. Similarly, persistence of the Moro response beyond 6 months of age or evidence of the crossed extensor response (Fig. 3.18) beyond 1 year of age suggests that motor damage has occurred preventing higher levels of control

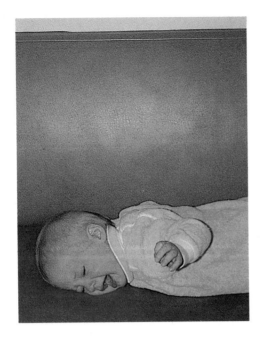

FIG. 3.19 Hemiparesis. Note that this child is unable to extend the involved arm forward to support weight in the prone position to lift chest off the mat.

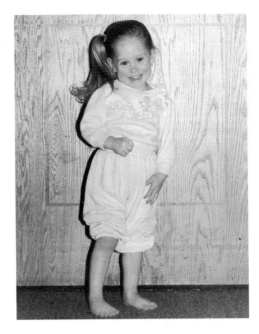

FIG. 3.20 Note the arm held in flexion and internal rotation and the leg circumducted on the involved side in this child with hemiplegic cerebral palsy.

from superseding the influence of the early reflexes. Along the same lines, a lack of development of lateral protective equilibrium reactions by 7 to 8 months of age or of the parachute reaction by 10 months of age should prompt similar concerns.

Hemiparesis

Asymmetric use of the upper or lower extremities is rare during the first 4 months of life, and when it is seen in resting activity or when it is elicited with the Moro or ATNR, peripheral problems such as congenital musculoskeletal abnormalities or neural plexus injuries should be considered.

Asymmetric motor development of CNS origin can be noted after 4 months of age, when hands should be opening and arms reaching and nearing the midline. The hand that remains fisted, the arm that remains caught beneath the infant when he tries to prop himself up in the puppy position (Fig. 3.19), and the infant's inability to use that arm in simple tasks by 6 months of age all suggest hemiparesis.

Later, during the first year, findings of concern would include failure to develop the protective response of lateral propping or the development of an asymmetric parachute response. In addition, crawling may be uneven with propulsion coming from one side while the opposite arm and leg are dragged behind.

ABNORMALITIES IN GAIT

Children with hemiparesis will have sufficient difficulty compensating for their lack of protective responses and for their uneven strength and poor balance, and typically will delay walking until 2½ to 3 years of age. In mildly affected children, walking may show little abnormality but when the child is asked to run, posturing of the upper extremity in flexion and internal rotation may emerge. Usually, the lower limb will rotate internally and the foot may be held in equinus, making it functionally longer on the swing-through part of the gait. To clear the foot from the floor, the child will compensate by swinging the leg farther out in abduction or by circumducting the affected side. These patterns, in some cases, also can be observed in standing (Fig. 3.20). Subtle changes in gait pattern may be heard or they may be observed in the wear pattern on the bottom of the child's shoes.

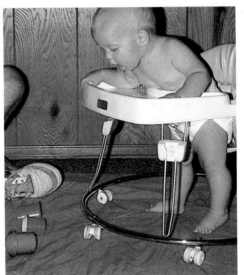

FIG. 3.21 This 6-month-old infant was able not only to track his toy through a vertical fall, but he continued to search for it on the floor even after his gaze had been interrupted. A stable mental picture of objects is developing.

FUNCTIONAL ABNORMALITIES

In children with hemiparesis, functional discrepancies often predate asymmetric changes in tone or reflexes. Increased resistance to supination at the wrist, limited flopping of one wrist when the upper extremities are gently yet passively shaken, or 2 to 3 beats of unilateral clonus elicited at the ankle are clues that can be found by the careful observer. In addition, the upper extremities usually will be affected more severely than the lower extremities.

Children with hemiparesis will neglect the visual field on their affected side. Parents should be aware of this phenomenon early, so they can position their infant in the crib to achieve maximal visual stimulation. Another consideration is that of abnormal bony stresses caused by asymmetric muscle strength. In children with hemiparesis, unequal stresses on the spine will result in a higher incidence of scoliosis seen especially during growth spurts.

Toe Walking

The child with spastic diplegia may present subtly, as with delayed crawling or walking, or the child may present with toe walking. The child with toe walking caused by cerebral palsy will have brisk deep tendon reflexes, limited range of

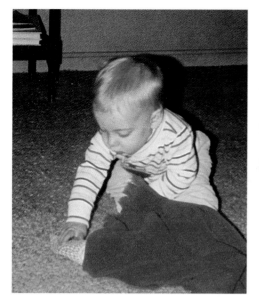 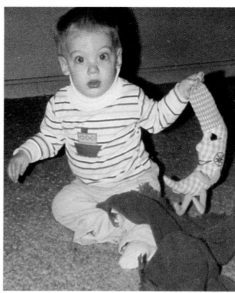

FIG. 3.22 A stable mental image of a toy has developed in this 9-month-old infant who can locate the partially hidden toy.

motion at the ankles, Babinski reflexes, and a normally proportioned muscle mass.

It is important for clinicians to recognize that the differential diagnosis of toe walking includes the muscular dystrophies, tethered spinal cords and spinal tumors, peripheral neuropathies, and fixed bony deformities of the feet. Each of these diagnoses will have different prognoses and therapeutic potentials that will differ markedly from that of cerebral palsy.

Abnormal Movements

In children with athetoid or ataxic cerebral palsy, ataxia or writhing movements do not present until after the first year of life. Likewise, the child who presents first with floppy tone and then with progressive rigidity may appear to have worsening symptoms. This rigidity, however, does not represent progressive deterioration but, rather, is a different expression of CNS dysfunction over time. Because cerebral palsy is a static lesion, if any question of progression is raised by the physical examination or by history, the presence of a degenerative disease or of another responsible pathology must be sought.

Miscellaneous Signs

Clumsiness or poorly developed motor coordination may be blamed appropriately on motor imbalance of the lower extremities, although the possibility of altered depth perception resulting from refractory errors or strabismus should not be ignored. Some physicians estimate that as many as 75 percent of children with diplegia or quadriplegia will have strabismus. Ophthalmologic referral for phorias and tropias that persist beyond 4 months of age is important, not only to prevent amblyopia but also to detect possible CNS dysfunction.

Motor deficits in children with cerebral palsy may not occur in isolation, and seizure disorders, mental retardation, and learning disabilities are found in this population with a greater than expected frequency. These children may require pharmacologic therapy and educational support. Furthermore, the development of behavioral problems that may result from the frustration of adjusting to disabilities can be prevented by matching the functional abilities of children with gross motor problems to appropriate developmental expectations.

COGNITIVE DEVELOPMENT

Sequential changes in the child's ability to process information from the environment were described at length by Piaget. During the first 2 years of life—the sensorimotor period of development—the young child's knowledge of the environment is increased through the senses and through the physical manipulation of objects. It is during this period that the child develops an understanding of object permanence and of the cause and effect nature of actions.

The child's understanding of object permanence enables him to recognize that an object exists even when it cannot be seen, heard, or felt; the child's understanding of cause and effect allows him first to practice predictable outcomes and then to experiment to produce novel outcomes that establish causality. Progress in the child's development of these concepts appears to be an important prerequisite to the development of symbolic language.

The Newborn

The world of the newborn appears to be one in which things that are out of sight are also out of mind. Familiar toys that are partially covered or seen from a different view may not be recognized by the infant. This type of "gestalt" recognition can be dramatic, as in the 4-month-old infant who becomes frightened by his parents if they are wearing hats or new glasses that obscure significant features. Gradually, a stable mental picture of objects develops, and the infant will continue to gaze expectantly, though briefly, at the site where a familiar toy or face has disappeared.

The Infant

Between 4 and 8 months of age, the child will begin to track an object visually through a vertical fall (Fig. 3.21), and to search for a partially covered toy (Fig. 3.22). At this point, the child also will begin to repeat actions that he has discovered will produce interesting results (e.g., continuously kicking the crib to shake the mobile). In these early months, the child's play consists of exploring toys to gain information about their physical characteristics. Activities such as mouthing, shaking, and banging can provide sensory input about an object beyond that of its visual features.

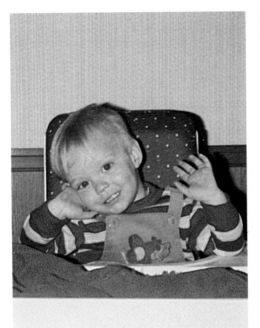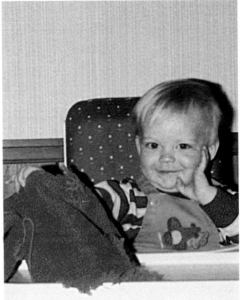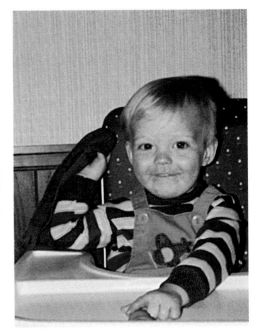

FIG. 3.23 *This 11-month-old child is able to locate this small object even if no part of the object remains visible. In doing* *so he is demonstrating his understanding that objects are permanent.*

At approximately 9 to 12 months of age, babies are able to locate objects that they have seen become hidden (Fig. 3.23), and peek-a-boo becomes an enjoyable pastime. Later, the baby can crawl away from his view of mom and recall where to return to find her. At this time infants begin to manipulate and to examine visually the details of new toys, as index fingers probe indentations and holes and investigate textures.

As children near a year of age, they begin to develop an interest in toys that extends beyond that of their physical properties. Through their play activities, children may demonstrate their awareness that different objects have different purposes. At this stage of development, a child might touch a comb to his hair in a "meaningful nonpretend action" typical of the 9- to 12-month age range (Fig. 3.24).

The Toddler

Beyond a year of age, children begin to vary their behavior to create novel effects, i.e., to experiment. They no longer need parents to show them how to work dials or knobs on a "busy box" nor do they need to hit something by accident to discover the interesting effect that will be created. At this point, genuine pretending begins, as the child engages in the playful representation of commonplace activities using objects for their actual purposes but accompanied by exaggerated sounds or gestures. While smiling at his audience, for example, a child might eat from an empty spoon using "mmm" sounds to distinguish his playfulness from the real activity. This period, referred to as the period of symbolic play, is centered around the child's own body.

Next, the child may begin to include others in his play activities as well as to include pretend actions he has learned from watching others. Along these lines, the 14- to 19-month-old child might be seen brushing the teddy bear's hair.

As the child's memory expands, he is able to locate objects

hidden through multiple changes in position. Piaget demonstrated this by hiding a candy in his hand and then by placing his hand under a hat and releasing the sweet. The younger child will not have developed the strategies needed to seek the multiply displaced object beyond the first hiding place. The early toddler, however, will first search in the hand, and then, upon not finding the sweet there, will persist in searching other sites. This child has developed a permanent image of the hidden object.

Soon the child can deduce the location of an object even if he has not seen the object hidden from his view. Mom will learn that she no longer can get away with putting "no-no's" in her purse while it is behind her back and out of the child's view.

The child's understanding of causality also has advanced, as the cause and effect relationship no longer needs to be direct to be appreciated. For example, a toddler at this stage can make the connection between the winding of a key and the music box playing (Fig. 3.25).

As the child nears 2 years of age, play advances as pretend actions are combined into a series of events. For example, the child may hold the phone to his ear and then put it to his doll's ear, or he may feed his teddy bear and then put the bear to bed.

The next development might be that of the child planning for his pretend activities in anticipation of the play theme to come. Preparing for play indicates an advancement in pretending that is beyond that of improvising with the objects at hand. For example, the child might be seen preparing the play area or searching for needed objects and announcing what the objects are meant to represent. This is evident in the child who upon finding a toy saw examines and discards a number of objects before finding those with appropriate log-like characteristics. This child might then move the saw over the pillows, stack them, and then announce "house" (Fig. 3.26).

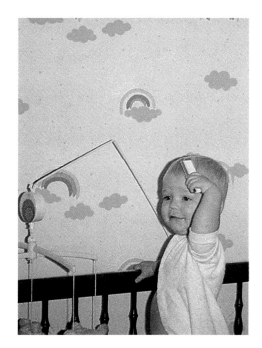

FIG. 3.24 Twelve-month-old child shows that the comb is used for some purpose related to the top of the head, demonstrating the awareness beyond 1 year of age that objects have different uses beyond banging and mouthing.

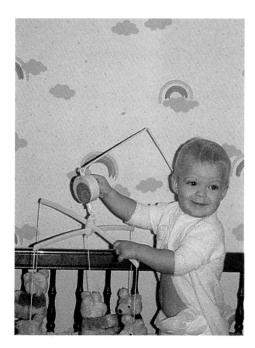

FIG. 3.25 Fifteen-month-old child turns the key of the music box (atop the mobile) to make it play. This child's understanding has advanced beyond that of direct causality (such as pulling a toy to bring it closer).

Assessing Cognitive Development

ASSESSMENT IN THE PREVERBAL PERIOD

Because the observations needed to assess cognitive abilities in the preverbal period are less well known by the general public than are the major motor milestones, parents often rely upon physicians to assess their child's development of cognitive skills. By simple observation of the child's use of toys or objects, the physician, while talking with the parent, can gain valuable information about the child's progress in cognitive development.

To parents, a delay in their child's attaining a well-known milestone may mean that the child is "mentally retarded." In many cases, parental concerns regarding the child's seemingly delayed progress in attaining a specific milestone can be put to rest when the physician has obtained enough information about the child's learning, to date, to determine that it is age appropriate.

On the other hand, if a child shows significant delays in cognitive development, then the parents should receive that information early enough to make informed decisions to maximize the type and degree of stimulation available for their child.

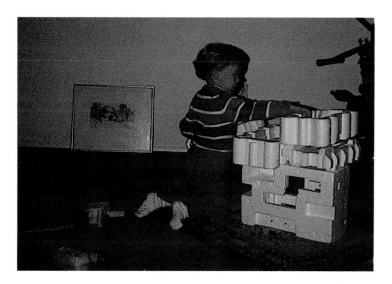

FIG. 3.26 Anticipation of play is demonstrated by this 3-year-old toddler who gathered packing material that he pretended to saw as he now builds a fort.

IQ SCORES

A number of methods have been devised for the formal assessment of mental achievement and almost all parents are familiar with the term "intelligence quotient," or "IQ." Although intelligence tests were designed as a means of identifying children who would fail in school (and not as a means of assessing all mental capabilities), normal IQ scores have not been found to be perfect predictors of which children will have the attention, social skills, intact perceptual abilities, as well as the intelligence to perform well in school.

On the other hand, low IQ scores may reflect a child's poor ability to grasp new concepts or they may indicate the presence of poor purposeful attending behaviors, such as those seen in depression or in attention deficit disorders. Low

IQ scores also may reflect poor social adjustment in obtaining the skills needed for test taking—namely, sitting in a chair at a table attempting a task requested by an unfamiliar authority figure while motivating oneself to do one's best.

When standard tests that have been normed on sighted hearing children with normal motor abilities are given to blind, deaf, or spastic children low scores often will be obtained. Frequently low scores will result from a combination of difficulties in all of the above areas. Conversely, some children who can perform easily in the normal range will not be able to learn to read.

Clearly, IQ tests cannot measure every skill needed to succeed in every task—a fact that is repeatedly borne out by children with specific learning disabilities. Different assessment techniques have been devised to circumvent specific

Type of Scale	Tests Used	Age Range
Standard Intelligence Scales	Stanford-Binet Form L-M	2–adult
	Wechsler Preschool and Primary Scale of Intelligence (WPPSI)	4–6 years
	Wechsler Intelligence Scale for Children— Revised (WISC-R)	5–15 years
Nonverbal Intelligence Scales	Leiter International Performance Scale	2–18 years
	Raven's Progressive Matrices	7–adult
Infant Development Tests	Gesell Developmental Schedules	0–5 years
	Bayley Scales of Infant Development	0–2½ years
	Cattell Infant Intelligence Scale	0–3 years
Developmental Scales for Visually Impaired	Raynell-Zinkin Scales	0–5 years
	Maxfield-Buchalty Social Maturity for Blind Preschool Children	0–6 years
Screening Instruments	Denver Developmental Screening Test (DDST)	0–5 years
	Peabody Picture Vocabulary Test (PPVT)	2–adult
	Vineland Social Maturity Scale—Revised	0–adolescence
	Draw a Person Test (DAP-Goodenough-Harris Drawing Test)	3–adult

FIG. 3.27 Tests Used in the Assessment of Cognitive Development.

disabilities while still obtaining information about a child's cognitive abilities. A variety of assessment tools are available and may be obtained through consultation with psychologists, child development specialists, and special educators (Fig. 3.27).

Abnormal Cognitive Development

DEFINING MENTAL RETARDATION

According to the American Association on Mental Deficiency, "mental retardation" is defined as "significantly subaverage general intellectual functioning existing concurrently with deficits in adaptive behavior and manifested during the developmental period." In this definition, significantly subaverage functioning refers to scores, obtained on standardized intellectual tests, that are at least two standard deviations below age-group norms; adaptive behaviors refer to the broader areas of functioning such as self-care, community survival skills (using the telephone, making change, using public transportation), and social interactions;

the developmental period refers to the period from birth to 18 years of age.

Some 3 percent of newborns will be classified as mentally retarded at some point in their lives. For those children who are so classified, gross estimates of their functional abilities may be obtained from the table in Figure 3.28, although exceptions to these guidelines should be expected.

The more significant the degree of retardation, the more likely that a specific etiology will be found. Mental deficiency that has occurred as a result of a congenital malformation during central nervous system development or from a severe neurological insult in the prenatal or perinatal period often will fall into the lower ranges of trainable mental retardation or into the range of severe/profound mental retardation.

The vast majority of children classified as mentally retarded, however, will function in the mild range, with no apparent evidence of malformation or deformity. The detection of disability in these more mildly affected youngsters may not occur until the child experiences school performance difficulties.

DEGREE OF MENTAL RETARDATION CORRELATED WITH FUNCTIONAL ABILITY

Degree of Mental Retardation in Terms of Educational Potential	IQ Scores on Stanford-Binet IQ Test	Level of Adaptive Functioning
Mild/Educable	67–52	Capable of reading and spelling with educational support and adaptations. With vocational training and community support programs, may become employed and live independently
Moderate/Trainable	51–36	Capable of self-care activities of daily living (feeding, dressing, hygiene, many household tasks). Capable of employment and residence in supervised setting, such as sheltered workshop or group home
Severe/Trainable	35–20	Requires increased supervision or assistance (in cutting meat or bathing, for example) even in performing activities of daily living
Severe/Profound	19–below	Unable to provide for own needs and dependent on others for self-care

FIG. 3.28 Degree of Mental Retardation Correlated with Functional Ability.

EVALUATION FOR ETIOLOGY

In children who present with global delays in all areas of functioning, the cause of mental retardation must be sought. This evaluation for etiology must be individualized, with assessment guided by findings from the patient's history and physical examination. Several excellent resources on diagnostic evaluation are listed at the end of this chapter (see Smith and Opitz). Specific features of the physical examination that deserve attention are discussed below.

Cranial Abnormalities

Head circumference provides an obvious clue to the presence of underdeveloped cerebral growth in microcephaly or of hydrocephalus in overgrowth. Aberrant patterning of scalp hair may be a clue to abnormal cerebral morphology as the direction of hair growth is dictated by pressures from the developing brain in early gestation. Similarly, abnormal skull shape (as with cranial synostosis) may indicate that the underlying nervous system has undergone unusual physical stresses.

The use of transillumination in young infants will aid in the diagnosis of porencephalic cysts or of other structural defects, if the defects are asymmetric. The presence of an intracranial bruit may indicate AV malformation although such bruits are sometimes heard in normal infants.

Facial Abnormalities

Facial features deserve study since the presence of certain characteristics may suggest a specific heritable syndrome. Findings of hypotelorism or hypertelorism, epicanthal folds, funduscopic evidence of congenital infection, or colobomata may help to identify a variety of disorders. However, isolated findings of auricles that are large, abnormally formed, or set low in comparison to the plane of the eyes may suggest only minor anomalies, rather than being a part of a major syndrome.

Nasal or preauricular pits are associated with some syndromes that have deficient mental development as a component. Likewise, a lengthened philtrum with a thin vermilion border to the lips is one clinical feature of the fetal alcohol

Findings Sometimes Present on History or Examination	Possible Disorder
Decreased vision or hearing	Specific sensory deficits
Startling spells, motor automatism	Seizure disorders
Lethargy, ataxia	Overmedication with anticonvulsants
Myxedema, delayed return on DTRs, thick skin and tongue, sparse hair, constipation, increased sleep, coarser voice, short stature, goiter	Hypothyroidism
Irritability, cold sweats, tremor, loss of consciousness	Hypoglycemia
Unexplained bruises (old and new), poor hygiene, failure to thrive	Child abuse and neglect
Short stature, weight below third percentile	Malnutrition or systemic illness producing failure to thrive
Poor purposeful attending in multiple settings	Attention deficit disorder
No specific findings	Environmental deprivation
Anemia	Toxin exposure (lead or other)
Absent venous pulsations or papilledema on funduscopic examination, morning vomiting, headaches, brisk DTRs in lower extremities	Increased intracranial pressure
Vomiting, irritability and seizures, failure to thrive	Some inborn errors of metabolism, e.g., methyl malonic acidemia
Hepatomegaly, jaundice, hypotonia, susceptibility to infection, cataracts	Galactosemia
Fair hair, blue eyes, "mousy" odor to urine	Phenylketonuria
Ongoing evidence of active or progressive disease	Chronic infection, inflammatory disease, malignancies

FIG. 3.29 Medically Remediable Disorders Associated with Global Developmental Delay.

syndrome. Similarly, teeth that are unusually shaped or that have discolored enamel may suggest congenital syphilis or a history of exposure to teratogenic medication. Along these lines, a high-arched palate may be secondary to abnormal motor activity of the tongue in utero, suggesting a prenatal origin to motor problems.

Other Physical Abnormalities

Webbing at the neck may suggest Turner or Noonan syndrome. Vertebral or scapular abnormalities may suggest known syndromes that include other more major anomalies. Widely set nipples as well as rib and sternal abnormalities should prompt careful examination for other minor or major anomalies that may lead to a specific diagnosis.

Hepatosplenomegaly in the neonatal period may suggest congenital infection, or, in the juvenile age range, may indicate a heritable storage disease affecting CNS and developmental functioning. Large testes are found in youngsters with fragile X chromosomal abnormalities, while hypogonadism

is a concomitant of the Prader-Labhart-Willi syndrome. About one half of the patients with this syndrome will be found to have an abnormality on chromosome 15.

Changes in the long bones of the limbs may show evidence of congenital infection; disproportionate bone length may suggest metabolic disorders such as homocystinuria or the osteochondrodysplasias. Errant toe proportions or changed crease patterns on the hands or soles of the feet may suggest early morphogenetic changes associated with certain defined syndromes.

Hirsutism occurs in both fetal alcohol and fetal hydantoin syndromes. Abnormal fingernail formation can signal teratogenic influences or ectodermal dysplasias. Other skin findings such as hemangiomas, café au lait spots, and sebaceous adenomas each may be evidence of an underlying neurocutaneous abnormality thereby providing a constitutional basis for a developmental delay.

Finally, aberrant growth patterns in themselves should prompt further evaluation. Obesity appears as part of a

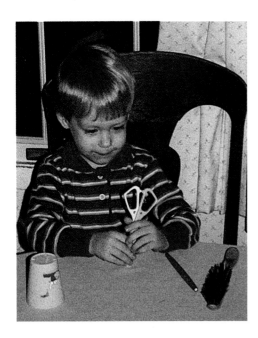

FIG. 3.30 Thirty-month-old child demonstrates his receptive language skills as he answers the question, "Which one do we use to cut?"

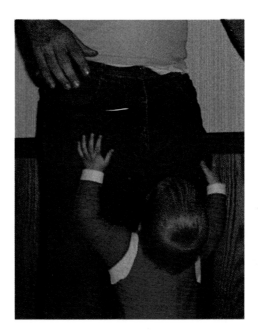

FIG. 3.31 Thirteen-month-old child couples gestures with emerging verbal language to indicate his needs. Use of a single word to represent broad general categories is common at this stage. Without this gesture the child's word "bup" may indicate the desire for other changes in position.

number of syndromes associated with mental deficiency, such as Laurence-Moon-Biedl syndrome and Prader-Labhart-Willi syndrome. Children who are exceptionally large may have endocrine disturbances or suffer from Sotos syndrome. Small-for-date infants deserve close study for evidence of anomalies or infection, as well as close follow-up because they are at risk for abnormal development.

Listed in Figure 3.29 are some of the disorders that may be the cause of delayed cognitive development, along with their associated physical findings.

EVALUATION AND MANAGEMENT

Overall then, findings of unusual features in any aspect of the physical examination may help to provide an explanation for abnormal or delayed cognitive development. In evaluating for the cause of developmental delay, the greatest need beyond that of assessing for the possibility of remediation is that of providing parents with effective genetic, behavioral, and educational counseling. Evidence that a child's lack of developmental progress is related to constitutional factors can help relieve parents of guilt feelings. In fact, in some cases, until the issue of cause has been thoroughly evaluated, families will be unable to progress in their emotional adjustment toward an exceptional child.

In contrast to severely delayed children who will be readily identified, mildly retarded children usually will present before their academic years with normal major motor milestones and will demonstrate delay only in adaptive areas such as self-care, language acquisition, or play—if at all. The extent of their disability will be most prominent during the school years or in times of life crisis beyond school age.

Careful historical documentation of the child's opportunities for interaction—with parents, with other children, and with stimulating environments—will help in determining the type and degree of intervention needed. Moreover, the benefits of intervention will be maximized by early identification. In this regard, the importance of careful screening of infant and preschool development by informed health professionals cannot be overemphasized.

LANGUAGE DEVELOPMENT

The use of symbolic language—that is, the ability to generate sounds or gestures that are reproducible and can be recognized by others as representative of concepts—develops largely during the first year of life. Given that this skill distinguishes humans from other animals, it is easy to understand the importance attached to the production of first words as well as the distress and anxiety produced in parents when their child's verbal expressive language is delayed.

Receptive and Expressive Language

Receptive language refers to the ability to receive information that is transmitted via speech and gestures while expressive language refers to the ability to communicate information.

Receptive language can be demonstrated as children follow increasingly complex commands. For example, one-step commands such as "throw the ball" will be understood by approximately 1 year of age. Understanding labeling of pictures is slightly more complex and may begin at approximately 1 year of age, whereas the ability to choose between two pictures when asked "show me the . . ." should be consistent between 18 and 24 months of age.

By 2½ years of age, receptive language skills have advanced beyond the understanding of simple labels, as the child is able to identify objects by their use (Fig. 3.30). Continued advances in receptive language occur during the preschool years and are highly susceptible to environmental stimulation or deprivation.

Even before word production begins, parents can be reassured that their child is communicating if the child's gestures have communicative intent. Many 9- to 10-month olds are able to communicate that their juice or cereal is "all gone" by putting their hands above their head in the "touchdown" signal. Even older children are encouraged to gesture to make themselves better understood, as gross and fine motor skills develop faster than does the oropharyngeal musculature used in articulation (Fig. 3.31).

RECEPTIVE AND EXPRESSIVE LANGUAGE MILESTONES

Age Range	Receptive Response	Expressive Response
0–1½ months	Startle, eye widening to sound	Range of cries (from hunger to pain)
1½–4 months	Quiets to voice, eye blinking to sound	Vocal contagion, two-syllable babble
4–9 months	Head turns toward sound, responds with raised arms when mom says "up" and reaches for child, responds appropriately to friendly or angry voices	Babbling, four-syllable babble, repeats self-initiated sounds
9–12 months	Listens selectively to familiar words, begins to respond to "no" and to one-step commands (usually accompanied by gesture), understands approximately ten words (no, bye-bye, clap, hat, own name)	Symbolic gestures, jargoning, repeats parent-initiated sounds
12–18 months	Points to three body parts (eyes, nose, mouth), understands up to 50 words, recognizes common objects by name (dog, cat, bottle, ball, book), follows one-step commands accompanied by gestures ("give me the doll," "hug your bear," "open your mouth")	Uses words to express needs, has ten words by 18 months, word usage may be inconsistent and mixed with jargon and echolalia
18 months–2 years	Points to pictures when asked "show me," understands "soon," "in," "on," and "under," begins to distinguish "you" from "me," can formulate negative judgments (a pear is not a cookie)	Telegraphic two-word sentences ("go bye-bye," "up daddy," "want cookie"), 25% intelligibility
30 months	Follows two-step commands, can identify actions in pictures and can identify objects by use	Jargon and echolalia decrease, average sentence of 2½ words, adjectives and adverbs appear, begins to ask questions, asks adults to repeat actions ("do it again")
3 years	Knows several colors, knows what we do when we are hungry, thirsty or sleepy, is aware of past and future, understands "today" and "not today"	Uses pronouns and plurals; can tell stories that begin to be understood; uses negatives ("I can't," "I won't," "I'm busy"); verbalizes toilet needs; can tell full name, age, and sex; forms sentences of three to four words
3½ years	Can answer such questions as "do you have a doggie," "which is the boy," "where is the dress," "what toys do you have," understands "little," "funny," "secret"	Can relate experiences in sequential order, can say a nursery rhyme, asks permission
4 years	Understands same versus different, can follow three-step commands, can complete opposite analogies (a brother is a boy, a sister is a . . .), understands why we have houses, stoves, umbrellas	Can tell a story, uses past tense, counts to three, names primary colors, enjoys rhyming nonsense words, enjoys exaggerations, asks up to 500 questions a day
5 years	Understands what we do with eyes and ears, understands differences in texture (hard, soft, smooth) understands "if," "because," "when," "why," identifies words in terms of use, begins to understand left and right	Can indicate "I don't know," can indicate "funny," "surprise," can define in terms of use, asks definition of specific words, makes serious inquiries ("how does this work," "what does it mean"), language is now complete in structure and form, all parts of speech are used as well as all types of sentences and clauses

FIG. 3.32 Receptive and Expressive Language Milestones.

PHONEMES AND INTELLIGIBILITY

Age Range*	Sounds Mastered	Percent Intelligibility (to a stranger)
2 years	. . .	50%
2½ years	. . .	75%
3 years	14 vowels and *p, b, m*	85%
4 years	10 vowel blends and *n, ng, w, h, t, d, k, g*	100%
5 years	*f, v, y, th, l, wh*	100%
6 years	*r, s, z, ch, j, sh, zh,* and consonant blends	100%

*The ages presented here are to be viewed as general guidelines, as authorities will differ with regard to the specific ages associated with articulation and intelligibility.

FIG. 3.33 Phonemes and Intelligibility.

Signing while speaking—the total communication approach—is used with some language-delayed children even though they may have normal hearing. In the child with normal language development, verbal utterances expand as two-word sentences begin, followed by the development of longer sentences. By age 3, the child has developed more complex language with the use of pronouns and prepositions. By age 5, the child is using all parts of speech, as well as clauses and sentences. Listed in Figure 3.32 are developmental milestones for receptive and expressive language.

Mastering Intelligibility and Fluency

Over and above language production and content are its intelligibility and fluency. For a variety of reasons that include control and coordination of oral musculature, the sounds required in our language are mastered at differing rates. The child who is attempting to say a word containing sounds he cannot yet produce has a variety of choices on how to proceed—by omission of the difficult sound ("ba" for bottle), by substitution of a different sound ("fum" for thumb), or by distortion ("goyl" for girl).

Some of these misarticulations are more difficult than others to interpret and hence are more damaging to intelligibility. Omissions, for example, are more damaging than are distortions. The information presented in Figure 3.33 provides an estimate of when mastery of particular sounds might be expected, along with estimates of overall intelligibility.

Delays in the development of intelligibility might include any of the following:

A lack of intelligible speech by 3 years of age

Frequent omission of initial consonants by age 4

Continued substitution of very easy sounds for harder ones after age 5

Persistent articulation errors after age 7

If any of these delays persist for 6 months or more, a referral should be initiated.

During the period in which articulation and vocabulary are being mastered, speech dysfluencies will be common. However, noticeable stuttering or rapid speech beyond age 4 should prompt further attention. The problems of nasality, inaudibility, and unusual pitch may sometimes be helped by a speech pathologist. Furthermore, the child of any age who is embarrassed by his or her speech is an appropriate candidate for referral.

Assessing Delayed Language Development

The differential diagnosis for delayed expressive language development includes impaired hearing, environmental deprivation, autism, emotional maladjustment, and global developmental delay. Keeping this in mind, the infant who fails to coo responsively, the 4- to 6-month-old infant whose babbling has diminished, the 9- to 10-month-old child who does not have reduplicated babbling, the 18-month-old child whose repertoire of words includes only "mama" or "dada," the 2-year-old child who does not use multiple real words, the 30-month-old child without two-word sentences, and the 3-year-old child without multiword phrases and sentences all should undergo evaluation for hearing loss as well as for cognitive and emotional impairment.

"Tongue tie" is not a sufficient cause for delayed speech development. Similarly, although there is a genuine need for parents to place communicative demands on their children to stimulate speech production, caution should be exercised before parents are told that their child is not talking "because he doesn't need to." Family patterns of delayed speech development are not uncommon.

In establishing the cause of delayed language development, clinicians and parents would do well to keep in mind that the child whose unusual pattern of language development is destined to be outgrown will not suffer from monitoring by a communications disorders specialist; in marked contrast, the child whose language impairment will *not* be outgrown has much to lose when help is delayed.

DISABLING EFFECTS OF HEARING LOSS

Average Hearing 500–2000 Hz (ANSI)	Description	Condition	Sounds Heard Without Amplification	Degree of Disability (if not treated in first year of life)	Probable Needs
0–15 dB	Normal range	Serous otitis, perforation, monomeric membrane, tympanosclerosis	All speech sounds	None	None
15–25 dB	Slight hearing loss	Serous otitis, perforation, monomeric membrane, sensorineural loss, tympanosclerosis	Vowel sounds heard clearly; may miss unvoiced consonant sounds	Mild auditory dysfunction in language learning	Consideration of need for hearing aid; lipreading; auditory training, speech therapy, preferential seating
25–40 dB	Mild hearing loss	Serous otitis, perforation, tympanosclerosis, monomeric membrane, sensorineural loss	Hears only some louder-voiced speech sounds	Auditory learning dysfunction, mild language retardation, mild speech problems, inattention	Hearing aid, lipreading, auditory training, speech therapy
40–65 dB	Moderate hearing loss	Chronic otitis, middle ear anomaly, sensorineural loss	Misses most speech sounds at normal conversational level	Speech problems, language retardation, learning dysfunction, inattention	All the above, plus consideration of special classroom situation
65–95 dB	Severe hearing loss	Sensorineural or mixed loss from sensorineural loss plus middle ear disease	Hears no speech sounds of normal conversation	Severe speech problems, language retardation, learning dysfunction, inattention	All the above; plus probable assignment to special classes
More than 95 dB	Profound hearing loss	Sensorineural or mixed loss	Hears no speech or other sounds	Severe speech problems, language retardation, learning dysfunction, inattention	All the above; plus probable assignment to special classes

FIG. 3.34 *Disabling Effects of Hearing Loss. (From Stewart JM, Downs MP: Medical management of the hearing-handicapped child, in Northern JL (ed): Hearing Disorders, 2nd ed. Little, Brown & Co., Boston, 1984, p. 271, with permission)*

Hearing Impairment

The presence of a hearing impairment can be a significantly disabling factor in the child's development of language skills. According to 1982 statistics from the Joint Committee on Infant Hearing, risk factors for hearing impairment in infants include the following:

1. A family history of childhood hearing impairment
2. Congenital perinatal infection (CMV, rubella, herpes, toxoplasmosis, and syphilis)
3. Anatomical malformations of the head or neck
4. Birth weight of less than 1500 grams
5. Hyperbilirubinemia with levels above those indicated for an exchange transfusion
6. Bacterial meningitis
7. Severe asphyxia (marked by Apgar less than 3, lack

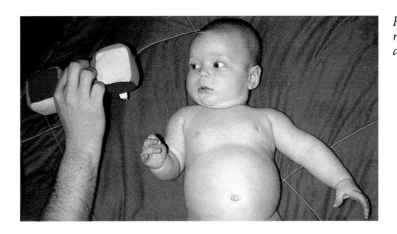

FIG. 3.35 Localizing sound. By 2 months of age, infants will respond to interesting sounds by looking in the general direction of the sound.

of spontaneous respirations by 10 minutes, hypotonia to 2 hours of age)

For those children who are at high risk for hearing impairment, clinicians need to maintain a high index of suspicion as well as to obtain early formal audiologic evaluation. Listed in Figure 3.34 are conditions associated with varying degrees of hearing loss, their disabling effects, and the interventions required for children with these conditions.

Some 60 percent of all cases of sensorineural hearing loss in preverbal children will not be associated with a known risk factor and will be of undetermined etiology. For these children, the absence of expected hearing behaviors will be the best clue to the presence of a hearing problem. Behavioral differences between healthy newborns and hearing impaired infants are described below.

EARLY HEARING BEHAVIORS

Healthy newborns will react to loud sounds with startle responses and with changes in their level of alertness. In the early months, eye widening and changes in activity level in response to new sounds can be observed and after 3 months of age, the infant should be able to turn toward the direction of a sound source (Fig. 3.35). The 3-month-old infant also will begin to enjoy musical toys and to respond to familiar voices with calming or cooing. By 6 to 9 months of age, the infant is able to achieve direct localization of a sound in any plane of space.

Qualitative differences in the early behaviors of hearing impaired children in comparison to those of their nonhearing impaired peers have been observed in the following five areas:

1. *Indifference to sounds or spoken words*—While hearing impaired children may respond to noise and become alerted to the vibrations of low-intensity high-frequency sounds, they will be far less responsive to the sound of the human voice.
2. *Less vocalization and sound production*—Hearing impaired children will produce less laughter, less sound play, and less squealing, and will display less pitch differentiation. Babbling in these infants cannot be initiated or prolonged by parental vocalizations.
3. *Increased visual attentiveness*—Hearing impaired infants seem to be more visually attentive as well as more vehement in their gestures and imitations.
4. *Altered social rapport*—Early observers have found hearing impaired children to be more interested in objects than in persons. They also may be less responsive to nursery rhymes and baby songs.
5. *Frustrations in communicating*—Hearing impaired children may use tantrums to call attention to their needs and may become distressed and irritable in their attempts to make themselves understood.

LATER SIGNS OF IMPAIRMENT

Given the subtleties with which hearing impairment presents itself, it is not surprising that often parents and physicians fail to recognize a hearing problem until speech delays occur. Even congenitally deaf children will coo and babble and up to a year or so will appear to develop speech, saying "mama" or "dada." Their speech acquisitions will then plateau. The 12-month-old child with no vocal imitation and no differentiated babbling deserves a hearing evaluation, as does the 18-month-old child who does not use single words.

Substantial delays in the rate of language acquisition and in the use of oral language can result even from mild sensorineural or conductive hearing impairments. Clinicians should take note that a hearing loss of only some of the speech frequencies may be enough to delay speech acquisition although there will still be a response to noises or to gross hearing screens. In this light, an infant's startling in response to clapped hands does not rule out the possibility of significant hearing loss.

Children with enough hearing to acquire language but with significant hearing loss at high or low frequencies may not appreciate ending sounds and thus they are particularly likely to articulate with omissions of *es, ing,* and *ed* as word endings. "Deaf speech" will have a nasal quality to it and often will lack the inflections and pitch variations of normal conversational speech.

Some of the difficulties in language interpretation are the result of an inability to hear tone changes that imply question or emphasis. Such difficulties will contribute to lags in receptive language development even in hearing impaired children with excellent lipreading capabilities.

Significant gains in expressive language development may be achieved by early intervention with hearing amplification or with alternative communication systems. Early intervention is dependent upon identification before age 3, and, to this end, careful history taking for risk factors and for hearing and speech behaviors is crucial. Examination for middle ear disorders; occluded external canals; congenital infection; or for congenital anomalies of the ear, nose, throat, mandible, head, face, or neck also will aid physicians in earlier identification of hearing impairment in children.

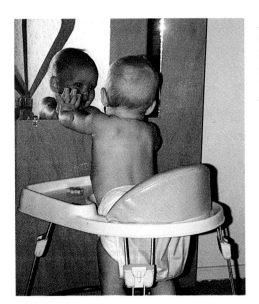

FIG. 3.36 Near 6 months of age, infants can be expected to show interest and pleasure in their mirror reflections.

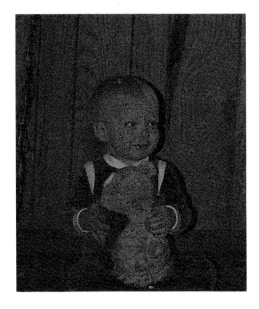

FIG. 3.37 Near 1 year of age, infants can demonstrate affection toward their parents as well as toward familiar toys.

SOCIAL DEVELOPMENT

Early Social Behaviors

The earliest social-developmental task of the newborn is to engage his caretaker and to convince her that it's a wonderful experience for her to awaken out of a sound sleep at his whimper to feed him on demand.

Neonates begin the social-developmental process by visually fixing on faces in preference to other sights—a skill that is evident during the first few days of life. At 2 weeks of age, the infant will track a bright object that is held within 6 to 10 inches of his view to the midline. Good eye contact is present by 1 month of age and the responsive smile develops soon thereafter.

Next the infant will track faces past the midline, and, by 3 to 4 months of age, can track a variety of objects through a 180° horizontal arc. During this time the infant has learned to associate his mom's voice with her face and so can be comforted by her voice. This infant will respond differently to different tones and may become distressed or excited by angry voices. Cooing in response to smiling or nodding adults also emerges.

The 4- to 6-month old becomes more involved with playthings but will reward people with giggles or laughter when he is tickled or bounced. This baby is beginning to enjoy socializing and can cough or click his tongue to gain notice, while later he can babble to attract attention. He wails when play is interrupted but is beginning to try to soothe himself or be calmed by his mom's voice when he is distressed.

A baby of this age will begin to display interest in his own mirror image (Fig. 3.36). Similarly, as this baby begins to recognize the faces of his parents, he may begin to squirm and cling in the company of others, exhibiting "stranger anxiety," the severity of which will vary with infant temperament.

A rising desire for independence is next to develop. The 7- to 8-month old is beginning to finger feed and may grab for the cup or spoon in an attempt to gain control of it. This infant also can hold his own bottle and may resist pressure to do something that he would rather not do (for example, he may fuss to stand when he has been placed in sitting). This child can tease too, and will begin to show humor.

As the child nears a year of age, his understanding of object permanence crystallizes and with it comes distress when his parents leave or separate from him. Similarly, this is the baby who wants to crawl and explore but who needs to crawl back to mom or dad for some verbal encouragement, eye contact, or some hugs before venturing farther.

This child also is becoming more sensitive to the moods of others and will cry if other babies are crying or will perform for a home audience if applauded. He is beginning to demonstrate moods of his own such as happiness, anger and playfulness. In addition, he is delighted by the sight of other children although his interactions with them are limited to an interest in the same toys or to vocalizing at them. This child also can show tenderness toward a familiar doll or stuffed animal (Fig. 3.37).

At the same time this child will begin to show guilt at wrongdoing and will seek approval for his actions. Although he is able to obey commands and understand "no," this child is not always cooperative.

The Toddler

Beyond a year of age, infants have become toddlers with a rapidly emerging sense of self. These children enjoy their own accomplishments and can clap for their own successes (Fig. 3.38). They are increasingly able to feed themselves and to manage a cup and spoon. Discipline will become more challenging in this group as temper tantrums begin. At about this time, a period of negativism emerges. During this time parents may need help in viewing their child's refusals to eat, nap or be washed as positive steps toward increased independence, as their child assumes a more active role in decision making.

Also at this time, sharper responses to separations may occur and the child displays a wider range of emotions. It is not uncommon for a child of this age to become attached to a familiar animal or blanket that is comforting in times of stress.

As the child nears 2 years of age, he is gaining increased independence in verbal abilities, in awareness of body sensations, in donning and doffing clothing (although still with assistance), and in locomotion. These developing skills combine with the child's desire to imitate adults and gain parental approval to allow for toilet training to occur, and may in fact be viewed as readiness signs. Children may differ sub-

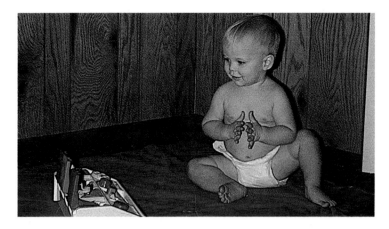

FIG. 3.38 Thirteen-month old demonstrates that toddlers beyond a year of age can take pride in their own accomplishments. This child is applauding his own success at having made the puppets appear.

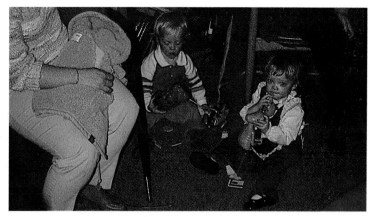

FIG. 3.39 Cooperative play begins near age 3.

stantially in their interest in achieving bladder and bowel control, and in some cases parents may benefit from counseling to help them maintain a relaxed approach toward their child's accomplishments in this area.

Play in this age group is still parallel in nature, and for parents to expect their child to interact or share with peers successfully would be inappropriate. In contrast, solitary play and apparent selfishness are to be expected. The pretending play in which 2 year olds engage allows them to explore the social roles of mom and dad as well as to practice what they have recently learned about the functions of various objects. While toddlers enjoy rough and tumble play with parents, they also will seek to engage their parents in activities that satisfy their growing curiosity—such as being read to or having their labeling questions answered. Parents are still all important to these children and separations from them will be met with distress.

The Young Preschooler

Near 3 years of age, children will begin to include one another in their pretending games (Fig. 3.39). At first both children may select the same role (two mothers, for example) while later the roles will become more interactive. The young preschooler is especially interested in imitating the parent of the same sex but shows no preference for play partners to be either boys or girls. As for playthings, a child of this age will tend to view possessions as extensions of himself, so that sharing will be thought of as giving away a part of oneself.

Taking turns also is fraught with difficulty since the preschooler possesses a very limited understanding of time. Impulse control also is just developing, so the parent/supervisor of new interactors will have plenty to keep him or her busy. Active goals for this age group may include learning to gain the cooperation of one's peers, learning to communicate ideas to new friends, and learning to handle conflicts.

It is important that children of this age group be supported in their attempts to initiate and control their own activities. To this end, parents should allow extra time in their interactions with children to help them practice their emerging self-care skills, such as zippering or buttoning their own coat. Should the child become frustrated or disappointed (or ask questions such as "why do I have to?") a response of

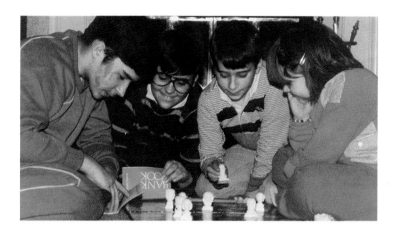

FIG. 3.40 These children, beyond preschool age, show interactive and complicated play.

empathy is likely to soothe more effectively than a response of reason, since rational reasoning does not occur during this preoperational cognitive period. Throughout childhood, the desire to grow up is in continued conflict with the desire to remain a child and the young preschooler is just beginning to address this issue.

It is likely that accomplishments in developmental tasks will backslide when new strains occur on the household equilibrium. As a result, in all young children, temporary regressions to earlier safer levels of functioning can be expected to occur. It is important that parents learn to view these lapses as expected components of development rather than as moral lapses on the part of the child.

The Older Preschooler

Social development in the 4- to 5-year old is characterized by increasing independence to allow for relatively trauma-free separations from parents, in preparation for school. Peer interactions grow increasingly cooperative and complicated at this time (Fig. 3.40) and pretend play activities may involve events occurring outside of the household as well as within—with pretend trips or parties as themes, for example.

The older preschooler enjoys helping with household tasks and is more interested in participating in gender-specific activities than he was at an earlier age. With the unfolding of the "Oedipal period" of development comes evidence of silliness or embarrassment in response to the intimacy of physical examination, and, as a result, increased sensitivity will be required on the part of the examiner.

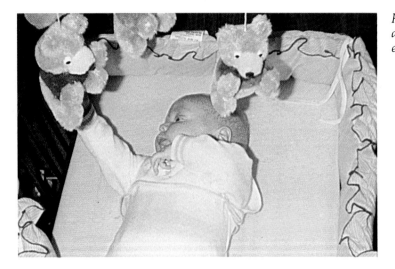

FIG. 3.41 Swiping. This infant uses his entire upper extremity as a unit in interacting with the toy. This activity is one of the earliest in fine motor development.

Abnormal Social Development

Because of wide variations in environmental variables, personality, temperament, and cultural norms, social-adaptive developmental disorders will require repeated extensive evaluation for definition. As a rule, the frequency, duration, and severity of interactional problems as well as the conditions under which they occur will require careful evaluation before an assessment and plan of action can be determined.

Childhood Autism

Among the children who present to physicians with developmental delay and unusual patterns of behavior are those with childhood autism. In general, the child who fails to develop normal relationships, who is upset by minor changes in the environment, and who shows unusual abnormalities in speech and language development may have this severely disabling developmental disorder.

Childhood autism is a behaviorally defined syndrome in which any of the following features may present prior to 30 months of age:

A disturbance in the rate and sequence of development

A lack of modulation in response to sensory stimuli

Abnormal patterns of speech, nonverbal communication, and cognitive development

Diminished capacity to relate appropriately to people, objects, and events

In the first 6 months of life, the autistic infant may demonstrate unusual sleep patterns—never resting for more than three or four hours—and unusual crying patterns, in which crying may not relate to needs. Hyperresponsivity to sights and sounds may alternate with hyporesponsivity, evoking questions of deafness or visual impairment.

One of the earliest warning signs of autism will be the baby's lack of social responsiveness marked by absent smiling, poor eye contact, and little response to maternal attention. Even in the second 6 months of life, the baby who is not babbling, who is disinterested in waving, imitating, engaging in baby games, or in playing with baby toys should be evaluated for autism and other related disorders.

In the second year of life, preoccupation with fingers and with repetitive motor activities such as whirling, rocking, or hand flapping may indicate aberrant sensorimotor patterns. It is also during this period that unusual language patterns emerge, such as the lack of meaningful speech or gestures or the noncommunicative use of sounds (as with echolalia or repetitive use of sounds).

Between 2 and 3 years of age, the autistic child may appear to be withdrawn and prefer to play alone, perhaps using toys in idiosyncratic ways, such as spinning them or lining them up in rigid patterns. This child later will fail to develop cooperative play. It should be noted that many autistic children will demonstrate very uneven development, with minimal speech or language skills, but with excellent memory or fine motor puzzle-solving skills.

PROGNOSTIC FACTORS

Although the pathogenesis of autism is poorly understood, it is now clear that this disorder is found in all parts of the world, in all races, and in all socioeconomic groups. While affected children will have normal life expectancies, about 75 percent of autistic patients will remain functionally retarded throughout their life and more than 90 percent will require lifelong social support systems because of continuing symptoms and severely handicapped development.

Patients who fail to develop communicative skills and appropriate use of toys by age 5 have a poor prognosis as do patients with concomitant seizure disorders or specific evidence of organic brain dysfunction. Children with fairly normal motor development who do develop communicative language before age 5 have a better prognosis. Although as adolescents these children are particularly shy and introvertive, in general they do not develop major thought disorders with delusions or hallucinations, and a tiny minority of these patients eventually are able to live semi-independently.

The autistic child with the best prognosis is one who is healthy and of average intelligence, who is identified by 3 to 4 years of age, and who is involved in a very structured and intensive behavioral training program. In general, a team approach to the pharmacologic, behavioral, and educational management of autism will be aided greatly by early identification of this disorder. Early identification also is important in that it will allow the physician to provide the family of an autistic child with accurate information regarding prognosis and management.

5 MONTHS RAKE	7 MONTHS RADIAL-PALMAR GRASP	9 MONTHS RADIAL-DIGITAL GRASP	10 MONTHS INFERIOR-PINCER GRASP	12 MONTHS FINE PINCER GRASP
Thumb adducted, proximal thumb joint flexed, distal thumb joint flexed	Raking object into palm with adducted totally flexed thumb and all flexed fingers, OR with two partly extended fingers	Between thumb and side of curled index finger, distal thumb joint slightly flexed, proximal thumb joint extended	Between ventral surfaces of thumb and index finger, distal thumb joint extended, beginning thumb opposition	Between fingertips or fingernails, distal thumb joint flexed

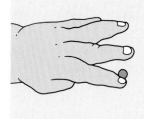 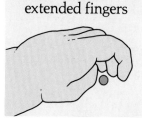 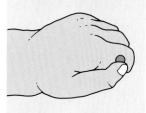 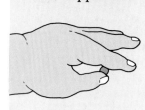 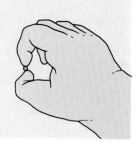

FIG. 3.42 Development of Prehension. (Adapted from Erhardt RP: Developmental Hand Dysfunction. Theory, Assessment, Treatment. RAMSCO Publishing Co., Laurel, Md, 1982, p. 61)

FINE MOTOR AND PERCEPTUAL DEVELOPMENT

The Neonate

At birth, a predominance of flexor tone is expected in the head, trunk, and extremities of the newborn. This physiologic flexion is included in the whole hand grasp reflex in which the infant's fingers and thumb are tightly fisted. Because of this grasp reflex, the infant's range of upper extremities motion is functionally reduced. This, in combination with the infant's distance limitations for clear vision, serves to limit the exploratory range of the neonate's hands to that of accidental contact with the world.

The beginning of fine motor development may be said to occur in the second or third month of life, when the infant begins to swipe at objects held in front of his shoulder but slightly off to the side (Fig. 3.41). Although swiping actually is a gross motor activity involving the entire upper extremity as a unit, it is through swiping that the infant increases his exploratory range. This allows for increased use and fine tuning of the small muscles of the wrist, hand, and fingers, which occurs in an expected progression.

Fine Motor Control in Infancy

With decreased influence of the hand grasp reflex, the 4-month-old infant usually is able to hold an object in either hand if it is placed there, although the infant cannot voluntarily grasp or release that object. At approximately 5 months of age, infants will begin to use their hands as entire units to draw objects toward them, although neither hand nor thumb movements are employed at this point and consequently the hand is used like a rake.

Next the child is able to bend the fingers against the palm (palmar grasp), squeeze objects, and obtain them independently for closer inspection. As the thumb begins to differentiate its plane of movement, a whole hand grasp develops with the thumb adducting and the fingers squeezing against the palm (radial-palmar or whole hand grasp). The next progression is for the thumb to move from adduction to opposi-

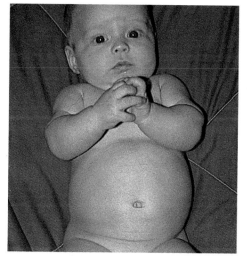

FIG. 3.43 A 4-month-old child achieves a major milestone in his use of upper extremities when he perceives that the two halves of his body are related as he discovers his midline.

tion and for the site of the pressure (of thumb against fingers) to move away from the palm toward the fingertips (inferior forefinger or radial-digital grasp).

By the time the infant has attained the position of thumb against distal interphalangeal joint (inferior-pincer grasp), usually he has attained voluntary release of objects as well (10 months). Soon thereafter, at 12 months, the fine pincer grasp between the tip of the thumb and the index finger has matured enough to allow for the precise prehension of tiny objects smaller than the child's fingers. Presented in Figure 3.42 is a table summarizing the development of prehension, along with schematic drawings to illustrate the different types of grasps. It should be noted that abnormalities in sensation and in muscle tone and control will delay or block this progression.

With improved fine motor control comes increased sensory input from the hands as well as the development of hand manipulation through space. By 2 to 3 months of age, the hands are no longer tightly fisted, and the infant may begin to choose a thumb or a digit to suck on for self-comfort, rather than the entire fist. Before 4 months of age, the infant will touch hands together in the midline (Fig. 3.43).

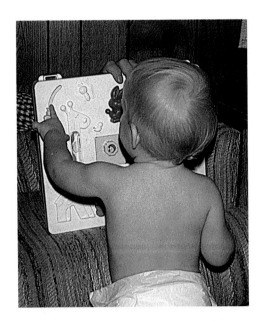

FIG. 3.44 In this child of 11 months the index finger is isolated from the others and can be used to explore fine details.

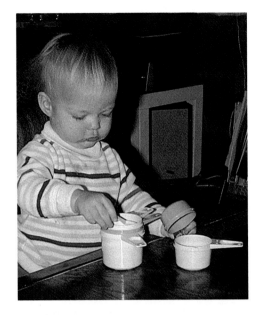

FIG. 3.45 Placing smaller objects inside larger ones can help in the perceptual development of spatial relationships in this 11-month-old child.

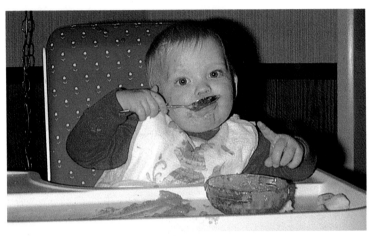

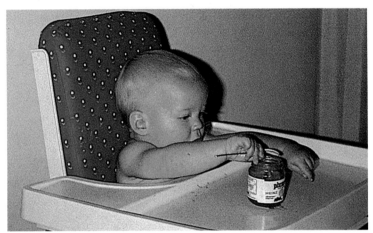

FIG. 3.46 By 15 months of age, parents should be encouraging their child to use his developing fine motor skills (left) to finger feed and (right) to use a cup and spoon independently.

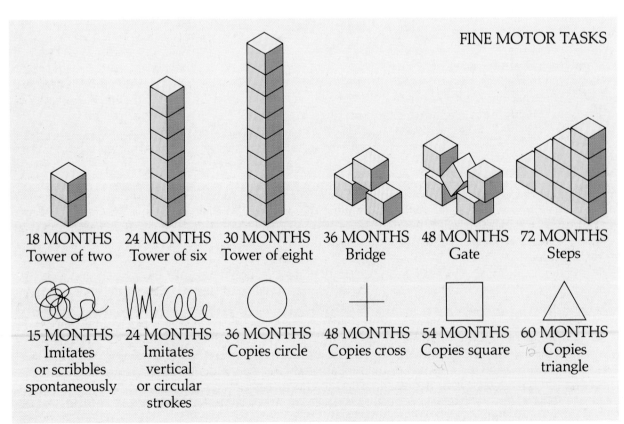

FINE MOTOR TASKS

FIG. 3.47 Fine Motor Tasks.

| 18 MONTHS Tower of two | 24 MONTHS Tower of six | 30 MONTHS Tower of eight | 36 MONTHS Bridge | 48 MONTHS Gate | 72 MONTHS Steps |

| 15 MONTHS Imitates or scribbles spontaneously | 24 MONTHS Imitates vertical or circular strokes | 36 MONTHS Copies circle | 48 MONTHS Copies cross | 54 MONTHS Copies square | 60 MONTHS Copies triangle |

VISUALLY RELATED BEHAVIORS

Age of Infant	Behavior
Term	Focuses on face, briefly tracks vertically and horizontally, turns toward diffuse light source, widens eyes to object or face at 8–12 inches
1 month	Blinks at approaching object "looming," tracks 60° horizontally, 30° vertically
2 months	Tracks across midline, follows movement 6 feet away, smiles to a smiling face, raises head 30° in prone
3 months	Eyes and head track 180°, looks at hands, looks at objects placed in hands
4–5 months	Reaches for object (12-inch cube) 12 inches away, notices raisins 1 foot away, smiles at familiar adult
5–6 months	Smiles in mirror
7–8 months	Rakes at raisin
8–9 months	Notes visual details, pokes at holes in pegboard and at elevator buttons
9 months	Neat pincer grasp
12–14 months	Stacks blocks, places peg in round hole

FIG. 3.48 Visually Related Behaviors.

Between 5 and 7 months of age, the infant can use his developing grasp to transfer objects across the midline.

Around 10 months, use of the index finger to explore the details of objects becomes prevalent (Fig. 3.44). By a year, the infant is positioning his hand in space to achieve vertical or horizontal orientation prior to grasping or releasing an object on target.

Manipulation of Objects

Early in the second year of life, the young child will begin to use his grasp to master tools and to manipulate objects in new ways. The "dropping and throwing game" and the movement of smaller objects into and out of larger ones (Fig. 3.45) will become favorite pastimes for children of this age as well as challenging ones to their parents. Mastery of the cup and spoon to supplement efficient finger feeding will become an active goal for this age group (Fig. 3.46).

Advancements in fine motor planning and control can be demonstrated by the child's manipulation of 1-in. cubes (in reproducing a structure that they have watched the examiner assemble) and by the child's ability to imitate a variety of drawings (Fig. 3.47). The sequence of drawings presented demonstrates how, as fine motor planning progresses, children are able to reproduce first vertical, then horizontal, then angulated, and then diagonal representations. In assessing performance, the examiner should distinguish between imitating (where the examiner demonstrates for the child) and copying (where the examiner presents the child with a completed drawing).

Fine Motor Evaluation and Testing

Fine motor testing as part of the physical examination frequently may uncover problems with vision, neuromuscular control or perception, in addition to difficulties with attention or cooperation. Of special concern is the child who develops consistent handedness prior to 18 months of age with neglect of the other limb. Likewise, the child who has not

developed use of the thumb and pincer grasp by 1 year of age deserves further evaluation.

To the preschooler, fine motor activities can be engaging and nonthreatening while providing the physician with the opportunity to make valuable observations and establish rapport. In the school-age child, inefficient performance of fine motor skills can impact significantly on the child's ability to compete with peers in timed tasks, even in the presence of sound academic conceptual skills.

Similarly, the child who lacks the dexterity to complete the simple activities of daily living (such as zippering, buttoning, or cutting meat) may suffer the lack of self-esteem that accompanies independence in self-care. Furthermore, the child who is continually dependent on parents or teachers in these areas may be viewed by his peers, his teachers, or perhaps, most damaging, by himself as less mature. For the child who generally is lacking in fine motor talent, the efforts of occupational therapists and special education teachers to help the child compensate can be of great benefit in terms of behavioral and emotional developmental gains.

Abnormal Fine Motor and Perceptual Development

Among the few children who present in the preschool age group with isolated fine motor delays are those with visual impairments. Development in these children deserves special comment.

VISION IN THE INFANT

The visual acuity of the full-term infant is estimated to be between 20/200 and 20/400, with improvement over the first year of life to 20/20. The full-term infant can fix on faces at close range and can track an object horizontally at 30 degrees. As the infant's visual skills develop, specific visually related behaviors emerge, as outlined in Figure 3.48.

Vision in the infant is a significant source of enjoyment, as well as a means of information gathering, attention attracting, and linking to one's caretaker. Not surprisingly, infants deprived of this sense will show a number of developmental aberrations and, in general, will probably experience delays in gross motor, social and language and/or conceptual development, as well as in early fine motor development.

Infants who do not develop horizontal and vertical tracking of objects, who do not look at the toys or faces they are involved with, and who hold their head in an unusual position deserve prompt evaluation for abnormal visual perception.

THE BLIND INFANT
Gross and Fine Motor Development
Apparently, much of the motivation for the sighted infant to raise his head 90° when he is in the prone position is to increase his visual field. Without the feedback of interesting sights however, the blind infant may not attain this milestone until 11 to 12 months of age. In contrast, rolling occurs in blind infants at close to the same age as in sighted infants and if sitting independently is an active goal, it occurs by 6 to 7 months of age. The transitional movements from lying to sitting or from sitting to standing will occur several months later, without the aid of visual reinforcement.

Protective reactions develop more slowly in blind than in sighted infants and are expected to appear in the 10- to 12-month age range. This delay, as well as the blind child's inability to integrate visual cues in attaining balance and equilibrium and the lack of a visual impetus for blind children to explore distant toys, may contribute to the delay in crawling or walking that typically occurs. Studies suggest that by presenting blind children with paired auditory-tactile cues to stimulate their interest in objects beyond their reach, gross motor development might be accelerated (see Fraiberg).

Regarding fine motor development, information gathering by index finger and manual manipulation may be more accurate in the blind child than in the sighted child. However, the blind youngster's acquisition of precise prehension is delayed and sometimes never develops, with raking favored as a more efficient means of exploration.

Social Development
The infant without sight lacks the opportunity to benefit from face to face contact with his caretaker, from the visual reinforcement of smiling, from the use of facial expressions to assist in the interpretation of voices or actions, or from the experience of tracking parents across the room to know that even when they cannot be heard or felt they are still there. These differences in sensory input will have significant impact on the blind child's social and emotional development, and parents of blind infants will need to be taught to use touch and sound to reinforce smiling and other desired behaviors in their infant.

At about the same time that sighted children smile at familiar faces, the blind child will smile in response to familiar touching and kinesthetic handling. Smiling in response to a familiar voice, however, may occur inconsistently up to a year of age. Furthermore, the blind infant will demonstrate attachment to the caretaker not by facial expression or by eye contact, but by calming to tactile exploration of the caretaker's familiar face or hands.

Blind children of about 1 year of age may present with stranger anxiety, although a greater hurdle for these children will be their reaction to separation. Because children without sight are limited in their capacity to track their caretakers, separations from them may induce "panic" states even in children up to several years of age. Similarly, the development of independent caretaking and play will be delayed in these children, and its achievement will require specific interventions.

Parents should be advised that, without purposeful stimulation, blind children may engage in nonpurposeful motor activities such as eye rubbing or rocking, and that these stereotypic behaviors (referred to as "blindisms") are difficult to extinguish. Examples of purposeful stimulation include directing the child's hands to exploration of a toy, with verbal reinforcement from the parent, and distracting the child with conversation or music. These efforts will serve to channel the child's activities in a more socially adaptive direction.

Cognitive Development
Given the importance of vision in stimulating the cognitive development of the normal child, the development of cognitive skills in the blind child must, of necessity, depend upon the use of other sensory modalities. For this reason, careful global evaluation of the child should be conducted early in infancy to assure that the child's other sensory modalities are intact. These modalities will have an even greater impact on development and intervention in the blind child than in the sighted child.

In the sighted child, for example, the understanding of object permanence develops through constant bombardment with the appearance and disappearance of an object so that objects will be perceived as permanent even when they cannot be felt, heard, sniffed, or tasted. For the blind child, however, the opportunities for object perception are fewer and thus the understanding of object permanence develops later and is stimulated by encouragement of the blind infant to reach for sound cues. Similarly, the blind child's understanding of conservation of continuous quantity—that a cup of water contains the same volume of liquid in a tall thin container as it does in a short fat one—also develops later than in the sighted child.

Haptic perception—the acquisition of information about objects or spaces by exploration with the hands—appears to be more important in the cognitive development of the blind child than in that of the sighted child. For this reason, tactile exploration in the blind child cannot be promoted at too early an age. In fact, without such encouragement, these children may be fearful and resistant to unfamiliar new feelings.

Language Development
Verbal imitation and receptive language skills develop at the same time for blind as for sighted children although the blind child will have somewhat better auditory attention. Not surprisingly however, blind children can be expected to encounter difficulties with words relating to visual concepts, such as "light," "dark," or "color." They also may have problems with words referring to large things that cannot be touched ("sky" or "stars"), things that change slowly ("age" or "growth"), or the concept "I." In fact, it is not unusual for a blind child to refer to himself in the third person.

In view of these difficulties then, one can see how standard IQ tests—with few exceptions—are culturally biased against blind children. Moreover, the use of measures normed on sighted children to assess the performance of blind children should be considered very carefully and the results interpreted only by experienced evaluators.

SUMMARY

As stated at the outset of this chapter, the task of developmental assessment and referral during infancy and in the preschool years falls largely and often exclusively to the primary care physician, who is most often a pediatrician. Throughout this chapter, an attempt has been made to provide the examining physician with gross estimates regarding the expected chronology of development. It must be stressed however that these estimates, presented here as developmental milestones, are to be viewed as guidelines rather than as fixed time frames within which behavior acquisition may be judged as normal or abnormal.

It is hoped that in evaluating a child, the physician will employ these guidelines in the light of his or her own clinical judgment, taking into account the child's own personality traits, experiences, and degree of cooperation with the behavior sample. Furthermore, in the presence of developmental disability, the importance of early intervention cannot be overemphasized in terms of its impact upon decision-making regarding further evaluation and treatment.

BIBLIOGRAPHY

American Academy of Pediatrics Joint Committee on Infant Hearing: Position statement 1982. Pediatrics 70: 496–497, 1982.

Diagnostic and Statistical Manual of Mental Disorders, 3rd ed. Washington, DC, American Psychiatric Association, 1980.

Fraiberg S: Insights from the Blind. Basic Books Inc, New York, 1977.

Grossman H: Manual on Terminology and Classification in Mental Retardation, American Association on Mental Deficiency special publication series No. 2, 1973.

Illingsworth RS: The Development of the Infant and Young Child Abnormal and Normal, 7th ed. Churchill Livingstone Inc, New York, 1980.

Knobloch H, Pasamanick B (eds): Gesell and Amatruda's Developmental Diagnosis, 3rd ed. Harper & Row, Publishers Inc, New York, 1974.

Levine M, Carey W, Crocker A, Gross R: Developmental-Behavioral Pediatrics. W B Saunders Co, Philadelphia, 1983.

Louick D, Baland T: Psychological tests: A guide for pediatricians. Pediatr Ann 7(12):86–101, 1978.

Northern JL, Downs MP: Hearing in Children. Williams & Wilkins, Baltimore, 1974.

Opitz JM: Mental retardation: Biological aspects of concern to pediatricians. Pediatrics in Review 2(2): 41–50, 1980.

Robinson N, Robinson H: The Mentally Retarded Child, 2nd ed. McGraw-Hill Inc, New York, 1976.

Rutter M: Autistic children: Infancy to adulthood. Seminars in Psychiatry 2:435–450, 1970.

Scheiner AP, Moomaw M: Care of the visually handicapped child. Pediatrics in Review 4(3):74–81, 1982.

Smith D: Recognizable Patterns of Human Malformation. W B Saunders Co, Philadelphia, 1976.

Smith DW, Simons FER: Rational diagnosis evaluation of the child with mental deficiency. Am J Dis Child 129:1285, 1975.

PEDIATRIC ALLERGY AND IMMUNOLOGY

David P. Skoner, M.D.
Paul K. Stillwagon, M.D.
Roger Friedman, M.D.
Philip Fireman, M.D.

CLASSIFICATION OF HYPERSENSITIVITY DISORDERS

		Interval Between Exposure and Reaction	Effector Cell or Antibody	Target or Antigen	Mediators	Examples
Type I	Anaphylactic a. Immediate b. Late phase	 <30 minutes 6 to 9 hours	 IgE IgE	Pollens, foods, drugs, insect venoms	a. Histamines b. Leukotrienes	Anaphylaxis Allergic rhinitis Allergic asthma Urticaria
Type II	Cytotoxic	Variable (minutes to hours)	IgG, IgM	Red blood cells Lungs	Complement	Immune hemolytic anemia Rh hemolytic disease Goodpasture syndrome
Type III	Immune complexes	4–8 hours	Antigen with antibody	Vascular endothelium	Complement Anaphyla-toxin	Serum sickness Poststrepto-coccal glomer-ulonephritis
Type IV	Delayed type	24–48 hours	Lymphocytes	*Mycobac-terium tuberculosis* Chemicals	Lymphokines	Contact der-matitis Tuberculin skin test reactions

From Gell PGH, Coombs RRA: Clinical Aspects of Immunology, 2nd ed., F.A. Davis Co, Philadelphia, 1968.

FIG. 4.1 Classification of hypersensitivity disorders.

Disorders of the immune system are diverse and range from mild to severe in their manifestations and impact on normal function. This chapter emphasizes physical findings and characteristic symptoms of disorders of hypersensitivity and immunodeficiency in the pediatric population, as well as diagnostic techniques and radiographic findings. Topics have been chosen on the bases of (1) their prevalence and importance in the pediatric population and (2) their association with characteristic physical findings.

IMMUNOLOGICAL HYPERSENSITIVITY DISORDERS

Hypersensitivity disorders of the human immune system have been classified by Gell and Coombs into four groups (Fig. 4.1) based on the different mechanisms by which immune reactions may initiate tissue inflammation. Type I reactions occur promptly after the sensitized individual is exposed to antigen and are mediated by specific IgE antibody.

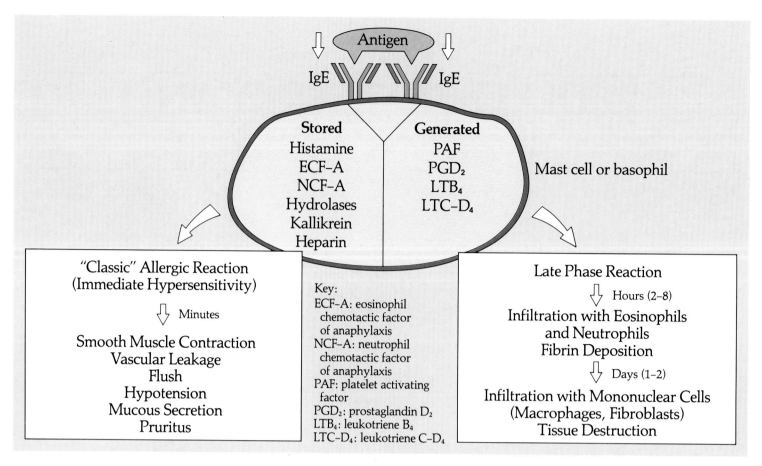

FIG. 4.2 Mechanism of antigen-induced mediator release in Type I hypersensitivity. Note that both an early (classic) and late phase reaction follow antigen exposure.

This mechanism is responsible for the common disorders of immediate hypersensitivity, such as allergic rhinitis and urticaria. Type II reactions involve antibodies directed against antigenic components of peripheral blood or tissue cells, resulting in cell destruction. Examples of this type include autoimmune hemolytic anemia, and Rh and ABO hemolytic disease of the newborn, which will be discussed in Chapter 14. In Type III reactions, antigen-antibody complexes are deposited in or near blood vessels, stimulating tissue inflammation mediated by complement or toxic leukocyte products. Examples of this type of reaction are hypersensitivity pneumonitis, serum sickness, and the immune-complex-mediated renal diseases (see Chapter 13). Type IV reactions occur 24 to 48 hours after antigen exposure and involve cell (T-lymphocyte)-mediated tissue inflammation. Examples of this type are tuberculin and fungal delayed cutaneous hypersensitivity reactions, and contact dermatitis (see Chapter 8).

Type I Disorders

Development of Type I or immediate hypersensitivity depends on hereditary predisposition, sensitization, and subsequent reexposure to specific antigens, known as allergens. The mechanism of antigen-induced mediator release in Type I hypersensitivity reactions is shown in Figure 4.2. Type I reactions may occur in one or more target organs, including the upper and lower respiratory tracts, the skin, conjunctivae, and gastrointestinal tract. Manifestations depend on the system(s) involved, as shown in Figure 4.3. Acuteness or chronicity of target organ manifestations depends on the particular allergen(s) to which the individual is sensitized.

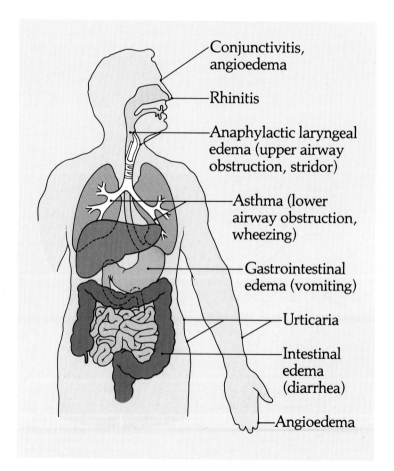

FIG. 4.3 Systemic manifestations of Type I hypersensitivity disorders. Note the characteristic physical findings of each affected organ system.

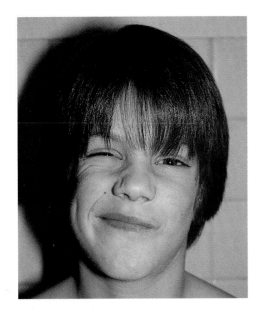

FIG. 4.4 Facial grimacing and twitching caused by nasal itching in patient with allergic rhinitis. These are frequently repeated and easily noted during patient evaluation.

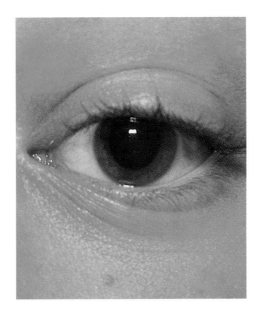

FIG. 4.6 Dennie's lines originate in the inner canthus and traverse one-half to two-thirds the length of the lower lid margin, in an arc nearly parallel to it.

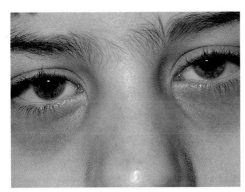

FIG. 4.5 "Allergic shiners" or dark circles beneath the eyes in patient with allergic rhinitis.

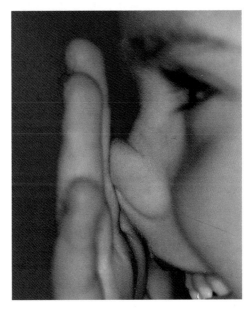

FIG. 4.7 The "allergic salute" is characteristic of children with allergic rhinitis and nasal itching, and is usually noticed by parents.

Inhalation of pollens such as ragweed (fall) or grass and trees (spring) produces seasonal symptoms, and inhalation of indoor molds, house dust, mite fragments, or animal danders produces year-round or perennial symptoms. Foods, insect venoms, and drugs produce intermittent symptoms depending on time of exposure.

ALLERGIC RHINITIS

Allergic rhinitis, characterized by inflammation, edema, and weeping of the nasal mucosa, is the most common of all allergic disorders and occurs in 10 to 20 percent of the population. Diagnosis is based on characteristic history, physical findings, and laboratory (skin test) results. Common presenting symptoms include nasal congestion and pruritus, clear rhinorrhea, and paroxysms of sneezing. Congestion may be bilateral or unilateral or may alternate from side to side. It is generally more pronounced at night. While older children blow their noses frequently, younger children do not. Instead, they sniff, snort, and repetitively clear their throats. Nasal pruritus stimulates grimacing and twitching (Fig. 4.4) and picking or rubbing the nose (allergic salute). Picking and repetitive sneezing and blowing may produce enough irritation to cause epistaxis.

Many patients have prominent itching and watering of the eyes in conjunction with nasal symptoms, and some experience pruritus of the throat or ears. Associated symptoms include (1) disturbed sleep and snoring; (2) morning dryness and irritation of the throat as a result of mouth breathing; (3) lassitude, fatigue, and irritability from sleep interruption; (4) early-nighttime cough; and (5) if maxillary, frontal, and ethmoidal sinuses are affected, a sensation of pressure over the cheeks, forehead, and bridge of the nose.

Many children with long-standing allergic rhinitis can be recognized by their facial characteristics. Ocular manifestations of the allergic disposition include the allergic shiner and Dennie's lines. Allergic shiners, bluish discolorations or dark circles beneath the eyes, are commonly observed in patients with allergic rhinitis (Fig. 4.5). This finding may represent chronic melanocyte stimulation due to repeated rubbing in response to itching. Dennie's lines are prominent folds or creases on the lower eyelid (Fig. 4.6), running parallel to the lower lid margin. While these lines were originally thought to indicate a predisposition to allergy, current data suggest that these signs may be present in any condition associated with periocular pruritus and scratching, and/or chronic nasal congestion. Frequent upward rubbing of the nose with the palm of the hand to alleviate itching (the allergic salute, Fig. 4.7) promotes development of a transverse nasal crease across the

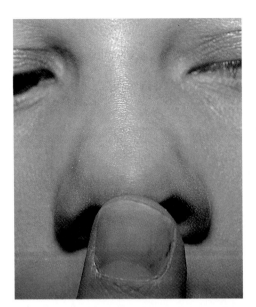

FIG. 4.8 The nasal crease across the lower third of the nose results from chronic upward rubbing of the nose with the hand (allergic salute). (Courtesy of Dr. Meyer B. Marks)

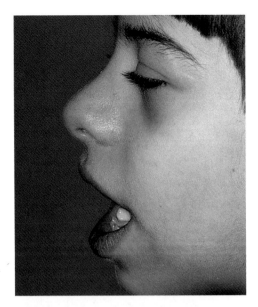

FIG. 4.9 Characteristic adenoid-type facies in a patient with long-standing allergic rhinitis. Note the open mouth and gaping habitus.

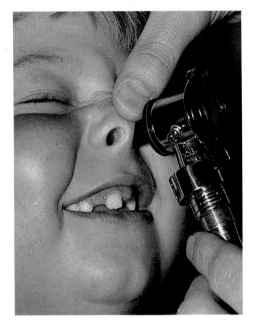

FIG. 4.10 To perform illuminated rhinoscopy, the nasal speculum is inserted into the anterior nares for magnified visualization of the nasal structures.

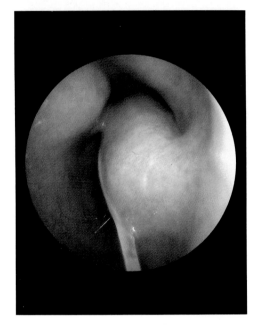

FIG. 4.11 Pale, edematous, inferior nasal turbinate of patient with allergic rhinitis, as seen through a fiberoptic rhinoscope. Even though this tool is not routinely used in evaluations, the physical findings are well illustrated, including watery nasal secretions.

lower third of the nose (Fig. 4.8). Chronic obstruction produced by nasal mucosal edema may result in the typical open-mouthed, adenoid-type facies (Fig. 4.9).

On rhinoscopy (Fig. 4.10), attention should be focused on position of the nasal septum, nasal patency, mucosal appearance, and presence and character of secretions, polyps, or foreign bodies (see Chapter 20). Use of a vasoconstrictor spray may be necessary to decrease edema and improve the rhinoscopist's view. The typical rhinoscopic findings in allergic rhinitis include a marked decrease in nasal patency due to swollen inferior turbinates, which appear wet and blue-gray in color (Fig. 4.11). Degree of nasal obstruction may be estimated by digitally occluding one nostril and maintaining normal breathing through the other with the mouth closed. It will be roughly proportional to the intensity of inspiratory nasal sounds, except when there is complete occlusion (no sounds). The mucosa appears edematous, and secretions are clear and watery or white. Examination of a Wright-stained smear of this discharge typically reveals eosinophils.

Depending on the specific allergies, allergic rhinitis may be acute, recurrent, or chronic, and must be distinguished from a number of nonallergic conditions. This necessitates a thorough medical and family history and careful

examination. In some instances, response to a trial of medication and/or observations over time may be necessary to confirm the diagnosis. When symptoms are seasonal or regularly associated with exposure to specific allergens, the distinction is generally clear. In evaluating patients with perennial or recurrent but nonseasonal symptoms, allergy, recurrent infection, eosinophilic nonallergic rhinitis, and vasomotor rhinitis must be considered.

Children with frequent upper respiratory infections and/ or persistent nasal congestion can present a major diagnostic challenge. In some cases the phenomenon is due to frequent or heavy exposure to pathogens. This is particularly true of children in their first year of day care or nursery school. In other patients, tonsillar and adenoidal hypertrophy provides favorable conditions for recurrent infections (see Chapter 20). Atopic children may have increased risk of infection by virtue of impaired flow of secretions stemming from mucosal edema, and infectious symptoms may be more protracted. They often have a history of frequent colds (more than the average of six to eight per year) which are unusually prolonged, lasting 1 to 2 weeks rather than the typical 3 to 5 days. During the course of infections, nasal eosinophilia disappears and the character of the nasal discharge often

COMPARISON OF ALLERGIC AND NONALLERGIC RHINITIS

	Allergic	Nonallergic ENR*	Vasomotor
Usual onset	Childhood	Childhood	Adulthood
Family history of allergy	Usual	Coincidental	Coincidental
Collateral allergy	Common	Unusual	Unusual
Symptoms			
Sneezing	Frequent	Occasional	Occasional
Itching	Common	Unusual	Unusual
Rhinorrhea	Profuse	Profuse	Profuse
Congestion	Moderate	Moderate to marked	Moderate to marked
Physical examination			
Edema	Moderate to marked	Moderate	Moderate
Secretions	Watery	Watery	Mucoid to watery
Nasal eosinophilia	Common	Common	Occasional
Allergic evaluation			
Skin tests	Positive	Coincidental	Coincidental
IgE antibodies	Positive	Coincidental	Coincidental
Therapeutic response			
Antihistamines	Good	Fair	Poor to Fair
Decongestants	Fair	Fair	Poor to Fair
Corticosteroids	Good	Good	Poor
Cromolyn	Fair	Unknown	Poor
Immunotherapy	Good	None	None

*ENR = eosinophilic nonallergic rhinitis

From Fagin J, Friedman R, Fireman P: Allergic rhinitis. Pediatr Clin North Am 28(4):802, 1981.

FIG. 4.12 Comparison of allergic and nonallergic rhinitis.

changes. With viral infections nasal discharge tends to be clear or white, but with bacterial infection it is often cloudy and yellow or green in color. Diagnosis of underlying atopy in these children is facilitated by obtaining a thorough past medical and family history with questions specifically directed at possible allergic symptoms and environmental allergens. Having the parents keep a symptom record with the patient on and off antihistamine therapy and reexamination at a time when the child is not acutely infected can be valuable as well. When atopy is strongly suspected and symptoms are perennial, requiring almost daily therapy with antihistamines, referral to an allergist for skin testing is indicated.

Other forms of rhinitis that must be distinguished from allergic rhinitis are enumerated in Figure 4.12. While characterized by eosinophilia, eosinophilic nonallergic rhinitis does not produce nasal pruritus, and patients lack specific IgE antibodies as measured by skin testing or serum RAST. Patients with vasomotor rhinitis do not complain of pruritus, have a clear discharge without eosinophils, and also lack specific IgE antibodies. Rhinitis medicamentosa is a condition seen in patients who have been using alpha-adrenergic vasoconstrictor nose drops as decongestants for more than a few days. The disorder is characterized by rebound vasodilation which produces an erythematous, edematous mucosa in association with profuse clear nasal discharge.

Some children with perennial allergic rhinitis have congestion that is so constant and severe as to produce signs of chronic nasal obstruction. This must be distinguished from other causes both acquired and congenital (see Chapter 20). Again history, physical findings, and results of nasal smears and therapeutic trials of antihistamine are major clues to diagnosis, which may then be confirmed by IgE testing.

The majority of patients with allergic rhinitis have mild symptoms which are easily controlled by intermittent antihistamine administration and/or environmental control. In many of these the pattern of symptoms suggests the probable responsible allergens, obviating the need for specific IgE testing. Those with severe symptoms only partially alleviated by antihistamines and those with perennial symptoms who require daily therapy should be referred for specific IgE testing and desensitization therapy.

ALGORITHM TO DETERMINE THE ETIOLOGY OF RESPIRATORY DISTRESS IN CHILDREN

Child with respiratory distress*

Inspiratory stridor† I:E ratio, 3:1 or 4:1

Yes = upper airway obstruction

No

Acute onset?

Yes

No (chronic) anatomic causes

Expiratory wheezing, I:E, 1:1, 1:2

No

Yes = lower airway obstruction

Toxic, quiet stridor, drooling

Loud stridor, no toxicity or drooling

Consolidation râles, egophony

Breath sounds & wheezing equal bilaterally?

Yes

Yes

No

Yes

| Epiglottitis (do not examine pharynx, recruit skilled personnel) | Croup Foreign body Laryngeal edema | Pneumonia Tumor | Foreign body Pneumonia Tumor Asthma | Asthma Cystic fibrosis Congestive heart failure |

*Tachypnea, with or without accessory muscle use, cyanosis, flaring or retractions. (Flaring and retractions are seen predominately in upper airway obstruction, also in late lower airway obstruction).

†Supraglottic-quiet stridor (may be audible only with stethoscope over mouth). Subglottic-loud stridor (may be audible across the room).

FIG. 4.13 Algorithm of differentiating features of upper and lower airway obstructive disorders in children.

RESPIRATORY DISTRESS

Respiratory distress in children (tachypnea with or without grunting, flaring, retractions, and cyanosis) of any etiology (allergic, infectious, anatomic) must be promptly evaluated and treated, since failure to do so may result in progression to respiratory failure, apnea, coma, and death. The first step in approaching respiratory distress is to differentiate upper from lower airway disorders. Once the level of involvement has been established, the cause can be promptly assigned on the basis of specific symptoms and signs. Appropriate therapy must be initiated without delay, based on the severity of distress and the type of disorder. At times, various degrees of upper and lower airway obstruction may coexist, as in laryngotracheobronchitis.

An algorithm for determining the etiology of respiratory distress in children is shown in Figure 4.13, demonstrating differences in physical findings between upper and lower airway obstructive disorders. Upper airway obstruction causes difficulty in moving air into the chest, whereas lower airway obstruction causes difficulty in moving air out of the chest. This difference results in the characteristic physical findings in each type. In general, lower airway obstruction produces prolongation of the expiratory phase of respiration and typical expiratory wheezing (Fig. 4.14). Wheezing is defined as musical or whistling auscultatory sounds, heard more often

on expiration than on inspiration. Inspiratory stridor, seen with upper airway obstruction, can mimic wheezing or both can be detected concomitantly, but their differentiation is seldom confusing to the experienced observer. Stridor is defined as a crowing sound, usually heard during the inspiratory phase of respiration. It tends to be loud when the obstruction is subglottic and quiet when obstruction is supraglottic.

All forms of acute upper airway obstruction present with suprasternal, supraclavicular, and subcostal retractions, which increase as the obstruction progresses. Mild to moderate increases in respiratory and heart rates are common. In lower airway disorders such as pneumonitis and asthma, retractions are primarily intercostal, and when present, usually indicate a significant degree of obstruction. Respiratory rate and heart rate are often markedly increased. Retractions are usually generalized in severe airway obstruction of any etiology.

In this chapter we will concentrate on disorders in which respiratory distress stems from hypersensitivity. These include anaphylactic laryngeal edema, in which upper airway obstruction is the result of an acute allergic reaction, and three lower airway disorders: asthma, hypersensitivity pneumonitis, and allergic bronchopulmonary aspergillosis. Infectious causes of acute upper airway obstruction and foreign body aspiration are discussed in Chapter 20.

Anaphylactic Laryngeal Edema

Anaphylactic (Type I hypersensitivity) laryngeal edema typically presents with symptoms and signs of subglottic obstruction such as stridor, dyspnea, and retractions. Onset is immediate and explosive following bee stings, drug administration, or food ingestion. Asphyxiation may result from delays in diagnosis or treatment. Frequently, other organ systems are also involved. Facial angioedema is common, and many patients have associated urticaria. Wheezing reflecting pulmonary involvement and vomiting due to gastrointestinal reaction may also be seen. In severe cases there is massive third spacing of fluid resulting in cardiovascular shock, with an initial phase of flushing and warm extremities due to vasodilation. This phase is superseded by pallor and cold due to vasoconstriction. Therapy depends on severity, and ranges from administration of antihistamines to use of epinephrine, steroids, volume expansion, and pressor agents.

Acute and Chronic Asthma

Type I hypersensitivity reactions can occur in large and small airways of the lungs and result in the disorder termed "asthma." Asthma is characterized by inherent hyperreactivity of the airways to one or more of several stimuli, including allergens, infections, exercise, chemical agents, cold or dry air, emotions, and weather changes. Hence in some cases asthma has an atopic basis and in others it does not. Specific allergens which have been implicated in atopic patients are pollens, molds, house dust, animal danders, drugs, food, and insect venoms. On exposure, these allergens, via Type I hypersensitivity, produce the characteristic features of asthma: mucosal edema, increased mucous production, and smooth muscle contraction which results in bronchoconstriction. These responses combine to produce obstruction of both large and small airways which, if recurrent and reversible with bronchodilator drugs, is the hallmark of asthma.

Affected individuals are usually aware of the specific stimuli that trigger their asthma. Viruses are the most common precipitants of asthma in children, especially respiratory syncytial virus, parainfluenza viruses, and rhinoviruses. These infections usually affect both upper and lower airways, producing rhinorrhea, nasal congestion, and fever in addition to wheezing, which tends to develop insidiously. In contrast, allergy-triggered episodes typically lack fever and have a more explosive onset of wheezing.

Asthma is one of the leading causes of pediatric morbidity. Peak incidence of onset is before the age of 5 years. In childhood, males are affected 30 percent more often than females and tend to have more severe disease. Beyond puberty, the sex distribution is equal. Asthmatic children with respiratory allergy and eczema usually have a more severe course than those who wheeze only with upper respiratory infections.

The diagnosis of asthma is frequently based on historical findings alone, indicating the importance of taking a thorough history. Even though asthma is a familial disorder, its clinical expression requires not only a hereditary predisposition but specific environmental factors as well. Family history often reveals affected siblings, parents, or first-degree relatives. Environmental survey can determine possible provocative factors, especially allergens, infections, occupational exposures, smoking, exercise, stress, climate, and medication use (aspirin, propranolol). The history should emphasize frequency, duration, and intensity of suspected episodes. A description of symptoms between acute episodes

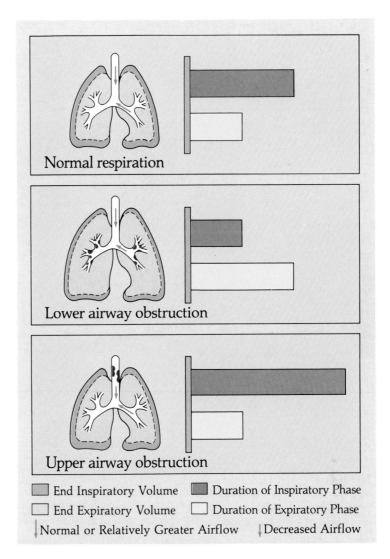

FIG. 4.14 Characteristic changes in lung volumes and duration of respiratory phases in upper and lower airway obstructive disorders. (Top) Normal respiration. On auscultation, the expiratory phase is prolonged in lower airway disorders (middle), and the inspiratory phase is prolonged in upper airway disorders (bottom). Note the increased lung volumes (hyperinflation) during both respiratory phases in lower airway disorders.

aids in determination of chronicity (night cough, exercise intolerance, fatigue, school absenteeism, social function). Individuals with asthma most commonly present with recurrent episodes of wheezing which, depending on the severity, may require emergency treatment. Episodes may be infrequent and/or seasonal, but may occur as frequently as every day. The spectrum of presenting complaints, however, is broad, and affected individuals may complain only of mild, occasional wheezing or shortness of breath with exercise and/or colds, or persistent dry hacking cough. The condition is diagnosed after three or more episodes have been successfully treated with bronchodilators.

Asthma should be considered as part of the differential diagnosis in any child with recurrent or chronic lower respiratory symptoms or signs. Even though a high index of suspicion must be maintained, excessive or erroneous diagnoses may result if they are made hastily without appropriate supportive evidence; normal children or those with potentially more severe disorders may be mistakenly labeled with the stigma of asthma and inappropriately treated. Parents must be instructed that physician assessment is essential during

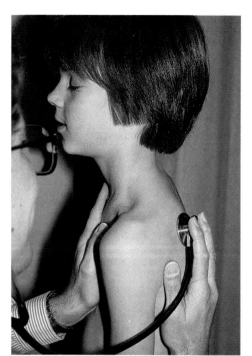

FIG. 4.15 Elicitation of compression wheezing. At the end of the expiratory phase of respiration, the physician's hand on the anterior chest gently compresses the chest, eliciting auscultatory wheezing over the posterior chest. This technique is useful in assessing asthmatics in whom wheezing is absent on routine auscultation.

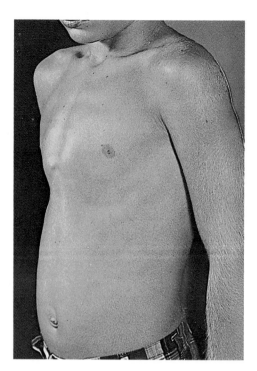

FIG. 4.16 The barrel-chest configuration of chronic asthma. Physical findings include an increased anteroposterior diameter of the chest and decreased repiratory excursion of the chest wall. (Courtesy of Dr. Meyer B. Marks)

suspected episodes of asthma, so that wheezing or other signs of lower airway obstruction and reversibility may be documented. If the diagnosis is unclear on clinical grounds, then specific laboratory studies must be performed to document asthma and rule out disorders that mimic asthma. Pulmonary function tests in asthmatic children older than 5 years show airways obstruction at baseline or after appropriate challenge, and document reversibility after administration of an aerosolized bronchodilator. In children younger than 5 years, or those in whom testing is unreliable, the diagnosis must be made on the basis of historical and physical findings, in conjunction with clinical response to bronchodilators. Lack of an immediate response to a bronchodilator does not eliminate asthma as a diagnostic consideration, however.

A thorough physical examination provides valuable information regarding the diagnosis of asthma and its severity and chronicity. The physical findings in asthma vary with the chronicity and state of activity of the disease process at the time of examination. The findings of acute asthma are markedly different from those of chronic and latent or quiescent asthma. Between episodes, the examination usually is entirely normal, but often by using the technique illustrated in Figure 4.15, compression wheezing may be elicited. If a patient with prolonged obstruction has not received appropriate therapy, signs of chronic lung disease may be present. These include a paucity of subcutaneous fatty tissue and a barrel-chest configuration (Fig. 4.16). Râles, wheezing, rhonchi, and decreased intensity and duration of the inspiratory phase of respiration are commonly noted on auscultation. Clubbing as a sign of chronic asthma is rare, and if present in a wheezing child suggests another chronic pulmonary disease.

During acute asthma, the following historical features should be noted: time of onset, possible triggers, present medications, comparison with previous episodes, and presence of complicating factors (vomiting, fever, chest pain). Examination should document the presence and degree of (1) dyspnea (the patient's own assessment of breathlessness), wheezing, accessory muscle use (visible contractions of the scalene and/or sternocleidomastoid muscles), and suprasternal, intercostal, or substernal retractions (visible depression in the chest wall during inspiration), all of which are graded as absent, mild, moderate, or severe; (2) cyanosis (central, involving the lips, and/or peripheral, involving the nail beds); (3) inspiratory breath sounds (normal or decreased); (4) air exchange (normal, decreased, or absent); and (5) abnormalities of the inspiration/expiration (I:E) ratio. In addition, râles are often heard, and pulse, respiratory rate and blood pressure are frequently elevated. Pulsus paradoxus, an exaggerated decrease in systolic blood pressure during inspiration (Fig. 4.17), correlates highly with the degree of airway obstruction and can serve as an indicator of severity and a guide to therapy. This phenomenon may result from physical forces on the pericardium that impede venous return and reduce cardiac output during forced inspiration. Normally, the inspiratory decrease in systolic blood pressure is less than 10 mmHg and not discernible during routine sphygmomanometry. In acute asthma, it is usually greater than 10 (up to 30 and 40) and easily detectable. The presence of pulsus paradoxus is correlated with a forced expiratory volume in 1 second of less than 20 percent predicted.

Individuals with asthma may be distinguished by their characteristic symptoms and signs during acute episodes, which typically change as the degree of airway obstruction increases. Symptoms usually consist of progressively increasing shortness of breath and difficulty breathing, with or without rhinorrhea, low-grade fever, and vomiting. On examination, expiratory wheezing or a prolonged expiratory phase may be the only manifestations of mild asthma. However, as the obstructive process progresses, the expiratory phase becomes longer and the wheezing louder. Eventually, airways collapse and signs of hyperinflation develop (low diaphragms, decreased lateral excursions of the chest wall with breathing, and hyperresonance to percussion). Subjectively, the patient experiences chest tightness and anxiety, and works harder to breathe. Accessory muscle use and retractions develop with or without a marked degree of wheezing

THE MEASUREMENT OF PULSUS PARADOXUS

Blood Pressure in Relation to Time and Respiratory Phase (mmHg)

	Expiration	Inspiration	Expiration	Inspiration	Expiration
Normal (no airway obstruction)	125 / 70	120 / 70	125 / 70	120 / 70	125 / 70
Asthma (airway obstruction)	125 / 70	100 / 70	125 / 70	100 / 70	125 / 70

Method

1. Pump sphygmomanometer cuff to occlude the peripheral pulse.
2. As the cuff pressure falls, listen carefully for the onset of the first Korotkoff sound.
3. Note the pressure at which the first Korotkoff sound is detected. This should be heard only during expiration. (In above example, 125 = normal and asthma.)
4. Continue to slowly decrease the cuff pressure until the first sound is detected during both inspiration and expiration. Note this pressure. (In above example, 120 = normal; 100 = asthma.)
5. When the difference between the two pressures is greater than or equal to 10, pulsus paradoxus is present. (In above example, 5 = normal, no pulsus paradoxus and 25 = asthma, pulsus paradoxus.)

FIG. 4.17 The measurement of pulsus paradoxus.

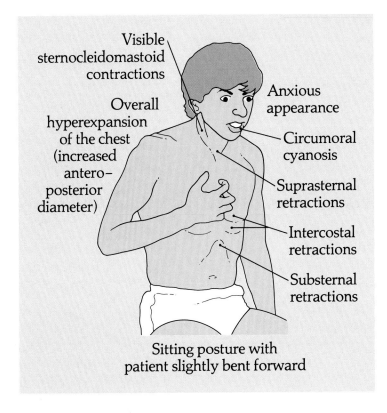

FIG. 4.18 Characteristic physical findings on inspection of a child with acute asthma. Note the posture, cyanosis, generalized retractions, prominence of sternocleidomastoid muscle, and increased anteroposterior diameter of the chest.

CLINICAL ASTHMA EVALUATION SCORE*

	0	1	2
PaO₂	70–100 in air	≤70 in air	≤70 in 40% O₂
Cyanosis	None	In air	In 40% O₂
Inspiratory breath sounds	Normal	Unequal	Decreased to absent
Accessory muscles used	None	Moderate	Maximal
Expiratory wheezing	None	Moderate	Marked or absent with ↓ airflow
Cerebral function	Normal	Depressed or agitated	Coma

*This score is designed for use in children with status asthmaticus. A score of 5 or more is thought to be indicative of impending respiratory failure. A score of 7 or more with an arterial carbon dioxide tension (PCO₂) of 65 mmHg indicates existing respiratory failure.

From Wood DW, Downes JJ, Lecks HI: A clinical scoring system for the diagnosis of respiratory failure. Am J Dis Child 123:227, 1972.

FIG. 4.19 Clinical asthma evaluation score.

on auscultation. The child usually assumes a characteristic posture to maximize air exchange (Fig. 4.18). Frequent examinations are warranted, and any change in sensorium requires prompt evaluation. As respiratory muscles tire, the patient becomes lethargic and cyanotic, even with supplemental oxygen. Maximum effort to breathe produces feeble air exchange, manifested by decreased intensity and duration or lack of inspiratory breath sounds. This is due to the decrease in audible sounds associated with respiration as air exchange decreases. Consequently, a patient with severe obstruction and impending respiratory failure may not be wheezing because he is moving too little air to do so. With extreme fatigue, respiratory muscles fail, retractions decrease, and respiratory failure is imminent unless appropriate therapy is promptly initiated. Following initial examination, serial assessment of the degree of respiratory distress, using the parameters outlined in Figure 4.19, facilitates determination of response to therapy.

The radiographic features of the hyperinflation, peribronchial cuffing, and atelectasis, characteristic of uncomplicated

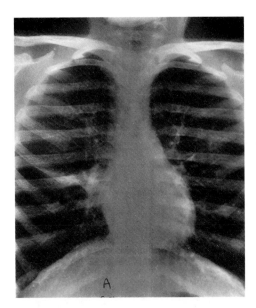

FIG. 4.20 Antero-posterior chest radiograph of child with acute asthma. Note the flattened diaphragms, hyper-inflation, peribron-chial thickening, and right middle lobe atelectasis.

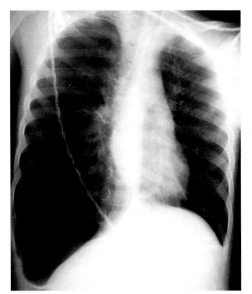

FIG. 4.21 Right-sided pneumothorax as complication of acute asthma. Clini-cal manifestations include pleuritic chest pain, dyspnea, cyanosis, tachypnea, and cough.

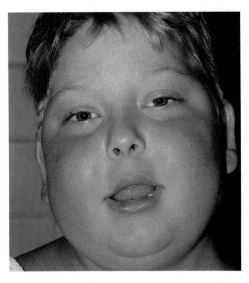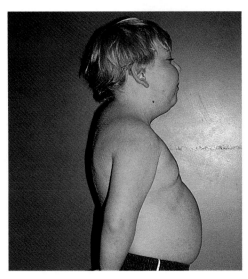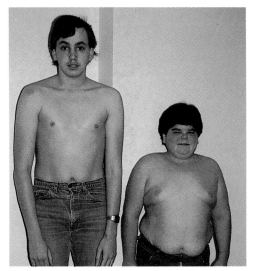

FIG. 4.22 Complications of corticosteroid therapy for chronic asthma. "Moon-type" facies (left) and buffalo hump (middle), both due to abnormal fat distribution. (Right) Short stature: a normal 16-year-old next to a 16-year-old steroid-dependent asthmatic.

acute asthma, are illustrated in Figure 4.20. Complications are generally diagnosed radiographically (Fig. 4.21), but may be suggested by symptoms and signs. Pneumothorax should be suspected in any asthmatic who develops pleuritic chest pain associated with dyspnea, cyanosis, tachypnea, and oc-casionally cough. Examination reveals respiratory distress, marked hyperinflation and decreased chest wall excursion, and decreased or absent breath sounds on the affected side. With tension pneumothorax, the trachea, mediastinum, and cardiac landmarks may be shifted to the opposite side. Pneu-momediastinum and subcutaneous emphysema, usually in-volving the neck and supraclavicular areas, are more com-mon than pneumothorax. When mild they may be asympto-matic and detected incidentally on chest radiograph. With more extensive air dissection the patient may complain of neck and chest pain, and the subcutaneous emphysema may be visibly evident as a soft-tissue swelling of the neck and chest which is crepitant (has a crunching sound) on palpation.

Other complications which are diagnosable on physical examination include those induced by chronic steroid use, such as weight gain, "moon-type" facies, hirsutism, polycy-themia (red, ruddy complexion), and short stature (Fig. 4.22). Such side effects of excessive steroid therapy for chronic asth-

ma should be avoidable complications.

In children with recent onset of wheezing, asthma must be differentiated from other disorders associated with wheez-ing. In the infant, this differentiation includes bronchiolitis, features of which are listed in Figure 4.23. Many asthmatic exacerbations are triggered by infection; 30 to 50 percent of children with recurrent bronchiolitis will later be diagnosed as having asthma. Even though these two entities may be dif-ferent manifestations of the same or a similar disease, the dis-tinction remains a clinically useful one for the following rea-sons: (1) the children with bronchiolitis who do not develop asthma may be inappropriately labeled with the stigma of asthma; and (2) children less than 2 years of age frequently may not respond to inhaled or injected bronchodilators. De-pending on response to a trial dose, the ongoing bronchodi-lator therapy characteristic of asthma management may or may not be indicated in children with bronchiolitis. While children with pneumonia (particularly of viral origin) may wheeze, they are more likely to have râles or normal findings on auscultation, with the diagnosis suggested by tachypnea in association with retractions, nasal flaring, or expiratory grunting. Other causes of wheezing are listed in Figure 4.24. Airway compression by anomalous vessels or mass lesions is

DIFFERENTIATING FEATURES OF ASTHMA AND BRONCHIOLITIS IN CHILDREN

	Asthma	Bronchiolitis
Primary etiologies	Viruses, allergens, exercises, etc.	Respiratory syncytial virus
Age of onset	50% by 2 years of age 80% by 5 years of age	<24 months
Recurrent wheezing	Yes (characteristic)	70% (≤2 episodes) 30% progress to asthma (≥3 episodes)
Onset of wheezing	Acute if allergic or exercise-induced	Insidious
Concomitant symptoms of upper respiratory infection	Yes, if infectious	Yes
Family history of allergy and asthma	Frequent	Infrequent in children with ≤2 episodes
Nasal eosinophilia	With allergic rhinitis	Absent
Chest auscultation	If viral, as in bronchiolitis Nonviral: high-pitched expiratory wheezes	Fine, sibilant rales, and coarse inspiratory and expiratory wheezes
Concomitant allergic manifestations	If allergic asthma	Usually absent
IgE level	Elevated (if allergic)	Normal
Responsive to bronchodilator	Yes (characteristic)	Unresponsive or partially responsive

FIG. 4.23 *Differentiating features of asthma and bronchiolitis in children.*

ASSOCIATED SYMPTOMS AND SIGNS IN THE WHEEZING CHILD WHICH ARE HELPFUL IN DIFFERENTIAL DIAGNOSIS

	Diseases Associated with Wheezing	
Symptoms/Signs	In Infants	In Older Children
Positional changes	Anomalies of great vessels, gastroesophageal reflux	Gastroesophageal reflux
Failure to thrive	Cystic fibrosis, tracheoesophageal fistula, bronchopulmonary dysplasia	Cystic fibrosis, chronic hypersensitivity pneumonitis, alpha₁-antitrypsin deficiency, bronchiectasis
Associated with feeding	Tracheoesophageal fistula, gastroesophageal reflux	Gastroesophageal reflux
Environmental triggers	Allergic asthma	Allergic asthma, allergic bronchopulmonary aspergillosis, acute hypersensitivity pneumonitis
Sudden onset	Allergic asthma, croup	Allergic asthma, foreign body aspiration, croup, acute hypersensitivity pneumonitis
Fever	Bronchiolitis, pneumonitis	Infectious asthma, acute hypersensitivity pneumonitis, croup
Rhinorrhea	Bronchiolitis, pneumonitis	Infectious or allergic asthma, croup
Concomitant stridor	Tracheal or bronchial stenosis, anomalies of the great vessels, croup	Foreign body aspiration, croup
Clubbing		Cystic fibrosis, bronchiectasis, bronchopulmonary dysplasia

FIG. 4.24 *Associated symptoms and signs in the wheezing child which are helpful in differential diagnosis.*

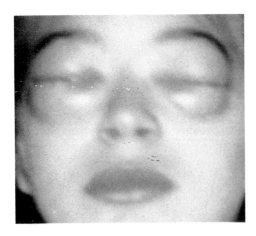

FIG. 4.25 Eyelid angioedema in child with inhalant allergies. Onset was explosive following exposure, and resolution was spontaneous and rapid.

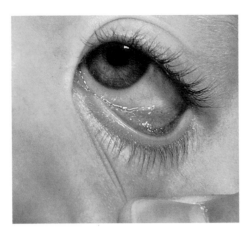

FIG. 4.26 Allergic cobblestoning of the conjunctivae in chronic allergic conjunctivitis. This granular appearance is due to edema and hyperplasia of the papillae.

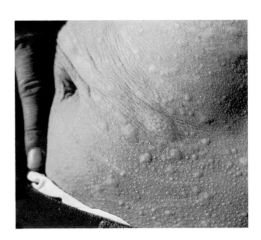

FIG. 4.27 Urticarial lesions. Note the well-demarcated borders, redness, elevation, and occasional confluence of the palpable lesions. (Courtesy of Dr. Michael Sherlock)

often distinguishable from bronchiolitis by virtue of absence of signs of infection, and from asthma by failure to respond to bronchodilators. History and presence of infiltrates help in diagnosis of aspiration which can mimic asthma closely, often responding to bronchodilator therapy. Radiographic studies such as barium swallow with fluoroscopy can be very helpful in distinguishing among these entities. pH-probe testing may be required to identify gastroesophageal reflux.

In older children who have sudden onset of wheezing and respiratory distress, the differential diagnosis includes respiratory infections, left ventricular failure, and aspiration. Respiratory infections such as croup may be distinguished by their characteristic histories and tendencies to involve the upper airways (see Chapter 20). Lower respiratory infections (pneumonia) generally produce fever and more localized findings of râles, decrease and change in quality of breath sounds, and egophony. Left ventricular failure, especially with pulmonary edema, may present with acute respiratory distress and wheezing. A history of cardiac disease and diffuse crackles or basilar râles and a third heart sound on auscultation help to distinguish this condition from asthma. Aspiration of a foreign body with lodgment in a mainstem bronchus may produce wheezing. A history of a choking episode and physical findings of unilateral wheezing and hyperresonance aid in distinguishing aspiration from asthma, but do not confirm the diagnosis. It is important to remember that wheezing due to foreign body aspiration may respond at least in part to bronchodilator therapy.

In the older child or adult with mild, infrequent episodes of wheezing that respond to bronchodilator therapy, asthma is readily diagnosed. However, with daily wheezing, frequent exacerbations, lack of response to bronchodilators, or poor growth, other diagnoses must be considered, including chronic obstructive pulmonary disease, cystic fibrosis, alpha₁-antitrypsin deficiency, carcinoid syndrome, and an associated immunological deficiency. Chronic obstructive pulmonary diseases, which include chronic bronchitis, emphysema, bronchiectasis, and bronchopulmonary dysplasia, are distinguished by their lack of significant reversibility with bronchodilator therapy. Cystic fibrosis may present with chronic cough, wheezing, and recurrent infections. Additionally, malabsorption with bulky, foul-smelling stools, failure to thrive, and clubbing of the nail beds are common. Alpha₁-

antitrypsin deficiency, an inherited autosomal-recessive disorder, is characterized by the onset of progressive emphysema in a young adult, and is one cause of neonatal hepatitis.

OCULAR ALLERGY

Ocular allergic reactions may involve the eyelid, the conjunctiva, or both. The eyelids have a rich blood supply and loose connective tissue. This facilitates edema collection in response to inflammation generated by histamine release in allergic conditions or by trauma. Immediate hypersensitivity reactions that produce eyelid angioedema may be triggered by a vast number of stimuli, including pollens, dusts, insect stings or bites, foods or drugs. They are characterized by sudden onset of periorbital edema, pruritus, and erythema following exposure to an allergen (Fig. 4.25). The disorder is distinguished from cellulitis by lack of induration, absence of tenderness and fever, and the fact that involvement is usually bilateral (see Chapter 20).

Allergic conjunctivitis may be acute or chronic and seasonal or perennial, depending on the allergen(s) to which the individual is sensitized. Commonly implicated allergens include weed, tree, and grass pollens; molds; dust; and animal dander. In the acute, seasonal form, onset may be explosive and coincident with the beginning of ragweed pollination. This condition frequently accompanies seasonal allergic rhinitis, and most commonly is due to ragweed and grass pollen. Itching and excessive tearing are the most prominent symptoms. Pruritus often interferes with sleep, and vision may be impaired by excessive discharge.

Physical findings depend on the degree of chronicity. In the acute form, these findings consist of diffuse bilateral conjunctival edema and hyperemia. Photophobia, profuse tearing, and mild lid swelling are commonly associated. In the chronic form, the conjunctivae appear pale, with mild edema and hyperplasia of the papillae. This may result in a fine, granular appearance of the conjunctivae, which is termed "allergic cobblestoning" (Fig. 4.26). More prominent cobblestoning is seen in vernal conjunctivitis. The clinical diagnosis may be confirmed by finding eosinophilia on smear of conjunctival secretions, and skin testing to the suspected allergen(s).

The differential diagnosis of allergic conjunctivitis includes atopic conjunctivitis, atopic keratoconjunctivitis, and vernal

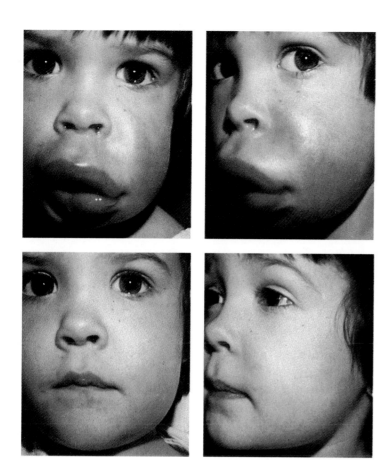

FIG. 4.28 (Top) *Angioedema involving the lips. Onset was sudden.* (Bottom) *Resolution was complete within 24 hours.*

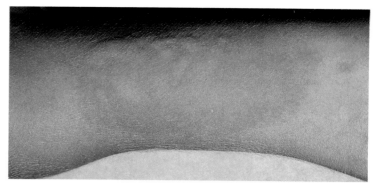

FIG. 4.29 *Positive ice cube test in child with cold urticaria. An ice cube placed on the arm for 10 minutes results in urticaria of the exposed skin. Onset is usually immediate, but may be delayed for up to 4 hours after cold exposure.*

conjunctivitis. Individuals with *atopic conjunctivitis* have a history of asthma, allergic conjunctivitis, or infantile eczema, and elevated serum IgE during active disease. The eyelids manifest a thickened, lichenified, red, exudative or dry rash. *Atopic keratoconjunctivitis* occurs in patients with atopic dermatitis, and is characterized by erythema and thickening of the conjunctivae. This may progress to scarring and vascularization of the cornea in severe cases. Ocular disease activity parallels that of cutaneous disease.

Vernal conjunctivitis is uncommon and chronic in nature. Its typical occurrence during the spring and summer is suggestive of an allergic etiology, but this is unproven. Young, atopic males are affected most frequently. Symptoms include severe itching, photophobia, blurring of vision, and lacrimation. Physical examination reveals white, ropy secretions containing many eosinophils. A palpebral form manifests hypertrophic nodular papillae that resemble cobblestones on the upper eyelids. These papillae consist of dense fibrous tissue with eosinophilic infiltrates. In the bulbar form, nodules appear as gelatinous masses called Trantas' dots, usually found at the corneal-scleral junction. This disease usually remits with maturity, and is rarely seen in adults. *Giant papillary conjunctivitis,* which clinically and histologically appears to be a mild form of vernal conjunctivitis, is associated with the use of hard and soft contact lenses. The stimulus is believed to be foreign material that accumulates on the surface of the contact lenses. Whether this material is antigenic and this represents an immune-mediated disease is not known.

URTICARIA/ANGIOEDEMA

Hypersensitivity reactions in which the skin is the major target organ are manifest clinically as diffuse erythema, urticaria, or angioedema. Type I hypersensitivity to inhalants, foods, insect venoms, and drugs is the most common mechanism, but urticaria and angioedema may also accompany Type II (transfusion reaction) or Type III reactions (cutaneous vasculitis, serum sickness). These disorders result from increased vascular permeability. The resultant edema collects in the dermis in urticaria, and primarily in the subcutaneous tissues in angioedema. While frequently seen in combination, urticaria and angioedema may also appear individually. Urticaria is most frequently an acute disorder that resolves spontaneously. When duration of recurrences exceeds 6 weeks, the condition is arbitrarily termed "chronic urticaria." In contrast to acute urticaria, extensive evaluations frequently do not reveal the cause(s) of chronic urticaria.

Urticarial lesions are well circumscribed, raised, palpable wheals that blanch with applied pressure (Fig. 4.27). They are usually erythematous, but may be pale or white with a red halo. Typically, the lesions are intensely pruritic; however, in some instances pruritus is mild. Angioedema is characterized by diffuse subcutaneous tissue swelling with normal or erythematous overlying skin. Itching is usually intense. The face, hands, feet, and perineum are the most commonly involved sites (Fig. 4.28).

Skin involvement may be generalized or localized to body parts exposed to a provoking stimulus. Careful history-taking concerning recent exposures and medications is often rewarding. In cases with associated fever and respiratory and/or gastrointestinal symptoms, infectious diseases due to viruses (including enterovirus, hepatitis B, and Epstein-Barr virus), group A beta-hemolytic streptococcus, and helminth infection should be considered. Generalized urticaria with or without angioedema may also be the initial manifestation of erythema multiforme or Henoch-Schönlein purpura. Thus, in cases in which specific etiology is unclear, parents should be informed of possible evolution and instructed regarding observation of signs and symptoms.

A subgroup of urticarial disorders results from hypersensitivity to physical and mechanical factors. These include cold urticaria, pressure-induced urticaria and angioedema, aquagenic and solar urticaria, and exercise-induced urticaria. History and distribution of lesions are often helpful in identifying the source, which can then be confirmed by challenge (Fig. 4.29).

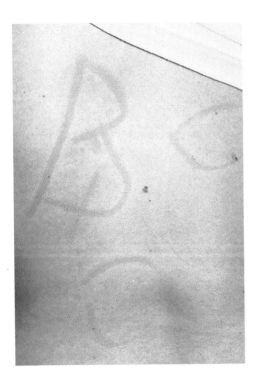

FIG. 4.30 Dermographism or writing on the skin is the most common type of urticaria induced by physical or mechanical factors. Firm stroking of the skin with fingernail or tongue blade will result in urticaria of the traumatized skin.

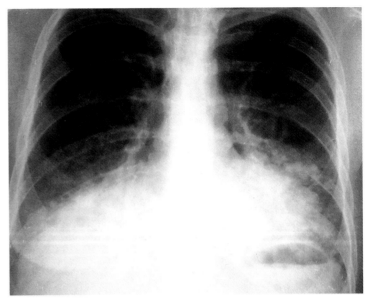

FIG. 4.31 Chest radiograph of patient with acute hypersensitivity pneumonitis. Note the soft, patchy coalescent infiltrates in both lower lung fields.

Dermographism, or the ability to write on the skin (Fig. 4.30), is a form of trauma-induced pressure urticaria. It is elicited by stroking the skin with a fingernail or tongue blade. The initial white line secondary to reflex vasoconstriction is supplanted by pruritic, erythematous linear swelling, as seen in a classic wheal and flare reaction. The condition is chronic and the etiology unclear. Patients with dermographism suspected of having an atopic disorder cannot be skin tested for specific IgE antibody because all tests appear positive.

Type III Disorders

HYPERSENSITIVITY PNEUMONITIS

Although IgE-mediated allergic respiratory diseases (allergic rhinitis, asthma) are the most common manifestations of inhalant sensitivities in humans, other immunological respiratory diseases, involving non-IgE immune mechanisms, may result from the inhalation of antigens present in the susceptible individual's environment. A wide variety of inhaled biological dusts may induce an inflammatory lung disease involving the interstitium, alveoli, and airways. The disorder is termed "hypersensitivity pneumonitis," "extrinsic allergic alveolitis," or "farmer's lung," and appears to be immune-complex-mediated.

Hypersensitivity pneumonitis is a syndrome with a broad spectrum of presenting symptoms and signs. The clinical features depend on several factors: (1) the nature of the inhaled dust, (2) the intensity and frequency of inhalation exposure, and (3) the immunological responsiveness of the exposed individual. A concomitant upper respiratory infection or other pulmonary insult may be an important factor in induction. Development of sensitization to the inhaled organic dust requires several months to years.

In the acute form, systemic and respiratory symptoms usually develop explosively, within 4 to 6 hours of exposure. These consist of cough, dyspnea, fever as high as 104°F, chills, myalgia, and malaise. Symptoms may persist up to 18

hours, subside spontaneously, and recur with each subsequent exposure. During such attacks, the patient appears acutely ill and dyspneic on physical examination. On chest auscultation, bibasilar end-inspiratory râles may be noted, and these may persist for weeks after the episode subsides. Chronic disease results from mild, continuous exposure. Progressive dyspnea, decreased exercise tolerance, productive cough, anorexia, and weight loss develop insidiously. Episodes of chills and fever are much less common than in the acute form. Physical findings in these patients include wheezing, cyanosis, and clubbing. Evidence of cor pulmonale develops as pulmonary inflammation and fibrosis progress.

Chest radiographs may be normal if attacks are widely spaced, but more commonly show characteristic findings which include fine, sharp nodulations, reticulation, and coarsening of bronchovascular markings. During an attack, soft, patchy, ill-defined parenchymal densities that tend to coalesce may be seen bilaterally (Fig. 4.31). Diffuse fibrosis with parenchymal contraction or honeycombing is a sign of end-stage disease. Pulmonary function tests reveal restrictive lung disease, especially in the chronic form, and challenge with the offending antigen may result in an immediate and a delayed response.

The differential diagnosis of hypersensitivity pneumonitis should include other conditions that cause interstitial lung disease and intermittent, explosive, and progressive pulmonary and systemic symptoms (drug-induced lung disease, recurrent pneumonias, allergic bronchopulmonary aspergillosis, sarcoidosis, collagen vascular diseases). Environmental (history, collection of antigenic materials) and immunological (serum IgG precipitins to thermophilic actinomycetes, Aspergillus species, or avian protein) studies, along with close observation of the patient during periods of exposure and avoidance, are useful in diagnosing this disorder.

ALLERGIC BRONCHOPULMONARY ASPERGILLOSIS

Aspergillus species, in addition to being one cause of hypersensitivity pneumonitis and allergic asthma, also cause a dis-

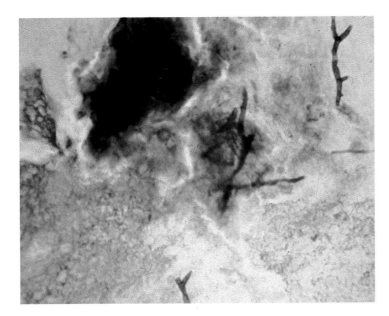

FIG. 4.32 Sputum smear from patient with allergic broncho-pulmonary aspergillosis. Note the fungal mycelia characteristic of this disorder. (Reproduced by permission from Slavin RG, Laird TS, Cherry JD: Allergic bronchopulmonary aspergillosis in a child. J Pediatr 76: 416–421, 1970)

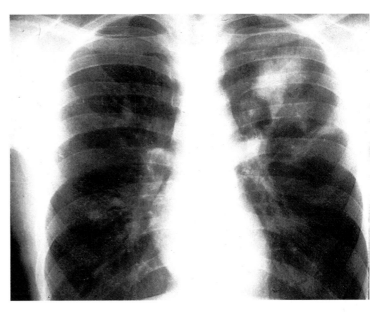

FIG. 4.33 Chest radiograph of patient with allergic broncho-pulmonary aspergillosis. These patients are frequently asympto-matic despite extensive areas of consolidation. (Courtesy of Dr. Raymond G. Slavin)

order termed "allergic bronchopulmonary aspergillosis." This entity is characterized by migrating pulmonary infiltrates and peripheral blood and sputum eosinophilia. Both Type I and Type III hypersensitivity are thought to be involved in pathogenesis. Most affected individuals are young; several under 2 years. Affected individuals are usually atopic and have a history of asthma. They present with anorexia, head-ache, generalized myalgias, loss of energy, temperature ele-vation, and acute episodes of wheezing and dyspnea. Spu-tum production is prominent and parents often report that their child's cough is productive of solid mucoid lumps of dif-ferent sizes, shapes, and colors, ranging from dirty green to brown or beige. Physical findings include the general signs of lower airway obstruction (see section on asthma). On aus-cultation, crepitant râles are frequently heard over areas of pulmonary consolidation.

Laboratory studies that assist in diagnosis include:

1. Direct examination of sputum plugs reveals fungal mycelia (Fig. 4.32) and large numbers of eosinophils in most patients. Cultures are not considered diag-nostic, as they may be negative during episodes of pulmonary consolidation and positive at other times.
2. Peripheral blood examination reveals eosinophilia, generally greater than 1000/mm³.
3. Serum IgE level (A. fumigatus specific and nonspe-cific) is markedly elevated and may be as high as 78,000 ng/ml.
4. Skin testing: Even though a positive immediate wheal and flare reaction to A. fumigatus is not con-sidered diagnostic of allergic bronchopulmonary as-pergillosis, a negative reaction makes the diagnosis unlikely. Most patients will also experience a secon-dary skin reaction (Arthus-type) at the injection site, first noted at 3 to 4 hours, consisting of erythema and poorly defined edema, reaching a peak at 8 hours and resolving by 24 hours.

5. Serum precipitating antibody (IgG) to A. fumigatus is found in most patients, but titer has a poor corre-lation with disease activity and intensity of the clini-cal picture.
6. Chest radiography most commonly shows a massive homogenous consolidation without fissure displace-ment. The upper lobes are most commonly involved and infiltrates characteristically shift rapidly from one site to the other. Remarkably, radiographic find-ings do not correlate well with clinical severity, and patients with extensive consolidation may be asymptomatic (Fig. 4.33).
7. Bronchography reveals the distinctive findings in al-lergic bronchopulmonary aspergillosis. These in-clude saccular bronchiectasis of proximal bronchi with normal filling of distal ones, in distinct contrast to usual forms of bronchiectasis.

Allergic bronchopulmonary aspergillosis is being recog-nized with greater frequency as awareness increases. The di-agnosis requires a high index of suspicion and should be considered in any asthmatic who has pulmonary infiltrates or suddenly uncontrollable disease. Allergic bronchopulmo-nary aspergillosis and hypersensitivity pneumonitis are fre-quently confused. Early diagnosis and corticosteroid treat-ment are necessary to prevent progression to severe, irrever-sible, end-stage lung disease.

IMMUNOLOGICAL DEFICIENCY DISORDERS

Normal Development of the Immune System

Integrity of the immune system is essential to maintain ap-propriate host defense mechanisms, which consist of hu-moral antibody, cell-mediated immunity, phagocytic, and complement systems. Defects of one or more of these host

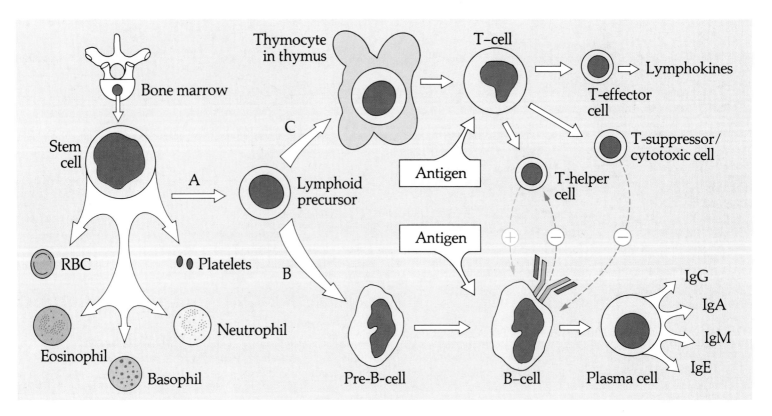

FIG. 4.34 Schematic representation of T- and B-cell ontogeny. Defects along pathway A result in combined immune deficiencies. Pathway B is responsible for normal antibody production, while normal cell-mediated immunity requires the integrity of pathway C.

defense mechanisms result in immunodeficiency disorders. In addition, skin and mucosal surface abnormalities may result in breakdown of the physical barriers that ordinarily prevent invasion of microorganisms.

Cellular and humoral immunity is dependent on the maturation of two distinct lymphoid cell lines, the T- and B-lymphocytes, both originating from a common bone-marrow stem cell. Both T- and B-lymphocytes undergo a complex series of maturational changes before arriving at a stage where they are capable of antigen-stimulated differentiation (Fig. 4.34). The thymus-dependent T-lymphocytes are responsible for cell-mediated immune responses directed against viruses, fungi, or less common pathogens, such as *Pneumocystis carinii*. Other functions of T-lymphocytes include graft rejection and tumor cytotoxicity. Subpopulations of T-lymphocytes also collaborate in immunoregulation by expression of helper and suppressor functional activities. On the other hand, the thymus-independent B-lymphocytes are precursors of plasma cells. Plasma cells produce the various classes of immunoglobulins that serve as functional antibodies for antigen recognition. Deficiencies of one or more of the immunoglobulin classes (IgG, IgA, IgM) constitute humoral or serum antibody immunodeficiency. Some patients, despite having normal numbers of B-cells and plasma cells and normal serum immunoglobulin levels, are nonetheless immunodeficient because they lack functional antibodies. Many of the immunodeficiency disorders described below are a result of either an arrest in cell maturation or a defect in the immunoregulatory cell interactions necessary for antigen recognition. Abnormalities in maturation of B- or T-lymphocytes result in humoral or cellular immunodeficiency, respectively. Abnormalities in maturation of both cell lines result in combined immunodeficiency.

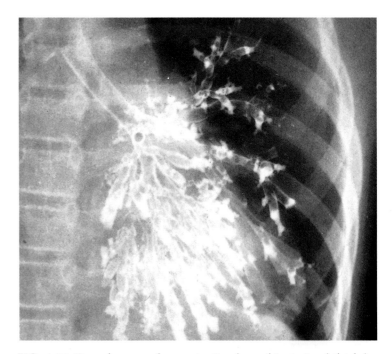

FIG. 4.35 Bronchogram demonstrating bronchiectasis of the left lower lobe in an older child with hypogammaglobulinemia. Symptoms consisted of chronic cough and sputum production.

Humoral Immunodeficiency (B-Lymphocyte)

CONGENITAL HYPOGAMMAGLOBULINEMIA
Congenital hypogammaglobulinemia may be X-linked (Bruton-type) or autosomal-recessive. Affected infants are clinically well for the first few months of life, due to placentally acquired maternal antibodies, but subsequently develop re-

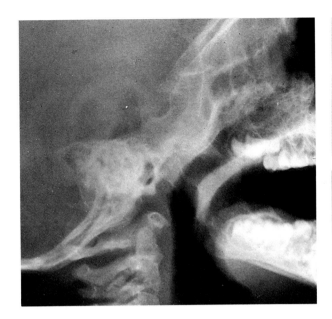
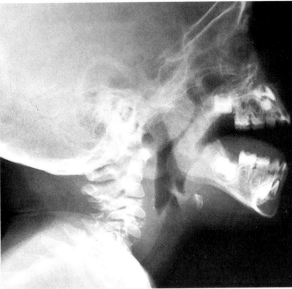

FIG. 4.36 (Left) Lateral neck radiograph showing absent adenoids in patient with congenital hypogammaglobulinemia. (Right) Radiograph showing normal adenoidal tissue.

current or chronic infections with virulent bacterial pathogens such as gram-positive cocci and *Hemophilus influenzae*. The infections may localize in the upper and lower respiratory tracts resulting in sinusitis, otitis media, and pneumonia. Sepsis, meningitis, and skin infections are also common. One of the complications of the chronic lower respiratory infections to which they are predisposed is bronchiectasis. This is characterized clinically by chronic cough with increased sputum production and by abnormal chest radiographs (Fig. 4.35). In the absence of chronic lung disease, growth is usually unimpaired and survival to adulthood is common with appropriate gammaglobulin and antibiotic therapy.

The physical findings are those of localized infection, with specific signs depending on the particular structure(s) infected. In addition, these children frequently manifest a paucity of adenoidal, tonsillar, and other lymphoid tissues (Fig. 4.36). The diagnosis of hypogammaglobulinemia should be considered in any child who has recurrent infections with virulent bacterial pathogens, and is confirmed by finding markedly decreased levels of the immunoglobulin classes (IgG, IgA, IgM) in the serum.

SELECTIVE IgA DEFICIENCY

Selective IgA deficiency, which affects 1:500 to 1:700 of the population, is the most common humoral antibody deficiency. Even though these patients are deficient in mucosal secretory IgA, only half of affected individuals manifest symptoms. Synthesis of IgG and IgM immunoglobulins is usually normal. Most cases are sporadic, but siblings with IgA or other immunodeficiencies have been frequently reported.

IgA deficiency has been associated with a variety of clinical syndromes. Chronic infections of the sinuses and middle ear are common, but severe or recurrent lower respiratory disease is unusual unless another form of immunodeficiency coexists with the IgA deficiency. Individuals with selective IgA deficiency may have severe malabsorption manifesting as chronic diarrhea, and have an increased incidence of autoimmune syndromes (collagen vascular disease) and of atopy. Therefore, the patient with a history of recurrent upper respiratory or sinopulmonary infections, malabsorption, or arthritis should be investigated for serum IgA deficiency.

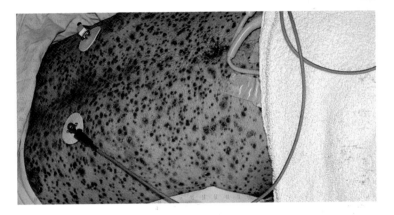

FIG. 4.37 Adolescent with abnormal T-cell function and disseminated varicella, in whom pneumonia resulted in respiratory failure.

Cellular Immunodeficiency (T-Lymphocyte)

Isolated defects of T-lymphocyte, or cell-mediated immunity, are rare. Since normal T-cell function is necessary for regulation of antibody production, many cellular immunodeficiencies are also associated with humoral immunodeficiencies. Patients with T-cell deficiencies experience an increased frequency of severe infections with viral agents such as herpes simplex and cytomegalovirus, certain fungi, intracellular parasites, and other organisms of relatively low virulence. Figure 4.37 demonstrates a severe disseminated varicella infection in a child with congenital cellular immunodeficiency.

DiGEORGE SYNDROME

DiGeorge syndrome is a pure T-cell immunodeficiency disorder characterized by absent T-lymphocytes with normal or near-normal B-lymphocyte numbers and function. Thymic hypoplasia, which results from abnormal development of the third and fourth branchial pouches during embryogenesis, is the hallmark of DiGeorge syndrome. The thymus provides the necessary microenvironment for maturation of lymphoid precursors into functioning T-lymphocytes. When the thymus is absent, this normal maturation does not pro-

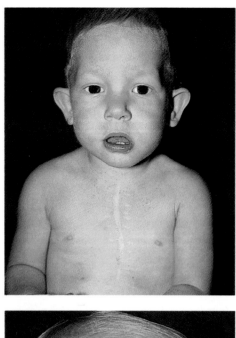

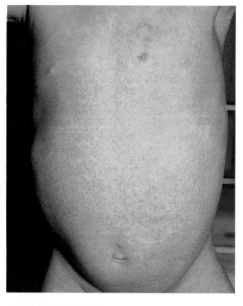

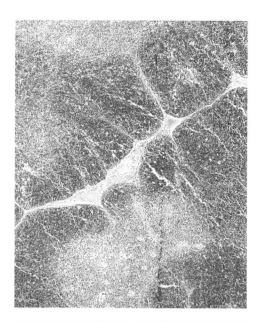

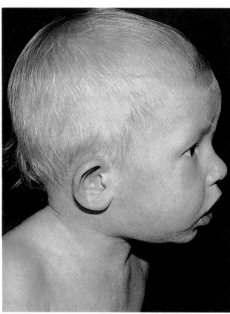

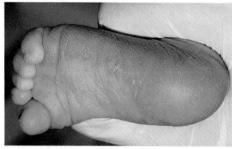

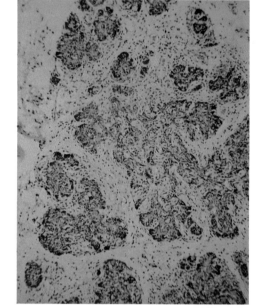

FIG. 4.38 Characteristic facial features of child with DiGeorge syndrome, frontal (top) and lateral (bottom) views. Note the micrognathia, hypertelorism, low-set malformed ears, and the midline sternotomy scar following repair of a congenital heart defect.

FIG. 4.39 Widespread fungal dermatitis with C. albicans over the trunk (top) and foot (middle) of child with SCID. (Bottom) Note the dystrophic changes of the nails secondary to chronic infection. Normal immune surveillance usually prevents persistent infection with this ubiquitous organism.

FIG. 4.40 Comparison of normal thymic architecture (top) with typical dysplastic thymus of SCID (bottom). Note the lack of normal lobulation and corticomedullary differentiation, and the decreased number of lymphocytes.

ceed, resulting in cellular immunodeficiency. Since major cardiovascular structures and the parathyroid glands are derived from the same branchial pouches, affected children frequently present with signs of congenital heart disease and hypocalcemic tetany or seizures within the first few days of life. Associated abnormalities include unusual facies (Fig. 4.38), esophageal atresia, and hypothyroidism. Even though the T-cell defect may be transient and resolve spontaneously, many of these infants succumb to overwhelming infections with bacteria, viruses, and fungi unless reconstituted with fetal thymus transplantation.

Combined T- and B-Lymphocyte Disorders

SEVERE COMBINED IMMUNODEFICIENCY DISORDERS

Severe combined immunodeficiency disease (SCID) is a heterogeneous group of disorders with varying etiologies. The consequent defects in stem cell maturation ultimately result in abnormalities of both humoral and cellular immunity (see Fig. 4.34). Inherited deficiency of the enzyme adenosine deaminase (ADA) is also associated with combined immunodeficiency. The mechanism involves the accumulation of

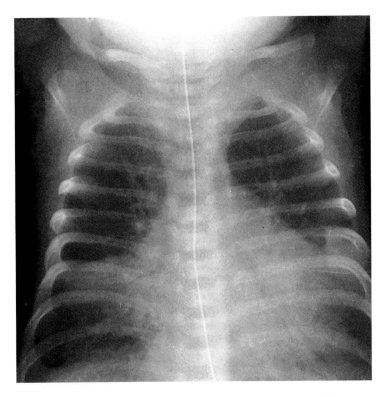

FIG. 4.41 Chest radiograph of infant with SCID. Note the absent thymic shadow and bilateral pulmonary infiltrates.

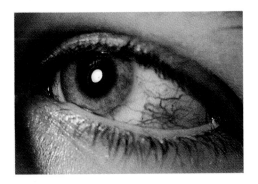

FIG. 4.42 Bulbar telangiectasia typical of ataxia-telangiectasia. Other characteristic findings in this disorder include variable immune deficiency and cerebellar ataxia.

metabolic substrates that are toxic to both T- and B-lymphocytes. ADA deficiency may be responsible for up to 25 percent of all cases of SCID.

Having deficiencies of both cell-mediated (T-lymphocyte) and humoral (B-lymphocyte) immunity, these infants present with recurrent, severe bacterial, viral, fungal, and protozoan infections. Manifestations typically appear in the first few months of life and are often associated with failure to thrive, diarrhea, and candidiasis (Fig. 4.39). Affected infants may be distinguished from normal babies by virtue of frequency and severity of infections, and of their recalcitrance to appropriate antimicrobial therapy. Presenting symptoms usually involve the respiratory tract, since pneumonia due to P. carinii or virulent bacterial pathogens is common. In addition to the clinical findings of infection, examination discloses hypoplastic or absent tonsils and lymph nodes. Laboratory abnormalities include peripheral blood lymphopenia; decreased serum IgG, IgA, and IgM; and defective lymphocyte responses to mitogens such as phytohemagglutinin. Histological examination of tonsillar, adenoidal, and lymph node remnants reveals immature lymphoid tissue. The thymus is typically dysplastic histologically (Fig. 4.40) and radiographically (Fig. 4.41).

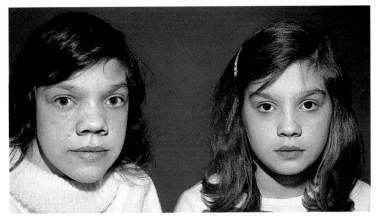

FIG. 4.43 Coarse facial features of female with hyper-IgE syndrome (left). Her sister (right) has IgA deficiency. Although distinct in etiology, these illustrate the frequency with which immune deficiencies are observed in family members of IgA-deficient individuals.

Once the diagnosis of SCID is considered, the child must be placed in protective isolation and given appropriate supportive therapy. All administered blood products must be irradiated to prevent the potential development of severe graft-versus-host disease.

PARTIAL COMBINED IMMUNODEFICIENCY DISORDERS
Congenital Disorders

Wiskott-Aldrich syndrome is an X-linked recessive disorder characterized by eczema, thrombocytopenia with cutaneous petechiae, and recurrent infections which begin in infancy. The immunodeficiency may result in infectious complications later in life. Inability to form antibody to bacterial capsular polysaccharide antigens is the most commonly reported immunological defect, but some patients also manifest a partial defect in T-lymphocyte responses.

Ataxia-telangiectasia is a complex and intriguing immunodeficiency disorder with autosomal-recessive inheritance. The pathogenesis is unclear, since no theory has been developed that explains the hallmark multisystem involvement characteristic of this disorder: telangiectasia, progressive ataxia, and variable immunodeficiency. Most patients develop ocular telangiectasia and ataxia during the first 6 years of life (Fig. 4.42). The ataxia is cerebellar in nature and characteristically progressive. Neurological involvement may be extensive, including abnormalities of speech, movement, and gait and mental retardation. The progressive, variable immunodeficiency consists most commonly of selective IgA deficiency and depressed T-cell function. Selective IgG subtype and IgG deficiencies have also been reported. Recurrent sinus and pulmonary infections, which may lead to bronchiectasis, are common and may be responsible for early death. These patients, in addition to those with other forms of immunodeficiency, have a higher incidence of neoplasia.

The hyper-IgE syndrome is a disorder of autosomal-recessive inheritance characterized by marked elevation of serum IgE. Clinical features include recurrent staphylococcal infections, a pruritic eczematoid dermatitis, and coarse facial features (Fig. 4.43). Recurrent staphylococcal skin infections, including impetigo and furuncles, are especially common and typically quite resistant to therapy. Staphylococcal

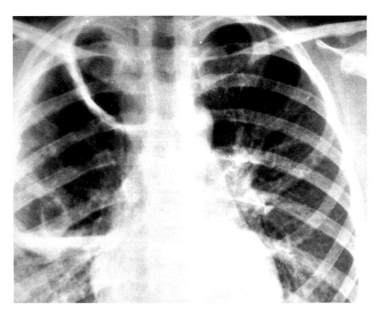

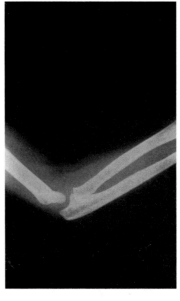

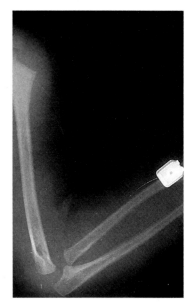

FIG. 4.44 Clearly outlined pneumatocele in the right lung of patient with hyper-IgE syndrome. This encapsulated lesion frequently complicates S. aureus pneumonia.

FIG. 4.45 (Left) Forearm radiograph of 3-year-old child with short-limbed dwarfism. Stenosis of the medullary cavity is evidenced by increased density. Bones are also of decreased caliber and length. (Right) Forearm radiograph of normal 3-year-old child.

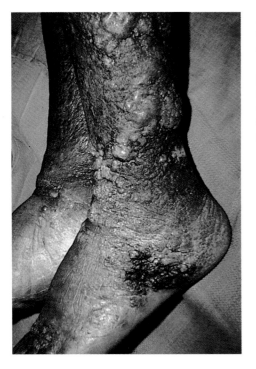

FIG. 4.46 Cutaneous manifestations of Kaposi's sarcoma. The purplish, hyperpigmented plaques and nodules, with edema of the lower extremities, are characteristic.

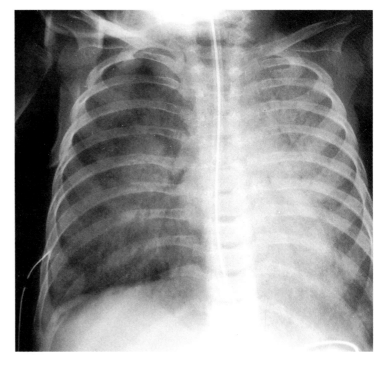

FIG. 4.47 Bilateral interstitial pneumonia in infant with severely compromised immunity. Diffuse haziness on chest radiograph and marked respiratory distress are typical of P. carinii pneumonia.

pneumonia complicated by pneumatocele formation (Fig. 4.44) and lung abscesses are not infrequent. Other organisms of relatively low virulence, including *Candida albicans*, may cause infection. Immunological findings include markedly elevated IgE levels (often greater than 10,000 IU/ml), eosinophilia, abnormal cell-mediated immunity, and in certain patients, abnormal polymorphonuclear leukocyte chemotaxis.

Short-limbed dwarfism is an autosomal-recessive disorder associated with metaphyseal or spondyloepiphyseal dyspla-

sia and immunodeficiency usually involving T-cell function. Since the immunodeficiency is variable, many affected children have no increase in frequency or severity of infections, while others develop fatal, overwhelming infections. At birth, the head size is normal, the hands and limbs are short, and elbow extension is limited. Radiographic abnormalities include flaring of ribs, sclerosis, and cystic changes of the widened metaphyses (Fig. 4.45). A variant consists of short-limbed dwarfism and cartilage hair hypoplasia in which fine, sparse hair is characteristic.

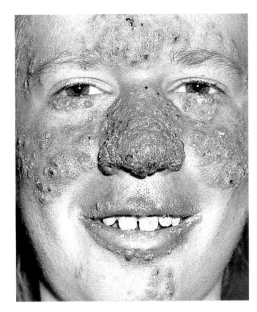 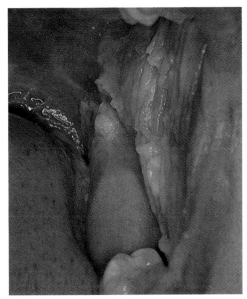 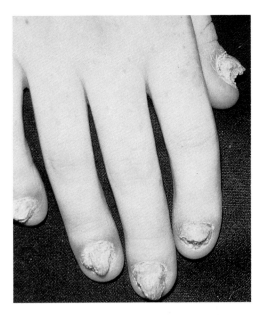

FIG. 4.48 Diffuse mucocutaneous involvement with C. albicans in older child with chronic mucocutaneous candidiasis. Lesions involving skin (left), oral mucosal surfaces (middle), and nail beds (right) are almost always present and recalcitrant to therapy with topical antifungal agents.

Acquired Disorders

Acquired immunodeficiency syndrome (AIDS) is a recently reported disorder caused by the HTLV III virus which illustrates the complexities of the immune system and the devastating consequences of defective immunoregulation. In 1981, the Centers for Disease Control noted a dramatic increase in the incidence of Kaposi's sarcoma and *P. carinii* pneumonia in young homosexual males without known congenital or acquired immunodeficiencies. Since then, over 10,000 cases, which now include infants and children, have been reported worldwide.

Persons at risk include homosexuals, intravenous drug abusers, Haitians, hemophiliacs, and infants born to infected mothers. The initial complaints are typically fatigue, malaise, weight loss, fever, and lymphadenopathy. These nonspecific symptoms may be present for up to 1 year before signs become apparent. Approximately 30 percent of cases present with skin lesions and tumors consistent with Kaposi's sarcoma (Fig. 4.46). The remaining 70 percent present with a variety of opportunistic infections, including those due to cytomegalovirus, Cryptococcus, Toxoplasma, Candida, Mycobacterium, and herpesviruses. The most frequent and devastating infection is due to *P. carinii*, which often leads to pneumonia (Fig. 4.47), disseminated disease, and death. Underlying these infectious and malignant complications is a severe, acquired cellular immune dysfunction. Immune abnormalities include lymphopenia, cutaneous delayed hypersensitivity anergy, a marked decrease in T-helper cells, and decreased lymphocyte proliferation responses to mitogens and antigens. Immunoglobulins are usually elevated.

A screening test to detect antibodies to the HTLV III virus was recently developed. A positive result only indicates prior exposure to the virus. As many antibody-positive individuals are totally asymptomatic, the percentage of exposed persons who will ultimately develop AIDS is as yet unknown.

Chronic mucocutaneous candidiasis is a T-cell disorder typified by superficial candidal infections of mucous membranes, skin, and nails (Fig. 4.48). This illness may be sporadic or familial. The disorder is often associated with an en-

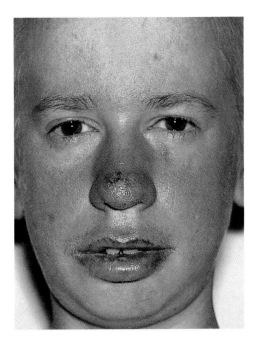

FIG. 4.49 Same patient as in Fig. 4.48 after treatment with oral ketaconazole.

docrinopathy, and variants of this syndrome may include hypoparathyroidism, hyperthyroidism, and polyendocrinopathy. Candidal infections typically begin in early childhood, but may be delayed for up to 20 years. Other manifestations of chronic mucocutaneous candidiasis result from the associated endocrinopathies, of which hypoparathyroidism is the most common. Abnormalities of the immune system include absent cutaneous delayed hypersensitivity to Candida and lack of lymphokine production by Candida-stimulated lymphocytes. Other mechanisms of host defense, including immunoglobulins, are normal. Treatment of chronic mucocutaneous candidiasis involves long-term antifungal therapy. Local application of nystatin and clotrimazole may prevent progression, but is rarely curative. Ketaconazole given orally has resulted in dramatic clinical improvement and decreased morbidity in affected patients (Fig. 4.49).

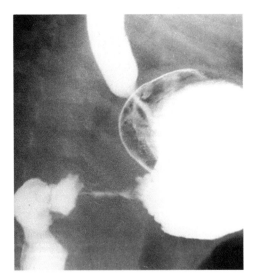

FIG. 4.50 Barium contrast radiograph demonstrating the "string sign," a thin line of barium which represents narrowing of the gastric antrum secondary to granuloma formation. This child presented with persistent vomiting, but none of the usual stigmata of chronic granulomatous disease.

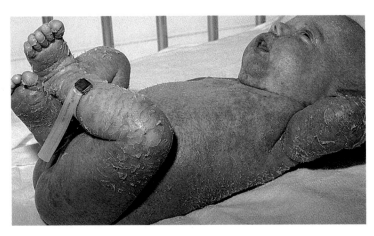

FIG. 4.51 Exfoliative dermatitis characteristic of severe seborrhea in an infant with Leiner syndrome.

Phagocytic Disorders

Polymorphonuclear leukocytes and mononuclear cells play vital roles in the defense against acute infections. Normal neutrophil numbers, intact neutrophil chemotaxis, phagocytosis, and killing are all necessary for the rapid elimination of microorganisms that invade skin or mucous membranes. Patients with neutropenia are highly vulnerable to bacterial infections, as are patients with disorders of phagocyte function. The neutropenias and Chediak-Higashi syndrome are discussed in Chapter 11.

Chronic granulomatous disease of childhood is one example of neutrophil dysfunction. Neutrophil chemotaxis and phagocytosis are intact, but killing of ingested microorganisms is defective. The responsible biochemical defect results in abnormal leukocyte oxidative metabolism, and inability to kill microorganisms. Intracellular survival of ingested bacteria, even those not typically associated with granuloma formation, can lead to development of granulomatous lesions. Because of its X-linked recessive inheritance, the disorder predominantly affects males; females are affected less frequently. Clinically, children with chronic granulomatous disease become symptomatic early in life. The most common presenting problems are severe, recurrent infections of the skin and lymph nodes with *Staphylococcus aureus*. The skin

infections often become chronic and heal slowly. Suppurative lymphadenitis often requires surgical drainage. Pneumonitis may progress to produce pneumatoceles (see Fig. 4.44). Osteomyelitis of the small bones of the hand and foot is common. Hepatosplenomegaly is a constant physical finding and presumably represents involvement of the reticuloendothelial system. Granulomas may also develop in other organ systems as well, and may or may not be palpable on examination. In the patient whose radiograph is seen in Figure 4.50, the diagnosis of chronic granulomatous disease was suggested by the finding of antral narrowing secondary to granulomatous involvement of the gastric antrum.

Complement System Disorders

The complement system is a complex system of nine distinct serum proteins, designated C1 through C9, which require serial activation, via either the classical or alternate complement pathways. Complement mediates and amplifies many of the biological functions of the immune system. These functions include: (1) enhancement of phagocytosis (opsonization) and viral neutralization, (2) mediation of inflammation via chemotaxis and alteration of vascular permeability, (3) cell lysis, and (4) modulation of the immune response. Defects of the complement system result from decreased levels of or absence of components, or from production of components which function abnormally. Although rare, inherited deficiencies of most complement components have been reported. Clinical presentation varies, depending on specific complement protein involved. Collagen vascular diseases and recurrent pyogenic infections predominate.

LEINER SYNDROME

Shortly after the turn of the century, Leiner described an infantile syndrome characterized by recurrent infections, severe seborrheic dermatitis, intractable diarrhea, and failure to thrive (Fig. 4.51). These children were subsequently observed to have a functional abnormality of C5 and an inability to opsonize yeast particles. Yeast opsonization has been used to identify individuals with Leiner syndrome, as other functional and antigenic assays of C5 are normal in these patients. Mothers of these children lack functional C5 in their breast milk; therefore, this disease occurs almost exclusively in breast-fed babies and not those fed cow milk formulas, which do contain functional C5. The disorder is self-limited, tending to resolve by age 2 months, coincident with appearance of endogenous functional C5.

HEREDITARY ANGIOEDEMA

Hereditary angioedema is an autosomal-dominant disorder characterized by absence or abnormal function of a protein in the complement cascade known as C1 esterase inhibitor. Inhibitors of the complement system are naturally occurring and are capable of blocking activated complement components. C1 esterase inhibitor binds to activated C1 and thereby prevents further activation of the classical pathway. In the absence of C1 inhibitor, complement activation proceeds unchecked. This results in increased vascular permeability and the observed clinical features of angioedema. Many clinicians do not consider hereditary angioedema an immunodeficiency disorder because these patients do not have recurrent infections. Nevertheless, a defect in the complement system is responsible for the clinical manifestations. This disor-

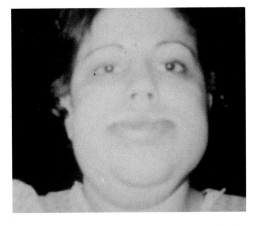
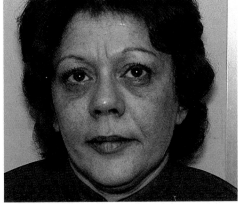
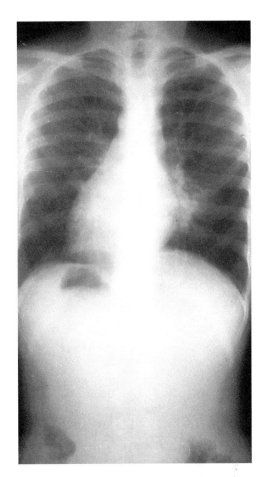
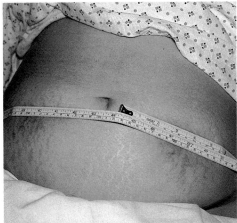
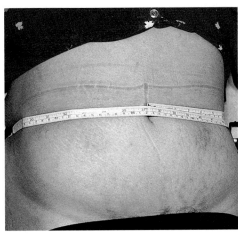

FIG. 4.52 Characteristic features of hereditary angioedema. (Top) Marked swelling of the lower face during acute episode in this adult followed by complete resolution a few days later. (Bottom)

Same patient exhibiting abdominal distention secondary to intestinal edema. Abdominal girth 44 in. at presentation and 36 in. at follow-up.

FIG. 4.53 Dextrocardia and situs inversus of abdominal organs in patient with Kartagener syndrome. Abnormal ciliary motion is thought to result in malrotation during embryogenesis.

der is characterized by recurrent bouts of swelling that involve any part of the body, but which most typically involve the face, extremities, and the respiratory and gastrointestinal tracts (Fig. 4.52). The swelling is generally self-limited and episodic. Laryngeal edema is a frightening, life-threatening complication that may result in asphyxiation. Involvement of the gastrointestinal tract is characterized by severe abdominal pain, bloating, vomiting, and rarely intestinal obstruction due to intussusception.

Mucosal Barrier Disorders

Intact mucosal barriers are of crucial importance in preventing the entrance of ubiquitous microorganisms into the host. The respiratory and gastrointestinal mucosa aid in host defense by secreting antibodies (predominantly IgA) into their lumina. In addition, physical factors such as saliva flow in the oral cavity, intestinal peristalsis, and the coughing reflex are important in the "washing out" effect on potential pathogens.

Immotile cilia syndrome is characterized by a defect in mucociliary transport, another component of the mucosal barrier. This disorder was first described as Kartagener syndrome, which consists of a triad of situs inversus viscerum (Fig. 4.53), chronic sinusitis, and bronchiectasis. These patients were also noted to be infertile, because their spermatozoa were poorly motile as a result of lack of dynein arms in the ultrastructure of their tails. Studies revealed similar defects in mucosal cilia and led to recognition of the fact that the

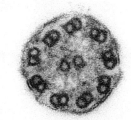
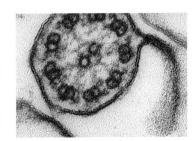

FIG. 4.54 (Left) Electron micrograph of cilia from patient with immotile cilia syndrome. Note the absence of dynein arms from the outer doublets. (Right) Normal cilia with dynein arms. (From Bluestone C, Stool S: Pediatric Otolaryngology, vol. 1, Saunders, Philadelphia, 1983)

phenomenon could exist in the absence of situs inversus viscerum. The resultant ciliary dysfunction impedes mucous clearance and produces a combination of the following signs and symptoms: (1) early onset of chronic rhinorrhea, (2) chronic otitis media, (3) chronic sinusitis with opaque sinuses on radiography, (4) chronic productive cough, (5) bronchiectasis, (6) digital clubbing, and (7) nasal polyps. The disorder should be suspected in any child with chronic or recurrent upper or lower respiratory tract infections. When situs inversus viscerum is not present, the diagnosis of immotile cilia syndrome requires confirmation by electron microscopic analysis of cilia obtained from biopsy of the nasal or tracheobronchial mucosa (Fig. 4.54)

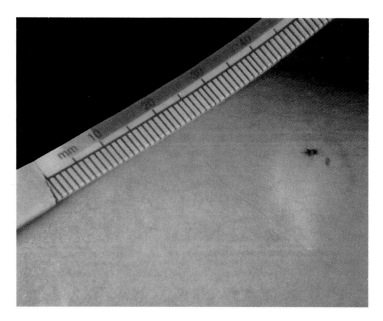

FIG. 4.55 *Positive wheal (greater than 5 mm in diameter) and flare (immediate hypersensitivity) 20 minutes after prick skin test. Note the pseudopod.*

COMMONLY USED SCORING SYSTEM FOR GRADING THE RESPONSE TO HYPERSENSITIVITY SKIN TEST

Grade	Wheal	Erythema
0(—)	<3 mm	0–5 mm
1+	3–5 mm	0–10 mm
2+	5–10 mm	5–10 mm
3+	10–15 mm	>10 mm
4+	>15 mm	>20 mm
	or with pseudopods	

FIG. 4.56 *Commonly used scoring system for grading the response to hypersensitivity skin testing.*

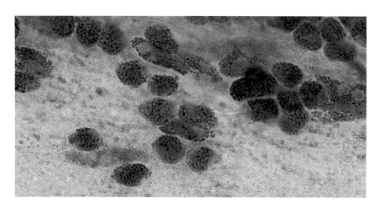

FIG. 4.57 *Eosinophilia on nasal smear from patient with allergic rhinitis.*

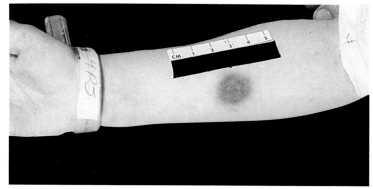

FIG. 4.58 *Reactive delayed hypersensitivity skin test 48 hours following intradermal injection of Candida. Note erythema over the area of induration, unlike the blanching associated with the wheal of immediate hypersensitivity skin testing.*

DIAGNOSTIC TECHNIQUES IN ALLERGY AND IMMUNOLOGY

Skin Testing: Immediate Hypersensitivity

For over 100 years, hypersensitivity skin tests have been used to confirm the diagnosis of allergy. This in vivo method detects the presence of IgE antibody specific to the test antigen. The prick skin test is the safest and most specific test, and correlates best with symptoms. It involves placing a drop of antigen solution on cleansed skin. A blunt needle is passed through the drop, punctures the skin, and is rapidly withdrawn without scratching the skin. The test site is "read" in 15 to 20 minutes by recording the presence or absence of a wheal surrounding flare and measurement of their sizes (Fig. 4.55). A typical scoring system is listed in Figure 4.56.

Although the prick skin test is very specific, it is less sensitive than intradermal skin tests. If prick tests are negative, then intradermal tests should be performed. This test involves injecting 0.02 ml of antigen solution intradermally and is also read in 20 minutes. The scoring system shown in Figure 4.56 is used for interpretation. Although more sensitive, the results of intradermal tests do not correlate as well with symptoms as do those of prick testing. Appropriate antigen solutions must be used to assure reliability, and results must be correlated with clinical symptoms. In addition, drugs that inhibit or suppress histamine action or release, such as antihistamines and cromolyn, must be discontinued 24 to 48 hours prior to skin testing. An in vitro correlate of skin testing is the serum RAST, which correlates well with history but is less sensitive than skin testing.

Nasal Smear

The nasal smear is another helpful tool in diagnosing allergic and nonallergic nasal disease. Mucus is obtained by having the patient sneeze into wax paper or by swabbing the posterior nares. The secretions are then applied in a thin layer onto a microscope slide. The slide is stained with either Wright's or Hansel's stain and the percentage of eosinophils is noted (Fig. 4.57). The presence of eosinophilia (greater than 25 percent), along with positive skin tests, is very suggestive of allergic disease. When skin tests are negative, the presence of nasal eosinophilia can differentiate eosinophilic nonallergic rhinitis from vasomotor rhinitis. This distinction has important therapeutic implications.

Skin Testing: Delayed Hypersensitivity

Traditionally, cell-mediated immunity has been assessed by the delayed hypersensitivity skin test. Intradermal injection of 0.1 ml of antigen solution in a sensitized individual is followed by the development of an indurated erythematous reaction over several hours. This reaction peaks at 24 to 48 hours and is recorded at 48 hours. A positive test occurs when 10 mm or more of induration and erythema is present (Fig. 4.58). Using an antigen such as *C. albicans*, the majority of children with intact cellular immunity will have positive tests after 6 to 12 months of age. Other antigens such as diphtheria and tetanus, if tested within 6 to 12 months of booster immunization, will frequently show delayed hypersensitivity. Purified protein derivative (PPD) is used to document exposure and sensitization to the tubercle bacillus. If delayed hypersensitivity skin tests are negative in a child with suspected immunodeficiency, a thorough evaluation of the T-lymphocyte system is indicated. For diagnosis of patients with contact dermatitis, delayed hypersensitivity skin testing is performed by the patch test technique (see Chapter 8).

BIBLIOGRAPHY

Buckley RH: Immunodeficiency. J Allergy Clin Immunol 72:627–644, 1983.

Ellis EF: Asthma in childhood. J Allergy Clin Immunol 72:526–539, 1983.

Ellis EF (ed): Pediatric allergy. Pediatr Clin North Am 30:1983

Henderson FW, Clyde WA, Collier AM, et al: The etiologic and epidemiologic spectrum of bronchiolitis in pediatric practice. J Pediatr 95:183, 1979.

Howard WA: Differential diagnosis of wheezing in children. Pediatr Rev 1:239, 1980.

Middleton E Jr, Reed CE, Ellis EF (eds): Allergy: Principles and Practice. Mosby, St. Louis, 1983.

Primer on Allergic and Immunologic Disease. JAMA 20:248, 1982.

Rosen FS, Cooper MD, Wedgewood RJ: The primary immunodeficiencies (Part 1). N Engl J Med 311:300–310, 1984.

Scott GB, Buck BE, Leterman JG, et al: Acquired immunodeficiency syndrome in infants. N Engl J Med 310:76–81, 1984.

Steihm ER, Fulginiti VA (eds): Immunologic Disorders in Infants and Children. Saunders, Philadelphia, 1980.

PEDIATRIC CARDIOLOGY

Cora C. Lenox, M.D.

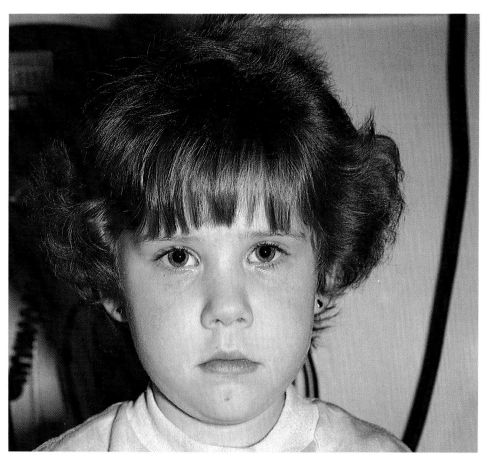 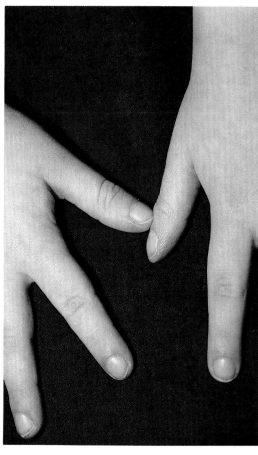

FIG. 5.1 *This child shows no obvious cyanosis of the face and lips, though the photograph at right demonstrates clubbing: loss of nail angle and curvature of nails, especially of the thumb. (Courtesy of Dr. L. B. Beerman)*

Careful physical examination for unusual characteristics in the skin, the nails, the mucous membranes, the face, and the body build may provide early clues in the diagnosis of certain heart defects in children. In addition to external examination, chest radiography and electrocardiography prove to be invaluable sources in the detection of certain abnormalities. Through their use the position and shape of the heart, the great vessels, and the lungs, as well as unusual shadows, or the absence of the usual shadows are seen.

PHYSICAL SIGNS OF CARDIAC DISEASE
Cyanosis and Clubbing

Even before mild desaturation is detectable, early clubbing may be seen (Fig. 5.1). The base of the nail, especially the thumbnail, may show loss of angle as early as 3 months of age. Elevated hemoglobin and hematocrit (H/H) and loss of nail angle indicate hypoxia, possibly a right to left shunt.

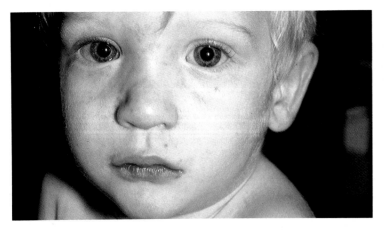

FIG. 5.2 *This child demonstrates moderate cyanosis of the lips (left) and nails (right). Note also the reddish discoloration of the* eyes *due to conjunctival suffusion.*

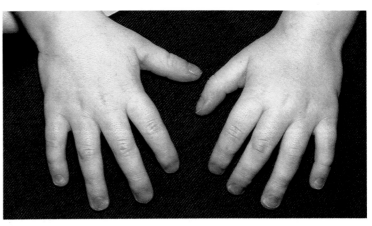

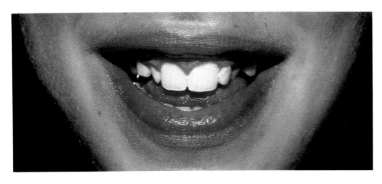

FIG. 5.3 *Severe cyanosis of the lips, tongue, and mucous membranes can be noted at left, associated with marked clubbing and* cyanosis *of nails at right.*

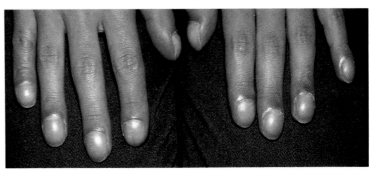

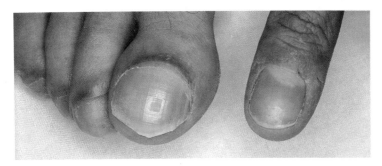

FIG. 5.4 *Differential cyanosis and clubbing due to reverse shunting through a patent ductus arteriosus in a patient with pulmonary vascular disease. Note marked cyanosis and clubbing of the toes, while the finger appears to be normal. (Courtesy of Dr. J. R. Zuberbuhler)*

Observation of the lips and mucous membranes for cyanosis is best done in good daylight (Figs. 5.2 and 5.3), since fluorescent light may produce a false cyanotic tinge. When the H/H is high (over 20 g hemoglobin per 60 percent hematocrit), the conjunctival blood vessels become engorged. This causes the eyes to take on a red discoloration (see Fig. 5.2).

Differential cyanosis between the upper and lower extremities occurs when there is right to left (reverse) shunting of venous blood across a ductus arteriosus as the result of pulmonary vascular disease and a patent ductus. A consequence of this will be clubbing of the toes but not of the fingers (Fig. 5.4). Normal pink toes with cyanotic and clubbed fingers may be seen where there is associated transposition of the great arteries.

SYNDROMES AND TRISOMIES, WITH THEIR ASSOCIATED CARDIOVASCULAR FINDINGS

Syndromes	Common Cardiac Defects
Down*	Septal defects, patent ductus, aortic arch findings
Holt-Oram	Atrial and ventricular septal defects, arrhythmias
Marfan	Dilatation and aneurysm of aorta, aortic and mitral valve insufficiency, mitral valve prolapse
Noonan	Atrial septal defect, pulmonic stenosis
Turner*	Coarctation of the aorta, bicuspid aortic valve
Williams	Supravalvular aortic stenosis, pulmonary artery stenosis

Trisomies	Common Cardiac Defects
13*	Patent ductus, septal defects, pulmonic and aortic stenosis (atresia)
18*	Ventricular septal defect, polyvalvular disease, coronary abnormalities

See Chapter 1 for detailed discussion.

FIG. 5.5 *Syndromes and trisomies, with their associated cardiovascular findings.*

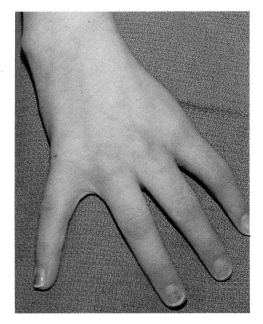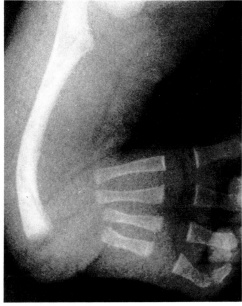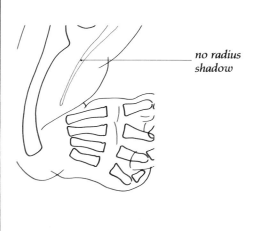

FIG. 5.6 Clinical photograph (left) reveals the absence of the radius and thumb in a patient with Holt-Oram syndrome. The associated cardiovascular abnormality is an atrial septal defect. Radiographic examination (right) demonstrates the absence of radius shadow; the missing thumb is apparent. (Clinical photograph courtesy of Dr. L. B. Beerman)

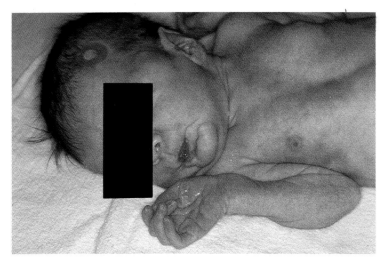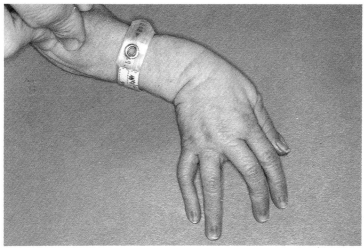

FIG. 5.7 Infant with Marfan syndrome. Note the narrow face, pectus, laxity, and long arms and fingers (left). At right is a close-up view of the infant's hand. (Courtesy of Dr. F. J. Fricker)

Syndrome-Associated Physical Findings

Inspection of the face may suggest certain syndromes. Figure 5.5 lists the syndromes and trisomies commonly associated with cardiac findings.

The typical facies in Down syndrome (trisomy 21) were demonstrated in Chapter 1. About 30 percent of children with this syndrome have heart disease; commonly seen are septal defects, a patent ductus arteriosus, and often, a minor aortic arch arrangement (right subclavian artery of distal origin). Possibly due to chronic upper airway obstruction, these infants quickly develop pulmonary vascular disease. Since the cardiac anomalies may be silent, it is important that all children with Down syndrome be thoroughly examined during infancy to rule out cardiac defects.

Holt-Oram syndrome, an autosomal-dominant disorder, causes prominent skeletal defects. Upper limb defects consist of narrow shoulders, hypoplasia of the radius, and sometimes phocomelia or proximal displacement of the thumb, or absence of both the radius and thumb (Fig. 5.6). In addition, there may be absence of the pectoralis major muscle. The commonly associated cardiovascular abnormalities are atrial septal defect, ventricular septal defect, and arrhythmias.

Marfan syndrome, an autosomal-dominant disorder, manifests as a connective tissue abnormality in which elastic fibers are disrupted, causing medial necrosis of large blood vessels, joint laxity, and dislocation of the ocular lens. Patients are characteristically tall and thin, and have long limbs, pectus excavatum or carinatum, a narrow face and palate, and hernias (Fig. 5.7). Cardiovascular problems are secondary to connective tissue laxity, and consist of dilatation and aneurysms of the aorta, aortic and mitral valve insufficiency, and prolapse of the mitral valve.

Patients with Noonan syndrome have some features characteristic of Turner syndrome, but possess normal chromosomes. Clinically, the condition manifests as webbing of the

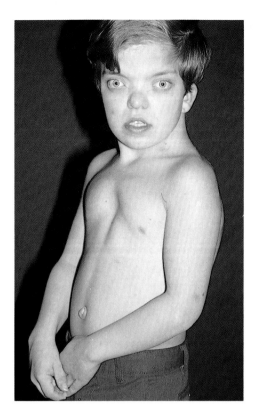

FIG. 5.8 Child displays characteristic features of Noonan syndrome: widely spaced eyes, low-set ears, webbing of neck, shield chest, pectus, and increased carrying angle of the arms.

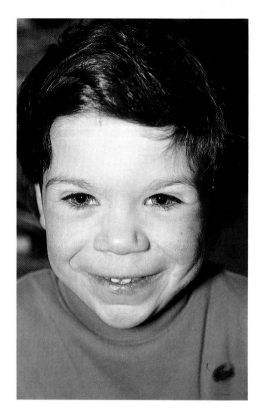

FIG. 5.9 Child with elfin facies (Williams syndrome). Note the wide-set eyes, upturned nose, large maxilla, thick lips, and pointed chin. (Courtesy of Dr. R. A. Mathews)

GENETIC SYNDROMES AND INBORN ERRORS OF METABOLISM, WITH THEIR ASSOCIATED CARDIOVASCULAR FINDINGS

Genetically Determined Diseases	Cardiac Findings
Metabolic — storage	
Pompe disease (glycogen storage)	Cardiomyopathy (storage of glycogen in myocardium)
Mucopolysaccharidosis	Storage of MPS in arteries, coronaries, and valves with insufficiency and stenosis Hurler MPS IH, Hunter II, Scheie IS, IHS, Morquio IV
Hyperlipoproteinemia, familial type II	Premature atherosclerosis of arteries, including coronaries
Neurologic	
Friedreich's ataxia	Cardiomyopathy (congestive or hypertrophic)
Muscular dystrophies	Myocardial degeneration and fibrosis

Inborn Error of Metabolism (no proven genetic basis)	Cardiac Findings
Progeria	Hypercholesterolemia, atherosclerotic changes in arteries, including coronaries

FIG. 5.10 Genetic syndromes and inborn errors of metabolism, with their associated cardiovascular findings.

neck, pectus, shield chest with widely spaced nipples, short stature, epicanthal folds, low-set ears, and skeletal abnormalities including increased carrying angle of the arms (Fig. 5.8). Mental retardation is often an associated finding. The commonly seen cardiovascular defects are atrial septal defect and dysplastic pulmonic valve with stenosis. Occasionally there may be dysplasia of other and possibly all valves.

The most common cardiac defects in Turner syndrome are coarctation of the aorta and bicuspid aortic valve. (See Chapter 1 for a detailed discussion of Turner syndrome.)

Patients with Williams syndrome characteristically have "elfin" facies: a broad maxilla and small mandible with full mouth and large upper lip, upturned nose and full forehead with hypertelorism, inner epicanthal folds, and large ears (Fig. 5.9). This syndrome has been associated with hypercalcemia in infancy and may be hereditary. Supravalvular aortic stenosis and pulmonary artery stenosis are the common cardiovascular manifestations.

In addition, there are many genetically determined diseases and inborn errors of metabolism with cardiac involvement, the most common of which are listed in Figure 5.10.

Visible Clues in Acute Rheumatic Fever

Examination of the skin in a patient with acute rheumatic fever may reveal the typical rash of erythema marginatum, though this rash is not specific for rheumatic fever. It is nonpruritic, has sharp serpiginous margins, and is found on the inner aspects of the upper arms, the thighs, and on the trunk (Fig. 5.11). The rash may be transient, brought out by application of heat or by a warm bath; treatment is unnecessary. Differential diagnosis should include: (1) drug rash, which is papular and pruritic; (2) rash of glomerulonephritis, which is macular and has no sharp margins; (3) rash of juvenile rheumatoid arthritis, which may be transient, but is pink and macular and lacks wavy margins; and (4) the skin findings of Kawasaki disease (see Chapter 12).

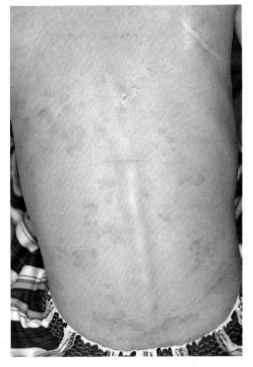

FIG. 5.11 Erythema marginatum rash in a child with acute rheumatic fever. Note the wavy margins and distribution on the trunk. (Courtesy of Dr. S. C. Park)

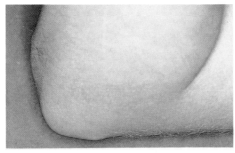

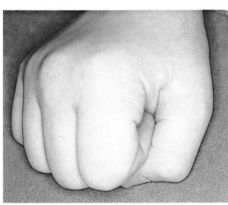

FIG. 5.12 Subcutaneous nodules over bony prominences of the elbow (top) and knuckles of the hand (bottom) in a patient with chronic rheumatic heart disease. (Courtesy of Dr. S. C. Park)

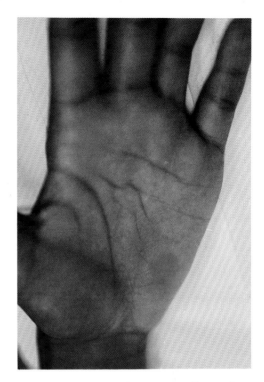

FIG. 5.13 Janeway lesions, small, painless nodules in the palm of a patient with bacterial endocarditis.

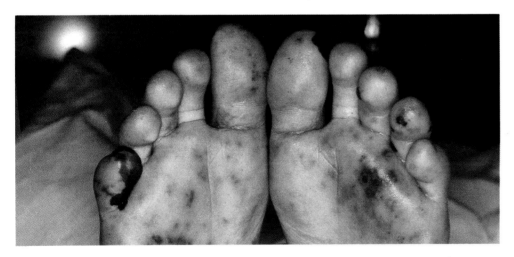

FIG. 5.14 Hemorrhagic lesions in a patient with acute bacterial endocard-itis. (Courtesy of Dr. W. H. Neches)

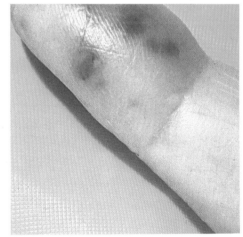

FIG. 5.15 Osler nodes, painful erythema-tous nodular lesions resulting from infec-tive endocarditis. (Courtesy of Dr. J. F. John, Jr.)

In chronic rheumatic heart disease, subcutaneous nodules may be found as a late sign and indicate severe carditis. These movable, nontender, cartilage-like swellings vary in size from 2 mm to 1 cm and are never transient. They are seen over the bony prominences of the large joints and external surfaces of the elbows and knuckles of the hands, knees, and ankles, and along the spine; they may also be found in the scalp. While difficult to photograph, they are easily palpated (Fig. 5.12).

Signs of Bacterial Endocarditis by Examination of the Skin

Bacterial endocarditis should be suspected whenever spiking fevers recur following antibiotic treatment for "infection," when a new heart murmur appears, and when classical skin lesions of bacterial endocarditis start to develop. These classical skin lesions include splinter hemorrhages of the nails, conjunctival hemorrhages, and Janeway lesions (Fig. 5.13); all of which are representative of embolic phenomena. Additional hemorrhagic involvement of the skin will occur in acute cases (Fig. 5.14). Osler nodes, which present themselves as small, tender, erythematous nodules, are found in both the intradermal pads of the fingers and the toes, or in the thenar or the hypothenar eminences (Fig. 5.15). All of the above findings are associated with an enlarged spleen, a spiking temperature, and a positive blood culture. Clubbing of the fingers may further be found in cases which are more chronic.

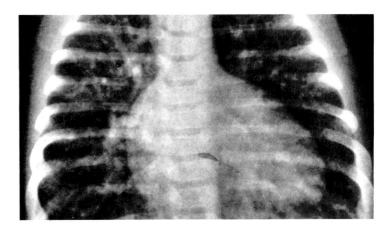

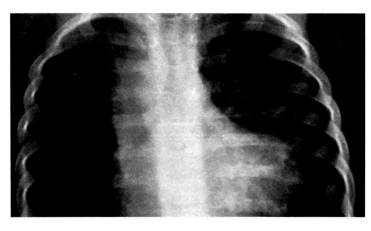

FIG. 5.16 "Egg on a string" heart shadow due to transposition of the great arteries. The main pulmonary artery is posterior and slightly to the left of the aorta, contributing to the narrow waist (the "string").

FIG. 5.17 Tetralogy of Fallot with pulmonic stenosis produces this "boot-shaped" heart. Due to right ventricular hypertrophy, the apex is tilted upward, and the small right ventricular infundibulum and small main pulmonary artery cause the concavity in the left upper border of the heart. Right aortic arch is present.

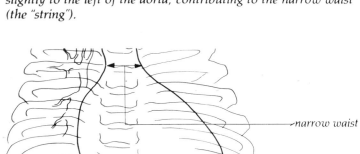

narrow waist

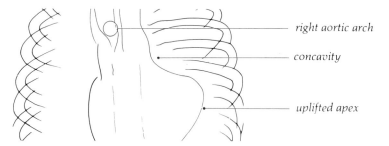

right aortic arch

concavity

uplifted apex

LABORATORY AIDS IN THE DIAGNOSIS OF CONGENITAL HEART DISEASE

In addition to the classical methods of physical examination, chest radiography and electrocardiography may provide clues in diagnosing heart defects. Many of these defects produce easily recognizable and characteristic heart shadows.

Transpositions of the Great Arteries

In the cyanotic and stressed newborn with transposition, the heart shadow has been likened to "an egg on a string" (Fig. 5.16). If the thymus shadow is not seen, the mediastinal shadow is narrowed by the posterior and medial position of the main pulmonary artery. This produces the "string." The apex of the "egg" points downward so that the heart appears to be held up by the string. Vascular markings are usually increased, and electrocardiography demonstrates right ventricular hypertrophy (RVH)—normal for the newborn. The second heart sound is loud and single at the high left sternal border. There may be no murmur or a nonspecific flow murmur along the left sternal border. Examination of the patient following a corrective procedure may show distended systemic veins, indicating systemic venous obstruction.

Tetralogy of Fallot (with Pulmonic Stenosis)

In this disorder the heart appears "boot-shaped," and is small because of the large right to left shunt at the ventricular level (Fig. 5.17). Right ventricular hypertrophy causes the apex (i.e., toe of the boot) to turn upward. The concavity of the left upper border is due to small right ventricular outflow and

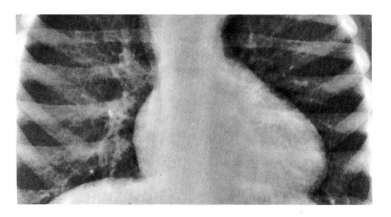

FIG. 5.18 Tetralogy of Fallot with pulmonary atresia produces this "egg on its side" appearance. Note the uplifted apex due to right ventricular hypertrophy. There is a concavity due to the absence of right ventricular outflow and pulmonary artery segments. Note also the right aortic arch.

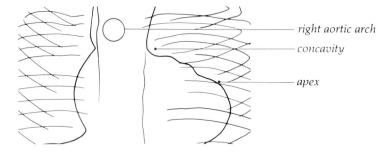

right aortic arch

concavity

apex

pulmonary artery segments, but it may be obscured by a large thymus. The murmur may resemble a small ventricular septal defect, when in fact it is a murmur of pulmonic infundibular stenosis. As this stenosis increases, the murmur becomes

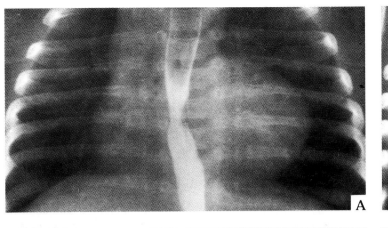

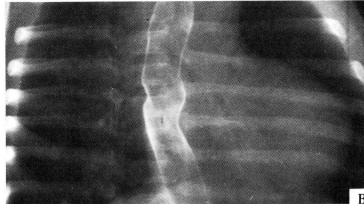

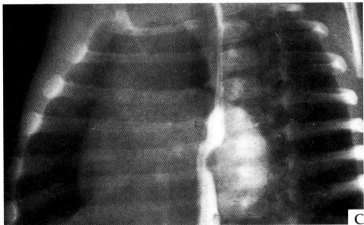

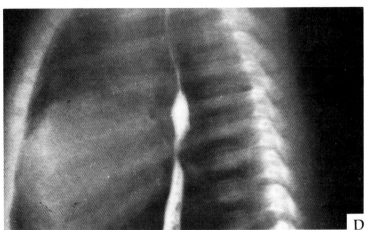

FIG. 5.19 Barium esophagraphy of a patient with tetralogy of Fallot with pulmonic atresia and systemic collaterals shows large collaterals to the lungs and indenting the esophagus. **A**, Frontal view; **B**, right anterior oblique view; **C**, left anterior oblique view; **D**, left lateral view.

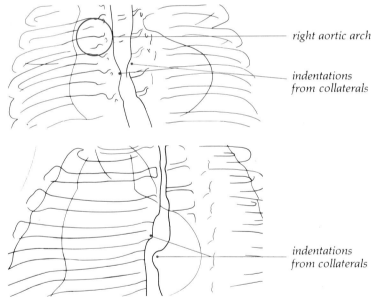

right aortic arch

indentations from collaterals

indentations from collaterals

indentations from collaterals

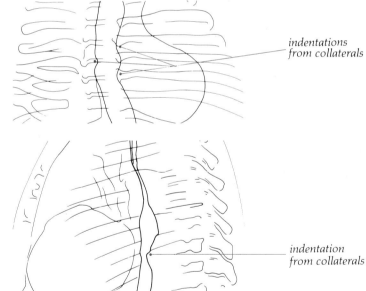

indentation from collaterals

shorter and softer and may even disappear in a hypercyanotic spell. Pulmonic valve closure is not audible. A right aortic arch is common, and pulmonary vascularity is usually decreased. The electrocardiogram is usually normal at first, but continues to show RVH.

Tetralogy of Fallot (with Pulmonic Atresia)

Here, the heart is shaped like "an egg on its side," with its transverse diameter wider than in tetralogy of Fallot with pulmonic stenosis (Fig. 5.18). Blood flow to the lungs may be supplied by a patent ductus arteriosus or by systemic collaterals to the pulmonary vessels. If a patent ductus is present, a continuous murmur may be heard in a localized area at the high left sternal border. If systemic collaterals supply the lungs, a louder continuous murmur is heard throughout the chest, but loudest posteriorly. Barium esophagraphy may demonstrate these collaterals indenting the esophagus (Fig. 5.19). When the blood flow to the lungs is increased and the left heart is normal in size, pulmonary vascularity is increased. With decreased flow via collaterals, the heart appears small and vascularity is decreased.

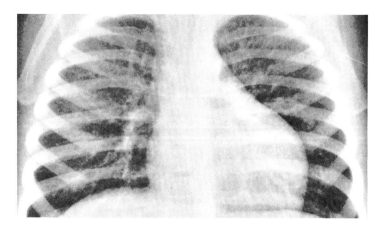

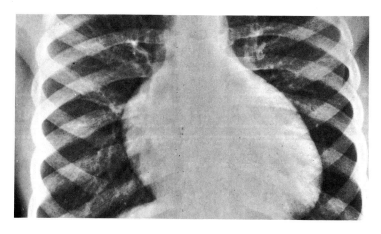

FIG. 5.20 Tricuspid atresia produces an "apple-shaped" heart due to the large left atrial appendage and the hypertrophied left ventricle.

FIG. 5.21 Radiograph demonstrates the "box-shaped" heart associated with Ebstein anomaly of the tricuspid valve. Note the large right ventricular outflow and the large right atrial shadow.

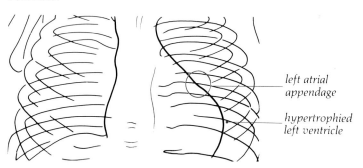

left atrial appendage

hypertrophied left ventricle

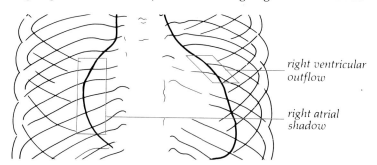

right ventricular outflow

right atrial shadow

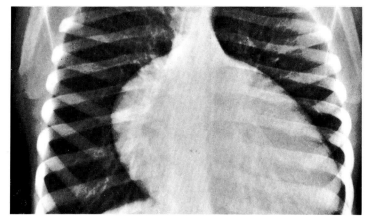

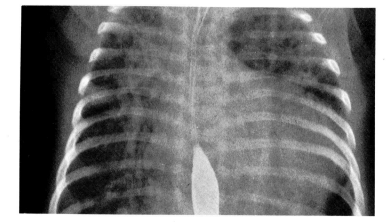

FIG. 5.22 Radiograph of a newborn with Ebstein anomaly demonstrates a marked decrease in vascularity. Note the large right ventricular outflow, as well as the narrow pedicle caused by small great arteries and the lack of a thymus.

FIG. 5.23 This radiograph of a child with persistent truncus arteriosus reveals a large right pulmonary artery well above the heart, presenting a "waterfall" appearance. Note also the right aortic arch.

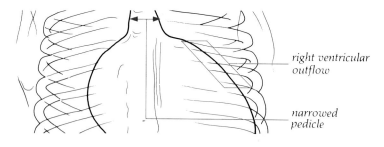

right ventricular outflow

narrowed pedicle

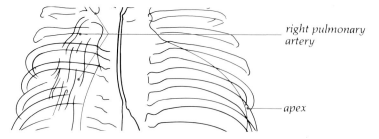

right pulmonary artery

apex

Tricuspid Atresia

Radiographic examination of a patient with tricuspid atresia reveals an "apple-shaped heart," the result of a large and hypertrophied left ventricle (Fig. 5.20). The upper enlarged left border is formed by the left atrium which accommodates the systemic venous return and the pulmonary venous return simultaneously. The apical shadow is the hypertrophied left ventricle. Vascularity depends on the presence of pulmonic stenosis and on the size of the ventricular septal defect. If transposition of the great vessels exists, vascularity is apt to be increased. The degree of cyanosis will also depend on the flow of blood to the lungs. The systolic murmur may be due to a restrictive ventricular defect or caused by infundibular stenosis (similar to tetralogy of Fallot). Electrocardiography will show left axis deviation and dominant left ventricular forces.

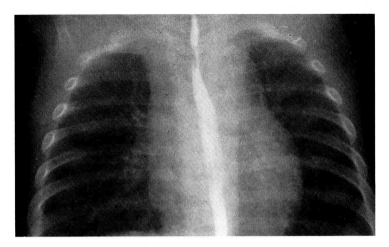

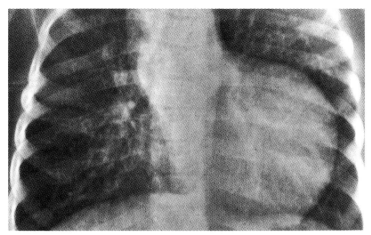

FIG. 5.24 Radiograph shows the "valentine-shaped" heart characteristically found in L-transposition. Note the ascending aorta on the left side.

FIG. 5.25 This radiograph demonstrates left juxtapositioned atrial appendages side by side above the ventricular mass, to the left of the great arteries. The right atrium is not visible and there is no right atrial shadow.

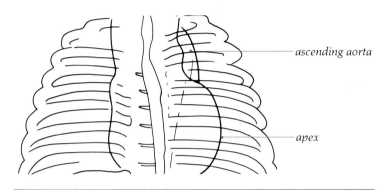

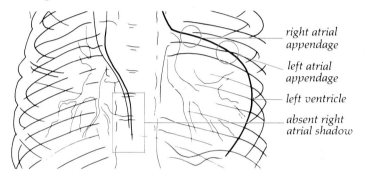

Ebstein Anomaly

In this disorder, the anterior leaflet of the tricuspid valve is large and redundant; and the septal and posterior leaflets, instead of being free from the ventricular wall to the valvular anulus, are attached at varying levels to the septal and posterior wall of the right ventricle. Cardiomegaly and decreased vascularity are common manifestations.

The heart appears "box-shaped" due to an enlarged right atrium and right ventricle, but especially due to the right large ventricular outflow tract (Fig. 5.21). On auscultation, a quadruple rhythm with a split first sound and second heart sounds is heard, and may be associated with a plethora or audible events in both systole and diastole secondary to restriction of tricuspid valve flow or stenosis. Phonocardiography can be helpful in sorting out these sounds. The typical electrocardiogram shows low voltage in the right chest leads, prolonged PR interval, right atrial enlargement, and increased duration of the QRS. In the newborn, vascularity may be markedly decreased, leading to extreme cyanosis (Fig. 5.22). Pulmonic atresia must be ruled out by echocardiography or catheterization.

Persistent Truncus Arteriosus

This condition occurs when the truncus fails to divide into aorta and pulmonary arteries. As a result, the patient presents with one large vessel, one large truncal semilunar valve which overrides the ventricular septum, and an outlet ventricular septal defect. The coronary and pulmonary arteries originate from this trunk, which continues as the aorta.

Radiographic examination of a child with this congenital anomaly will demonstrate a "waterfall" appearance in the

right lung due to the large right pulmonary artery positioned above the level of the heart shadow (Fig. 5.23). A right aortic arch is also commonly observed. Vascularity and degree of cyanosis depend on blood flow to the lungs. On examination an early ejection sound and a systolic murmur along the left sternal border are heard. Increased pulses are palpated. A high-pitched decrescendo diastolic murmur along the left sternal border indicates truncal insufficiency.

Corrected Transposition

In corrected transposition (i.e., L-transposition or ventricular inversion) the heart takes on a "valentine" shape, with the apex pointing down just to the left of the midline (Fig. 5.24). The fullness in the upper left border is the ascending aorta. The electrocardiogram may show a Q wave in the right chest leads, but never in the left. A loud, single, second heart sound at the high left sternal border may be the only clinical sign in this disorder, unless there are associated defects.

Juxtapositioned Atrial Appendages

This alignment occurs when the right atrium is rotated posteriorly, causing the right atrial appendage to rotate behind both great vessels and lie adjacent to the left atrial appendage. Associated heart defects such as transposition, double-outlet right ventricle, and/or tricuspid atresia may be associated findings (Fig. 5.25). The right atrium is displaced posteriorly, therefore no right heart border can be observed radiographically. The heart will have an uplifted apex and shelflike high left border, with the atrial appendages above the shelf. The clinical findings depend on the intracardiac abnormalities.

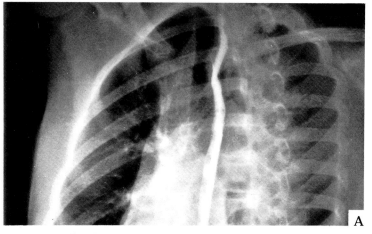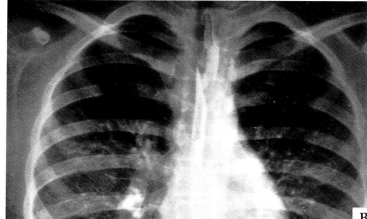

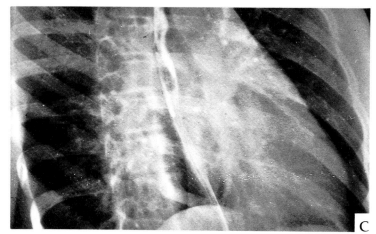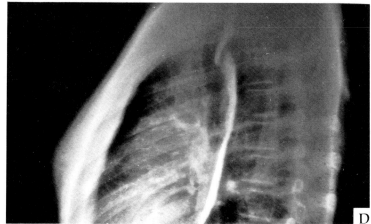

FIG. 5.26 Barium esophagraphy reveals anomalous right subclavian artery of distal origin. Note the shadow where the artery crosses behind the barium-filled esophagus as it slants upward to the right shoulder. In the drawings below, the arrows course through the indentations and indicate the path of the subclavian artery. **A**, Left anterior oblique view; **B**, frontal view; **C**, right anterior oblique view; **D**, left lateral view.

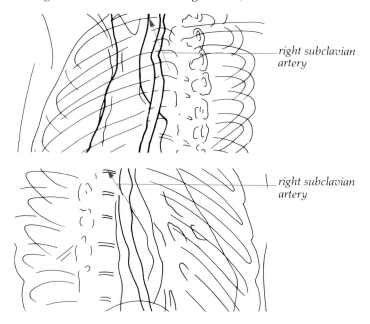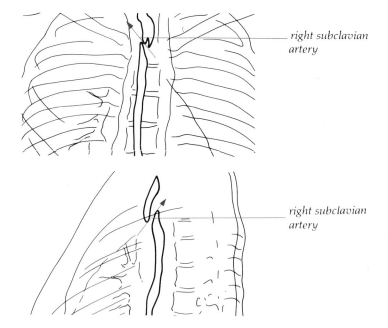

Radiographic Anomalies of the Great Vessels

Some relatively common arrangements of the arch vessels are easily diagnosed radiographically; these may or may not be clinically significant. Anomalous right subclavian artery (of distal origin from the arch) occurs with left aortic arch and is not uncommon. This is, in fact, a common finding in Down syndrome. Barium esophagraphy demonstrates an indentation which slants upward toward the right as the vessel courses up toward the right shoulder (Fig. 5.26).

Anomalous left subclavian artery is associated with a right aortic arch and gives, on barium esophagraphy, the mirror image appearance of the anomalous right subclavian as it courses toward the left shoulder (Fig. 5.27). It is not uncommon to find a left ductus arteriosus; and if it originates from the descending aorta, it will form a vascular ring composed of

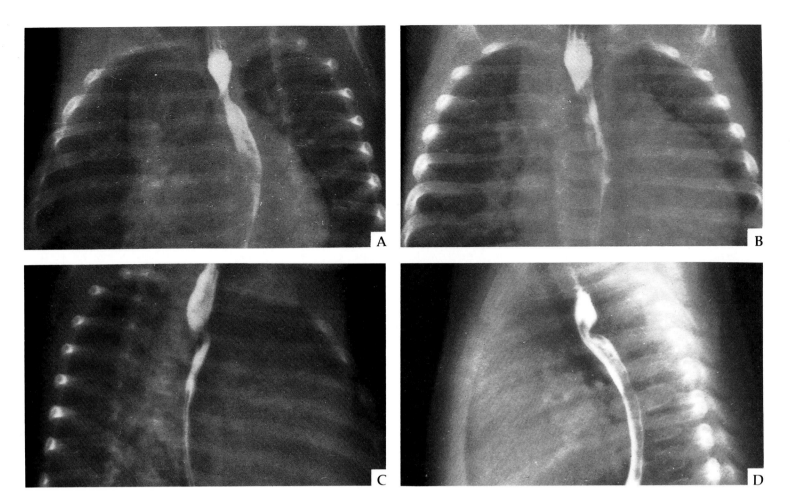

FIG. 5.27 Barium esophagraphy reveals anomalous left sub-clavian artery of distal origin. Note the mirror image of the shadow where the artery crosses behind the esophagus when compared to the shadow in Fig. 5.26. Again, the arrows represent the path of the artery.

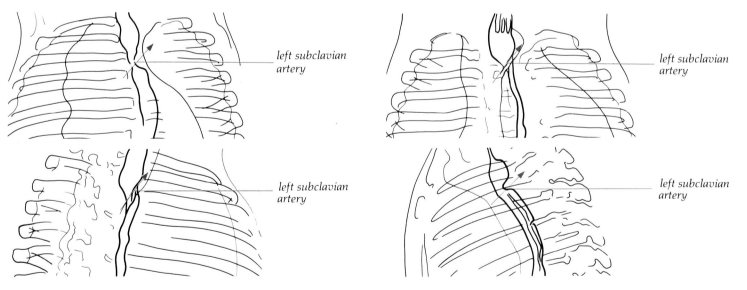

the aorta, the ductus, and the main pulmonary artery. Fortunately, many of these rings are not tight enough to cause symptoms of stridor and respiratory distress.

Coarctation of the aorta is usually found at the junction of the aortic isthmus and the descending aorta, and may be encountered at any age. It may be difficult to visualize radiographically in the young infant, especially when coarctation occurs with intracardiac defects. Congestive heart failure as well as stronger pulses and higher blood pressure in the upper extremities than in the lower usually lead to cardiac catheterization and diagnosis. However, when there is a patent ductus arteriosus and pulmonary hypertension, the pulse differential may not be found. If the pulmonary artery pressure is higher than that in the descending aorta, differential cyanosis (pink in the upper body, cyanotic in lower) should be seen.

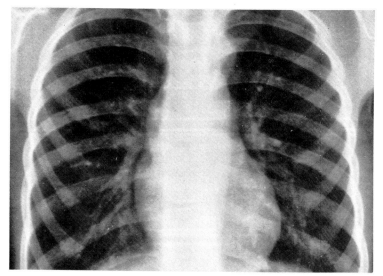

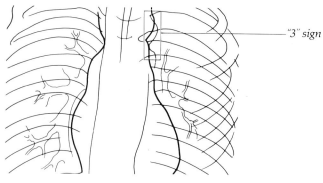

FIG. 5.28 Radiograph of a 5-year-old child reveals the characteristic signs of coarctation of the aorta. The site of stenosis can be observed at the center of the "3" sign with pre- and poststenotic dilatation of the aorta.

"3" sign

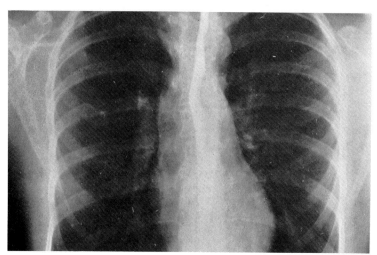

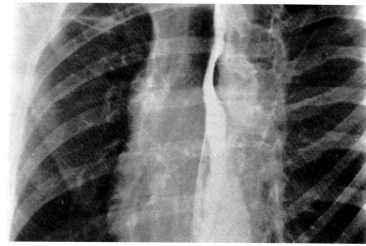

FIG. 5.29 Frontal (left) and left anterior oblique (right) barium esophagrams reveal indentations on the esophagus, indicative of coarctation of the aorta.

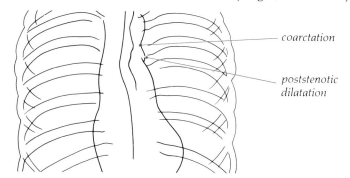

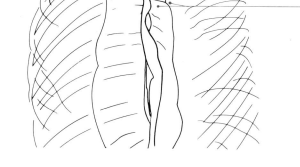

coarctation

poststenotic dilatation

coarctation

FIG. 5.30 Rib notching can be observed here, resulting from coarctation of the aorta in the older child.

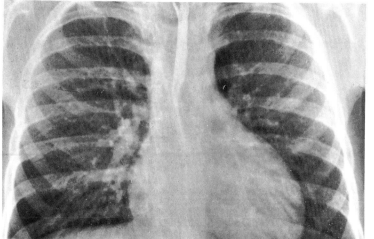

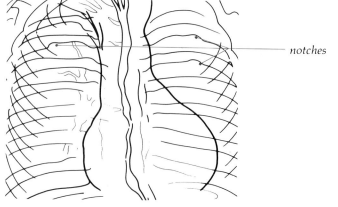

notches

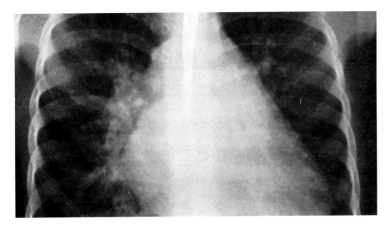

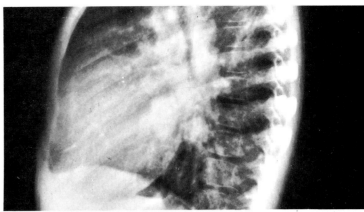

FIG. 5.31 *Frontal (left) and lateral (right) radiographic views demonstrate azygos vein continuation of the inferior vena cava*

to the superior vena cava. Note on the lateral view that there is no inferior vena cava shadow, as would be expected.

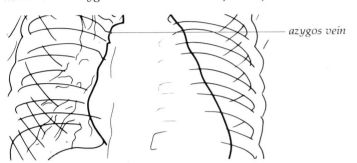

— azygos vein

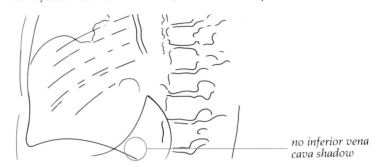

no inferior vena cava shadow

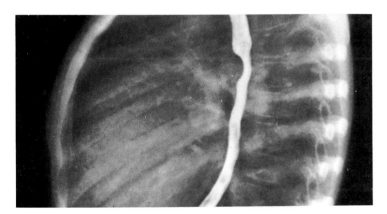

FIG. 5.32 *Anomalous left pulmonary artery (the pulmonary artery sling) can be observed as a rounded shadow between the barium-filled esophagus posteriorly and air-filled trachea anteriorly.*

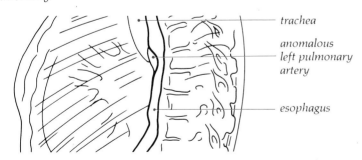

— trachea

anomalous left pulmonary artery

— esophagus

In the older child with a small thymus, examination of the plain X-ray reveals a "3" sign just below the aortic knob (Fig. 5.28). This can also be well demonstrated in some children by barium esophagraphy on the frontal and left anterior oblique projections (Fig. 5.29). On these views, the indentations on the esophagus are the mirror image of the aorta and represent coarctation and poststenotic dilatation. Rib notching is rarely seen before 6 years of age (Fig. 5.30). A long systolic murmur

from the collateral vessels should be heard in the axilla and over the back along the intercostal spaces.

Radiographic Anomalies of the Systemic Veins

In the absence of the hepatic segment of the inferior vena cava, there is loss of continuity between the inferior vena cava and the right atrium. The systemic venous blood returns from the lower part of the body by way of the azygos vein which drains behind the heart to the superior vena cava. Enlargement of the azygos vein as it arches toward the superior vena cava produces, radiographically, a rounded shadow adjacent to the upper mediastinum (Fig. 5.31). This finding is most often associated with an atrioventricular defect and, sometimes, polysplenia. In dextrocardia, the inferior vena cava may join the hemiazygos system and empty into a left superior vena cava. This gives a similar rounded shadow, but on the left side.

Radiographic Anomalies of the Pulmonary Arteries

Anomalous left pulmonary artery is often associated with respiratory problems early in life, especially atelectasis of the right middle or right lower lobe. Auscultation may reveal respiratory problems only. The left pulmonary artery originates from the right pulmonary artery and arches above the right mainstem bronchus. It then passes between the trachea and esophagus, coursing to the left lung. If there is obstruction of the vessel as it passes between these two structures, a systolic or even a continuous murmur may be heard. Lateral radiographs and, more so, barium esophagraphy will confirm the diagnosis by demonstrating the abnormal position of the pulmonary artery between the trachea and the esophagus (Fig. 5.32).

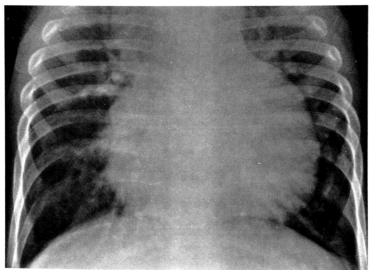

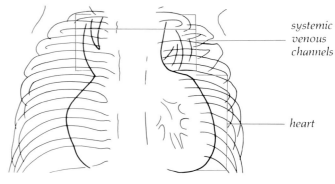

FIG. 5.33 The "snowman" shadow seen here is formed by the enlarged left superior vena cava, the innominate vein, and right superior vena cava.

systemic venous channels

heart

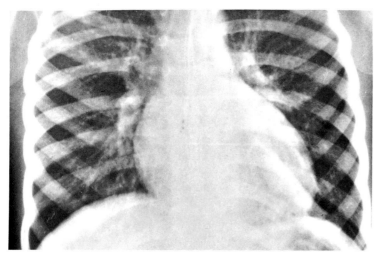

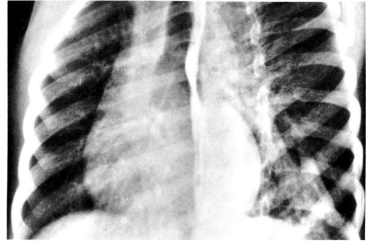

FIG. 5.34 Frontal (left) and left anterior oblique (right) views demonstrate large pulmonary veins bringing increased

pulmonary venous blood to the left atrium from the sequestered segment in the left lower lobe.

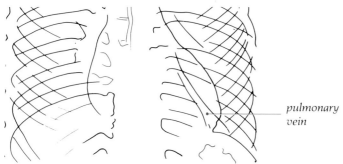

pulmonary vein

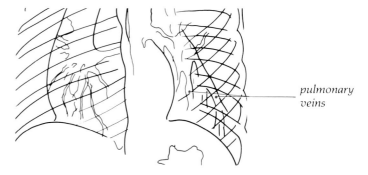

pulmonary veins

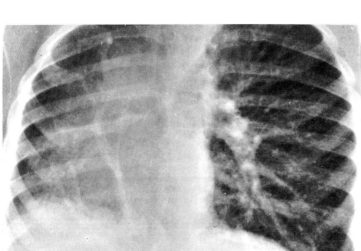

FIG. 5.35 Radiographic appearance of scimitar syndrome with a hypoplastic right lung. The scimitar-shaped shadow is formed by pulmonary veins draining the sequestered segment and connecting to the inferior vena cava. Note also the systemic artery coursing diagonally upward from the abdominal aorta to the sequestered lobe.

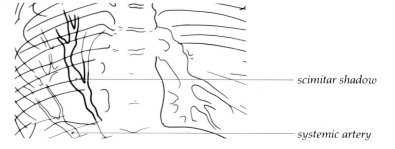

scimitar shadow

systemic artery

Radiographic Anomalies of the Pulmonary Veins

The abnormal connection of the common pulmonary vein to a systemic vein may be observed radiographically. Most commonly seen is anomalous pulmonary venous return to the left superior vena cava, producing a "snowman" appearance. This may not show up well in the very small infant, but as the systemic venous channels enlarge, a typical picture develops (Fig. 5.33). The heart is large, with increased pulmonary vascular markings. The electrocardiogram shows right ventricular hypertrophy. The older child's electrocardiogram may demonstrate a right bundle branch block. The findings of this anomaly resemble those of a large atrial septal defect. On examination there is a right ventricular thrust along the left sternal border, as well as a systolic murmur along the left sternal border which is transmitted over the pulmonary arteries, especially to the left axilla and back. In addition, there may be an associated diastolic tricuspid valve flow murmur. If there is stenosis in the anomalous connection, a high-pitched, continuous murmur may be heard over that site.

With sequestration of the lung, pulmonary venous return is usually to the left atrium. This is best observed on frontal and oblique views (Fig. 5.34). The physical findings may be essentially normal unless there is stenosis of the systemic collateral vessel. When this is the case, a continuous murmur will be heard in the axilla or posteriorly at the base of the lung.

Sometimes, in association with a sequestered lobe, pulmonary veins may connect with a systemic vessel. This occurs in scimitar syndrome, where the pulmonary veins form the configuration of a scimitar (Turkish sword) as they course down to the inferior vena cava, and hypoplasia of the right lung usually occurs (Fig. 5.35). Treatment may be unnecessary; however, if the lung is supplied by a systemic artery, the child may receive a large flow to the lung at high pressure, causing respiratory distress. Early intervention is then required.

BIBLIOGRAPHY

Markovitz M, Gordis L: Rheumatic Fever, 2nd ed. Volume II in Schaffer AJ (ed.) Major Problems in Clinical Pediatrics. Saunders, Philadelphia, 1972, pp. 61–79.

Nora JJ: Etiologic aspects of congenital heart disease. In Moss AJ, Adams FH, Emmanouilides GC (eds.) Heart Disease in Infants, Children and Adolescents, 2nd ed. Williams & Wilkins, Baltimore, 1978, pp. 3–11.

Park SC, Mathews RA, Zuberbuhler JR et al: Down syndrome with congenital heart malformation. Am J Dis Child 131: 29–33, 1977.

Tonkin IL, Kelley MJ, Bream PR, Elliott LP: The frontal chest film as a method of suspecting transposition complexes. Circulation 53: 1016–1025, 1976.

Zuberbuhler JR: Clinical Diagnosis in Pediatric Cardiology. Churchill-Livingstone, Edinburgh, 1981.

CHILD ABUSE AND NEGLECT

Holly W. Davis, M.D.

Child abuse and neglect constitute a pediatric public health problem of enormous magnitude. Their relative contribution to morbidity and mortality is especially prominent in developed nations where sanitation, immunization, and high standards of medical care have substantially reduced the sequelae of infectious diseases.

Although, within the last century, the incidence of abuse and neglect appears to have increased, stepped up and improved reporting must also be considered. The attention first brought to the problem by Caffey in the late 1940s and then continued through the efforts of Kempe and coworkers in the early 1960s fostered a marked increase in the recognition of the real needs and problems of child abuse. Subsequent passage of legislation mandating reports of suspected cases has further improved the rate and accuracy of reporting. Thus, while some of the increasing incidence is real, much is probably due to these developments. Additionally, societal standards have changed, for much of what is presently regarded as abuse was once sanctioned as discipline.

Statistics for the United States in 1982 (courtesy of the American Humane Society) underline the extent of the problem: 929,310 reports (substantiated and unsubstantiated) were filed involving 1.4 million children. Only 24 states report deaths resulting from abuse so statistics on mortality are incomplete, but those states recorded a total of 484 deaths. These figures are thought to significantly underestimate actual numbers, for in 1981 the National Incidence Study in collaboration with the National Center for Child Abuse and Neglect and the American Humane Association found that for every case reported at least two went unreported.

Four major forms of abuse have been delineated: active physical abuse, sexual abuse, physical neglect, and emotional abuse. Not infrequently an individual child is found to be the victim of more than one form. For purposes of reporting under abuse laws, the abuse or neglect generally must result from the acts or omissions of a parent, guardian, or custodian of the child. In addition to recognition of pertinent physical findings, the diagnosis of abuse is facilitated by an appreciation of its epidemiology and of certain risk factors.

EPIDEMIOLOGY

The incidence of child abuse, per capita, is greatest in lower socioeconomic groups, probably due in part to chronic stress and problems of socialization. Nevertheless, abuse is a phenomenon found in all socioeconomic, cultural, racial, and religious subsets of society.

Parental Risk Factors
1. Past history of being an abused child
2. Poor socialization and lack of trust in others—such people have difficulty with relationships and are thus poorly able to develop and utilize support systems
3. Limited ability to cope with stress, anger, and frustration
4. Alcoholism, addiction, or psychosis
5. Occupation in the military—frequent moves hinder development of support systems, and occupational interest may predispose to violence

Child Risk Factors
1. Age less than 3 years—young children are unable to escape attack, are incapable developmentally of meeting many expectations, and frequently are negativistic and stubborn
2. Infants separated from their mothers at birth because of illness or prematurity (perhaps due in part to impaired bonding)
3. Infants born with congenital anomalies, and children with chronic illness (possibly due to parental grieving and guilt compounded by the chronic stress of caring for a handicapped child)
4. Adopted children

A common thread underlying all of these risk factors appears to be unmet expectations: either unrealistic parental expectations of the child or the child's inability to meet realistic expectations. With the preceding as background, the approach to diagnosis of the major forms of abuse can now be addressed more specifically.

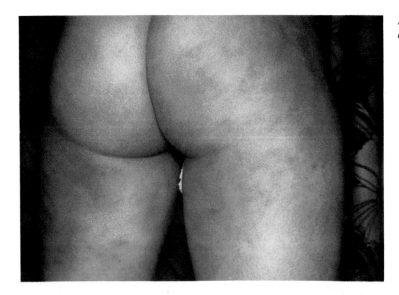

Fig. 6.1 Extensive contusions, inflicted with a belt, can be observed over the buttocks and thighs.

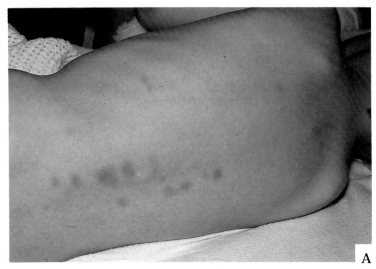

A

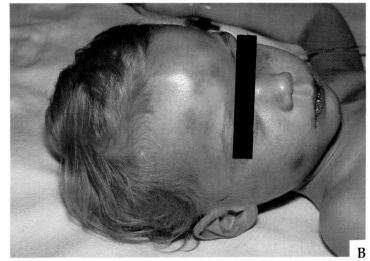

B

*Fig. 6.2 **A** Multiple ecchymoses are evident over the back and upper chest of this child who presented poorly nourished but with normal coagulation studies. **B** The same patient with multiple bruises of the face and forehead.*

ACTIVE PHYSICAL ABUSE

In cases of physical abuse, diagnosis is based on a constellation of factors including historical, physical, and behavioral observations. Radiographs and laboratory studies are often useful in confirming injuries and in ruling out other differential diagnostic possibilities.

Historical Factors
In many instances, one or more of the following historical red flags provides the first clue to the possibility of abuse.
1. The history is incompatible with the type or degree of injury; e.g., the distribution of lesions or type of injury doesn't fit the story, or the history suggests a minor injury but major trauma is found.
2. The history of how the injury occurred is vague, or the parent has no idea of how it happened.
3. The history changes each time it is told to a different health care worker.
4. The parents, when interviewed separately, give contradictory histories.
5. The history is impossible. The child may be said to have done something developmentally impossible; e.g., having climbed and fallen when yet unable to sit.

Behavioral Factors
1. There is often a significant delay between the time of injury and the time medical care is sought.
2. The parent may not show the degree of concern appropriate to the severity of the child's injury.
3. A pathologic parent-child interaction. Here unrealistic expectations, inappropriate demands, or angry impulsive behavior are expressed by the parent to the child. Such parents are often unaware of their child's needs and insensitive to behavioral cues.

Miscellaneous Observational Red Flags
1. Repeated visits for accidents or injuries
2. Repeated fractures
3. Repeated ingestions

Whenever one's index of suspicion is aroused by historical or observational findings, the physician should seek more detailed information concerning the family's current living situation, stresses, and emotional support systems. This and the history in general should be obtained in a supportive, nonjudgmental manner, as interrogation will only serve to alienate the parent, limiting the value of the data obtained. It is helpful to bear in mind that many of these parents truly want help for the child and want to stop abusing him. They

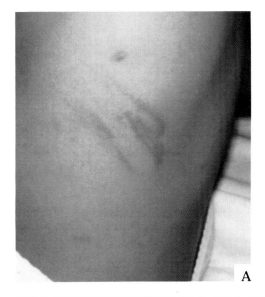

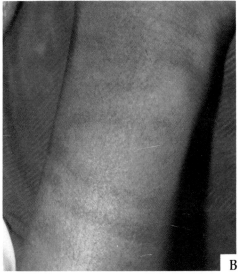

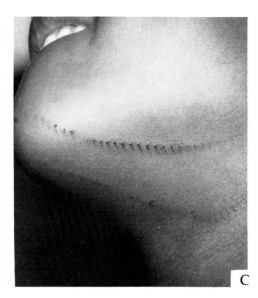

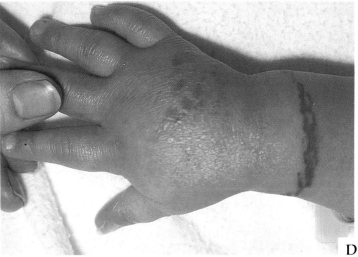

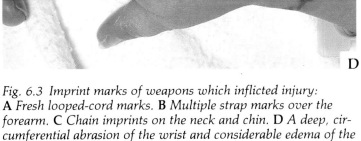

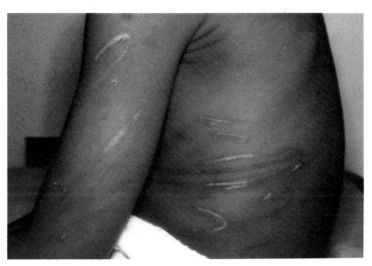

Fig. 6.3 Imprint marks of weapons which inflicted injury:
A Fresh looped-cord marks. **B** Multiple strap marks over the
forearm. **C** Chain imprints on the neck and chin. **D** A deep, circumferential abrasion of the wrist and considerable edema of the
hand are seen as a result of restraint with a rope.

Fig. 6.4 Multiple scars produced by a prior whipping with a
looped cord are seen in this patient.

typically feel very alone, guilt-ridden, and inadequate as persons and parents, and their own abusive behavior often
evokes painful memories of having been abused themselves.

In approaching the child, one must recognize that his parents are the only ones he knows, that he loves them, and may
feel in some way deserving of abuse. Young children rarely
acknowledge that a parent has injured them, especially when
questioned directly, and may have been sworn to secrecy. If
they can be interviewed alone (when old enough to give a history) in pleasant nonthreatening surroundings, helpful historical information can often be obtained via indirect questions.

Physical Findings and Patterns of Injury

SURFACE MARKS: BRUISES, WELTS, AND SCARS
Inflicted injuries are often found in locations such as the back,
buttocks, upper arms, chest, and face (Figs. 6.1 and 6.2). This
is in contrast to the "usual" small bruises found on the shins,
extensor surfaces of the forearms, and the forehead of a normally active child. In order to avoid errors in diagnosis, children presenting with multiple bruises in unusual locations
should be thoroughly examined for evidence of an underlying

coagulopathy, and screening coagulation studies should be
performed before arriving at a final diagnosis.

In many instances the surface marks are recognizable imprints of the weapon used to inflict injury. Those most commonly seen include looped-cord marks; belt, buckle, or
switch marks; finger, thumb, and hand prints; or strangulation and restraint marks (Fig. 6.3).

Resolution time of a bruise depends on the degree of force
used to produce it and varies widely. It is therefore impossible
to determine accurately the ages of ecchymotic lesions other
than to say that they are fresh or old. However, the presence
of old scars reflecting prior use of a weapon in a child with
acute injuries can be helpful in identifying abuse or confirming prior abuse (Fig. 6.4). All external signs of trauma
should be carefully documented both in writing and by
photography.

BURNS
While generally accidental, burns are a fairly common mode
of abusive injury. Here too, inconsistency of history, the pattern of injury, and delay in seeking medical attention are
valuable clues.

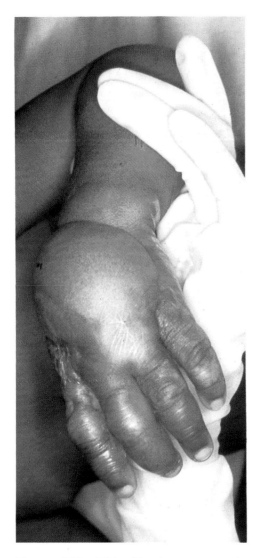

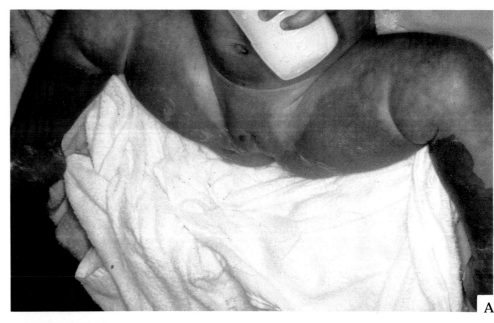

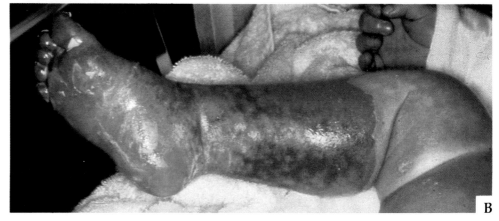

Fig. 6.5 This child suffered severe second-degree dip burns of both hands and wrists. (Courtesy of Dr. Thomas Layton, Mercy Hospital, Pittsburgh)

Fig. 6.6 **A** Patient seen 2 days after receiving dip burns to the lower extremities and perineum. **B** Close-up of

severe second-degree burn of the foot and lower leg. (Courtesy of Dr. Thomas Layton, Mercy Hospital, Pittsburgh)

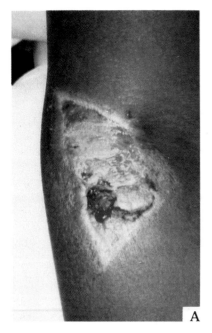

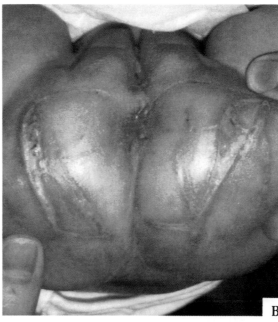

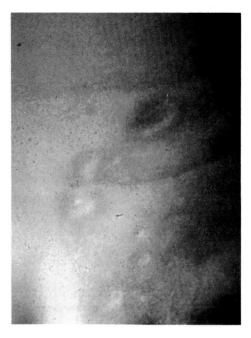

Fig. 6.7 **A** The pattern of this full-thickness burn to the arm reflects that a hot iron was used on this patient. **B** This

infant received multiple, linear, full-thickness burns when she was forced to sit on the hot grill of a space heater.

Fig. 6.8 These full-thickness punched-out scars resulted from cigarette burns. (Courtesy of Dr. Marc Rowe, Children's Hospital of Pittsburgh)

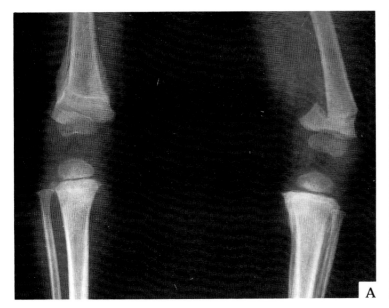
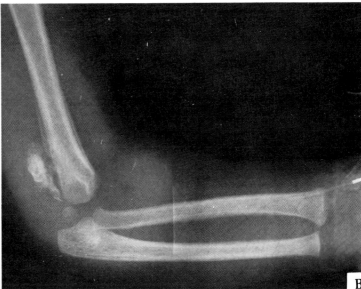

Fig. 6.9 **A** This young child presented with multiple fractures of the lower extremities. Radiographic examination reveals a non-displaced healing fracture of the right distal femur, with subperiosteal new bone formation. The left distal femur has a fresh displaced fracture, and the proximal left tibia is also rimmed with periosteal new bone. **B** This same child was also found to have an old fracture of the distal humerus, with vigorous callus formation and soft-tissue swelling. (Courtesy of the Dept. of Radiology, Children's Hospital of Pittsburgh)

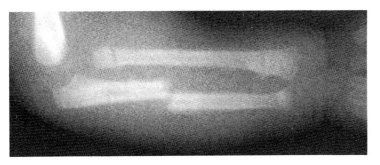

Fig. 6.10 This radiograph reveals a healing transverse fracture of the distal radius, a recent fracture of the proximal radius, and a fresh fracture of the midulna in the right forearm of an abused infant. (Courtesy of the Dept. of Radiology, Children's Hospital of Pittsburgh)

Immersion scalds are among the more commonly seen forms of inflicted burns. Typical patterns include symmetrical burns of both hands (Fig. 6.5), of both feet, or of the lower legs and perineum (Fig. 6.6), produced by dipping the infant or child in scalding water. Despite claims to the contrary, such burns are rarely accidental.

Other types of burns may reflect the instrument used to inflict them. For example, one may see the imprint of a hot iron or of the grill of a heater used to inflict full-thickness burns (Fig. 6.7). No child with normal sensation would remain in contact with these objects long enough to incur such a severe burn. Cigarettes produce a sharply circumscribed full-thickness burn, approximately 5 mm in diameter. When seen acutely this burn will have a black central eschar, and on healing will leave a deep punched-out scar (Fig. 6.8). This presentation is in contrast to some impetiginous lesions which may appear to have a thick brown eschar. When the latter eschar is lifted off, the lesion will be found to be very superficial.

SKELETAL INJURIES

The finding of multiple unexplained fractures of varying ages involving the long bones and ribs of an infant or young child is a paradigm of child abuse (Figs. 6.9 to 6.11). The degree of

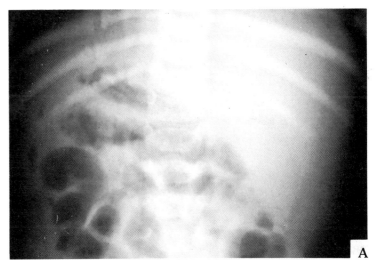
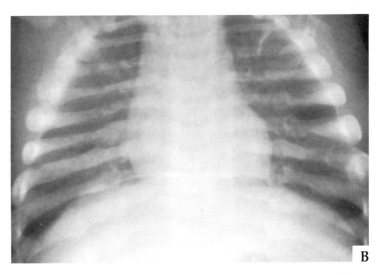

Fig. 6.11 Rib fractures. **A** This abdominal film of an infant who presented with symptoms of colic reveals a normal bowel gas pattern and multiple rib fractures in various stages of healing. **B** Chest radiograph of this same infant taken 2 months later demonstrates in excess of 20 healing rib fractures. (Courtesy of the Dept. of Radiology, Children's Hospital of Pittsburgh)

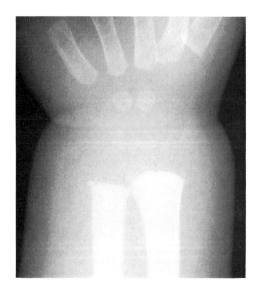

Fig. 6.12 These metaphyseal chip fractures of the distal radius and ulna were produced by vigorous shaking. (Courtesy of the Dept. of Radiology, Children's Hospital of Pittsburgh)

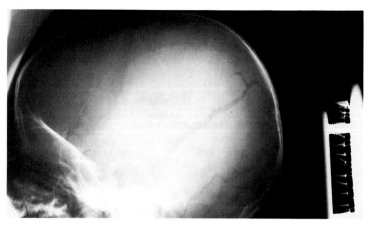

Fig. 6.13 A large, temporoparietal linear skull fracture can be seen radiographically in this abused child. (Courtesy of the Dept. of Radiology, Children's Hospital of Pittsburgh)

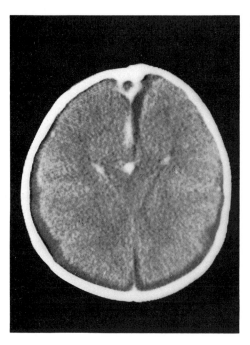

Fig. 6.14 CT scan reveals a subdural hematoma, caused by trauma to this infant. This is seen as a dark rim between the bony calvarium and the brain substance. (Courtesy of the Division of Neuroradiology, University Health Center of Pittsburgh)

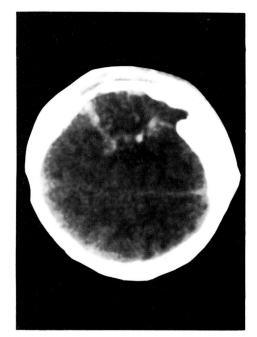

Fig. 6.15 CT scan demonstrates a skull fracture and an underlying cerebral contusion. Note the subgaleal hematoma, bony discontinuity, and cortical contrast enhancement. (Courtesy of the Division of Neuro-radiology, University Health Center of Pittsburgh)

callus formation and the extent of subperiosteal new bone and remodeling help in determining fracture age. Often the child is brought in for a single injury or for a totally unrelated complaint such as a rash or cold.

Another common constellation is the "shaken baby" syndrome, which consists of subdural hematoma, without evidence of skull fracture, in association with multiple chip fractures of the metaphyses of long bones (Fig. 6.12). These injuries result from shearing forces generated by repetitive vigorous shaking while the child is held by the hands or feet.

While the above patterns are pathognomonic of inflicted injury, other pictures are probably more common, especially if abuse is detected before multiple episodes occur. Long-bone fractures, particularly those involving the humerus or femur, and rib fractures are highly suspect in infants, especially when there is no reasonable explanation.

The frequency of skeletal injury necessitates that examination of the suspected abuse victim include careful palpation of *all* bones for evidence of tenderness, crepitus, or callus formation. Because of the greater probability of multiple occult fractures in the infant and toddler, a skeletal survey is advisable in suspected cases where the child is less than 2 years of age. In older children, careful physical examination should reveal areas requiring radiographic evaluation.

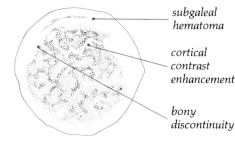

subgaleal hematoma

cortical contrast enhancement

bony discontinuity

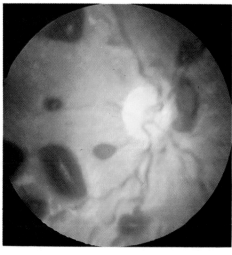

Fig. 6.16 Multiple retinal hemorrhages are seen on funduscopic examination of this infant who was a victim of the "shaken baby syndrome." Subdural hematoma and multiple metaphyseal "shake" fractures are typical associated findings. (Courtesy of Dr. Stephen Ludwig, Children's Hospital of Philadelphia)

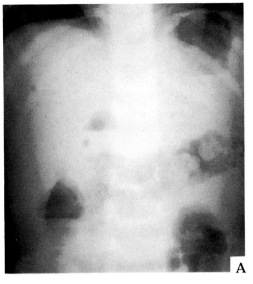
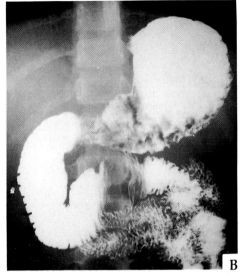
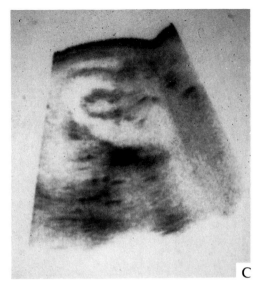

A **B** **C**

Fig. 6.17 Duodenal hematoma. **A** *Abdominal film reveals an air-fluid level in the dilated duodenal loop proximal to the duodenal hematoma.* **B** *This upper GI series shows narrowing of duodenal lumen and widening of duodenal wall at the site of hematoma. Obstruction is partial, as some barium has passed through the* *narrowed segment.* **C** *Ultrasonography demonstrates distention of the duodenal wall by the hematoma. (**A** and **B** courtesy of the Dept. of Radiology, Children's Hospital of Pittsburgh; **C** courtesy of Dr. Marc Rowe, Children's Hospital of Pittsburgh)*

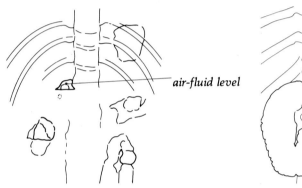

air-fluid level

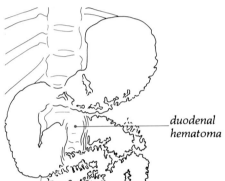

duodenal hematoma

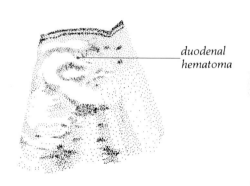

duodenal hematoma

CNS INJURIES

Both the head and the central nervous system are frequent sites of pathology resulting from child abuse. This is especially so for infants. Injuries range from surface hematomas and linear fractures (Fig. 6.13) to subdural hematomas (Fig. 6.14) and cerebral contusions (Fig. 6.15). Blunt trauma is the major mode of injury, although, as noted earlier, shaking can cause tearing of the bridging veins and produce a subdural hematoma in the absence of a fracture or any external sign of trauma.

Given the wide range of severity of injury, there are many possible modes of presentation. Patients seen acutely may present with irritability, vomiting, altered state of consciousness, seizures, or sudden onset of shock (the latter is seen in the infant with massive subgaleal and/or intracranial hemorrhage). Infants with chronic subdural hematomas may present with rapidly increasing head circumference, split sutures and a full fontanelle, or with recurrent vomiting and failure to thrive. Diagnosis is further complicated by the fact that, in the absence of external signs of injury, the possibility of trauma is often denied. Careful external, general, neurologic, and funduscopic examinations are therefore warranted. The latter is often quite helpful in revealing retinal hemorrhages in patients seen soon after injury (Fig. 6.16). Neurologic examination may reveal altered level of consciousness, signs of increased intracranial pressure, alterations in tone, or, on occasion, focal abnormalities. Routine skull radiographs may also

be helpful, but CT scans are generally more useful for delineating the nature and extent of the trauma.

INTRA-ABDOMINAL INJURIES

While less common than surface and skeletal trauma, abdominal injuries may be observed and can be quite severe. Typically, the injury is due to blunt trauma resulting from being hit or thrown. External evidence is often minimal or absent, and trauma is frequently not reported. The major types of pathology are duodenal hematomas, small intestinal and/or mesenteric tears, and lacerations of the liver or spleen. Patients with duodenal hematoma typically present with signs of intestinal obstruction (e.g., vomiting and abdominal pain). Plain radiographs may reveal an air-fluid level in a dilated duodenal loop proximal to the hematoma, while an upper GI series and sonar studies reveal narrowing of the lumen and thickening of the duodenal wall (Fig. 6.17). Children with small intestinal or mesenteric tears generally complain of diffuse abdominal pain and have signs of diffuse tenderness, distention, and peritoneal irritation. Splenic and hepatic lacerations may present similarly or may produce severe shock which is often unexplained by history.

In most instances of inflicted abdominal trauma, abuse is not confirmed until special radiographic studies including sonar and CT scan have been obtained or surgery has been performed.

CHILD ABUSE AND NEGLECT

MOST COMMON SUBSTITUTE COMPLAINTS IN SEXUAL ABUSE CASES

Any Age	Preschool Age	School Age	Adolescence
Abdominal pain	Excessive clinging	Decreased school performance	Same as school age
Anorexia	Thumbsucking	Truancy	plus
Vomiting	Speech disorder	Lying, stealing	Runaway behavior
Constipation	Encopresis/enuresis	Tics	Suicide attempts
Sleep disorders	Excessive masturbation	Anxiety reaction	Sexual offenses
Dysuria		Phobic and obsessional states	
Vaginal discharge		Depression	
Vaginal bleeding		Conversion reaction	
Rectal bleeding		Encopresis/enuresis	

Fig. 6.18 Most common substitute complaints in sexual abuse cases.

SEXUAL ABUSE

Of all the forms of abuse, sexual abuse is probably the most underreported, yet may be the most prevalent. As a result, incidence and prevalence statistics are speculative at best. Estimates of incidence range as high as 360,000 cases per year. Prevalence studies suggest that as many as 20 to 30 percent of all women will have experienced at least one episode of sexual abuse by age 18. While females are most frequently the victims, males are by no means immune to the problem.

Sexual abuse may involve visual exposure to exhibitionistic or masturbatory behavior; fondling, masturbation, and digital manipulation; orogenital contact; and direct genital contact including penetration or attempted penetration of the vagina or anus. Studies of perpetrators suggest that between 30 and 37 percent are parents, parent surrogates, or close relatives; between 26 and 60 percent are known to the victim but are unrelated (neighbors, babysitters, nursery school or day care personnel); and between 11 and 37 percent are strangers. When the perpetrator is a family member or acquaintance, the encounter is generally nonviolent with persuasion, bribery, or threats used to cajole the victim. Not infrequently, these experiences are repetitive and occur over long periods of time. The victim is sworn to silence, bearing both the guilt of engaging in unwanted sexual activity and the pressure of keeping it a secret. Lack of violence or injury does not imply consent, as the offender is usually in a position of power over the victim, making it difficult for the child to refuse. Episodes involving strangers are more likely to be isolated incidents and frequently involve physical violence, adding the emotional stress of being in a potentially life-threatening situation.

Forensic requirements for a detailed history, physical examination, and multiple laboratory specimens (all carefully documented) necessitate a lengthy evaluation which, if not handled sensitively, can compound the existing emotional trauma. This can be minimized if the physician approaches the patient and family with patience, gentleness, and tact.

Because physical findings are often nonspecific or even normal in molestation and incest cases, the history is often the most important aspect of the evaluation. When possible the parent or parents should be interviewed first, separately from the child. During this interview, information about the child's emotional status, present and past history, family psycho-social situation, and terms used by the child for body parts can be obtained. When the chief complaint is not sexual abuse, but findings on examination point to molestation, a detailed psychosocial history should be obtained and parents should be questioned about persons caring for the child or in the home who might have unwitnessed access to the child.

In approaching the child one should convey an understanding that she or he may have been sworn to secrecy, but that the person who asked that has a serious problem and can't be helped to stop unless the child tells you just what has happened. Calmness, empathy, and gentleness in questioning are essential. If the child is willing and able to give a history, it should be documented verbatim. If she or he is unwilling to discuss the episode or episodes, it can be deferred to a later appointment or to a play therapy session with a psychiatrist or psychologist. It must be remembered that when young children do give detailed descriptions of sexual experiences they are not fantasizing, for they are not capable developmentally of imagining such activities.

A thorough and complete physical examination is warranted for all such patients, with examination of the genitalia and rectum deferred until last (see Chapter 16 for techniques of examination). Each part of the examination should be explained as the examiner proceeds. Where possible, and when desired by the child, a parent or supportive nurse should be present. If an attempt to examine the perineum provokes anxiety which cannot be allayed, this should be deferred. Where injuries or venereal disease are obvious or likely, the patient should be admitted and examined (and specimens obtained) under general anesthesia. If the patient is asymptomatic and there is no evidence of violence or trauma, the procedure can be postponed for a follow-up visit. Observance of these cautions is important so that the child does not feel she is being assaulted yet again.

Mode of Presentation

In cases of sexual assault involving violence and resulting in injury, the patient typically seeks medical care promptly, and directly acknowledges the true nature of the problem. Victims of incest or molestation, or their parents, may occasionally report sexual abuse as their chief concern, but more often do not. The majority present with substitute complaints gener-

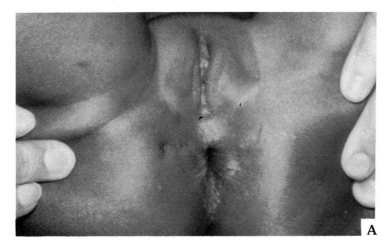

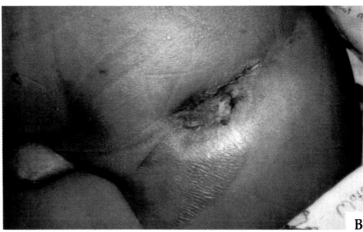

Fig. 6.19 Physical signs of sexual abuse. **A** Abrasions, contusions, and punctate tears of the perineum and perianal area can be observed in this prepubescent girl. **B** Severe perianal lacerations, contusions, and abrasions are apparent in this prepubescent boy subjected to sodomy.

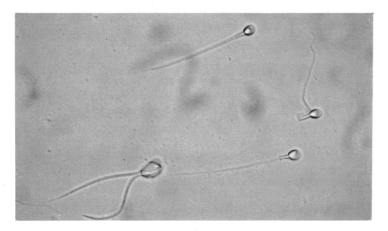

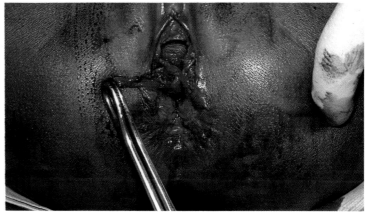

Fig. 6.20 This is the microscopic appearance of seminal fluid removed from a young rape victim. When a vaginal discharge is found in a patient presenting within 72 hours after sexual abuse, a wet mount may reveal sperm. A portion of the discharge should also be collected for acid phosphatase, blood grouping, and enzyme studies.

Fig. 6.21 Severe genital trauma in a prepubertal girl, resulting from forcible rape. Inspection reveals a hymenal tear at 6 o'clock extending posteriorly through the perineal body to the rectum. On examination under anesthesia, a 1-inch vaginal tear was discovered along with a rectal tear and complete disruption of the external anal sphincter. (Courtesy of Dr. Kamthorn Sukarochana, Children's Hospital of Pittsburgh)

ated by either physical or emotional sequelae, making diagnosis of the actual problem very difficult unless there are unequivocally positive physical findings. Such alternate complaints are myriad, somewhat age-dependent, and generally have a number of possible alternative causes (Fig. 6.18). While there may be a wide range of differential diagnostic possibilities in patients presenting with these problems, sexual abuse should be considered and addressed when other sources have been ruled out.

Physical Findings

Victims of sexual assault almost inevitably show evidence of physical and genital injury. Bruises and abrasions of the head, face, neck, chest, forearms, knees, and thighs are commonly present. Occasionally, even more severe nongenital injuries are encountered.

Genital and rectal examination may reveal contusions, erythema, abrasions, or lacerations (Fig. 6.19); at times, evidence of seminal products in the form of a vaginal discharge will be observed (Fig. 6.20). Seminal fluid has been reported to fluoresce under Wood's lamp, but in our tests we found only weak fluorescence when wet and none when dry. Under normal light, the seminal products are practically invisible after drying. When external contusions or tears are seen, internal injury must be suspected. The prepubescent child is particularly vulnerable to severe internal trauma as a result of forceful penetration of either the vagina or rectum (Fig. 6.21). This stems from the fact that the structures are relatively small, and the tissues more delicate and rigid. Young children with mild external injuries may in fact have major internal tears including perforation of the peritoneum and damage to pelvic vessels, mesentery, and intestine. Signs of internal pathology may be subtle, but such patients will have hymenal tears or vaginal bleeding and may have lower abdominal rebound tenderness or evidence of occult blood loss. Therefore, evidence of external injury generally necessitates examination under general anesthesia (EUA) in this population. The postpubescent female can usually be adequately assessed by careful pelvic examination, unless she is emotionally unable to tolerate the procedure, in which case an EUA would also be advisable. Rectal examination is necessary for assessment of internal tears, pelvic tenderness, sphincter tone, and for bimanual palpation (see Chapter 16).

GUIDELINES FOR SPECIMEN COLLECTION IN SEXUAL ABUSE EXAMINATION
(at Children's Hospital, Pittsburgh)

Orogenital Contact	Genital Contact		Anal Contact
	No Evidence of Penetration	Evidence Consistent with Vaginal Penetration	

1. Swabs: use two at a time‡
  a. For wet mount for sperm*
  b. For two air-dried slides*
  c. For GC culture
2. Baseline RPR (repeat in 4–6 weeks if initial test is negative)
	1. Urinalysis for occult blood
	2. Vaginal aspirate† (swabs may be used in postpubescent patients‡)
	  a. For wet mount for sperm, trichomonas, Gardnerella, and Candida
	  b. For two air-dried slides*
	  c. For GC and routine culture
	  d. For Gram stain if vaginal discharge present
	3. Baseline RPR (repeat in 4–6 weeks if initial test is negative)
		1. Urinalysis for occult blood
		2. If external tears seen:
		  a. Consult surgeon for possible EUA
		  b. If EUA done, collect specimens
		3. Vaginal aspirate† (swabs may be used in postpubescent patients‡)
		  a. For wet mount for sperm, trichomonas, Gardnerella, and Candida
		  b. For two air-dried slides*
		  c. For GC and routine cultures
		  d. For Gram stain if vaginal discharge present
		4. Baseline RPR (repeat in 4–6 weeks if initial test is negative)
			1. If external tears seen:
			  a. Consult general surgeon for possible EUA
			  b. If EUA done, collect specimens
			2. Swabs: use two at a time‡ (must be done before rectal examination)
			  a. For wet mount for sperm*
			  b. For two air-dried slides*
			  c. For GC and routine culture
			3. If no tears:
			  a. Rectal exam
			  b. Stool guaiac: if positive consult general surgeon
			4. Baseline RPR (repeat in 4–6 weeks if initial test is negative)

*Omit if seen > 72 hours after the last incident, except in patients with vaginal discharge.

†In prepubescent patients, vaginal specimens are best obtained by aspiration using a syringe attached to either a #3 French feeding tube or a soft 18- or 20-gauge intracatheter. If nothing is obtained on aspiration, a small amount of sterile nonbacteriostatic saline may be instilled and then aspirated back. Aspiration is less painful and less traumatic to prepubertal mucosa. In postpubescent patients, GC culture and Gram stain specimens should be obtained from the cervical os after cleaning the area with a dry swab. A cervical swab for chlamydia culture should also be considered when a cervical discharge is present.

‡Two of the swabs used to obtain specimens should be air-dried and placed in a sterile test tube for acid phosphatase, blood group, and enzyme studies. When specimens are obtained by vaginal aspirate, a small amount of aspirate should be applied to two swabs which should then be processed in the same manner.

Fig. 6.22 Guidelines for specimen collection in sexual abuse examination (at Children's Hospital of Pittsburgh).

In cases of molestation or incest, findings on examination are often totally normal. Other patients may have no symptoms yet have suggestive findings. In cases of previous or repeated intercourse, well-healed circumferential hymenal tears, rounded hymenal tags, or a healed laceration may be noted. The introitus may appear spacious or patulous in such patients as well as in children subjected to repeated digital penetration. Patients repetitively sodomized may have reflex relaxation of the anal sphincter on perineal stimulation. Forceful orogenital contact may result in perioral and intra-oral injuries. While such oral lesions are unusual, the patients may have asymptomatic gonococcal infections.

Many victims are identified upon presenting with vaginal discharge that is positive for a venereal pathogen, particularly gonorrhea (see Chapter 16). It is important to realize that while nonvenereal transmission of venereal pathogens lies within the realm of possibility, the vast majority of prepubescent children presenting with venereal disease (whether gonorrhea, trichomonas, venereal warts, or another form) have acquired their infection as a result of sexual abuse. Nonspecific vaginal discharges, especially when chronic or recurrent, are also suspect. All should be tested for the presence of sperm.

Laboratory Evaluation

Laboratory studies are designed to augment the physical assessment of injury, identify venereal pathogens, and docu-

ADDITIONAL SPECIMENS NEEDED IN RAPE CASES
(Seen within 72 hours)

Specimens may be obtained by the physician or nurse. All containers used in evidence collection should be paper and must be labeled with:

Patient's name	Body site	Initials of collector
Type of specimen	Date and time	

Clothing If the patient is wearing the same clothes, they should be collected along with debris, as this may provide valuable clues regarding the assailant. The patient should disrobe while standing on a towel or sheet. Each article including the towel or sheet should then be placed in a separate paper bag. Avoid shaking the articles. Each bag is then labeled and sealed.

Fingernail scrapings* These may provide bits of skin, fiber, and debris from the assailant. Scraping from beneath the nails or nail clippings should be obtained. Specimens from each hand should be collected over separate sheets of paper, and placed in separate paper envelopes, sealed, and labeled.

Hair samples* Any loose or suspected foreign hairs should be collected, placed in an envelope, and labeled. If patient is postpubescent, comb pubic hairs onto a sheet of clean paper, fold, place in an envelope with the comb, label, and seal. Then, gently pull a small clump of the patient's pubic hair (12 hairs are needed), place on clean paper, fold, put in envelope, and label "standard pubic hair." Then, comb and obtain head hairs in this same manner.

Blood sample 5 cc of blood should be drawn for blood grouping and enzyme typing, and placed in a purple top tube.

Saliva sample This enables testing of the patient's secretory status. The specimen should be obtained either by wiping the patient's oral mucosa with a gauze pad or by having the patient expectorate onto a gauze pad. The pad is then placed in an envelope, sealed, and labeled.

Destination of Specimens

The following specimens are handled by the hospital laboratories or performed in the ER:

Urinalysis	Gram stains	RPR
Wet preps	Stool guaiac	Cultures

All other specimens are to be signed over to police custody for transport to the crime laboratory.

Maintaining an Unbroken Chain of Evidence

Evidence should be packaged and labeled upon collection. All evidence should be kept together and must remain under the direct supervision of the physician, the nurse, or the security guard until signed over to the police. Receipt for release of evidence to police should be signed before evidence is given over to the police.

Omit if patient has already bathed and shampooed.

Fig. 6.23 Additional specimens needed in rape cases (seen within 72 hours).

ment the presence of seminal fluid (when appropriate). The sites of specimen collection and the studies performed depend in part on the history and the time interval between the last reported episode and the medical visit. The likelihood of finding evidence of seminal fluid is so small after 72 hours that these studies can be eliminated if the patient seeks attention 3 or more days after the last incident. Cultures should be obtained regardless of time of presentation or lack of symptoms, as infections may be asymptomatic.

Adolescents and prepubescent victims with possible internal injuries require pelvic examination, which in the latter case can be performed under anesthesia. If an exam under anesthesia is indicated, all required specimens beyond the urinalysis may be obtained at that time. The possibility of pregnancy must also be considered in the postmenarchal patient.

Figure 6.22 outlines our current protocol for specimen collection in sexual abuse patients. Figure 6.23 enumerates the additional specimens required by authorities in rape cases. Because the examination is for the purpose of gathering evidence in addition to assessing the patient's physical status, the procedures must be meticulous. The patient or parent must sign a consent form prior to collection of evidence. Each specimen for the crime lab should be packaged and labeled immediately after collection. All evidence should then be kept together, and must remain under the direct supervision of the physician or nurse who was present at collection until it is handed over to the authorities. Finally, police should sign a receipt for release of evidence upon accepting the specimens.

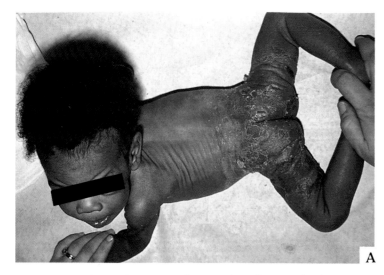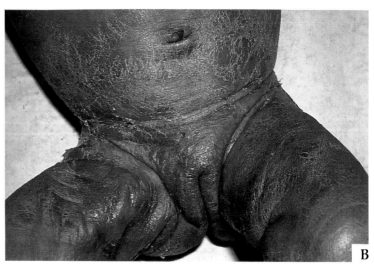

Fig. 6.24 Findings of severe neglect: **A** Note decreased subcutaneous tissue, particularly over the thighs and buttocks, but also over the thorax and upper arm. The patient also manifests a serious worried expression and severe diaper rash. **B** Close-up view reveals the grossly neglected chronic nature of the diaper rash. (Courtesy of Dr. Michael Sherlock)

PASSIVE ABUSE OR NEGLECT

This type of abuse is by far the most commonly reported, accounting for over 50 percent of cases each year. In its mildest form, this may be seen as a lack of vigilance and safeguarding of the young child who is thereby at greater risk for accidents and ingestions. In its more severe form, the patient presents with failure to thrive and developmental delay as a result of inadequate or ineffective nurturing. Typically, in infancy, the patient has been fed irregularly and inadequately, given little interactional attention, and received minimal basic care. In some cases it appears that the infant may have picked up on maternal anxiety and depression and developed secondary anorexia and autonomic disturbances of intestinal motility. Some of these infants actually begin to resist contact and become difficult to feed.

Risk factors are similar to those seen in cases of active physical abuse, with a few additions. More of these infants were unwanted, and often little or no prenatal care was sought during pregnancy. Mothers of such infants are more likely to be frankly depressed or mentally dull and to have difficulty caring for the children they already have. There may be significant historical clues or red flags as well. Frequently, the parent appears relatively unconcerned about the child's failure to thrive, having brought the child for a minor unrelated problem such as a cold or rash, or for vomiting or constipation. Some present with a history of colic, crying "all the time," or a feeding problem. There are often glaring inconsistencies in the feeding history (e.g., "he takes 6 ounces every 4 hours" and "he takes 16 ounces in 24 hours"). A high percentage of these infants have received little or no professional well-child care and are behind on their immunizations.

On examination, the child is usually found to be significantly undergrown. Weight may be below the 3rd percentile, or there may be evidence of plateauing of weight gain. In long-standing cases, height and head circumference are abnormally low as well. Comparison with birth parameters and measurements made at prior visits (if any) reveal that the child has "fallen off his curve." The more severe case presents with decreased subcutaneous tissue (most notable over the buttocks and thighs), a pinched face, and sunken prominent eyes (Fig. 6.24). The child tends to look serious, smiling infrequently and often appearing watchful. Vocalization is sparse, and development is delayed and uneven. Many of these infants appear withdrawn and resist cuddling. We have even seen some who have had abnormal tone, scissoring, and posturing suggestive of a neurologic problem, which promptly abated within a few days of hospitalization. Poor hygiene, dirty clothes, and badly neglected diaper rashes are common additional findings suggestive of neglect (Fig. 6.24B).

The easiest, least traumatic way to confirm the diagnosis of psychosocial failure to thrive is to remove the infant from his home environment and observe his growth in a nurturing situation. Milder cases will gain weight promptly, while marasmic infants may take 1 to 2 weeks before resuming growth.

It is important to remember that psychosocial failure to thrive is the most common form of growth failure in infancy, accounting for over 50 percent of cases. Therefore, in evaluating the infant with failure to thrive, obtaining a thorough psychosocial and family history is as important as a detailed medical history. The latter should include information regarding duration of the problem, mode of onset, and pattern of growth. A complete review of systems — gastrointestinal, cardiorespiratory, neurologic, genitourinary, and endocrine — emphasizing intake and output is often helpful. A thorough general physical examination will reveal gross abnormalities in patients with underlying CNS, cardiopulmonary, and genetic problems. A few basic screening tests (CBC and differential; urinalysis and culture; sedimentation rate; stool pH, reducing substance, and fat stain; and urea nitrogen, electrolytes, and creatinine) will rule out most other organic causes of failure to thrive. Figure 6.25 presents the most common causes of infantile growth failure and their major findings on evaluation.

EMOTIONAL ABUSE

This form of abuse accompanies all of the others previously described, but can also occur in isolation and can range from inattentiveness to frank rejection, scapegoating, or even terrorization. Emotional abuse is very difficult to document since it leaves no visible stigmata. Victims may present with

FAILURE TO THRIVE IN INFANCY

Cause	Approximate Percent of All Cases	History	System-specific Physical Findings	System-specific Laboratory Studies
Psychosocial	50% or >	Vague inconsistent feeding history	None. May have soft neurologic signs	None
Central Nervous System	13%	Poor feeding, gross developmental delay, vomiting	Grossly abnormal neurologic examination	Frequent gross abnormalities on EEG and CT scan or grossly abnormal neuromuscular function testing
Gastrointestinal	10%	Chronic vomiting and/or diarrhea, abnormal stools	Often negative, may have abdominal distention	Abnormal barium studies or abnormal stool examination (pH-reducing substances, fat stain, Wright stain)
Cardiac	9%	Slow feeding, dyspnea and diaphoresis with feeding, restlessness and diaphoresis during sleep	Often cyanotic, or have signs of congestive heart failure	Abnormal cardiac series, EKG, catheterization
Genetic	8%	May have positive FH or developmental delay	Often have facies typical of a syndrome, skeletal abnormalities, or neurologic abnormalities, visceromegaly	May have typical radiographic findings, chromosomal abnormalities, abnormal metabolic screens
Pulmonary	3.5%	Chronic or recurrent dyspnea with feeding, tachypnea	Grossly abnormal chest examination	Abnormal chest radiograph
Renal	3.5%	May be negative or may have history of polyuria	Often negative, may have flank masses	Abnormal urinalysis, frequently elevated BUN and creatinine
Endocrine	3.5%	With hypothyroidism, constipation and decreased activity level; with diabetes, polyuria, polydipsia	With hypothyroidism, no wasting but mottling, umbilical hernia, often open posterior fontanelle. With diabetes, often without specific abnormality, but may have signs of dehydration, ketotic breath, and hyperpnea. With hypopituitarism and isolated GH deficiency, growth normal until 9 months or later, then plateaus, but normal weight for height; delayed tooth eruption	Decreased T4, increased TSH; glucosuria and hyperglycemia; abnormal pituitary function studies

Fig. 6.25 Findings for failure to thrive in infancy.

chronic severe anxiety, agitation, hyperactivity, depression, or frank psychotic reactions. Many are socially withdrawn, have trouble relating with peers, and generally perform poorly in school. Low self-esteem is the rule. When suspected, psychological testing and psychiatric examination may prove helpful.

CONCLUSION

While treatment and follow-up are beyond the scope of an atlas of physical diagnosis, a few additional points bear emphasis. Use of a team approach including physician, nurse, and social worker greatly facilitates evaluation of victims of abuse and their families, and reduces the burden of any one health care worker. Reporting requirements necessitate only *reasonable* grounds for suspicion, and place the onus of full investigation on state agencies. Close follow-up, while highly important, is often neglected, especially when patients get caught up in large bureaucratic systems. Having improved our performance on identification and documentation of cases, we must increasingly address ourselves to facilitating better long-term outcome.

BIBLIOGRAPHY

Bauer CH (ed.): Failure to thrive. Pediatric Annals 7(11), Nov. 1978.

Berdon WE, et al: Caffey's Pediatric X-ray Diagnosis, 8th ed. Yearbook, Chicago, 1985.

Green FC (ed.): Incest and sexual abuse. Pediatric Annals 8(5), May 1979.

Helfer RE, Kempe HC (eds.): The Battered Child, 3rd ed. University of Chicago Press, Chicago, 1980.

Helfer RE, Kempe HC (eds.): Child Abuse and Neglect: The Family and the Community. Ballinger, Cambridge, Mass., 1976.

Huffman JW: Gynecology of Childhood and Adolescence, 2nd ed. Saunders, Philadelphia, 1981.

Woodlong BA, Kossosis PD: Sexual misuse. Pediatr Clin N Amer 28:481–499, 1981.

PEDIATRIC RHEUMATOLOGY

Andrew H. Urbach, M.D.

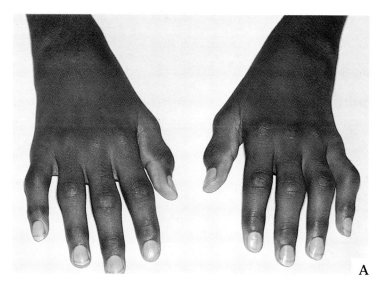

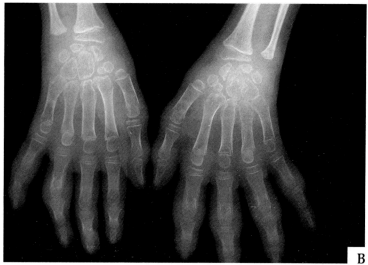

FIG. 7.1 *Swelling and inflammation of the small joints of the hands in a patient with polyarticular juvenile rheumatoid arthritis (JRA). Note the inability to fully extend the fingers* (**A**).

On x-ray, fusiform swelling of the PIP joints with demineralization, and diffuse soft-tissue swelling are seen (**B**).

The collagen vascular diseases are a diverse group of disorders associated with inflammation of the connective tissues. Their etiologies and pathogenesis remain largely unknown at this time. Despite advances in the laboratory diagnosis of these entities, most of the collagen vascular diseases are diagnosed by the clinical constellation of physical findings with which they present.

Most of the collagen vascular diseases manifest themselves as distinct clinical entities and can be diagnosed as such; however, overlap is common. This chapter illustrates the more distinctive clinical features of these rather unique disorders.

Specifically, we discuss juvenile rheumatoid arthritis, dermatomyositis, systemic vasculitis, scleroderma, and systemic lupus erythematosus, and the clinical presentations peculiar to each disorder.

JUVENILE RHEUMATOID ARTHRITIS

Juvenile rheumatoid arthritis (JRA) is the most common of the collagen vascular diseases in children. Its true incidence is not known, though it is estimated that there are approximately 250,000 affected persons in the United States alone.

The first clear description of this entity was presented by George Still in 1897. He postulated multiple etiologies for JRA, and this concept is still supported today. JRA can present as systemic, polyarticular, or pauciarticular disease, all having inflammation of the synovial tissue as one of their cardinal features. Synovium is usually hypertrophied and joint effusions may occur, as well as an increase in the amount of joint fluid. On physical examination one will note joint swelling (Fig. 7.1), with loss of normal anatomical landmarks as well as joint pain, decreased motion, warmth, and

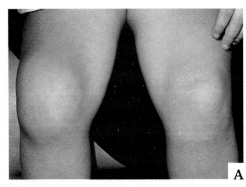
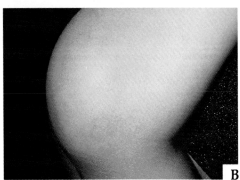
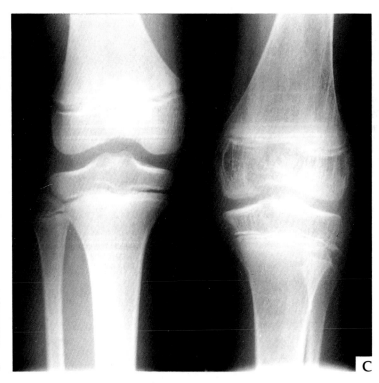

FIG. 7.2 **A** *This toddler with pauci-articular JRA has unilateral knee swelling with slight erythema. A closer examination of the right knee (**B**) demonstrates loss of the normal anatomical landmarks. Demineralization of the right femur and tibia with soft-tissue swelling and hyper-trophy of the epiphyses secondary to hyperemia are demonstrated in **C**.*

CLASSIFICATION OF JRA

Type	%	Characteristics	Sex Ratio	Rheumatoid Factor/ANA	Iridocyclitis	Severe Arthritis
Systemic	20	Systemic symptoms; large (L) & small (S) joints affected	M > F	− / −	−	25%
Polyarticular						
RF−	25	Early or late onset of symptoms; L/S	F > M	− /25%	−	10–15%
RF+	10	Late onset of symptoms; L/S Rheumatoid nodules	F > M	+ /50–75%	−	Majority
Pauciarticular						
Early onset	25	Few joints; hips & SI joints not involved	F > M	− /60%	50%	Not usually severe
Late onset	15	Few joints; SI, hips involved, HLA B27 75%	M > F	− / −	Occasional	Ankylosing spondylitis sometimes present

FIG. 7.3 *Classification of JRA. (Adapted from Schaller, 1980)*

erythema (Fig. 7.2). Extreme pain, intense erythema, and very warm joints should suggest not JRA, but rather an infectious etiology for this dramatic presentation. Despite objective arthritis, the child may not present with arthralgia. When inflammation persists for a long enough period of time, destruction of the articular surface and bony structures may occur. Due to the poor regenerative properties of articular cartilage, these deformities may be permanent. Fortunately, most cases of JRA do not have permanent joint deformity associated with them.

Because of the variability of the diseases grouped under the heading JRA, three distinct categories (with subgroups) exist:

1. Systemic onset disease
2. Polyarticular disease: rheumatoid factor negative and positive
3. Pauciarticular disease: early childhood onset and late childhood onset

This classification of disease is based on its presentation during the first 6 months of illness (Fig. 7.3).

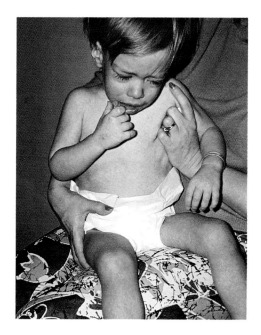

FIG. 7.4 A preschool child with systemic onset JRA displaying the typical irritable demeanor of Still disease.

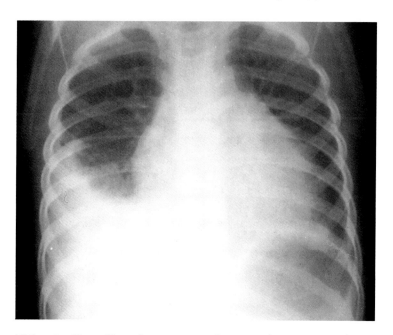

FIG. 7.5 Typical fever curve of a child with systemic onset JRA. Daily fever spikes occur with intermittent temperatures in the normal range. The patient was not receiving antipyretics.

FIG. 7.6 Rash of systemic onset JRA is erythematous, macular, and often evanescent. It can be more prominent during periods of fever. The rash was pruritic in this patient.

FIG. 7.7 Chest film of a patient with pericarditis associated with JRA. Note the right pleural effusion with fluid in the fissure and blunting of the right costophrenic angle. The cardiothoracic ratio is increased.

Systemic Onset JRA

Systemic onset JRA represents 10 to 20 percent of all children with JRA. Fever, rash, irritability (Fig. 7.4), arthritis, and visceral involvement dominate the clinical presentation. The fever usually spikes greater than 39°C and often can occur twice daily. Chills are associated with fever, but rigors do not occur. Though the late afternoon is a typical time for a temperature spike, many other patterns may occur (Fig. 7.5). Other manifestations of systemic onset JRA such as rash and joint symptoms may be evanescent with fever.

The rash of JRA is macular, 2 to 6 mm in diameter, evanescent, salmon or red with slightly irregular margins (Fig. 7.6). There is often an area of central clearing. The rash occurs on the trunk and proximal extremities but may also be distal in

distribution with palms and soles affected. Though the rash generally does not produce discomfort, some patients report pruritus. Superficial mild trauma to the skin or exposure to warmth and stress may precipitate the rash. While the rash is seen with polyarticular JRA, it does not occur with pauciarticular disease.

Arthritis and arthralgia almost invariably occur at some time during the presentation and often will secure the already suspected diagnosis. Myalgia can be prominent early, as can hepatosplenomegaly and lymphadenopathy. Serositis, pleuritis, pericarditis (Fig. 7.7), hyperbilirubinemia, transaminase elevations, leukocytosis, and anemia have also been seen with this illness. Only 25 percent of this group of JRA patients progress to have chronic joint symptoms.

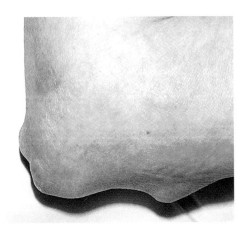

FIG. 7.8 Subcutaneous nodules over the pressure points of the elbow.

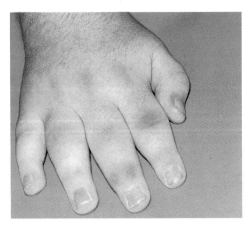

FIG. 7.9 Swelling of the PIP and MCP joints in this patient with polyarticular JRA produces spindle-shaped fingers.

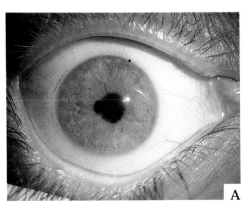

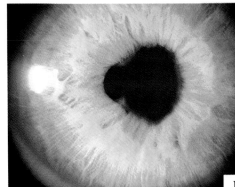

FIG. 7.10 Iridocyclitis with an irregular pupil in a patient with pauciarticular JRA (A). Note synechiae projecting posteriorly toward the lens (B).

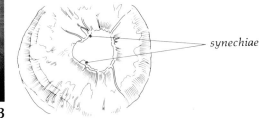

synechiae

Polyarticular Onset JRA

Polyarticular onset of disease accounts for 35 percent of all children with JRA. Five or more joints need to be involved in the absence of prominent systemic signs and symptoms. There appear to be two subgroups within this category: rheumatoid factor seropositive and seronegative. The seropositive group is felt to be nearly identical to the adult entity of rheumatoid arthritis (RA). Onset usually occurs after age 8 and, as with seronegative disease, females predominate; 80 percent of all adult RA patients are seropositive.

In addition to the joint findings of warmth, swelling, erythema, and tenderness seen in both subgroups, seropositive disease provides some additional clues to diagnosis. The subcutaneous nodules which occur in seropositive onset disease are firm, nontender nodules on the skin surface with a predilection for pressure points (Fig. 7.8). The most common location is the elbow, but the nodules also occur on the heels, hands, knees, ears, scapulae, sacrum, and buttocks. Other features of seropositive disease may include cutaneous vasculitis, Felty syndrome (leukopenia and splenomegaly), and Sjögren syndrome (keratoconjunctivitis sicca and parotitis).

The onset of polyarthritis may be either insidious or acute. While the seropositive group progresses to destructive sinovitis and a prolonged chronic course in more than half of the patients, children with seronegative disease often have remarkably little permanent joint destruction relative to their duration of symptoms. Any synovial joint may be involved in the inflammatory process, including the knees, wrists, elbows, ankles, the small joints of the feet, the proximal interphalangeal (PIP) joints, and the metacarpophalangeal (MCP) joints (Fig. 7.9). The lumbosacral spine is usually spared.

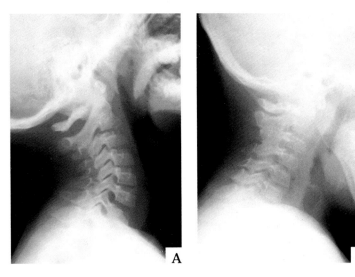

FIG. 7.11 Ankylosing spondylitis with fusion of C2, C3, C4 occurring during an 18-month period between A and B.

Pauciarticular Onset JRA

Pauciarticular onset JRA is strictly defined as onset of disease in fewer than five joints, though clearly children with additional joints may informally belong in this category. The large joints (knees, ankles, and elbows) are often asymmetrically involved. Two subgroups seem to exist under this heading: early and late onset. In early-onset pauciarticular disease there is female predominance, the ANA is positive in 25 percent, and onset is usually before the fifth birthday. As

FIG. 7.12 Extra-articular manifestations of JRA. (From Cassidy, 1982)

	Polyarthritis (%)	Oligoarthritis (%)	Systemic Disease (%)
Fever	30	0	100
Rheumatoid rash	10	0	95
Rheumatoid nodules	10	0	5
Hepatosplenomegaly	10	0	85
Lymphadenopathy	5	0	70
Chronic uveitis	5	20	0
Pericarditis	5	0	35
Pleuritis	1	0	20
Abdominal pain	1	0	10

with polyarticular disease, systemic symptoms do not dominate the clinical picture. If the disease does not progress to polyarticular involvement within the first half-year of illness, the patient often will maintain the pauciarticular pattern. While joint disease may be cosmetically evident, pain is rarely severe. This disease entity is particularly unique because of its 50 percent association with chronic iridocyclitis (Fig. 7.10). In its earliest stages, diagnosis often depends on slit-lamp examination, though photophobia and eye pain can occur. The importance of routine eye examinations cannot be overemphasized, as severe visual handicap can result from undetected inflammation.

While fulfilling the criteria of JRA, later onset of pauciarticular disease may be more logically placed among the spondyloarthropathies (Fig. 7.11). These patients are generally males, older than 8 years, with involvement of hips, knees, ankles, and foot joints. Onset can be acute and of a more prolonged nature in children with a family history of spondyloarthropathies or associated conditions. In the child who progresses to lumbar and sacral joint disease, the designation spondyloarthropathy is appropriate. Other children will manifest findings of Reiter syndrome (a seronegative asymmetric arthropathy associated with urethritis, cervicitis, dysentery, inflammatory eye disease, or other mucocutaneous disease) and some will go on to have limitation of spinal flexion. Still others will never progress to a spondyloarthropathy, and hence the designation of JRA will continue to be more appropriate.

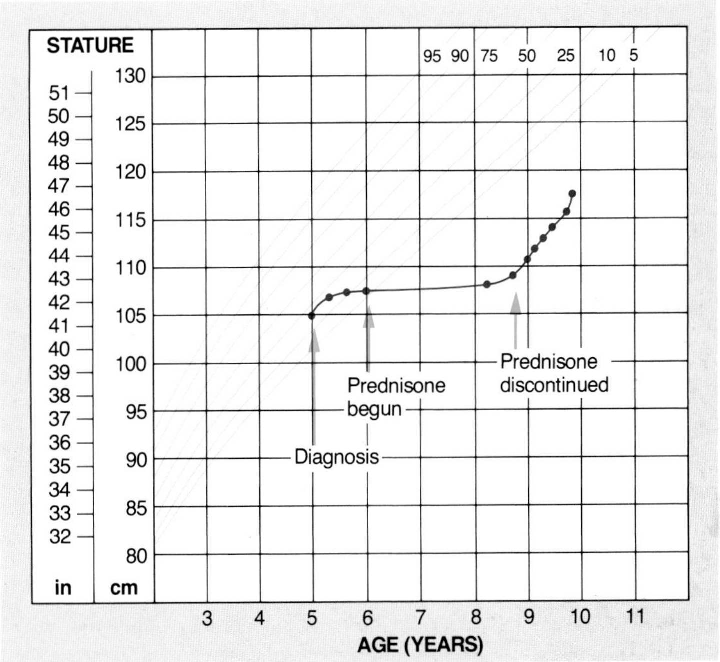

FIG. 7.13 Growth curve of a patient with JRA. Note the persistent fall-off in height during the period of active disease before prednisone therapy. Poor growth persisted during therapy, but the patient exhibits good growth when off prednisone and in clinical remission.

Extra-articular Manifestations of Disease

Many extra-articular features of JRA have been reported. The more common ones are listed in Figure 7.12. Linear growth retardation is well known to occur in the child with active JRA (Fig. 7.13). The degree of retardation and the ultimate prognosis for reaching adult height are related to the severity and duration of inflammation. During early illness, bony development may be advanced while later in the course of the illness the opposite may be true. Premature epiphyseal fusion may occur. In addition, steroids themselves may inhibit linear growth. Careful use of standardized growth curves will assist in the early detection of growth failure. This may in turn guide one's long-term therapeutic approach.

Chronic uveitis is an entity of considerable importance in JRA patients because of the visual impairment that may accompany prolonged inflammation. It is seen most commonly in pauciarticular onset, occurring rarely in polyarticular disease and almost never in systemic onset disease. Onset is usually without symptoms and can often only be detected by

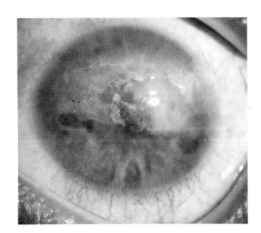

FIG. 7.14 Band keratopathy in a patient with JRA. Note the calcium deposits in Bowman's layer.

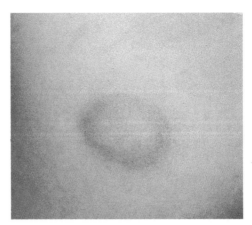

FIG. 7.15 Erythema chronicum migrans in a patient with Lyme arthritis. The lesion may be a large erythematous macule with central clearing, occurring singly or multiply.

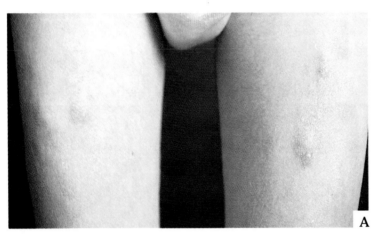

A

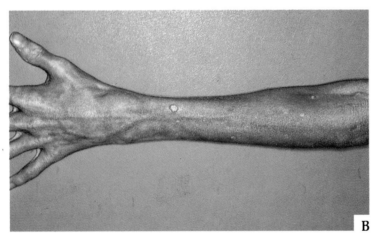

B

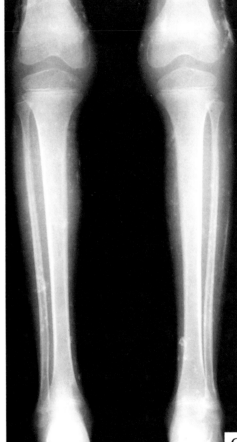

C

FIG. 7.16 **A** Nodular calcific densities in thighs of patients with dermatomyositis (DM). **B** Atrophy, hyperpigmentation, and subcutaneous calcium deposits in the arm of a patient with burned-out DM. **C** Radiologic evidence of soft-tissue calcification in a patient with DM.

careful slit-lamp examination. Ophthalmic complications may not parallel activity of the arthritis. The first clinical sign is cellular exudate in the anterior chamber. If the uveitis is left untreated, synechiae (adhesions) between the iris and lens may develop, leading to an irregular and poorly functioning pupil (see Fig. 7.10). Further along in the clinical course, band keratopathy (calcium deposits in the cornea) (Fig. 7.14) may occur as well as cataracts or glaucoma. For these reasons, eye examinations three to four times yearly are recommended early in the disease's course for high-risk patients.

Cardiac involvement occurs in over one-third of systemic onset JRA patients. Pericarditis, myocarditis, and endocarditis all occur, with pericarditis being the most common. The presence of chest pain, a friction rub, tachycardia, dyspnea, and supportive x-ray findings may all occur. These episodes

may occur for weeks to months and usually are associated with a generalized flare of disease.

A variety of other extra-articular manifestations are also known to occur. Hepatosplenomegaly and lymphadenopathy are particularly common in systemic disease. Tenosynovitis and myositis (without enzyme elevation) occur, as does a generalized vasculitis. Many clinicians report hematuria and proteinuria as well.

Differential Diagnosis

Because JRA is largely a clinical diagnosis, very strict clinical criteria have been set to make the diagnosis of JRA. Most authors suggest the presence of objective joint findings (arthritis) for a minimum of 6 consecutive weeks coupled with

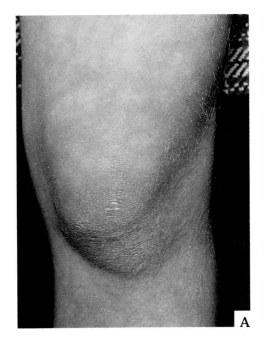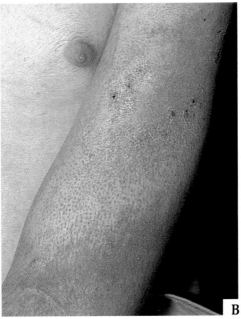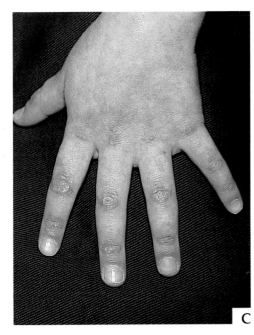

FIG. 7.17 *Typical rash of DM over the extensor surfaces of the knee* (**A**), *elbow* (**B**), *and PIP and MCP joints* (**C**), *showing* erythema and atrophic skin changes.

the exclusion of other causes of arthritis in children. The extra-articular features of JRA, as discussed earlier, may solidify the diagnosis purely because of their distinctiveness, that is, uveitis and rheumatoid nodules.

Because of its destructive nature, pyogenic arthritis (Staphylococcus, Streptococcus, *Haemophilus influenzae*, etc.) must be ruled out in any child with active joint disease. The intensely red and tender joint, well beyond the degree one usually sees with JRA, should raise one's suspicion of a bacterial pathogen. This combined with systemic symptoms of infection (fever, chills, malaise) should prompt one to perform an arthrocentesis early in the course of the illness. If the joint in question is the hip, one's suspicion should be even higher because of the rarity with which the hip is the first affected joint in JRA. Other infectious etiologies include Lyme arthritis. This spirochetal form of arthritis is tick-borne and usually affects the knee, elbow, or wrist. Malaise, fever, myalgia, and weakness may also occur in addition to a rather distinctive rash. The rash, known as erythema chronicum migrans (Fig. 7.15), begins as an erythematous macule or papule. After this clears, the borders of the lesion expand to form an erythematous circular lesion which can be as large as 30 cm in diameter. Salmonella, Shigella, Yersinia, and Campylobacter should also be considered. Viral diseases such as rubella, mumps, hepatitis B, varicella, and adenovirus can also mimic JRA.

Malignancies such as neuroblastoma and leukemia may present with joint disease. Sickle cell disease, particularly in the form of dactylitis, can have prominent joint involvement. Inflammatory bowel disease, hemophilia, trauma, psoriasis, and Henoch-Schönlein purpura must also be thought of in the patient with arthritis. All of the collagen vascular diseases can have significant joint disease; however, their clinical features and laboratory tests can usually distinguish them from JRA.

DERMATOMYOSITIS

Dermatomyositis (DM) is an uncommon but distinctive disease which accounts for approximately 5 percent of all collagen vascular diseases in children. Though it was first described in 1887, its etiology remains largely unknown. The hallmarks of this entity are various skin manifestations coupled with nonsuppurative inflammation of muscle. Dermatomyositis affecting the adult generally carries a worse prognosis than if encountered in the pediatric age group. There is no association with malignancy in pediatric DM patients, as there is in adults. Nevertheless, vasculitis of varying severity is often seen earlier in the course of the illness in children and there is a relatively high incidence of calcinosis (nodular calcium deposits) in nonvisceral tissues such as muscle (Fig. 7.16).

Though the age range for DM is broad, the 4- to 10-year-old child is particularly at risk. Females predominate by a 2:1 ratio. There is no racial bias nor is there any evidence of a familial predisposition.

Clinically, patients usually present with proximal muscle weakness, particularly affecting the hip girdle and legs. Though shoulders and arms are often involved, this may not be as easily detected in the child. The first complaints are often inability to climb stairs and disturbances of gait. Dysphagia, dysphonia, and dyspnea may occur if the respective muscles for these functions are affected. The affected muscles may be tender and indurated with a superficially edematous appearance. A distinctive rash seen in three-quarters of DM patients can confirm the diagnosis. Even in the absence of this distinctive rash, all patients will have some degree of cutaneous disease. The rash is symmetrical and erythematous with atrophic changes located over the extensor surfaces of the knees, elbows, and PIP and MCP joints (Fig. 7.17). Other features of the rash include a violaceous discoloration of the

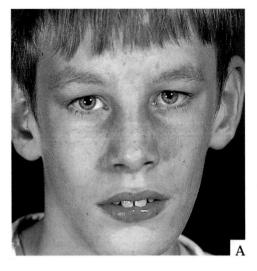
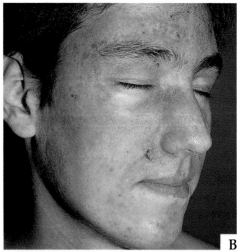

FIG. 7.18 **A** *Facial rash of DM with a violaceous color around the eyes and malar region.* **B** *More severe, erythematous, scaly rash involving almost the entire face.*

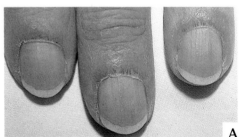
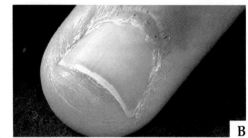

FIG. 7.19 *Nail bed telangiectasia. Note the erythema around the nail edge* (**A**) *and the pinpoint telangiectasia that may require a magnifying lens to identify* (**B**).

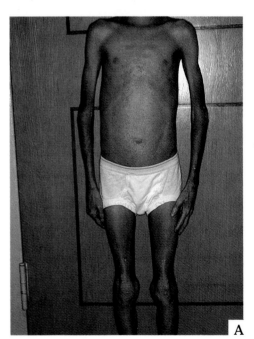
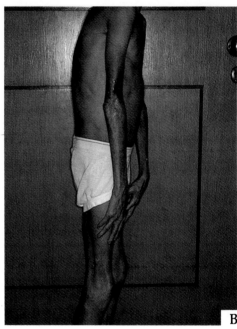

FIG. 7.20 *Burned-out chronic DM. Limbs are thin, with muscle and skin atrophy* (**A**) *and diffuse contractures have occurred* (**B**).

eyelids, a scaly red rash in a malar distribution (Fig. 7.18), and the very characteristic dystrophic skin changes. With these changes one sees nailbed telangiectasia (Fig. 7.19) and hyper- or hypopigmentation of the skin. The rash may precede muscle disease. However, because of the pathognomonic features of the rash, the diagnosis of DM can often be suspected before other overt symptoms occur. Constitutional symptoms such as anorexia, malaise, weight loss, and fever may be present with this entity. The illness may progress at variable rates in different patients; however, the majority of patients have a more insidious rather than acute course. Unfortunately, long delays in diagnosis can occur, particularly in the insidious group. Other more uncommon findings are

mouth ulcers, retinitis, hepatosplenomegaly, pulmonary infiltrates, myocarditis, and pericarditis. Though calcinosis occurs in 40 percent of children with dermatomyositis, it does not occur during the acute phase of the illness. On the other hand, in chronic indolent disease, it may be the presenting complaint.

The clinical diagnosis of DM can be supported by an abnormal EMG, muscle biopsy, elevated muscle enzymes [creatine phosphokinase (CPK), SGOT, aldolase], elevated ESR, and occasionally a positive ANA. Steroids are the mainstay of therapy and their early use will often preserve muscle function and minimize the potentially destructive nature of this illness (Fig. 7.20).

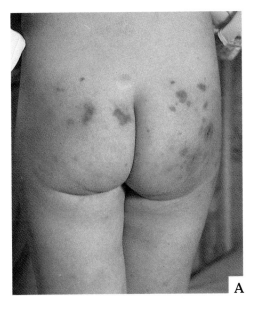
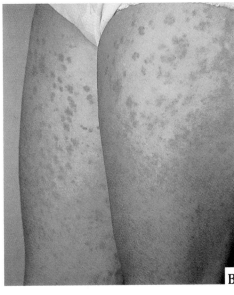

FIG. 7.21 The distinctive rash of Henoch-Schonlein purpura (HSP) characteristically involves the buttocks (**A**) and lower extremities (**B**), with purpuric coalescent lesions.

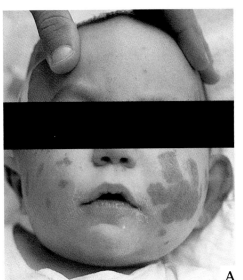
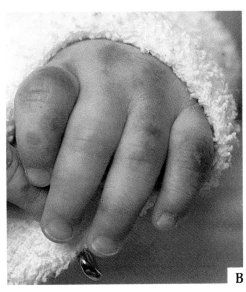
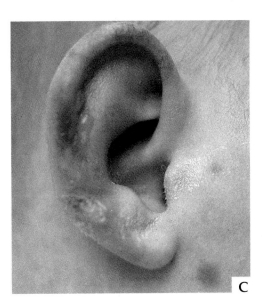

FIG. 7.22 An infant with HSP. The rash may occur on the face along with edema (**A**) and rash and edema of the extremities (**B**), as well as ulceration (**C**).

SYSTEMIC VASCULITIS

The vasculitides are a broad group of disorders which can be classified into a number of different categories: medium- and small-vessel disease, small-vessel disease, and giant-cell arteritis. Polyarteritis nodosa, infantile polyarteritis nodosa, and Kawasaki disease are examples of medium- and small-vessel disease. Cranial arteritis and Takayasu arteritis are examples of giant-cell arteritis. These entities remain relatively unusual in the pediatric age group. Henoch-Schönlein purpura (HSP), a small-vessel vasculitis, however, is occasionally encountered by the practicing pediatrician. Its unique rash and constellation of signs and symptoms can make the diagnosis rapid for the experienced observer.

Henoch-Schönlein syndrome consists of nonthrombocytopenic purpura, arthritis and arthralgia, gastrointestinal symptomatology, and a variety of renal findings. Seventy-five percent of cases occur in children less than 10 years of age with the median age being 5 years. Most authors feel that this syndrome occurs after an upper respiratory infection or other viral illness, though HSP has been reported following insect bites, dietary allergens, and numerous drugs. There does not appear to be a familial predilection, and all races have been affected.

The clinical picture of HSP is that of a previously well child who acutely develops a distinctive skin rash, arthritis, and abdominal pain. The skin rash allows for definitive diagnosis and hence it is said to occur in all patients with HSP. The rash usually involves the buttocks, lower extremities, and the hands (wrist-down distribution) with the trunk and face generally being spared (Fig. 7.21). The lesions begin as petechial or approximately 0.5 cm purpuric areas which coalesce and become confluent with nearby lesions. They begin as red macules or papules and progress with time to purplish and then brownish areas. On occasion ulceration will occur. Some patients will have lesions that mimic urticaria and about 25 percent will have subcutaneous edema (Fig. 7.22). The edema is nonpitting, painless, and most commonly affects the hands and feet. The child less than 2 years of age is most likely to have edema as a feature of this illness.

Approximately 85 percent of patients will display some

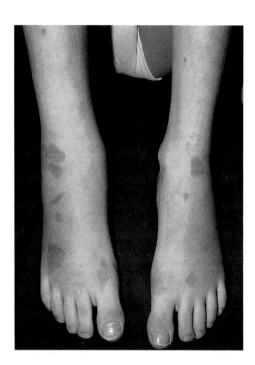

FIG. 7.23 The arthritis of HSP. Note the swelling of the right ankle in addition to the rash.

FIG. 7.24 Forms of morphea. A Hypopigmented plaque of scleroderma with skin atrophy. B "Salt and pepper" appearance of a plaque in a patient with scleroderma. Note the hyperpigmentation within the hypopigmented lesion.

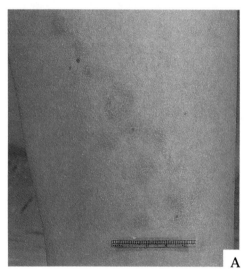

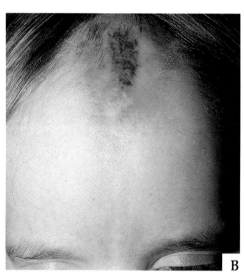

FIG. 7.25 A Linear scleroderma. Localized involvement of a dermatome with hyperpigmentation. B An unusual form of morphea affecting the scalp, termed "coup de sabre" (stroke of the saber) or linear scleroderma.

form of gastrointestinal symptomatology. Simple abdominal pain can be the only symptom, but its severity can cause the physician to become concerned about the more severe abdominal complications. Massive gastrointestinal hemorrhage or intussusception occurs in 5 percent of patients and complete perforation rarely occurs. Melanotic stools, vomiting, ileus, and hematemesis may be present as well. In rare circumstances abdominal pain can precede the other features of HSP, making diagnosis impossible until the characteristic rash appears.

Arthritis is a part of HSP in three-quarters of reported cases. Knees and ankles are the most common sites of involvement (Fig. 7.23). Warmth and erythema are not usually associated with the pain and swelling that occur. The joints are never affected permanently and this feature of HSP generally resolves in several days. As with the gastrointestinal symptoms, arthritis can precede the rash. For this reason, one needs to consider HSP in the child with acute onset of arthritis.

While renal involvement is detected in only half of HSP patients, it is important because the degree of renal pathology generally affects the patient's ultimate prognosis. Renal manifestations can be as mild as hematuria or proteinuria, but they may be as severe as nephrotic syndrome, nephritis, and, in 5 percent of patients, end-stage renal disease. Patients will usually declare themselves within several months but cases of renal failure and hypertension have occurred many years after the initial illness.

Other features of HSP include low-grade fever, malaise, scrotal swelling with pain, cerebral vasculitis, nosebleeds, parotitis, pancreatitis, and cardiopulmonary disease.

The course of the illness varies with age. The majority of patients are over their initial illness in 4 weeks; however, 50 percent will have at least one recurrence. Recurrences generally are limited to cutaneous and mild abdominal symptomatology.

Clotting functions and platelet counts in these patients are normal. Since there are no specific laboratory examinations diagnostic of this syndrome, the history and physical examination provide clues to the successful recognition of HSP.

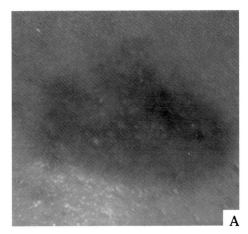

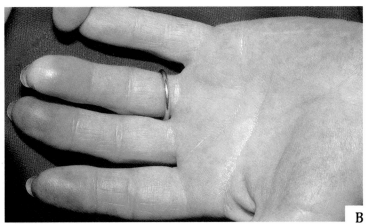

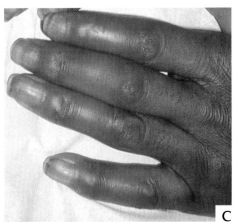

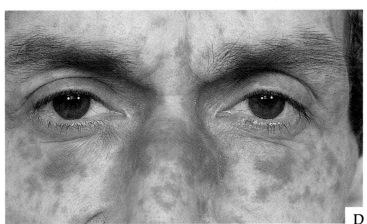

FIG. 7.26 CREST syndrome: Cutaneous calcinosis (**A**) and Raynaud's phenomenon (note cyanosis as well as pallor of the fingertips) (**B**), sclerodactyly (**C**) and telangiectasia (**D**). Esophageal dysmotility may also occur.

SCLERODERMA

Scleroderma is an uncommon collagen vascular disease which involves the skin, gastrointestinal tract, heart, lungs, and kidneys as well as a variety of other organ systems. Scleroderma, or "tight skin," remains an enigmatic entity with no known etiology and no consistently effective therapy. In recent years, increasing numbers of patients with scleroderma have been described in the pediatric literature; however, prior to 1960, only 12 children with generalized scleroderma were described. Presently less than 5 percent of patients with collagen vascular disease carry this diagnosis. There appears to be a female predominance, but no racial or genetic predisposition has been reported.

The cutaneous manifestations of scleroderma and the presence or absence of systemic involvement guide the clinician in classifying scleroderma. Local disease or morphea may present in the form of plaques, drops (the "guttate" variety), or with diffuse cutaneous involvement (Fig. 7.24). Linear scleroderma affects a single dermatome (Fig. 7.25). Systemic scleroderma or progressive systemic sclerosis is notable because visceral organ involvement occurs. Variants of systemic scleroderma are the CREST syndromes, which are comprised of *c*alcinosis cutis, *R*aynaud's phenomenon, *e*sophageal abnormalities, *s*clerodactyly, and *t*elangiectasias (Fig. 7.26). Often, mixed connective tissue disease is considered under the same classification.

In 1980 the American Rheumatism Association developed criteria for the clinical diagnosis of scleroderma. The single major criterion is the presence of proximal scleroderma or the typical cutaneous manifestations of the disease proximal to the wrists. The three minor criteria decided upon are sclerodactyly, digital pitting ulcers (Fig. 7.27), and, lastly, bilateral pulmonary fibrosis. In order to diagnose scleroderma one must confirm the presence of one major and two minor criteria.

Many organ systems may be involved in the child afflicted with scleroderma. Cutaneous manifestations frequently

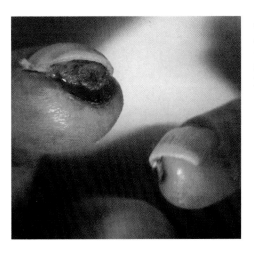

FIG. 7.27 Digital pitting ulcers, one of the three minor diagnostic criteria for scleroderma.

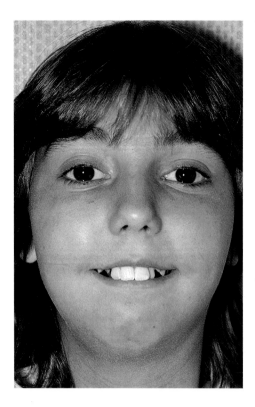

FIG. 7.28 Facial features of scleroderma. The skin appears tight and drawn, without evidence of wrinkles. (Courtesy of Dr. J. Jeffrey Malatack)

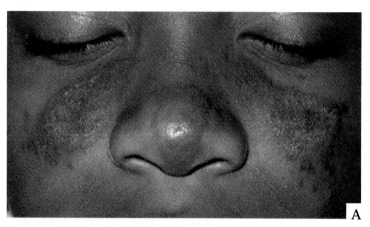

A

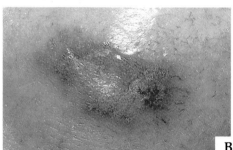

B

FIG. 7.29 Typical malar rash of SLE (**A**), with erythema, erosion, and atrophy (**B**).

bring children to medical attention. Early in the clinical course, the skin is edematous with a particular predilection for the distal extremities; rarely, more proximal limb, face, and trunk involvement is present. The induration phase, for which scleroderma is named, is characterized by loss of the natural pliability of the skin and the presence of a palpable thickness to the skin. The skin will take on a shiny, tense appearance with distal tapering of the fingers (see Fig. 7.26C). The visual impression that movement might be impaired is, in fact, supported by the lack of flexibility in the hands and the typical scleroderma facies. Tight skin and skin atrophy produce the appearance of a fixed stare, pinched nose, thin pursed lips, small mouth, prominent teeth, and characteristic grimace (Fig. 7.28). Further along in the clinical progression of scleroderma the skin may become very soft and atrophic. Subcutaneous calcium deposits (calcinosis cutis) may occur at pressure points and will occasionally extrude through the skin in a fashion similar to DM (see Fig. 7.16). These lesions may be painful and not uncommonly may ulcerate. Often, generalized hyperpigmentation occurs with punctuated areas of hypopigmentation or vitiligo (complete depigmentation) (see Figs. 7.24 and 7.25). Telangiectasias of three varieties are known to occur: linear telangiectasias of the cuticles, well-defined macules of various sizes and shapes, and the reddish-purple papules typical of Osler-Weber-Rendu disease (tiny circular lesions positioned eccentrically from their telangiec-tatic spokes) (see Fig. 7.26D).

Because of the involvement of the digital arteries in sclero-derma, patients often develop the clinical picture of Ray-naud's phenomenon (see Fig. 7.26B). Patients will develop intense pallor secondary to cold or emotion. This is followed by cyanosis and erythema and is often associated with pain or paresthesias. In its most severe form, ischemia may lead to necrosis and eventual gangrenous destruction of tissue.

Gastrointestinal symptoms occur in approximately half of the children, though more detailed investigation often indi-cates the presence of abnormalities in a larger percentage.

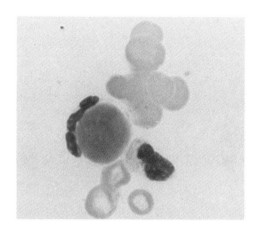

FIG. 7.30 LE cell. Antibody-coated nuclear debris phagocytized by a healthy neutrophil. (Courtesy of Professor A.V. Hoff-brand, Royal Free Hospital, London)

Esophageal dysmotility associated with gastroesophageal reflux often leads to dysphagia and symptoms of esophagitis. In more severely affected individuals, aspiration and cough may occur while esophageal strictures can develop if the process of reflux is chronic. If the small bowel is involved, diarrhea and constipation may result from peristaltic dys-function. Bacterial overgrowth, steatorrhea, weight loss, volvulus, and even perforation can occur. Colonic disease occurs in the form of wide-mouth diverticula and a loss of the normal colonic architecture.

As might be expected, mortality and morbidity often are the results of the cardiorespiratory stigmata of the disease. In addition to pulmonary fibrosis, one may see cough, dyspnea with exertion, findings of pulmonary hypertension, and pleural effusion. Cardiac involvement includes heart block, congestive heart failure, ECG changes, and pericardial effu-sion.

Other manifestations of disease are arthritis, arthralgia, systemic hypertension, proteinuria, azotemia, Sjögren syndrome, and various CNS findings such as sensory cranial nerve dysfunction and decreased vibratory sensation.

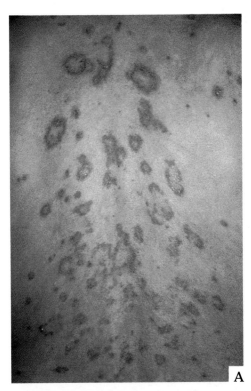

FIG. 7.31 The localized erythematous rash of SLE in a nonmalar distribution (**A**). The rash of SLE often has a slight white scale (**B**).

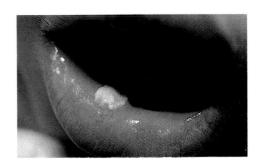

FIG. 7.32 Mucosal ulceration of the lip as evidence of vasculitis in SLE.

SYSTEMIC LUPUS ERYTHEMATOSUS

Systemic lupus erythematosus (SLE) is a complex autoimmune disease with a myriad of clinical presentations. SLE may present in an insidious fashion and hence escape early diagnosis, or it may present acutely and progress rapidly, leading to the patient's demise. As with other collagen vascular diseases, its etiology is unknown. The disease may involve just one organ system or, more commonly, it may be a multisystem disease. Because of the large number of serologic markers known to occur in SLE, it is considered by many to be the prototype of autoimmune disease.

The word "lupus," which means wolf, alludes to the erosive nature of the rash of SLE —"wolf bite" (Fig. 7.29). This feature of the disease was critical to the diagnosis of SLE until the discovery of the LE (lupus erythematosus) cell in 1948. The LE cell represents a healthy neutrophil which has phagocytized the nuclear debris of a nonliving cell that has been coated with antibody (Fig. 7.30). This antibody is directed against deoxyribonucleoprotein (DNP), which is made up of both DNA and histones. The presence of this serologic marker for lupus greatly expanded the recognized clinical entity of SLE. With the recognition of milder cases of SLE and the advent of new therapies, the prognosis has improved substantially.

While SLE comprises 10 percent of the group of patients with collagen vascular disease, its incidence is approximately 1 in 200,000 in children, with 80 percent of its victims being female. The incidence of other connective tissue diseases is higher among family members of patients with SLE. Hematologic malignancies and immunodeficiencies are also reported in increased frequency among SLE relatives. These well described phenomena may reflect a genetic alteration of immunity or, as some researchers suggest, the effects of a transmissible agent. Drugs are known to induce a lupus-like reaction, and their withdrawal leads to a resolution of this syndrome. Among the more common offenders are the anticonvulsants, hydralazine, oral contraceptives, and several antibiotics. The high incidence of disease in females, SLE's common exacerbation during pregnancy, and the induction of disease by birth control pills support the role of hormonal factors as contributing to the pathogenesis of SLE. Other investigators suggest the influence of viruses, sunlight, and emotional stress on those developing lupus.

While immunologic markers have made the diagnosis of SLE considerably easier, one must still have a high index of suspicion to obtain these studies. The early symptoms are often nonspecific and, in fact, sometimes unrecognized as a harbinger of serious disease. Fever, fatigue, malaise, anorexia, and weight loss may be all that the clinician is provided with to suspect the diagnosis. In the adolescent population, these symptoms may be all the more difficult to interpret. Conversely, this multisystem disease may present with a plethora of physical findings and the presentation may be so dramatic that clues to diagnosis are quite readily apparent. Among the more commonly involved organ systems are skin, joints, reticuloendothelial, renal, cardiac, and pulmonary.

Cutaneous manifestations of SLE are present at some time during the course of the disease in 80 percent of affected individuals. The classic butterfly rash in the malar distribution is seen about one-third of the time (see Fig. 7.29A). The rash of lupus is often reddish-purple, raised with a whitish scale (Fig. 7.31). When the scale is removed, the underlying skin often has produced "carpet tack"-like fingers on the unexposed side of the scale itself. Carpet tacking is caused by the contouring of the scale into the skin follicles. These fingerlike projections on the scale strongly suggest the diagnosis of lupus. Purplish-red lesions which are urticarial in character also occur but these do not produce scale and do not cause atrophy as other lupus lesions do. If the skin manifestations are left untreated, the cosmetic results are marred by hypo- and hyperpigmentation. Mucosal erosions and ulcers of both the oral cavity and nasal mucosa are part of lupus as well (Fig. 7.32).

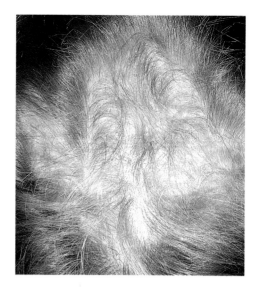

FIG 7.33. Scarring alopecia seen in SLE.

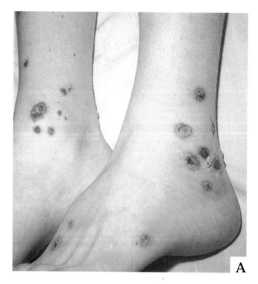

FIG. 7.34 Cutaneous vasculitis in SLE. Purpuric, ulcerative, and necrotic skin

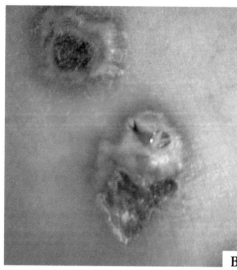

lesions of active disease (**A**). Closeup of necrotic lesions (**B**).

Alopecia (Fig. 7.33) is seen in 20 percent of patients and may occur as broken hair shafts or patchy, red, scaling areas on the scalp which may eventually scar and yield permanent hair loss. Other reported mucocutaneous findings are livedo reticularis (blotchy cyanotic areas in a lacy pattern), urticaria, atrophy, and telangiectasia. Though rare in children, discoid lupus refers to the absence of systemic disease in the presence of typical lupus dermatologic pathology.

The vasculitis of lupus, a small-vessel vasculitis, is responsible for a number of easily recognized clinical findings. The skin may be purpuric, or in more severe instances necrotic lesions may result (Fig. 7.34). The vasculitic component of lupus may also present with full-blown Raynaud's phenomenon. With repeated tissue injury, one may see glossy, atrophic, ulcerated skin and distorted nail architecture.

The heart is often significantly involved in patients with lupus. While the pericardium is most commonly involved, the myocardium and the endocardium may also be of clinical importance. Pericarditis can be nonpainful and present only as cardiomegaly on chest radiograph or as pericardial effusion on echocardiogram. However, one might also see chest pain or auscultate a friction rub. The myocardium, when affected, can lead to the life-threatening complications of arrhythmia, heart failure, and infarction. "Libman-Sacks endocarditis" is the term given to the verrucous projections of fibrinoid necrosis of the endocardium. These lesions rarely cause clinical symptoms, though the presence of a murmur should raise one's suspicion of endocardial disease.

Pulmonary manifestations of lupus are particularly difficult to diagnose noninvasively. Migrating pneumonitis, particularly involving the lung bases, suggests "lupus lung;" however, distinguishing these densities from infection may be impossible without invasive procedures. Typically, patients have atelectasis, pleural effusions, interstitial pneumonitis, or hemorrhage (Fig. 7.35). These sequelae may present as cyanosis, dyspnea, or almost any other form of respiratory distress.

Unlike the destructive arthritis of JRA, lupus arthritis is more transient and does not commonly result in loss of function. The fact that arthralgia is more predominant than

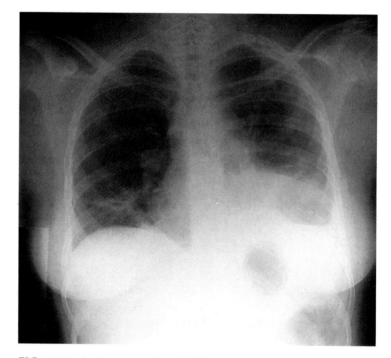

FIG. 7.35 Atelectasis, pleural effusions, and pulmonary infiltrates in a black teenage girl with SLE.

arthritis has been noted consistently. Myalgia and weakness also occur as a feature of lupus, but do not dominate the clinical picture as they do in DM.

CNS signs and symptoms of lupus present a great challenge to physicians. A wide range of neurologic and psychiatric manifestations of the disease have been described. Further complicating the spectrum of CNS lupus is the difficulty in distinguishing the disease itself from side effects of therapy, emotional response to the disease, and a non-CNS etiology for CNS pathology (e.g., hypertension). It is estimated that approximately one-quarter of all lupus patients have some form of CNS disease. The findings range from mononeuritis multiplex (inflammatory lesions of multiple nerves located in anatomically unrelated parts of the body) to chorea, ataxia, peripheral neuropathy, seizures, headaches, psychosis, pseudomotor cerebri, and intellectual impair-

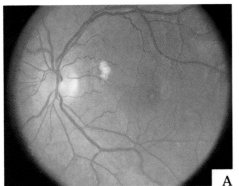

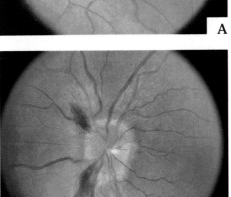

FIG 7.36. **A** A white exudate (cotton-wool spot) between the disc and macula. **B** Papilledema with flame hemorrhages.

ANTIBODIES FOUND IN SLE PATIENTS

Antibody	Percent of Patients
Native DNA (double-stranded)	50 to 60
DNP (DNA and histone protein)	Up to 70 (usually high titer)
RNP (RNA and non-histone protein)	30 to 40
Histones	
All SLE patients	60
Drug-induced lupus patients	95
SS-A (Ro)	30 to 40
SS-B (La)	15
Sm	30

FIG. 7.37 Antibodies found in SLE patients. (Adapted from Tan, 1983)

ment. In fact, the thorough investigation of a large number of neurologic disorders mandates screening serologies for lupus. As a direct extension of the brain, the retina not surprisingly may also show evidence of disease. Perhaps best known of the ocular manifestations is the cotton-wool spot, an exudative whitish lesion of the retina. Hemorrhage and papilledema are also seen (Fig. 7.36). As might be expected, the CNS effects of lupus are responsible for much morbidity as well as mortality.

At least as important as CNS disease in determining ultimate prognosis is the degree of renal involvement. Approximately three-quarters of all children with SLE will have some degree of clinically apparent renal disease. This often manifests itself in the first 2 years of illness, but can also appear many years after the initial diagnosis of lupus. The type of pathology seen largely relates to the nature of immune complex deposition at various sites in the kidney. At a histologic level, renal involvement may be classified as membranous nephritis, focal or diffuse nephritis, or mesangial nephritis. Other than the glomeruli, the tubules, interstitium, and blood vessels may be involved. From the clinician's point of view, these lesions are difficult to distinguish clinically. More importantly, one must search for the presence of renal involvement at frequent intervals. This is best accomplished by urinalysis looking for protein, hematuria, red cell casts, and abnormalities in the specific gravity patterns over time. One must also obtain BUN and creatinine, 24-hour urine for creatinine clearance and protein at periodic intervals. Hypertension may also direct the clinician to the presence of renal disease.To complicate the clinical picture, histologic evidence of renal pathology may be present even when all the above clinical parameters are normal. Early biopsy is advocated by many rheumatologists, as is the careful serologic evaluation of these patients.

Additional clinical findings in SLE include lymphadenopathy with or without hepatosplenomegaly, hepatitis, anemia, leukopenia, thrombocytopenia, disorders of esophageal motility, pancreatitis, malabsorption, diarrhea, and abdominal pain. Lupus is also reported to occur in infants of mothers with the disease. IgG is passed by the placenta to the fetus leading to positive serologies and findings of lupus. The presence of rash, thrombocytopenia, hemolytic anemia, and congenital heart block should suggest the diagnosis. Fortunately, neonatal lupus is short-lived, lasting only a few months.

Perhaps more than any other collagen vascular disease, the clinical diagnosis of lupus can be confirmed serologically. The ANAs represent a group of antibodies found in serum which are directed against antigens within the cellular nuclei of lupus patients. These antibodies combine with their respective nuclear antigens to form immune complexes. Many of these immune complexes go on to cause the histopathology and symptomatology of lupus. The well described lupus erythematosus (LE) cell is simply a reflection of this pathologic mechanism. Because the ANA test can now directly detect DNP, the LE cell is only significant from a historical perspective.

Other antibodies found in SLE patients are listed in Figure 7.37. Anti-native DNA (NDNA) antibodies are detected in 50 to 60 percent of lupus patients, but of note is the fact that they are rarely found in non-lupus patients. Antibodies to single-stranded DNA (SSDNA) are also present in SLE; however, their presence in many other entities limits their clinical utility. Ribonucleoprotein (RNP), while better known for its presence in high titers in mixed connective tissue disease, is also seen in low titers in 30 to 40 percent of lupus patients. Other SLE antibodies include SS-A and SS-B (Sjögren syndrome), also known as Ro and La, respectively. Lastly, one finds antibodies to Sm antigen, a nonhistone antigen which appears to be very specific for lupus.

In summary, SLE is a chronic disease with a variable course and with periods of varying degrees of activity. While the mortality and morbidity remain high, marked improvement in prognosis has occurred in recent years.

ACKNOWLEDGMENTS

Thanks to Bernard Cohen, John Zitelli, A'Delbert Bowen, Basil Zitelli, J. Carlton Gartner, Jr., Jeffrey Malatack, Joseph McGuire, Holly Davis, Virginia Steen, Joseph Warnicki, Albert Biglan, Susan Gelnett, and Mary Killian for their valuable assistance with photographs and text.

BIBLIOGRAPHY

Cassidy JT: Textbook of Pediatric Rheumatology. Wiley, New York, 1982.

Kelley WN et al: Textbook of Rheumatology. Saunders, Philadelphia, 1981.

Schaller JG: Juvenile rheumatoid arthritis. Pediatrics in Review 2(6): 163–174, 1980.

Silber D: Henoch-Schoenlein syndrome, Pediatr Clin North Am 19(4), 1972.

Tan EM: Antinuclear antibodies in diagnosis and management. Hosp Prac Jan: 79–84, 1983.

Wedgewood RJ: The pediatric arthritides. Hosp Prac June: 83–97, 1977.

PEDIATRIC DERMATOLOGY

Susan B. Mallory, M.D.
John A. Zitelli, M.D.

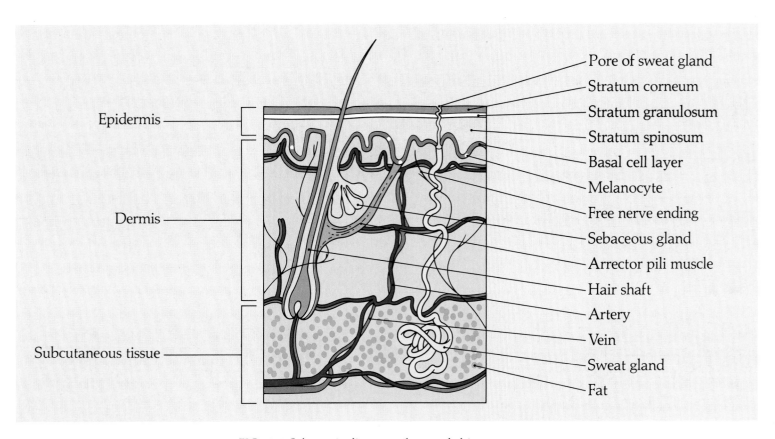

Epidermis

Dermis

Subcutaneous tissue

Pore of sweat gland
Stratum corneum
Stratum granulosum
Stratum spinosum
Basal cell layer
Melanocyte
Free nerve ending
Sebaceous gland
Arrector pili muscle
Hair shaft
Artery
Vein
Sweat gland
Fat

FIG. 8.1 Schematic diagram of normal skin anatomy.

Most of us think of our skin as a simple, durable covering for our skeleton and internal organs. However, the skin is actually a very complex organ, consisting of many parts and appendages (Fig. 8.1). The outermost stratum corneum is an effective barrier to the penetration of irritants, toxins, and organisms, as well as a membrane that holds in body fluids. The remainder of the epidermis manufactures this protective layer. Melanocytes within the epidermis are important in protecting us from the harmful effects of ultraviolet light, and Langerhans' cells are one of the body's first lines of immunologic defense. The dermis (largely fibroblasts and collagen) is a tough, leathery, mechanical barrier against cuts, bites, and bruises, and it also holds sebaceous glands and other vital appendages. Hair follicles are important not only for cosmetic purposes, but provide protection from sweat and particulate matter that would otherwise cause a constant visual problem. Nails are specialized organs of manipulation that also protect sensitive digits. Thermoregulation of the skin is accomplished by eccrine (sweat) glands as well as changes in the cutaneous blood flow, regulated by glomus cells. The skin also holds specialized receptors for heat, pain, touch, and pressure. Beneath the dermis, in the subcutaneous tissue, fat acts as stored energy and as a soft, protective cushion.

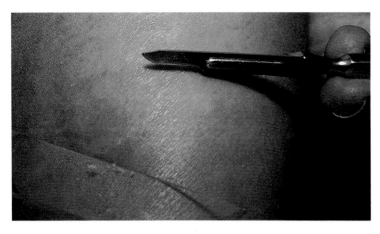
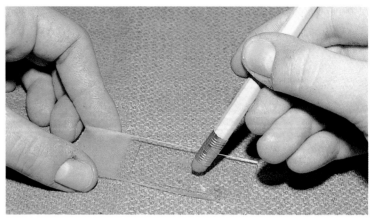

FIG. 8.2 Potassium hydroxide (KOH) preparation. (Left) Small scales should be scraped from the edge of lesion onto a micro-scope slide. (Right) Crush the scales to make a thin layer of cells, in order to easily visualize the fungus.

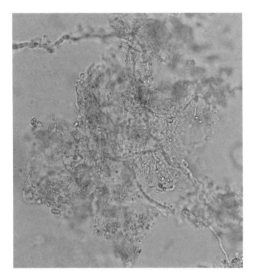
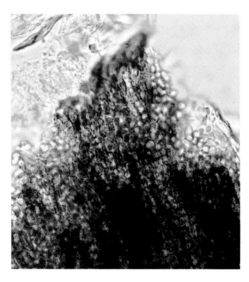
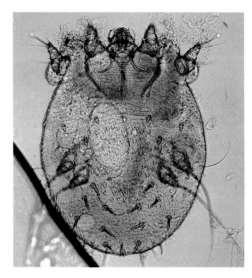

FIG. 8.3 Microscopic appearance of skin scrapings prepared with KOH. Fungal hyphae are long, branching rods at the margins and center of the scales.

FIG. 8.4 Microscopic appearance of a hair shaft infected with fungus. Note the tight packing of fungal arthrospores that causes hair shaft fragility and breakage (KOH mount – endothrix).

FIG. 8.5 Microscopic appearance of adult scabies mite. Note the small oval egg within the body.

Defects or alteration in any component of the skin may result in serious systemic disease or death. Each and every part of the skin can be affected by congenital, inflammatory, infectious, and degenerative disorders and tumors. For example, an altered stratum corneum is seen in ichthyosis, melanocytes are selectively destroyed in vitiligo, the epidermis proliferates in psoriasis, excess collagen is produced in connective tissue nevus of tuberous sclerosis, hair is preferentially infested by certain fungi, and the list goes on.

In addition, the skin is affected by many systemic diseases and may thus be a marker for internal disorders. A skin examination may show vasculitis, explaining a child's hematuria, or the white macules of tuberous sclerosis may give insight into the cause of seizures.

The skin is the most accessible and easily examined organ of the body, and is the organ of most frequent concern to the patient. Therefore, all physicians should be able to recognize basic skin diseases and dermatologic clues to systemic disease, understand the pathophysiology, and know where to turn for treatment.

DIAGNOSTIC TECHNIQUES
Potassium Hydroxide Preparations

There are a number of simple, noninvasive, definitive diagnostic techniques in dermatology. One of the most useful tests is a wet mount of skin scrapings for microscopic examination. Twenty percent potassium hydroxide (KOH) is used to change the optical properties of the material and make the scales more transparent. The technique requires practice and patience. The first step is to obtain material by scraping the loose scales at the margin of a lesion (Fig. 8.2), subungual debris, or the small pearly globules within a molluscum papule. Hair stubs or root ends of easily removed hairs should be removed with a forceps or the point of a scalpel. Scales should be mounted onto the center of the slide, and one or two drops of 20 percent KOH added. Next, apply a glass coverslip and gently press it with the eraser end of a pencil to crush the scales. Warm the slide with a match, taking care not to boil the KOH solution, and again crush the scales. View under a microscope, with the condenser and light at low levels to maximize contrast, and with the objec-

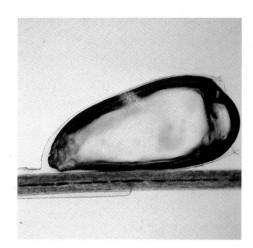

FIG. 8.6 Microscopic appearance of the nit of a head louse attached to scalp hair. Microscopic examination distinguishes nits from hair casts and other artifacts.

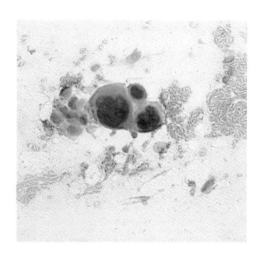

FIG. 8.7 Tzanck preparation. Note the multinucleated giant cells characteristic of viral infection.

tive at 10×. Focus up and down continuously. True hyphae are long-branching rods of uniform width that cross the borders of epidermal cells (Fig. 8.3). They often contain septa. False positives may be vegetable fibers, cell borders, or other artifacts. Yeast infections show both budding yeast cells and pseudohyphae. Molluscum bodies are oval discs that have homogeneous cytoplasm and are slightly larger than keratinocytes. The microscopic appearance of fungi in the hair consists of packed spores within or surrounding the hair shaft (Fig. 8.4). Hyphae are less commonly seen on the hair.

Scabies Preparation

A skin scraping showing a mite, egg, or feces is necessary to diagnose infestation with *Acarus scabiei*, because many other skin diseases resemble scabies clinically. The most important factor for obtaining a successful scraping is choice of site. Burrows and papules are most likely to be identified on the wrists, finger webs, or elbows. A fresh burrow can be identified as a 5- to 10-mm raised mound, with a small dark spot, resembling a fleck of pepper, at one end. This spot is the mite, and it can be lifted out of the burrow with a needle or the point of a scalpel. If a scalpel is used to scrape the burrow, it is worthwhile to place a drop of mineral oil onto the skin to ensure adherence of the scrapings to the scalpel. The scrapings are placed on a slide, another drop of mineral oil is added, and a coverslip is applied. Mites are eight-legged arachnids easily seen with the scanning power of the microscope (Fig. 8.5). Care must be taken to focus through thick areas of skin scrapings, so as not to miss camouflaged mites. The presence of eggs (smooth ovals, approximately one-half the size of an adult mite) or feces (red-brown pellets, often seen in clusters) is also diagnostic.

Lice Preparation

Lice are six-legged insects visible to the unaided eye; they are commonly found on the scalp, eyelashes, and pubic areas. Pubic lice are short and broad, with claws spaced far apart to grasp the sparse hairs on the trunk, pubic area, or eyelashes. Scalp lice are long and thin, with claws closer together to grasp the denser hairs found on the head. These lice are best identified close to the skin, where eggs are more numerous and more obvious. Diagnosis can be made by identifying the louse, or by plucking hairs and confirming the presence of nits by microscopic examination (Fig. 8.6).

Tzanck Smear

The Tzanck smear is an important diagnostic tool in the evaluation of blistering diseases. It is most commonly used to distinguish viral diseases, such as herpes simplex, varicella, and herpes zoster, from nonviral disorders. The smear is obtained by removing the roof of the blister with a scalpel or scissors, and scraping the base of the blister to obtain the moist, cloudy debris. The debris is spread on a glass slide with a small drop of saline, air-dried, and stained with Giemsa or Wright stain. The diagnostic finding of viral blisters is the multinucleated giant cell (Fig. 8.7). The giant cell is a syncytium of epidermal cells, with multiple overlapping nuclei; it is much larger than other inflammatory cells. A giant cell may be mistaken for multiple epidermal cells piled on one another.

Wood's Light

Wood's light is an ultraviolet source that emits at a wavelength of 365 nm. Formerly, its most common use was in screening patients for fungal alopecia, because the most common causative organism, *Microsporum audouini*, was easily identified by its fluorescence under Wood's light. Today, *Trichophyton tonsurans* is the fungus that most often causes hair loss, but it does not fluoresce. Currently, the only important alopecic fungus that fluoresces is *M. canis*; hair infected with this organism fluoresces bright blue-green. However, the most useful diagnostic test for fungal disease of the scalp is the KOH smear.

Wood's light is still of value in diagnosing a number of other diseases. Erythrasma is a superficial bacterial infection of moist skin in the groin or axilla. It appears as a brown or red flat plaque, and is caused by Corynebacterium that excretes a pigment. This pigment fluoresces coral red or pink under Wood's light. Tinea versicolor, a superficial fungal infection with hypopigmented macules and plaques on the trunk, also fluoresces under Wood's light with a green-yellow color. Pseudomonas infection of the toe web spaces will fluoresce yellow-green. Patients with porphyria cutanea tarda excrete uroporphyrins in their urine, and examination of a urine specimen will show an orange-yellow fluorescence. Adequate blood levels of tetracycline produce yellow fluorescence in the opening of hair follicles, while lack of fluorescence indicates poor intestinal absorption or poor patient compliance.

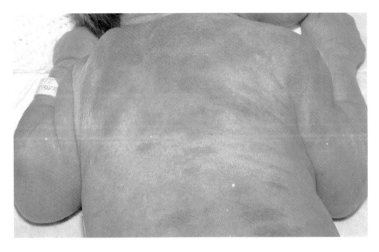

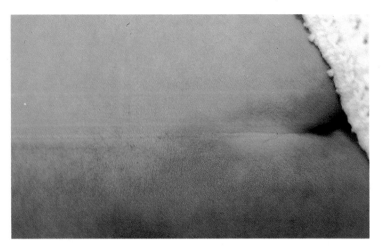

FIG. 8.8 Erythema toxicum neonatorum. Tiny central yellow pustules surrounded by intense erythema.

FIG. 8.9 Mongolian spot. Typical slate-gray lesion is located over the lumbosacral area of this black infant.

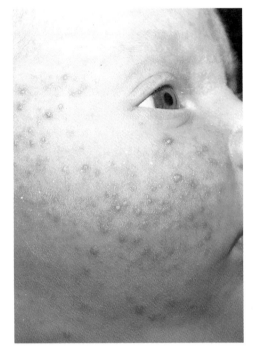

FIG. 8.10 Neonatal acne. Red papules and pustules are present over the nose and cheeks of this infant.

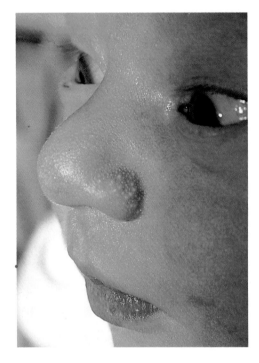

FIG. 8.11 Sebaceous gland hyperplasia. Note the yellowish papules on the nose of this infant.

NEONATAL DERMATOLOGY

The skin of the newborn differs from that of the adult in several ways: It is less hairy, has fewer sweat and sebaceous gland secretions, is thinner, and has weaker intercellular attachments. During the neonatal period (the first 4 weeks of life), common rashes or skin abnormalities may develop which need to be differentiated from the more serious cutaneous disorders. Transient phenomena include erythema toxicum neonatorum and transient neonatal pustular melanosis. More serious diseases include Letterer-Siwe disease, because it involves other organ systems, and staphylococcal scalded skin syndrome, because of potential fluid and electrolyte disturbances and life-threatening infection.

Erythema toxicum neonatorum (Fig. 8.8) is a benign, self-limited asymptomatic disorder of unknown etiology. It occurs in up to 50 percent of term infants, and there is no racial or sexual predisposition. Lesions usually begin 24 to 48 hours after birth, but may appear from birth up to the tenth day of life. Erythema toxicum neonatorum has been described as

"flea-bite" dermatosis of the newborn because the intense erythema with a central papule or pustule resembles a flea bite. Composed of blotchy macules, the lesions are typically 2 to 3 cm in diameter. There may be a few to several hundred lesions on the back, face, chest, and extremities, while the palms and soles are usually spared. The eruption fades within 5 to 7 days. A smear of material from the central pustule reveals numerous eosinophils; a circulating eosinophilia may also be present in up to 20 percent of patients. No treatment is necessary. Differential diagnosis includes transient neonatal pustular melanosis, staphylococcal folliculitis (see Chapter 12), milia neonatorum, miliaria rubra, and herpes simplex (see Chapter 12).

Mongolian spots are flat, slate-gray to blue-black, poorly circumscribed lesions. They are most commonly located over the lumbosacral area and buttocks (Fig. 8.9), although they can be seen anywhere on the body. The spots may be large or small, single or multiple. Ninety percent of black infants, 81 percent of Oriental infants, and 9.6 percent of white newborns have these spots, which are accumulations of melano-

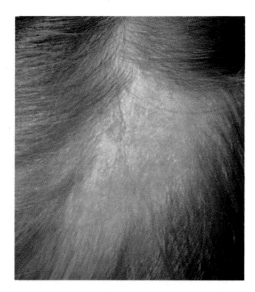

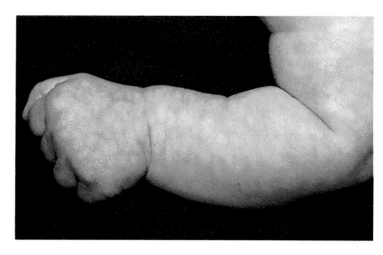

FIG. 8.12
Sebaceous nevus of
Jadassohn. A
yellowish hairless
plaque has been
present since birth.

FIG. 8.13 Cutis marmorata. Note the reticulated bluish mottling of this infant's arm.

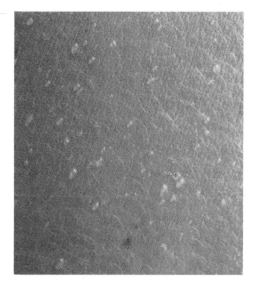

FIG. 8.14 Miliaria
crystallina. Tiny,
thin-walled vesicles
quickly desquamat-
ed when the child
was in a cooler en-
vironment.

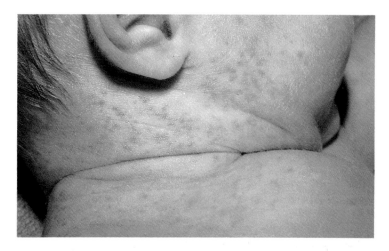

FIG. 8.15 Miliaria rubra. The red papules of prickly heat are clearly visible on this infant.

cytes deep within the dermis. Because this is a benign condition, therapy is not necessary; the spots usually fade by age 7.

Neonates can develop **acne vulgaris** in the first few weeks of life. This condition is thought to be secondary to stimulation of the sebaceous glands and induction of abnormal keratinization of the hair follicles by maternal androgens. Lesions appear as comedones, papules, and pustules over the cheeks, forehead, and upper chest (Fig. 8.10). Therapy is rarely required; the acne usually resolves spontaneously over 4 to 8 weeks. The likelihood of developing adolescent acne in these children is unknown.

Sebaceous gland hyperplasia is a common entity consisting of multiple 1- to 2-cm papules, usually located over the nose and cheeks of term infants (Fig. 8.11). It is a normal physiologic response to maternal androgenic stimulation of sebaceous gland growth. Lesions resolve spontaneously by 4 to 6 months.

Sebaceous nevus of Jadassohn is characterized by a hairless, well circumscribed skin-colored or yellowish plaque located on the scalp (Fig. 8.12), face, or neck. The lesion is usually solitary, and may be linear or round. It is most often present at birth, although at puberty the plaque may become more verrucous, raised, and nodular. Approximately 10 to 15 percent of these nevi develop secondary neoplasms; the most

common associated tumor is basal cell carcinoma, although other appendageal tumors have been reported. Long-term regular observation or prophylactic full-thickness excision is necessary.

Cutis marmorata (Fig. 8.13) is a net-like reddish-blue mottling of the skin due to vascular contraction and dilatation. It is a normal response to chilling, and upon rewarming, normal skin color returns. The discoloration is seen primarily over the trunk and extremities in infants. In neonates the condition is benign; if mottling persists beyond 6 months of life, it may be a sign of congenital hypothyroidism.

Miliaria crystallina are clear, very superficial 1- to 2-mm vesicles (Fig. 8.14), resulting from obstruction of the eccrine glands, with sweat retention in the epidermis. The lesions can develop in neonates over the head, neck, and upper trunk, and in older children within areas of sunburn. The lesions rupture spontaneously and leave a tiny white scale.

Miliaria rubra (prickly heat) is characterized by 2- to 4-mm erythematous papules or papulovesicles (Fig. 8.15). It is caused by deeper obstruction of the eccrine ducts, and leakage of sweat into the surrounding dermis, with subsequent inflammation. The rash is more commonly found in flexural areas. Avoidance of excessive heat and humidity will prevent new lesions; existing lesions heal spontaneously.

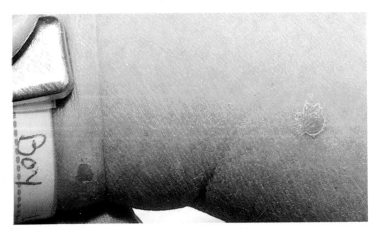

FIG. 8.16 Transient neonatal pustular melanosis. Characteristic hyperpigmented lesion with a tiny collarette of scale on the extremity.

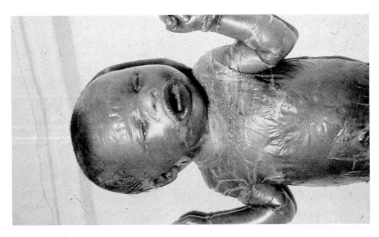

FIG. 8.17 Collodion baby. A shiny transparent membrane covered this baby at birth; she later developed lamellar ichthyosis. Note the ectropion and eclabium.

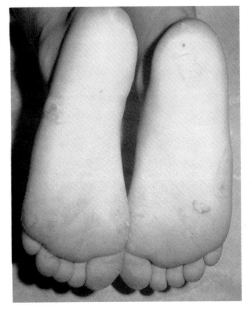

FIG. 8.18 Epidermolysis bullosa (simplex). Numerous blisters form easily in pressure areas.

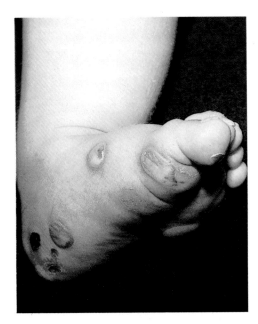

FIG. 8.19 Epidermolysis bullosa (mild junctional form). Areas of friction develop recurrent blisters, some with hemorrhage and secondary infection.

Transient neonatal pustular melanosis (TNPM) (Fig. 8.16) is a self-limited dermatosis of unknown etiology. The rash usually presents at birth with 1- to 2-mm vesiculopustules or ruptured pustules which disappear in 24 to 48 hours, leaving pigmented macules with a collarette of scale. Lesions may appear anywhere on the body, but are most often seen on the neck, forehead, lower back, and legs. Wright stain of a pustular smear shows numerous neutrophils, and Gram stain and culture are negative for bacteria. The hyperpigmentation fades in 3 weeks to 3 months; TNPM is a benign disorder and requires no therapy. Differential diagnosis is similar to that of erythema toxicum neonatorum.

The **collodion membrane** is a rare disorder in which at birth the entire skin is encased in a a thin, parchment-like membrane (Fig. 8.17). The membrance dries out and is shed in large sheet-like layers within a few days. Fluid and electrolyte losses can occur, and there is usually residual erythema and hyperkeratosis. In addition, ectropion and eclabium may develop. Most infants born with a collodion membrane develop lamellar ichthyosis after the membrane is shed.

Epidermolysis bullosa (EB) is a group of inherited mechanobullous disorders characterized by the development of blisters following mild friction or trauma. There are three general types: simplex, junctional, and dystrophic (scarring). These types are classified according to where blister formation takes place. Each type has several subgroups, and all types typically present in the newborn with blistering.

Epidermolysis bullosa simplex (Fig. 8.18) can present with mild or marked blistering. It can be generalized over the entire body, or localized to the hands and feet. It is inherited as an autosomal-dominant trait, and there is no scarring. Secondary infection is the most common complication. Blister formation takes place in the basal cell layer of the epidermis.

Junctional epidermolysis bullosa is inherited as an autosomal-recessive trait and usually presents at birth with bullae and erosions in a generalized distribution. The most common form is usually fatal within the first year due to sepsis and fluid loss. A milder subtype resembles generalized EB simplex (Fig. 8.19). Blisters form at the junction of the epidermis and dermis.

The scarring forms of EB are divided into dominant and recessive types. In both types, scars form after the blisters heal, and milia are common. The dominant form results in

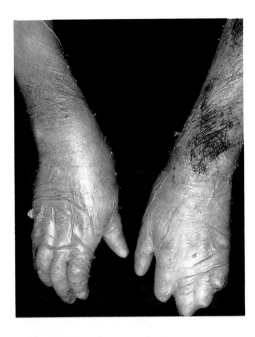

FIG. 8.20 Epidermolysis bullosa (recessive dystrophic form). The fingers are encased with epidermis, with resulting syndactyly.

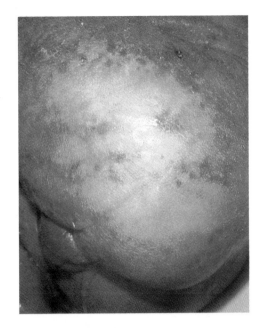

FIG. 8.21 Incontinentia pigmenti (papular phase). Linear streaks of red papules often overlap the bullous and hyperpigmented phase.

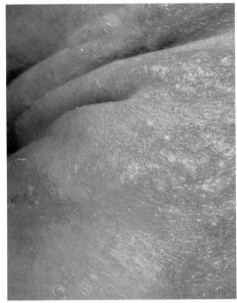

FIG. 8.22 Incontinentia pigmenti (bullous phase). Blisters and crusts that were not induced by trauma.

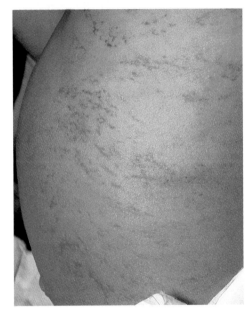

FIG. 8.23 Incontinentia pigmenti (hyperpigmented phase). Swirled hyperpigmented lesions on the trunk of an older girl.

much less scarring than the recessive form; patients with the latter show retardation in growth and development, severe oral blisters, loss of nails, and sometimes syndactyly (Fig. 8.20). The plane of cleavage is in the upper portion of the dermis. A skin biopsy is helpful in distinguishing among the three general types, and is also helpful in determining prognosis. Treatment is symptomatic and supportive, and genetic counseling is advised.

Incontinentia pigmenti (IP) is an X-linked dominant disorder that affects the skin and can involve the central nervous system (CNS), eyes, and skeletal system. It is seen predominantly in females and thus is thought to be fatal to males in utero. Clinically, the disorder may present in any of three general phases, which usually overlap. In the first phase, inflammatory vesicles or bullae appear on the trunk and extremities (Fig. 8.21), generally within the first 2 weeks of life. There is usually a circulating peripheral eosinophilia present. The blistering episodes can recur over the first 3 months of life. A skin biopsy shows characteristic inflammation with intraepidermal eosinophils. The blistering phase is usually present with the second phase, which is marked by irregular papular lesions (Fig. 8.22), usually located over the extremities. These lesions resolve spontaneously within several months. A characteristic swirling or streaking brown to blue-gray pigmentation on the trunk or extremities marks the third phase (Fig. 8.23), which is most often located in a different area from the first two phases. The pigmentation lasts for many years, and then gradually fades.

Systemic manifestations are seen in many patients with IP. Thirty percent have CNS abnormalities, such as seizures, mental retardation, and spasticity. Ophthalmic complications are seen in 35 percent of IP patients. Pegged teeth, delayed dentition, and other skeletal defects are seen in 65 percent. Cardiac and skeletal malformations have also been reported.

Differential diagnosis of IP in the blistering stage includes herpes simplex, bullous impetigo, and EB. Warts or epidermal nevi may mimic the warty phase. The swirled pigmentation of the third phase is very characteristic and not likely to be confused with other hyperpigmentation disorders. No specific therapy is required for IP, but genetic counseling is advised.

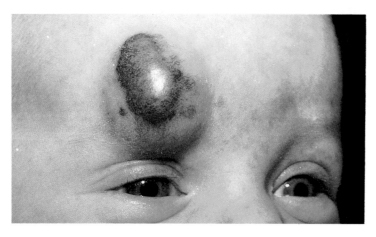

FIG. 8.24 Capillary hemangioma. This lesion, which was not present at birth, became raised in the first few months of life.

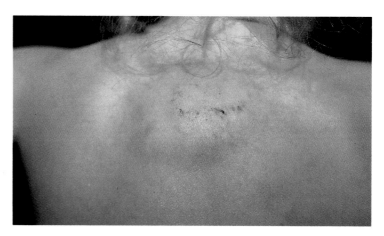

FIG. 8.25 Cavernous hemangioma. Note deep blue color in this large cavernous hemangioma.

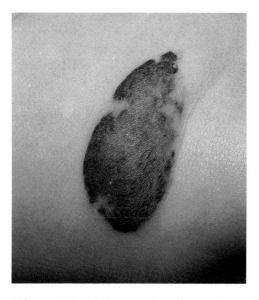
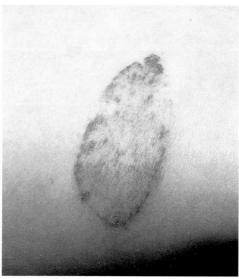
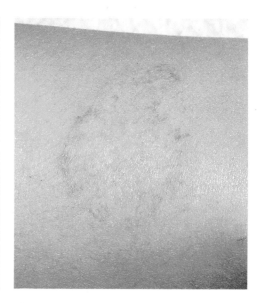

FIG. 8.26 Resolving capillary hemangioma. (Left) Appearance at age 5 months. (Middle) Appearance at 2½ years. (Right) Almost total resolution at age 5 years.

VASCULAR LESIONS

Congenital vascular malformations (**hemangiomas**) are the most common neoplasms of childhood, occurring in 10 to 40 percent of newborns. These lesions arise when islands of angioblastic tissue fail to reestablish normal communication with the vascular system. Hemangiomas can be divided into two groups, raised and flat, depending on their architecture. They are of developmental origin, and although family members may be affected, hemangiomas are not thought to be inherited.

Skin overlying the capillary hemangioma (sometimes called "strawberry hemangioma") is usually normal or slightly red at birth. Within the first few months of life, there is marked vascular overgrowth with definite elevation above the skin's surface (Fig. 8.24). Lesions are soft and compressible, and range in size from 0.5 to 4 cm, though they can be much larger, involving the entire face or extremity.

Cavernous hemangiomas, another type of raised hemangiomas, are so named because the vessels they comprise are deep beneath the surface of the skin and appear bluish in color (Fig. 8.25). The borders are usually indistinct. The lesion feels like a doughy mass and is only partially compres-

sible. Combined capillary and cavernous hemangiomas are common.

The natural history of raised hemangiomas is one of rapid growth for approximately 1 year, followed by a plateau period during which the lesion remains the same size, and then slow involution (Fig. 8.26). Fifty percent of raised hemangiomas disappear by age 7, and 90 percent have vanished by age 9. The skin overlying the resolved lesion shows mild redundancy with telangiectasis.

Unless the hemangioma involves a vital structure, watchful waiting is the best therapy. Steroids or surgical intervention may be indicated if the lesion is life-threatening or if it interferes with vital functions, for example, vision. Complications such as ulceration, bleeding, or infection occur infrequently. Ulcers can be treated with wet compresses and topical antibacterial ointments. Ulceration frequently hastens resolution of the lesion as it heals.

Port wine stains are flat hemangiomas present at birth. Unlike capillary hemangiomas, these lesions do not enlarge rapidly in the first few months of life, but tend to remain stable and flat. In adults, small angiomatous papules may develop within the lesion over time. The discoloration is a permanent dilatation of mature capillaries. Most commonly,

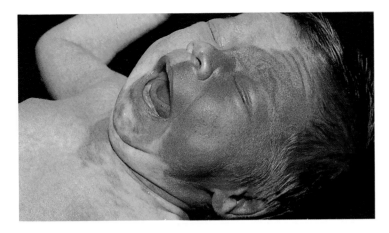

FIG. 8.27 *Port wine stain. The unilateral reddened area on the face was present at birth; it darkens with crying.*

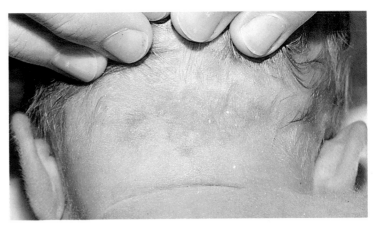

FIG. 8.28 *Nevus flammeus. A typical, light red splotchy area is seen at the nape of the neck.*

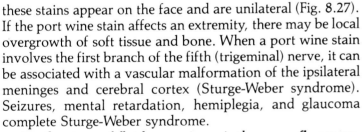

FIG. 8.29 *Pyogenic granuloma. A quickly growing friable lesion is present between the fingers.*

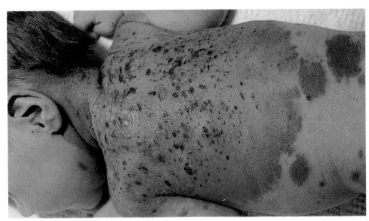

FIG. 8.30 *Giant congenital nevocytic nevus. The CNN in this infant shows speckled pigmentation and numerous small satellite nevi.*

these stains appear on the face and are unilateral (Fig. 8.27). If the port wine stain affects an extremity, there may be local overgrowth of soft tissue and bone. When a port wine stain involves the first branch of the fifth (trigeminal) nerve, it can be associated with a vascular malformation of the ipsilateral meninges and cerebral cortex (Sturge-Weber syndrome). Seizures, mental retardation, hemiplegia, and glaucoma complete Sturge-Weber syndrome.

Another type of flat hemangioma is the **nevus flammeus,** or "salmon patch" (Fig. 8.28). This lesion is seen in 40 percent of newborns, and is usually located at the nape of the neck, glabella, forehead, or upper eyelids. The patches represent distended capillaries and tend to fade within the first year of life. They may become more apparent during episodes of crying, breath-holding, or physical exertion.

Pyogenic granuloma (Fig. 8.29) is a common, benign vascular tumor resembling a small hemangioma; it is usually seen in children and young adults. Lesions are 5- to 6-mm solitary, bright red, soft nodules; they are often pedunculated. The surface is friable and bleeds easily. The rapid growth of these tumors causes them to be confused with malignancies such as melanomas. Pyogenic granuloma is thought to be induced by trauma, with vascular overgrowth of the granulation tissue. Treatment consists of electrodesiccation of the blood vessels at the base; occasionally, the lesion will recur, and repeat surgery is recommended.

CUTANEOUS NEVI

The term "nevus" has two meanings in dermatology. The more common use refers to a nevocytic nevus, a benign tumor composed of nevus cells (melanocytes); the less common use refers to a congenital skin lesion composed of mature or nearly mature structures (hamartoma), without the presence of nevus cells. Examples of this latter type of nevus are eccrine nevus, nevus sebaceous, and epidermal nevus.

Nevocytic Nevi and Melanomas

Nevocytic nevi can be congenital or acquired. Congenital nevocytic nevi (CNN) are pigmented plaques, usually with dense hair growth (Fig. 8.30). At birth, the lesion may be tan or light pink with only soft vellus hairs. During infancy the nevus darkens, and hair becomes prominent. Small dark macules eventually appear within the large plaque. Giant CNN over large areas of skin are associated with a 10 to 15 percent incidence of melanoma. Early treatment is recommended by full-thickness, prophylactic excision and grafting. It is not sufficient to delay treatment and observe for signs of melanoma, because melanomas may occur in early childhood, arising deep within the skin without visible surface changes. Small CNN may also be associated with a higher than normal risk of developing melanoma, but the in-

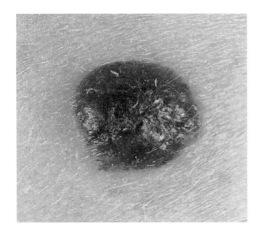

FIG. 8.31 *Acquired compound nevus. This typical acquired compound nevus shows a regular border and uniform pigmentation.*

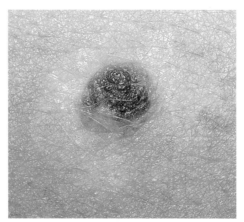

FIG. 8.32 *Halo nevus. The ring of depigmentation surrounds a normal compound nevus. This reaction is often followed by disappearance of the nevus and eventual repigmentation of the surrounding skin.*

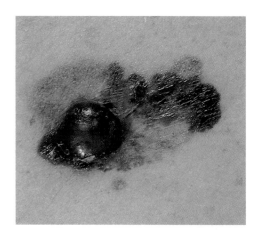

FIG. 8.33 *Melanoma. This lesion shows variation in outline, color, and thickness, typical of a melanoma.*

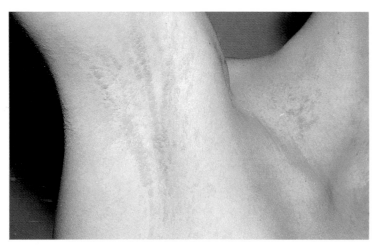

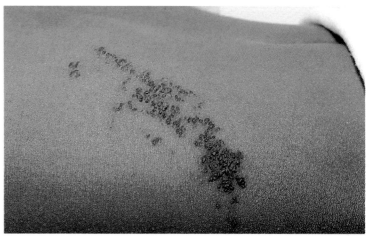

FIG. 8.34 *Localized epidermal nevus.* (Left) *Light color in whites.* (Right) *Darker color in blacks. More extensive nevi may be associated with systemic abnormalities (epidermal nevus syndrome).*

cidence is unknown, and there are no uniformly accepted guidelines for treatment.

All CNN must be differentiated from the congenital pigmented spots such as urticaria pigmentosa, lentigines, café au lait spots, and mongolian spots.

Nevocytic nevi acquired after birth are often referred to as "moles;" these begin in early childhood as small flat macules 1 to 2 mm in diameter, most common on sun-exposed areas. At this stage, the nevus cells are limited to the epidermal–dermal junction and are called junctional nevi. The lesions enlarge slowly and become papular or even pedunculated (Fig. 8.31). These elevated nevi represent a proliferation of nevus cells into the dermis (either intradermal or compound nevi). Noticeable darkening and increase in size may be noted during puberty, but normal nevocytic nevi rarely exceed 1 cm in diameter. They are less common on the soles, palms, legs, genitalia, and mucous membranes; typical nevi in these locations need not be removed if they can be distinguished clinically from melanoma. Sudden enlargement of a nevus with redness and tenderness may alarm the patient and necessitate dermatologic evaluation. This change often occurs because of infection of a hair follicle within the nevus, or the rupture of a follicular cyst with acute foreign body in-

flammation. Another, slower change causing concern in patients is the appearance of a hypopigmented ring and mild local pruritus around a benign nevus. This is called a halo nevus (Fig. 8.32), and is caused by a cytotoxic T-lymphocyte reaction against both the nevus cells and the innocent melanocytic bystanders. The nevus may disappear partially or completely, and the halo eventually repigments. As long as the clinical appearance of the nevus is not atypical, excision is unnecessary.

Other changes in pigmented lesions may portend the development of melanoma (Fig. 8.33). The most important clinical features of melanoma include:

1. A change in size, shape, or outline, with scalloped irregular borders
2. A change in the surface characteristics, such as development of a small, dark, elevated papule or nodule within an otherwise flat plaque; or flaking, scaling, ulceration, or bleeding
3. A change in color, with the appearance of black, brown, or mixing of red, white, or blue
4. Burning, itching, or tenderness, which may be an indication of the body's immune reaction to malignancy

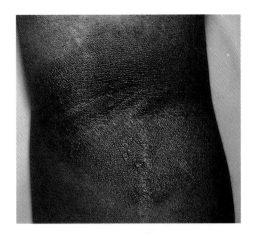

FIG. 8.35 Postinflammatory hyperpigmentation following chronic atopic dermatitis and trauma from persistent scratching.

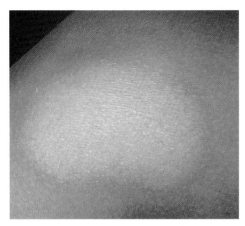

FIG. 8.36 Postinflammatory hypopigmentation following chronic dermatitis. Note the narrow rim of hyperpigmentation at the margin.

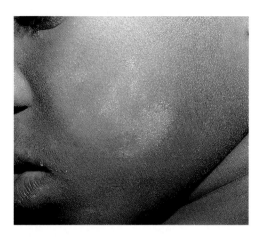

FIG. 8.37 Pityriasis alba. Fine superficial scales can be seen on the cheeks.

Fortunately, melanomas are very rare in children; but the incidence of melanoma is increasing, and curative treatment is contingent on early diagnosis. Therefore, an awareness of diagnostic features is important.

Melanomas in children may occur de novo, or they may develop within a giant congenital nevus; the latter is the most common cause of melanoma in children. Another cause of melanoma in the pediatric age group is transplacental transfer of maternal melanomas. Thus, neonates born to mothers with a history of melanoma should be examined and followed carefully. Likewise, mothers of infants with melanoma should be examined thoroughly for signs of the lesion.

Differential diagnosis of childhood melanoma includes congenital and acquired nevocytic nevi; blue nevus, a small, firm, blue papule of the deep nevus cells; traumatic hemorrhage, especially under the nails or in mucous membranes; vascular lesions, such as pyogenic granuloma or angiokeratoma; Spitz nevus (benign juvenile melanoma), a red and rapidly growing nevocytic nevus that can be confused clinically and histologically with melanoma.

Hamartomatous Nevi

Developmental defects of the skin can result in abnormal growth of skin appendages. When the defect is limited to the epidermis, it is called an epidermal nevus. Hamartomatous nevi can affect the hair follicles (nevus pilosis), apocrine and eccrine glands (apocrine and eccrine nevi), fibroblasts (connective tissue nevi), blood vessels (nevus flammeus), and multiple components (nevus sebaceous). The epidermal nevus (Fig. 8.34) is not a rare pediatric finding and must be distinguished from nevus sebaceous. The lesion presents at birth or during childhood as a slightly hyperpigmented and papillomatous or verrucous growth. It may be small and localized, linear, dermatomal, or generalized. The numerous clinical presentations are reflected in the number of descriptive synonyms: nevus verrucosus for localized disease, nevus unius lateralis for linear or unilateral involvement, and ichthyosis hystrix for bilateral involvement with irregular geometric patterns. Important associations with extensive epidermal nevi are seizures, mental retardation, and ocular and skeletal defects (epidermal nevus syndrome).

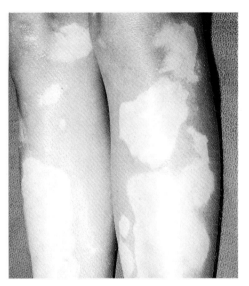

FIG. 8.38 Vitiligo. Depigmented patches on the legs. Occasionally, macules of repigmentation arise from epidermal appendages within the white patches. A characteristic distribution helps to distinguish vitiligo from other causes of hypopigmentation.

PIGMENTATION DISORDERS

Childhood disorders of pigmentation are usually of cosmetic importance only, although some pigmented lesions are markers of multisystem disease.

The most common pigmentation disorder is postinflammatory **hyperpigmentation** (Fig. 8.35) or **hypopigmentation** (Fig. 8.36). This alteration in normal pigmentation follows some inflammatory disorders of the skin, such as dermatitis, infection, or injury. It usually resolves spontaneously in a few months. Melanocytes are normal in these areas, although the dispersion of melanin and pigment to other cells is disturbed. A common form of hypopigmentation in children is seen on the cheeks or trunk as one or more large patches, 2 to 4 cm in diameter, with a fine surface scale. This scaling white patch is known as **pityriasis alba** (Fig. 8.37) and is a mild form of dermatitis that responds slowly to topical steroids. Tinea versicolor may also present with hypopigmented patches with a fine scale, but KOH examination will confirm the correct diagnosis by demonstrating typical "spaghetti and meatballs" organisms. Postinflammatory hypopigmentation must be distinguished from vitiligo, which is not usually associated with scaling or prior inflammation. **Vitiligo** (Fig. 8.38) appears as completely depigmented ma-

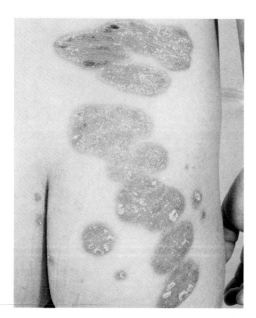

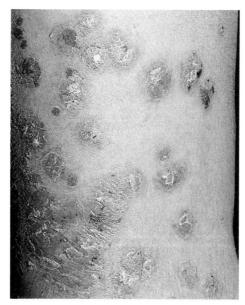

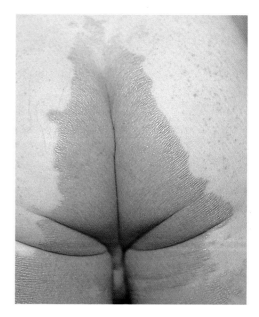

FIG. 8.39 Psoriasis. Typical erythematous plaques are topped by a silver scale.

FIG. 8.40 Guttate psoriasis. Small plaques with typical scales quickly developed in a generalized distribution after a streptococcal pharyngitis.

FIG. 8.41 Psoriasis. Persistent diaper dermatitis that did not resolve with routine treatment. Note the lack of scale in the diaper area.

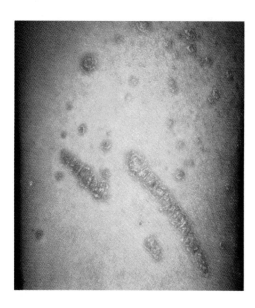

FIG. 8.42 Koebner's response in psoriasis. Lesions frequently develop in areas of trauma, as in these scratch marks.

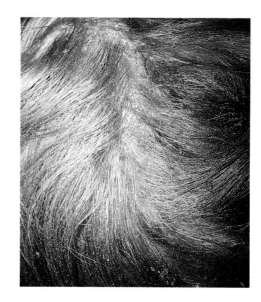

FIG. 8.43 Seborrhea. Typical "cradle cap" with greasy scale.

cules in a characteristic distribution around the eyes, mouth, genitals, elbows, hands, and feet. Spontaneous, but slow, repigmentation may occur in areas beginning around the opening of a hair follicle, resulting in a speckled appearance. Melanocytes in areas of vitiligo are absent, and evidence suggests destruction by an immune mechanism.

White oval macules (**ash leaf macules**) are a valuable early marker of tuberous sclerosis. These macules appear at birth or shortly thereafter as 1- to 3-cm lesions on the trunk; they are not as sharply demarcated or ivory white as the lesions of vitiligo, and their distribution is different (see Chapter 14).

Cafe au lait spots are tan macules and patches that can be an indication of neurofibromatosis (von Recklinghausen disease) or Albright syndrome with polyostotic dysplasia. Swirled hyperpigmentation may be a marker of IP, and diffuse hyperpigmentation may be seen in Addison disease, hemochromatosis, and other systemic disorders. Peutz-Jeghers syndrome includes lentigo-like pigmentation of the lips, oral mucosa, hands, and fingers and benign, small-intestinal polyps in children.

SCALING DERMATOSES

Scaling dermatoses share a single feature: scaly areas of skin. The pathophysiology of the scales varies from disorder to disorder. For example, increased epidermal mitotic rate leads to red papules and plaques, with a thick adherent scale, as seen in psoriasis. In contrast, generalized scaling occurs in spite of normal epidermal turnover in lamellar ichthyosis. In the latter disorder, stratum corneum cells are more adherent and do not shed normally, creating a thick scale. It is important for the clinician to understand that scaling disorders are produced by different mechanisms in order to ensure proper diagnosis and therapy.

Psoriasis is a common inherited disorder characterized by red, well demarcated plaques with a silvery scale (Fig. 8.39), which have a predisposition for the extensor surfaces of the extremities, scalp, and buttocks. There may be a single lesion or many drop-like (guttate) lesions scattered over the body (Fig. 8.40). Psoriasis in the infant may present as a persistent diaper dermatitis (Fig. 8.41). Nail changes include psoriatic

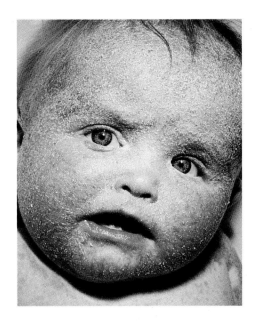

FIG. 8.44
Seborrhea. A more
generalized form of
seborrhea involves
the scalp, face, and
trunk of this child.

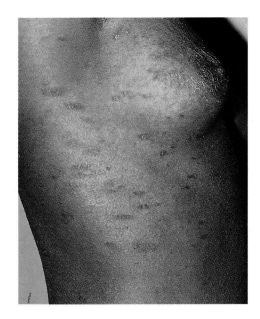

FIG. 8.46 Pityriasis
rosea. Numerous
oval lesions on the
trunk. The lesions
can appear in a fir
tree distribution on
the back.

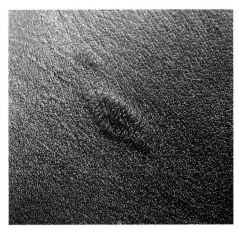

FIG. 8.45 Pityriasis
rosea. The herald
patch in this black
patient is oval and
raised, with a
slightly hyperpig-
mented center.

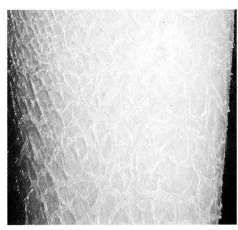

FIG. 8.47 Ichthy-
osis vulgaris.
Typical fish-scale
appearance on the
lower extremities.

plaques in the nail bed with a red-brown discoloration (oil-drop changes), surface pitting, and distal hyperkeratosis. Lesions of psoriasis may be induced in areas of local injury, such as scratches, surgical scar, or sunburn. This response is called Koebner's phenomenon (Fig. 8.42).

The factors initiating the rapid turnover in epidermal cells that causes the plaques is unknown, although an inherited predisposition, in addition to upper respiratory tract or streptococcal infections, may precipitate lesions. The increased epidermal growth causes thickening of the skin in the psoriatic plaque; however, there are also areas between the epidermal ridges where the skin is very thin and the scale is close to the subepidermal vessels. Thus, when the scale is removed, small bleeding points are often seen. This is called the Auspitz sign, and is the hallmark of psoriasis.

The course of psoriasis is chronic and unpredictable, marked by remissions and exacerbations. Although psoriasis is thought to be rare in childhood, 37 percent of adults with the disorder first develop lesions before the age of 20.

Seborrheic dermatitis is characterized by a red scaling eruption which occurs predominantly on the scalp, eyebrows, eyelashes, and perinasal, presternal, and postauricular areas. Intertriginous folds can also be affected. In infants, the scalp can be affected with a greasy, salmon-colored, scaly dermatitis called cradle cap (Fig. 8.43). A severe type may be more generalized (Fig. 8.44). In adolescents, the dermatitis may manifest itself as dandruff or flaking of the eyebrows, postauricular areas, or flexural areas.

The dermatitis is usually nonpruritic and mild in nature; most cases respond to topical steroids and many clear spontaneously. Antiseborrheic shampoos may also be helpful. In infants and young children, atopic dermatitis can have a greasy, scaly appearance, and may be confused with seborrhea. Differential diagnosis also includes Letterer-Siwe disease and tinea.

Pityriasis rosea is a benign, self-limited disorder of unknown etiology. It can occur at any age, but is more common in adolescents and young adults. A prodrome of malaise, headache, and mild constitutional symptoms may precede the rash.

The typical eruption starts as a single, isolated, pink, oval, slightly scaly lesion called a "herald patch" (Fig. 8.45), which may occur anywhere on the body. From 5 to 10 days later, crops of oval 2- to 10-mm lesions appear on the body, frequently concentrated on the trunk. The lesions often run parallel to the skin lines of the thorax, creating a "fir tree" pattern (Fig. 8.46). The rash reaches its peak in several weeks and then slowly fades over 4 to 6 weeks. Ultraviolet light may hasten the disappearance of the eruption.

The herald patch is often mistaken for tinea corporis. Other eruptions that can resemble pityriasis rosea are guttate psoriasis, viral exanthems, measles-like (morbilliform) drug eruptions, and secondary syphilis (see Chapter 12).

Ichthyosis vulgaris can range from a very mild, dry scaling to prominent, large, plate-like scales (Fig. 8.47). The disorder is inherited as an autosomal-dominant trait; it is not present

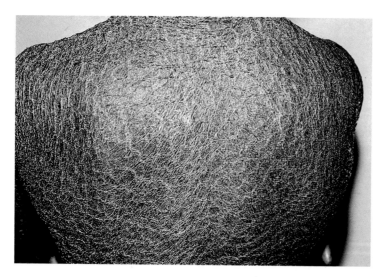

FIG. 8.48 Lamellar ichthyosis. Note the thick brown scales covering the entire skin.

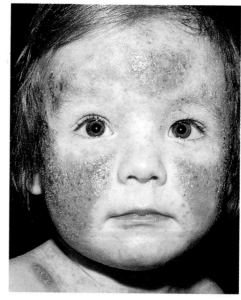

FIG. 8.49 Infantile atopic dermatitis. This infant has an acute weeping dermatitis on the cheeks and forehead.

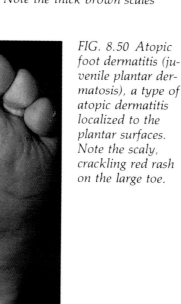

FIG. 8.50 Atopic foot dermatitis (juvenile plantar dermatosis), a type of atopic dermatitis localized to the plantar surfaces. Note the scaly, crackling red rash on the large toe.

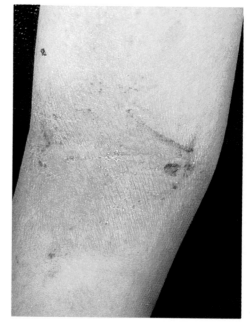

FIG. 8.51 Adult atopic dermatitis. Erythematous excoriated plaques with indistinct borders are seen in the antecubital areas. Note the blood from recent excoriation.

at birth, but is usually noted in the first year of life. Scales are most prominent on the extensor surfaces of the extremities, particularly the lower legs, and are exacerbated by dry weather. The flexural areas are usually spared. Other associated conditions are keratosis pilaris (horny follicular papules, see Fig. 8.53), hyperlinearity of the palms, atopic dermatitis, and other atopic skin disorders. Treatment consists of hydrating the skin with ointments and moisturizers.

Lamellar ichthyosis is an autosomal-recessive disorder seen in babies born with a collodion membrane (see Fig. 8.17). The infants slough the membrane in a few days; many then develop broad dark scales on a background of red skin, and later brownish-gray sheet-like layers of scales with raised edges (Fig. 8.48). There is prominent scaling over the face, trunk, and extremities. In contrast to ichthyosis vulgaris, the flexor areas are involved. Ectropion is common and can lead to drying of the cornea. Palms and soles can show a thick keratoderma with fissuring. There is some improvement of the scaling with age.

INFLAMMATORY DERMATOSES

Inflammatory dermatoses (dermatitis) are characterized clinically by redness, swelling, scaling, and itching. These disorders may be caused by activation of the immune system through antibodies, complement, chemotactic and vasoactive substances, and cellular immunity.

Microscopically, these dermatoses show infiltration of the skin with inflammatory cells. The inflammation may center around sebaceous follicles, as in inflammatory acne; in the dermis and epidermis, as in atopic dermatitis; or it may be mediated by Type I (IgE) immune response, as in the wheal and flare of an insect bite.

Atopic dermatitis (eczema) is one of the most common skin disorders in children. This entity can be divided into three phases based on the age of the patient. Each type has a different distribution.

The infantile form of atopic dermatitis (Fig. 8.49) begins between 1 and 6 months of age and lasts about 2 or 3 years.

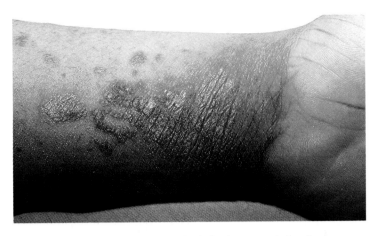

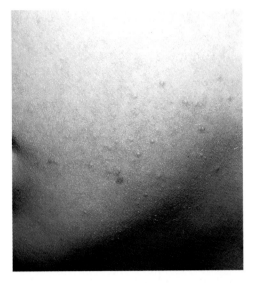

FIG. 8.52 Lichenification. Marked thickening of the skin in an area of chronic scratching. In addition, this patient had postinflammatory hyperpigmentation.

FIG. 8.53 Keratosis pilaris. Follicular papules can be seen on the cheek of this atopic patient. Some lesions are more inflamed than others.

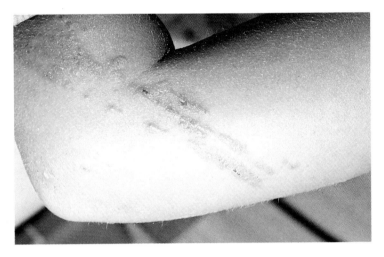

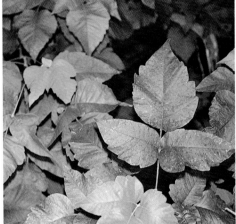

FIG. 8.54 Poison ivy dermatitis. (Left) Linear streaks of pruritic vesicles are typical of contact dermatitis to a plant. (Right) Poison ivy plant with characteristic shiny "leaves of three."

Characteristically, the rash is composed of red, itchy papules and plaques, and there is oozing and crusting. The lesions are located on the cheeks, forehead, scalp, trunk, or extremities; the patches are often symmetrical.

The childhood phase of atopic dermatitis occurs between ages 4 and 10 years. The dermatitis is typically dry, papular, and intensely pruritic. Circumscribed scaly patches are distributed on the wrists, ankles, and antecubital and popliteal fossae; these areas are frequently secondarily infected. Crackling, dryness, and scaling of the plantar surfaces are also common (Fig. 8.50). Remission may occur at any time, or the disorder may evolve into a more chronic type of adult dermatitis.

The adult phase of atopic dermatitis begins about age 12 and continues indefinitely. Major areas of involvement include the flexural areas of the arms, neck, and legs (Fig. 8.51). Eruptions are sometimes seen on dorsal surfaces of the hands and feet and between the fingers and toes. Marked lichenification can occur (Fig. 8.52).

Seventy-five percent of children with atopic dermatitis improve by age 10 to 14 years; the remaining children may have a chronic dermatitis. Other associated disorders include xerosis (dryness), keratosis pilaris (Fig. 8.53), hyperlinearity of the palms, Dennie-Morgan folds (double skin creases under the lower eyelid), and altered cellular immunity, which is manifested by an unusual susceptibility to certain cutaneous infections, such as warts, herpes simplex, and molluscum contagiosum.

The cause of atopic dermatitis remains unknown. However, it is thought by many that there is an underlying predisposition to pruritus; the resultant scratching leads to chronic cutaneous change typical of atopic dermatitis.

Differential diagnosis of atopic dermatitis includes seborrheic dermatitis, contact dermatitis, psoriasis, scabies, Letterer-Siwe disease, and acrodermatitis enteropathica (see Chapter 10).

Treatment entails reducing skin dryness and pruritus with lubricants, topical steroids, and oral antihistamines. Systemic steroids should be used only in extreme cases, and only for short periods of time.

Allergic contact dermatitis is a T-cell–mediated immune reaction to an antigen coming in contact with the skin. It presents with the acute onset of erythema, vesiculation, and pruritus, and is limited to the area of contact with the offending substance. Usually, the irritant is obvious, such as poison ivy or nickel jewelry. Initial allergic contact dermatitis develops within 7 to 10 days of exposure to a sensitizing substance. Reexposure to the allergen will also provoke a reaction. This is a classic example of Type IV (delayed) hypersensitivity. The most common type of allergic contact dermatitis in the United States is reaction to poison ivy. This frequently appears as linear streaks of vesicles (Fig. 8.54). Direct contact with the sap of

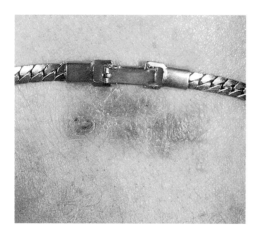

FIG. 8.55 Nickel contact dermatitis. Location of the rash is helpful in determining the cause of a contact dermatitis.

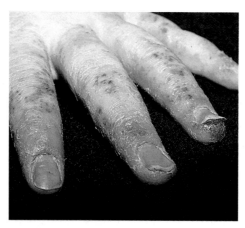

FIG. 8.56 Dyshidrosis. Chronic crackling, oozing, and scaling seen after the tiny pruritic vesicles have been scratched.

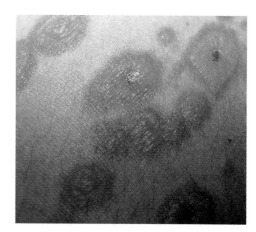

FIG. 8.57 Erythema multiforme. Typical target lesion with central dusky area. These lesions become blisters.

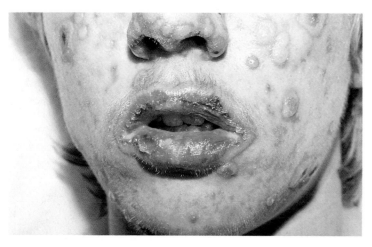

FIG. 8.58 Stevens-Johnson syndrome. Severe oral mucous membrane involvement, with typical target lesions and bullae on the face.

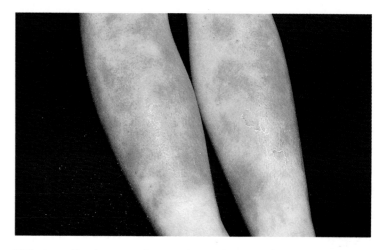

FIG. 8.59 Erythema nodosum. Note the typical, red, raised, tender nodules overlying the anterior surfaces of the legs.

the plant is necessary to produce the dermatitis. Other common offending allergens are nickel (Fig. 8.55), rubber in shoes, ethylenediamine, neomycin, and topical anesthetics.

Dyshidrosis (Fig. 8.56) is a severe, recurrent, chronic vesicular eruption affecting the palms, soles, and lateral aspects of the fingers. Characteristically, the vesicles are symmetrical, 1 mm, and pruritic. The cause of this disorder is unknown; however, frequent exposure to water or chemicals on the hands exacerbates the condition. Treatment includes topical steroids and avoidance of irritants.

Erythema multiforme (EM) is a distinctive, acute hypersensitivity syndrome that may be caused by several different agents, including drugs, viruses, bacteria, foods, immunizations, and connective tissue disorders. Infectious diseases and medication are the most common causes in children.

The classic eruption is symmetrical and may occur on any part of the body, although it typically appears on the distal surfaces of the palms and soles. The initial lesion is a dusky red macule or erythematous wheal that evolves into an iris or target lesion, the hallmark of EM (Fig. 8.57). These lesions may become bullous. The eruption continues in crops which last from 1 to 3 weeks. Rarely, the condition progresses to Stevens-Johnson syndrome or toxic epidermal necrolysis (TEN), with large areas of epidermal shedding secondary to necrosis.

TEN begins as erythema (either confluent or patchy) and a positive Nikolsky's sign (lateral thumb pressure on intact skin causes the epidermis to slide off the dermis). Later, the full-thickness epidermis necroses and spontaneously sloughs off, leaving a denuded base. The eruption is usually caused by a drug, but other etiologic agents have been reported.

The mortality rate for TEN is high because of fluid and electrolyte imbalance, bacterial pneumonia, and sepsis. TEN must not be confused with staphylococcal scalded skin syndrome (SSSS): TEN is associated with a full-thickness loss of epidermis, while SSSS produces a superficial subcorneal skin separation with low mortality. A skin biopsy can easily distinguish the two. The clinician may have difficulty distinguishing TEN from Stevens-Johnson syndrome. Patients with Stevens-Johnson syndrome have severe constitutional symptoms, including high fever, cough, sore throat, vomiting, diarrhea, chest pain, and arthralgias. There is involvement of the mucous membranes, particularly the oral, conjunctival, and urethral mucous membranes (Fig. 8.58). Sequelae of Stevens-Johnson syndrome can be severe, especially when corneal ulceration leads to blindness.

Erythema nodosum (Fig. 8.59) is characterized by symmetrical, red, tender nodules, 1 to 5 cm in diameter, usually located on the pretibial surfaces. It most likely represents a hypersensitivity eruption caused by streptococcal infection, medication, sarcoidosis, tuberculosis, or another bacterial or

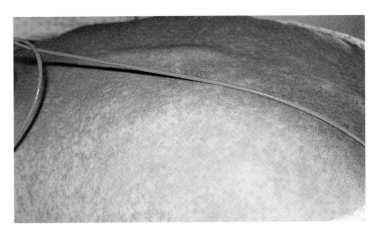

FIG. 8.60 A drug eruption. Generalized urticarial eruption in a patient taking ampicillin.

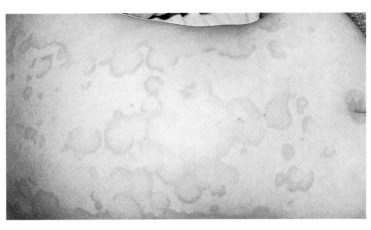

FIG. 8.61 Urticaria. Gyrate urticarial plaques have formed from individual plaques that became confluent.

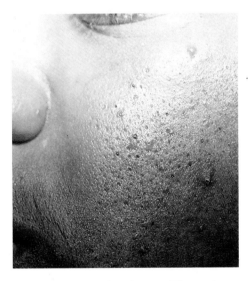

FIG. 8.62 Comedonal acne. The major components of this acne are blackheads and whiteheads, easily seen over the cheek.

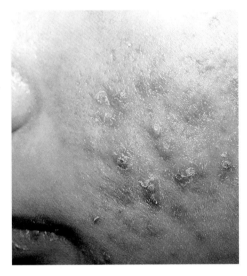

FIG. 8.63 Papulopustular acne. Inflamed papules and pustules over the cheeks responded well to antibiotics.

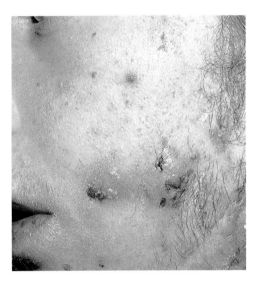

FIG. 8.64 Cystic acne. Deep cysts with marked erythema can cause severe scarring after the acne has resolved.

fungal infection. Noninfectious disorders such as ulcerative colitis and regional ileitis have also been implicated.

Erythema nodosum is most often seen in children older than 10 years. The lesions begin as red, tender, slightly elevated nodules and develop into brownish-red or bruise-like lesions within a few days. The rash usually lasts between 2 and 6 weeks, but recurrences are common. Treatment of the underlying cause and bedrest are beneficial. Differential diagnosis includes cellulitis, insect bites, thrombophlebitis, ecchymosis, and vasculitis.

Many different types of **drug eruptions** are seen in children: macular or papular rashes can develop after the ingestion of a drug. The rash is frequently morbilliform or urticarial. Ampicillin (Fig. 8.60) and phenytoin are two of the more common offenders in children. The eruptions are generally diffuse and widespread, and appear 5 to 14 days after starting a medication. Most patients with infectious mononucleosis who are given ampicillin develop a distinct, purpuric erythematous eruption over the trunk and extremities.

Urticaria (hives) (Fig. 8.61) is characterized by the sudden appearance of transient, well-demarcated erythematous wheals that are intensely pruritic. Lesions usually last 1 to 2 hours, but can persist up to 24 hours.

Urticaria can be caused by a variety of immunologic mechanisms, including IgE antibody response, complement activation, or abnormal levels of or sensitivity to vasoactive amines. Most commonly, acute urticaria (lasting less than 6 weeks) is caused by a hypersensitivity reaction to food, drugs, insect bites, infections, contact allergens, or inhaled substances. Chronic urticaria (lasting more than 6 weeks) can be a sign of an underlying disorder, such as occult infection, hepatitis B, or connective tissue disease.

Acne vulgaris is a disorder of the pilosebaceous apparatus; it usually begins in the second decade of life and is the common skin problem of the adolescent years. There are three major types of acne. In the first type, comedonal acne, lesions appear as open and closed comedones (Fig. 8.62). These are caused by the retention of dead keratinocytes with distention of the follicle.

The second type of acne is the papulopustular type, with more inflammatory papules (Fig. 8.63). In this type of acne, bacterial proliferation causes secretion of metabolic by-products that attract leukocytes and disrupt the follicular wall.

Cystic acne (Fig. 8.64), the third type, is typified by nodules and cysts scattered over the face, chest, and back. These lesions frequently lead to severe scarring.

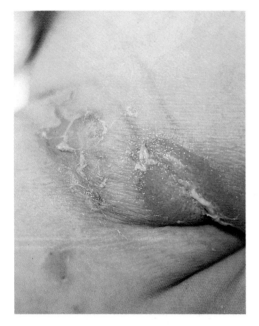

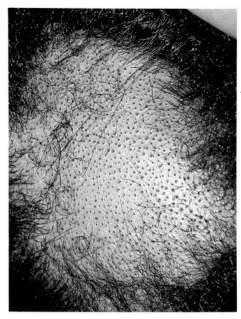

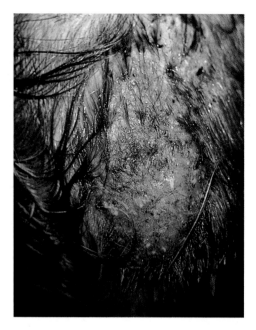

FIG. 8.65 Staphylococcal scalded skin syndrome. Early denudation of the skin in the intertriginous area of the neck. Exfoliation of the surrounding skin occurred the next day.

FIG. 8.66 Tinea capitis. Typical patches of alopecia with broken-off hairs. There is mild associated scaling.

FIG. 8.67 Kerion. Extensive inflammatory kerion that was mistaken for a bacterial infection.

INFECTIONS AND INFESTATIONS

Bacterial, fungal, parasitic, and viral eruptions are common in childhood. The cutaneous barrier protects the host from the outside world; when this barrier is broken, through a wound or a hair follicle, organisms may invade. Some infections, such as tinea capitis, are much more common in children than in adults, perhaps because of the higher content of fungistatic fatty acids in the sebum of postpubertal individuals. Viral infections such as warts and molluscum contagiosum cause localized growth of virus-laden cells and their products. Other viral infections such as herpes simplex and varicella cause blistering eruptions. Parasites and insects cause eruptions by trauma or toxins, and may also produce allergic reactions.

FIG. 8.68 Tinea corporis. Annular scaly patch on the face typical of tinea corporis.

Staphylococcal Scalded Skin Syndrome

Staphylococcal scalded skin syndrome (SSSS) is characterized by a coagulase-positive staphylococcal infection and superficial exfoliation of the skin. The staphylococcus produces an exfoliative toxin, causing separation of the stratum corneum from the underlying layers.

The syndrome begins as a generalized erythema with a fine sandpaper appearance. It frequently first appears in the intertriginous (Fig. 8.65) and periorificial areas in infants. Children are extremely uncomfortable and irritable. The next phase of the infection evolves into a generalized redness; the upper layer of the epidermis becomes wrinkled, and there is a positive Nikolsky's sign, leaving a shiny red surface. The final stage is desquamation of the upper layers of the epidermis. The disease is usually self-limited, although it may be serious in neonates. Appropriate antistaphylococcal antibiotic therapy is indicated.

Fungal Infections

Tinea capitis is a fungal infection of the scalp characterized by scaling and patchy hair loss; it is most common in prepubertal children. The lesion typically presents as a patch of short, broken-off hairs (Fig. 8.66). Sometimes this breakage results in marked inflammation with a boggy patch and pustules called a kerion (Fig. 8.67). Tinea capitis caused by Trichophyton species does not fluoresce under Wood's light; however, disease caused by Microsporum species does fluoresce with a greenish-yellow color. Hair loss is temporary, even with the inflammatory kerions. Diagnosis is made by observing spores and hyphae within the remaining hair (see Fig. 8.4) and by demonstrating the organisms on culture. Treatment is with systemic antifungals.

Tinea corporis is a superficial fungal infection of the nonhairy (glabrous) skin. It has been labeled "ringworm" because of the characteristic round lesions with central clearing and a

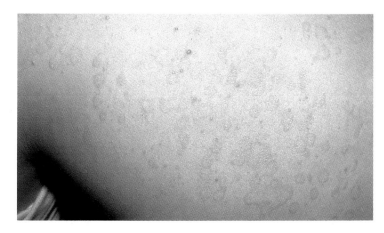

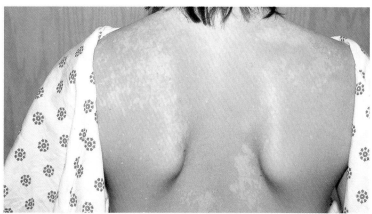

FIG. 8.69 Tinea versicolor. (Left) *Red scaling annular patches on the back of a teenager.* (Right) *Hypopigmented patches on* the upper back with a superficial scale that was noted when the lesion was scraped.

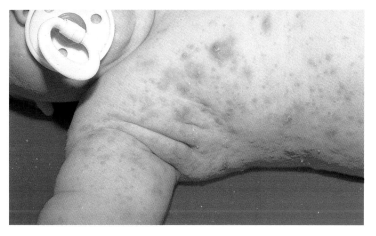

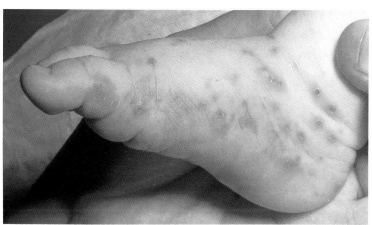

FIG. 8.70 Scabies. (Left) *Extremely pruritic erythematous papules and vesicles cover the arm and trunk of this infant.*

(Right) *Lesions on the soles and feet of infants are common.*

scaly annular border (Fig. 8.68). Multiple lesions may be present. Tinea infection can be found in any age group and is usually acquired from an infected domestic animal or through direct human contact. Examination by KOH reveals hyphae, confirming the diagnosis. Differential diagnosis includes nummular dermatitis, pityriasis rosea, granuloma annulare, psoriasis, contact dermatitis, seborrheic dermatitis, tinea versicolor, vitiligo, and lupus erythematosus. Treatment is with topical antifungal agents.

Tinea versicolor is a common dermatosis characterized by multiple oval scaly lesions measuring 1 to 3 cm in diameter, usually located on the upper chest and trunk (Fig. 8.69). They may be hyperpigmented or erythematous, giving rise to name "versicolor." Tinea versicolor is caused by the dimorphic fungus *Pityrosporum orbiculare*. It is most commonly seen in adolescents and young adults and is usually asymptomatic. Diagnosis is made by observation of hyphae and spores on microscopic examination of scrapings.

Infestations

Scabies is a contagious disorder caused by the itch mite *Acarus scabiei*. It is contracted by direct contact with infested humans. The characteristic eruption (Fig. 8.70) appears approximately 4 to 6 weeks after the initial contact and is thought to be a hypersensitivity reaction to the mite. Pru-

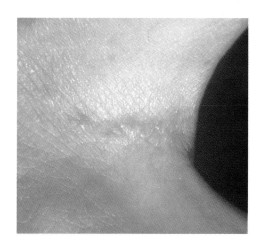

FIG. 8.71 Scabies burrow. *Linear lesion in the finger web is characteristic of a burrow.*

ritic papules, vesicles, pustules, and linear burrows appear in the finger webs, axillae, wrists, waist, nipples, and genitals. In infants, the palms, soles, head, and neck can also be affected. The burrow is the pathognomonic sign of scabies. It consists of a small, scaly, linear lesion with pinpoint vesicles at the end, in which the female mite lives (Fig. 8.71). Diagnosis is made by scraping an unexcoriated papule or burrow, examining the tissue microscopically, and observing a mite, egg, or feces (see Fig. 8.5).

Pediculosis capitis is an infestation of head lice frequently

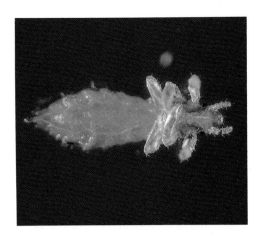

FIG. 8.72 Head louse. The long, thin body distinguishes this louse from the pubic or crab louse.

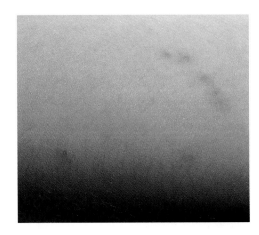

FIG. 8.73 Papular urticaria. Erythematous excoriated papules are characteristically seen in groups, where insects repeatedly bite the victim.

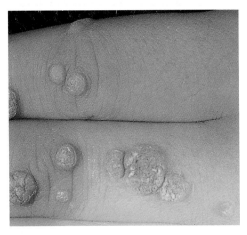

FIG. 8.74 Wart. Typical dry, rough finger lesions.

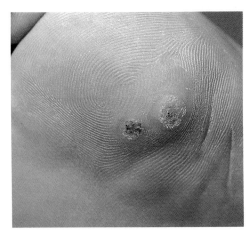

FIG. 8.75 Plantar wart. Two painful lesions on the plantar surface.

seen in children (Fig. 8.72). Pruritus is the principal symptom. Nits are seen as oval, white, 0.5-mm dots glued onto the hair shaft about 0.5 to 1 cm from the scalp (see Fig. 8.5). These nits are firmly attached onto the hair, and do not move along the hair shafts as do the hair casts for which they are frequently mistaken. Nits may be seen along the entire length of the hair, although they are deposited by the lice only near the scalp. Nits far from the root end indicate a span of perhaps months between infestation and examination. Nits are difficult to remove, and may in fact be nonviable shells. Patients adequately treated for lice will still have nonviable shells attached to the hair until removal with a weak vinegar wash and fine-toothed comb or until the hair is cut. The persistence of these dead nits is a common cause of misunderstanding by school health care workers who insist on re-treating the children or sending them home from school. New or viable nits rarely occur in a previously treated child; reports of lice resistant to treatment are rare and poorly documented. Active disease is present only if a viable organism or new nits attached close to the scalp are identified.

Papular Urticaria (Insect Bites)

Papular urticaria is a sensitivity reaction to the bite of a mosquito, flea, bedbug, or other insect. It usually occurs in infants and children in the spring and summer months. Lesions tend to be grouped in clusters (Fig. 8.73) and are 3- to 10-mm urticarial wheals with a central punctum; they can be excoriated or secondarily infected. The lesions recur in crops and may persist for 2 to 10 days. Therapy consists of insect con-

trol, topical corticosteroids, and oral antihistamines for symptomatic relief.

Viral Infections

Warts are a common viral disorder in children, most often seen on the fingers, hands, and feet. The incubation period of warts ranges from 1 to 6 months, and the majority of lesions disappear spontaneously over a period of 5 years. Local trauma promotes inoculation of the papilloma virus; thus periungual lesions are common in cuticle-pickers and nail-biters. Warts appear as round, discrete, skin-colored lesions with a papillomatous (roughened) surface (Fig. 8.74). The characteristic black dots are due to thrombosed superficial capillaries. Filiform warts are seen as thread-like projections on the face.

Plantar warts (Fig. 8.75) frequently cause pain when the patient walks. These lesions can be confused with corns, calluses, or scars; but plantar warts are distinguished by the interruption of normal skin lines (dermatoglyphics) and superficial red-brown dots.

Molluscum contagiosum is characterized by single or multiple, skin-colored, dome-shaped papules with umbilicated centers (Fig. 8.76). This contagious disease is caused by a poxvirus. Lesions are seen on the trunk, axillae, face, and genitals. They usually begin as pinpoint elevations of the skin, and rapidly increase in size to 2 to 5 mm. Frequently, a curd-like core can be expressed; microscopic examination of this material reveals typical molluscum bodies. Removal of lesions is curative, although spontaneous regression is eventual.

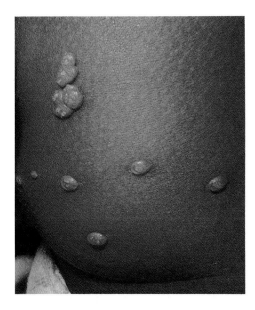

FIG. 8.76 Mollus-
cum contagiosum.
Typical shiny skin-
colored papules
with central umbil-
ication.

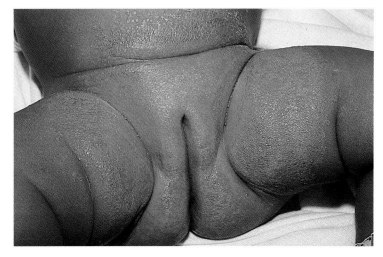

FIG. 8.77 Irritant diaper dermatitis. Note the erythema of the
convex surfaces and the sparing of the creases.

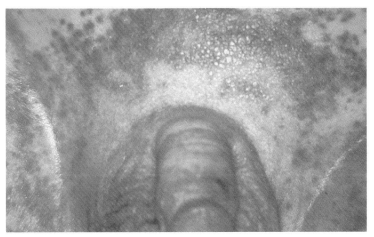

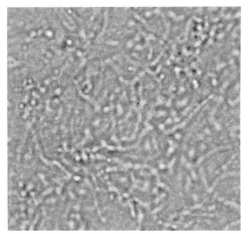

FIG. 8.78 Candidal
diaper dermatitis.
(Left) Note erythe-
matous satellite
papules characteris-
tic of candidal in-
fection, and in-
volvement of the
intertriginous
areas. (Right)
KOH preparation
of a candidal infec-
tion. Note the
pseudohyphae and
spores.

DIAPER DERMATITIS

Diaper dermatitis is the most common skin disorder of childhood. The diaper area is a prime target for infection because
it is often bathed in urine and feces and is usually occluded
by plastic diaper covers. This environment causes a breakdown of natural stratum corneum defense, allowing irritants, bacteria, and yeasts to invade the skin. Persistent
diaper dermatitis that does not resolve with conservative
therapy may be due to other disorders, such as psoriasis. Irritant contact diaper dermatitis is usually confined to the convex surfaces of the perineum, lower abdomen, buttocks, and
proximal thighs. The intertriginous creases are spared (Fig.
8.77). This disorder may be attributed to contact with prote-
olytic enzymes of bacteria, irritant chemicals, urine or feces,
harsh soaps, and detergents.

Candidal diaper dermatitis appears as a bright red eruption with sharp borders and pinpoint satellite papules and
pustules (Fig. 8.78). Examination of a pustule by KOH preparation reveals the typical budding yeasts and pseudohyphae
of Candida. Candidal diaper dermatitis is occasionally associated with oral thrush and is a common sequela of systemic
antibiotic therapy. Secondary invasion by *C. albicans*
should be considered whenever a diaper rash fails to respond
to symptomatic treatment.

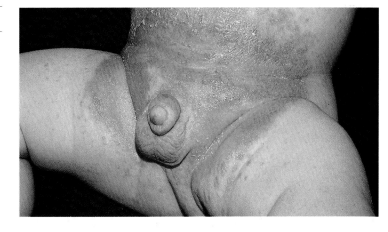

FIG. 8.79 Seborrheic diaper dermatitis. Yellowish greasy scale in
the diaper area involving the intertriginous folds.

Seborrheic diaper dermatitis (Fig. 8.79) is characterized by
salmon-colored greasy lesions with a yellowish scale. The
rash is most commonly seen in the intertriginous areas. The
disorder is commonly associated with seborrheic dermatitis
of the scalp, face, and postauricular areas (see Figs. 8.43 and
8.44).

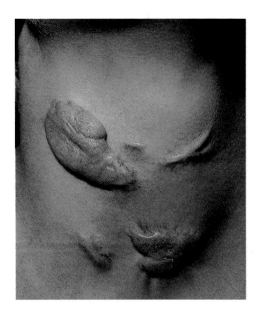

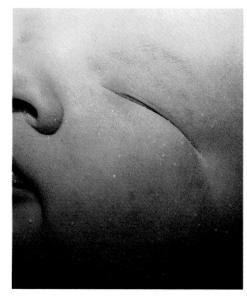

FIG. 8.80 Keloids. An abnormal reparative reaction to skin injury characterized by proliferation of fibroblasts and collagen extending beyond the original injury.

FIG. 8.81 Milia. Small, white-yellow papules close to the skin surface, particularly common around the eyes and midface.

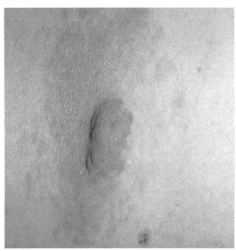

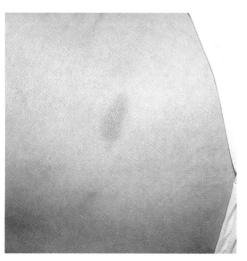

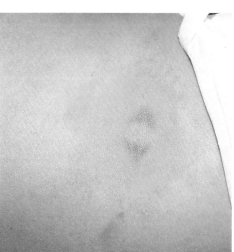

FIG. 8.82 Neurofibromatosis. Soft pink neurofibroma arising within a cafe au lait spot. Usually, neurofibromas arise from normal skin.

FIG. 8.83 Mastocytoma. (Left) An infiltrated plaque is present on the trunk of this infant. (Right) Darier's sign is demonstrated by the wheal and flare following slight pressure on the lesion.

TUMORS AND INFILTRATIONS

Persistent lumps and bumps in the skin often bring fears of skin cancer. Fortunately, primary skin cancer is very rare in children, and most tumors and infiltrated lesions are benign. Hemangiomas, warts, molluscum contagiosum, and various nevi are the most common lumps and were discussed earlier in the chapter.

Keloids (Fig. 8.80) are common growths following injury to the skin, such as ear piercing or laceration. They are rubbery nodules or plaques that result from the proliferation of fibroblasts and deposition of collagen. The lesions can be pruritic or tender, especially during the active growing phase, and may extend well beyond the margins of the original wound. This latter trait distinguishes keloids from hypertrophic scars, which remain confined to the wound margins and disappear spontaneously within 6 months of the injury. Keloids may arise spontaneously or occur in a familial form. They are most common in blacks, and occur most often on the ear lobes, upper trunk, and deltoid areas; for-

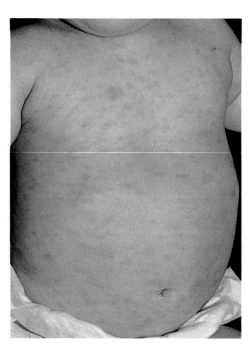

FIG. 8.84 Urticaria pigmentosa. Numerous pink and slightly hyperpigmented macules, papules, and plaques infiltrated with mast cells. Firm striking releases histamine granules and causes a wheal and flare.

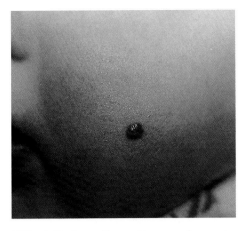

FIG. 8.85 Juvenile xanthogranuloma (JXG). Biopsy of this yellow-red papule showed typical JXG. Multiple lesions are common.

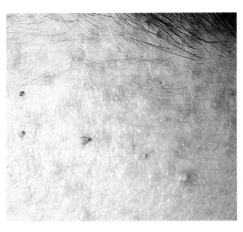

FIG. 8.86 Letterer-Siwe disease. The skin manifestations of the histiocytosis syndrome are similar and show the infiltrated scaling papules with petechiae, resembling seborrheic dermatitis.

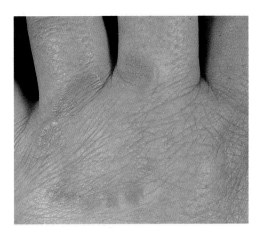

FIG. 8.87 Granuloma annulare. Grouped papules forming a large ring, commonly located on hands, feet, and elbows.

tunately, they are not seen on the midface. Keloids regress with intralesional steroids, alone or in combination with surgical excision.

Milia (Fig. 8.81) are small (1 to 2 mm), whitish-yellow papules commonly seen on the face in neonates. They are firm and not easily removed by pressure, unlike pustules. Milia are epithelial-lined cysts arising from hair follicles. They are persistent, although they may resolve spontaneously after months to years. Milia usually arise without any apparent cause, although they are often seen after superficial skin injury, such as blistering eruptions or dermabrasion.

Neurofibromas are solitary or multiple growths of neural tissue, presenting as soft, skin-colored or pink dermal nodules (Fig. 8.82). The central portion of an early lesion is particularly soft, and fingertip pressure creates the illusion of pressing in a buttonhole. Von Recklinghausen disease (neurofibromatosis) is a syndrome of multiple neurofibromas, cafe au lait spots, and various systemic disorders. When considering this diagnosis it is important to remember that the neurofibromas usually appear after puberty; in prepubertal children, café au lait spots are the most important cutaneous marker of von Recklinghausen disease. Solitary neurofibromas without other skin lesions are not suggestive of neurofibromatosis. Lumps and bumps of the skin can also be caused by infiltration of the skin by cells that produce indurated papules or plaques. Because many of the lesions are red or skin-colored nodules, subtle clues are important in making the proper diagnosis.

Cutaneous mastocytosis is an infiltrating disease where subtle clues are valuable. Isolated mastocytomas (dermal accumulations of mast cells) may be seen in neonates and infants. The mastocytomas are usually skin-colored, slightly indurated plaques 1 to 2 cm in size (Fig. 8.83). The clue to diagnosis is a wheal and flare following firm stroking of the lesion (Darier's sign). This response is caused by physical release of histamine from infiltrating mast cells and the effects of the histamine on the local vasculature. Occasionally, enough histamine will be released from a large mastocytoma to cause localized blistering or systemic symptoms of flushing, wheezing, or diarrhea. Mastocytomas can be located

anywhere on the body, and usually resolve by puberty.

Urticaria pigmentosa (Fig. 8.84) is another form of cutaneous mastocytosis that presents with numerous small papules or plaques, most commonly on the trunk. The disorder may be congenital or noted later in childhood with similar findings. Hyperpigmented macules overlying mast cell infiltrates are common; these macules will sometimes react to stroking with a wheal and flare. Urticaria pigmentosa in children is usually limited to the skin, and often resolves by adolescence.

Infiltration of the skin by other types of cells can occur. For example, local infiltration and proliferation of histiocytes in an isolated plaque or nodule or in groups of small nodules is seen in **juvenile xanthogranuloma** (JXG) (Fig. 8.85). These asymptomatic red or yellow-brown lesions grow very rapidly in infants and young children, but resolve spontaneously later in childhood. They are not associated with abnormalities of circulating lipids. When multiple lesions are seen, ocular involvement may occur and is the most common cause of nontraumatic hyphema in children. Ophthalmologic evaluation is important in patients with multiple or diffuse xanthogranulomas.

Histiocytosis syndromes are more serious proliferative disorders of Langerhans' cells. This group of disorders includes Letterer-Siwe disease, Hand-Schüller-Christian disease, and eosinophilic granuloma. Skin infiltration is most common in Letterer-Siwe disease. This entity begins in infants with a diffuse papular and scaly eruption with small petechiae, and differs from the usual seborrheic dermatitis by the presence of infiltrated, crusted papules and petechiae (Fig. 8.86). Diagnosis is confirmed when systemic abnormalities and skin biopsies show characteristic Langerhans' granules within the cytoplasm of infiltrating mononuclear cells.

Granuloma annulare (Fig. 8.87) is an example of dermal infiltration by lymphocytes around altered collagen. This disease presents with a ring of small, nonscaling, skin-colored or red papules. Granuloma annulare is most commonly confused with tinea corporis (ringworm). The annular plaques of granuloma annulare are seen on the dorsal surfaces of the hands and feet. They are asymptomatic and resolve spontaneously after a few months to a year.

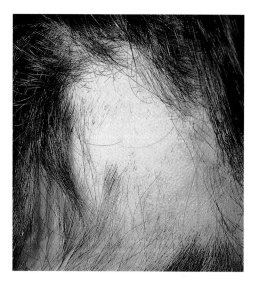

FIG. 8.88 Alopecia areata. Patches of hair loss with typical small broken hairs at the margins. In contrast to trichotillomania, these short hairs are easily removed.

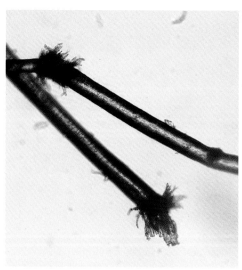

FIG. 8.89 Trichorrhexis nodosa. A brittle hair shaft defect usually caused by overmanipulation of the hair or chemical use. The frayed broom appearance is typical.

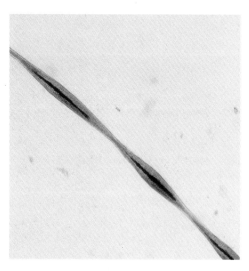

FIG. 8.90 Monilethrix. Beaded hairs are quite brittle and often break off close to the scalp, causing noticeable hair loss.

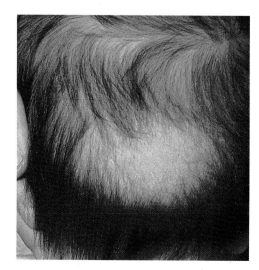

FIG. 8.91 Frictional alopecia. Hair loss on the occiput from rubbing the head on sheets and pillows.

DISORDERS OF HAIR AND NAILS

Diseases of the hair and nails are an integral part of dermatology. Both hair and nails are composed of keratin, produced by the epidermal structures of hair follicles and nail matrix. Some diseases are specific to these structures, while others affect the skin as well. In many cases, important diagnostic clues to skin disease can be found in related abnormalities of the hair and nails.

Hair

The most common diseases of the hair manifest as hair loss (alopecia). Evaluation begins by determining whether scarring is present. Nonscarring alopecia can be caused by growth defects causing the hair to be lost by the roots (effluvium) or defects of the hair shaft causing breakage.

Normal hair cycles through a growth phase lasting 3 years or more (anagen phase) to a resting phase of 3 months (telogen phase), after which the hair is shed. The cycle then begins again. Telogen effluvium is one form of partial, temporary alopecia rarely causing more than 50 percent hair loss, and is seen 3 months after a severe illness, surgery, or high fever. The initial systemic insult induces more than the normal 20 percent of hairs to enter the telogen phase, and 3 months later, these hairs are shed simultaneously, producing marked thinning of scalp hair until new anagen hairs regrow. Anagen effluvium is the sudden loss of the growing hairs (80 percent of normal scalp hairs), and is caused by the cessation of the anagen phase, with tapering of the shaft and loss of adhesion to the follicle. This type of hair loss is most common after systemic chemotherapy.

Alopecia areata (Fig. 8.88) is a form of localized anagen effluvium, presenting with round patches of alopecia anywhere on the scalp, eyebrows, lashes, or body, or even diffuse hair loss. The injury causing the cessation of growth is presumably of immunologic origin. A clue to diagnosis is finding short 3- to 6-mm easily epilated hairs at the margins of alopecia. Microscopically, these hair stubs resemble exclamation points. Another finding in many patients with alopecia areata is Scotch plaid pitting, rows of pits crossing in a transverse and longitudinal fashion (see Fig. 8.96). The clinical course of alopecia areata is difficult to predict. The disorder may resolve spontaneously, may persist with the appearance of new patches while the old patches regrow, or it may progress to total scalp or body alopecia that can be permanent.

Alopecia caused by hair shaft breakage is due to structural defects and is easily diagnosed by microscopic examination.

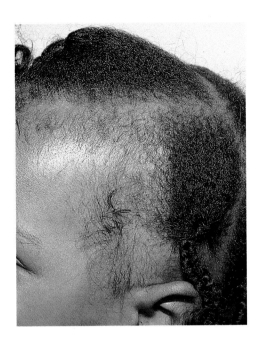

FIG. 8.92 Traction alopecia. Hair thinning and loss due to prolonged and repeated pulling.

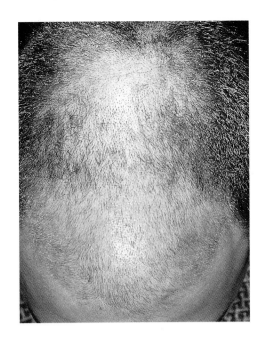

FIG. 8.93 Trichotillomania. Extensive hair loss on the vertex due to intentional pulling and breaking.

The most common structural defect is acquired trichorrhexis nodosa. This presents at any age as brittle short hairs that are perceived by the patient as nongrowing. By gently pulling the hair, one can show many hairs easily broken. Microscopically, the distal ends of the hairs are frayed, resembling a broom (Fig. 8.89). Other hairs may show a nodule resembling two brooms stuck together. The fragility is caused by the damage to the outer cortex of the hair shaft, resulting in a loss of structural support. Without this support, the weaker fibrous medulla frays like an electrical cord with broken insulation. This disorder is most common in blacks, due to the trauma of combing tightly curled hairs. It is also seen after repeated or vigorous chemical damage to the cortex from hair straighteners, bleach, and permanents. Since hair growth is normal, the disorder is self-limited, and normal hairs regrow when the damage is discontinued.

Fungal infection of the hair shaft weakens the shaft and causes breakage. Tinea capitis is easily diagnosed by microscopic examination with KOH.

Other structural defects may be congenital or associated with heritable syndromes. **Monilethrix** is a developmental hair defect that produced brittle, beaded hair. It is autosomal-dominant and usually appears after 2 to 3 months of age, when the fetal/neonatal vellus hairs are replaced by abnormal beaded hairs. The scalp is most severely affected, although hair on any part of the body can be involved. The disease is generally permanent. Microscopically, there is regular periodic narrowing of the hair shafts (Fig. 8.90). Breakage commonly occurs in the constricted areas close to the scalp. Care must be taken not to confuse monilethrix with pili torti, which is another structural defect in which the hair shaft is twisted on its own axis. Pili torti may be localized or generalized and also appears with the first terminal hair growth of infancy. It may be associated with Menkes kinky hair syndrome, and is due to defects in copper metabolism, affecting the central nervous and cardiovascular systems.

Other common causes of hair loss associated with shaft abnormalities include frictional alopecia, traction alopecia, and trichotillomania. All are caused by external trauma and breakage of an otherwise normal hair shaft. **Frictional alo-**pecia (Fig. 8.91) is common on the posterior scalp of neonates and infants, where the scalp rubs on the pillow or bed clothes. Although worrisome to parents, this disorder is self-limited. **Traction alopecia** (Fig. 8.92) is common in young girls whose hairstyles, such as ponytails or cornrowing, maintain a tight pull on the hair shafts. This tight traction causes shaft fractures, as well as follicular damage; if it is prolonged, permanent scarring alopecia can result. **Trichotillomania** (Fig. 8.93) is a common disorder in school-aged children that mimicks many other types of alopecia. It presents with bizarre patterns of hair loss, often in broad linear bands on the vertex or sides of the scalp, where the hair is easily twisted and pulled out. Rarely, the entire scalp, eyebrows and eyelashes are involved. Parents and children usually vigorously deny that the alopecia could be caused by the child, and thus diagnosis rests on a high index of suspicion and recognition of the clinical findings. The most important clue is the finding of short, broken-off hairs at the scalp and often stubs of different lengths in adjacent areas. This is caused by easy pulling and fractures of the longer shafts; once broken, the hairs are too short to be rebroken until they grow longer. Trichotillomania is often confused with alopecia areata because there are patches of hair loss with short hairs and involvement of the eyebrows and eyelashes. However, in trichotillomania, the hair shafts are normal anagen hairs and are usually difficult to remove from the scalp. In addition, there are no associated nail abnormalities. Trichotillomania is often seen in middle-class families with marital or social problems, and is a clue that some form of family counseling may be necessary to prevent abnormal child development.

Scarring alopecia in children is less common than nonscarring alopecia and may be caused by a number of disorders. Aplasia cutis congenita is an ulceration of the vertex of the scalp of a newborn that heals with a hairless scar. Morphea (localized scleroderma) may involve the scalp with indurated hairless plaques. Scarring alopecia may result from severe infection or trauma, such as oil burns from hot-comb straightening of the hair. A scalp biopsy is often helpful in determining the cause of scarring alopecia.

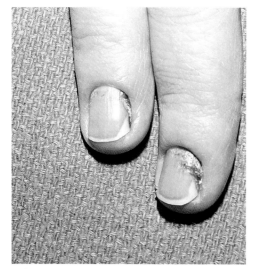
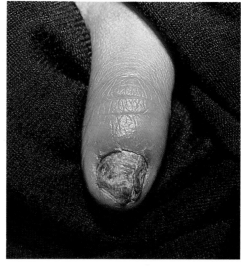

FIG. 8.94 *Candidal paronychia and nail dystrophy.* (Left) *Early presentation with lateral and proximal nail fold involvement.* (Right) *Late presentation with dystrophy of the entire nail.*

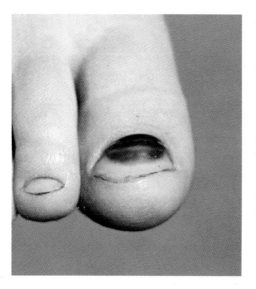

FIG. 8.95 *Traumatic subungual hemorrhage. Discoloration due to traumatic hemorrhage under the toenail is common in children and athletes. It is a result of jamming the toe into the end of the shoe while running or stopping (turf toe).*

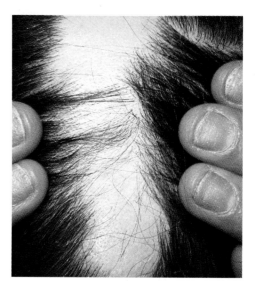

FIG. 8.96 *Alopecia areata, nails. Note the broad shallow pitting. This condition is associated with alopecia areata.*

Nails

Patients may seek the advice of a physician for nail disorders because of pain or cosmetic concern. For the physician, knowledge of nail disorders is helpful in detecting clues to systemic disease.

Paronychia is a common childhood disorder. It presents as a red, swollen, tender nail fold, usually on the side or base of the nail. The acute form with sudden swelling and marked tenderness is often caused by bacteria invading after trauma to the cuticle or after dermatitis that damaged the stratum corneum barrier. Chronic paronychia is more common and involves more than one nail (Fig. 8.94). There is usually a history of chronic dermatitis or frequent exposure to water. The tenderness is mild, with a small amount of pus and often some nail dystrophy. The causative organism is Candida species, usually *C. albicans.* Paronychia resolves with the use of topical antimycotics and the avoidance of water.

Onychomycosis, or infection of the nail plate with fungus, is very rare in children before puberty. Thus, nail dystrophy should not be treated as a fungal infection unless proven by microscopic examination or fungal culture.

Trauma to the nail may cause subungual hemorrhage, resulting in a brown-black discoloration (Fig. 8.95). Usually the diagnosis is simple unless trauma is subtle and frequent. Pigmentation at the base of the great toenail caused by jamming the toe into the end of the shoe at a sudden stop is called "turf toe" and results in mild subungual hemorrhage. This must be distinguished from melanoma. Hemorrhage can be identified by the presence of small splinter hemorrhages at the margin of pigment and outgrowth of pigment with the nail, along with the appearance of a normal proximal nail plate.

Nail disorders may provide clues to other dermatologic or pediatric syndromes. For example, alopecia areata is associated with a characteristic Scotch plaid pitting of the nails (Fig. 8.96). Similarly, psoriasis affects the nails in a number of ways that may help to distinguish it from other scaling disorders. Psoriasis affecting the nail matrix results in scattered pits that are larger, deeper, and less numerous than those found in alopecia areata (Fig. 8.97). Psoriasis of the nail bed, especially the bed under the distal nail, causes separation of the nail from the underlying skin (onycholysis) and oil-drop discoloration with heaped-up scaling. Onycholysis alone, without pits or discoloration, may be caused by trauma, infection, nail-polish hardeners, or phototoxic reactions to drugs such as tetracycline.

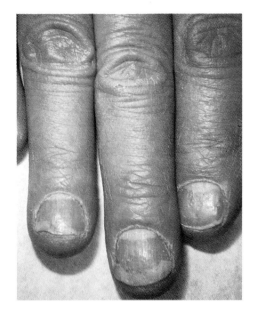

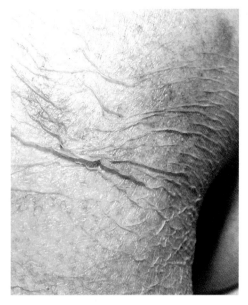

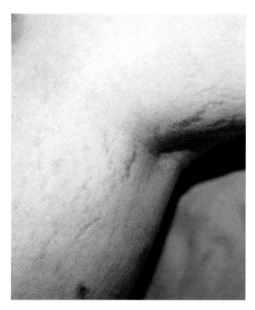

FIG. 8.97 Psoriasis, nails. Psoriasis affecting the nails results in onycholysis and pitting.

FIG. 8.98 Steroid atrophy. Topical steroids may cause marked atrophy and fragility of the skin, especially if used under occlusion regularly for more than 1 month.

FIG. 8.99 Striae distensae. Prolonged use of potent fluorinated steroids may cause permanent striae distensae.

COMPLICATIONS OF TOPICAL SKIN THERAPY

An important rule in medicine is "do no harm." To follow that rule, the physician must recognize the adverse effects of therapy.

The most commonly used topical medications are steroids. These may be classified as high or low potency, according to their biological activity. Generally, fluorinated steroids are more potent than nonfluorinated steroids, and steroids in ointment bases are more active than those in cream or lotion bases. High-potency steroids should be used for short durations or major side effects may develop. These include skin atrophy (Fig. 8.98), telangiectases, and increased skin fragility; acneiform eruptions; permanent skin striae (Fig. 8.99); and masking or delayed recognition of infections and infestations such as tinea corporis and scabies. Fluorinated steroids are rarely used on the face, genitals, or intertriginous areas, because absorption is greater and side effects are more common. Injection of steroids into fat may cause subcutaneous atrophy (Fig. 8.100). Adrenal suppression may occur from absorption of potent steroids through the skin if the medication is applied to large areas or if the treated area is occluded.

Other complications, such as contact dermatitis, can be easily prevented. Allergic contact dermatitis is frequently seen as a reaction to both prescribed and over-the-counter drugs. The most common allergens are neomycin, "-caine" topical anesthetics or antipruritics, and ethylenediamine (a preservative in Mycolog cream). It is important to remember that anaphylaxis may occur to topical medications, especially if applied to broken skin, so a history of drug allergies is important before prescribing topical medication.

Fortunately, most complications of therapy can be avoided if the doctor has knowledge of the disease and its treatment.

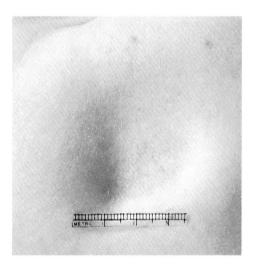

FIG. 8.100 Subcutaneous atrophy. Injection of steroids into fat instead of muscle often produces subcutaneous atrophy. This usually resolves in 6 months to a year.

BIBLIOGRAPHY

Eaglstein WH: Office Techniques for Diagnosing Skin Disease. Year Book, Chicago, 1978.

Hurwitz S: Clinical Pediatric Dermatology. Saunders, Philadelphia, 1981.

Rasmussen J: Pediatric Dermatology; Pediatric Clinics of North America, vol. 30, no. 3. Saunders, Philadelphia, 1983.

Verbov J, Morley N: Color Atlas of Pediatric Dermatology. Lippincott, London, 1983.

Weinberg S, Leider M, Shapiro L: Color Atlas of Pediatric Dermatology. McGraw-Hill, London, 1975.

Weston W: Practical Pediatric Dermatology. Little, Brown, Boston, 1979.

PEDIATRIC ENDOCRINOLOGY

David Finegold, M.D.

Clinical presentations of endocrine disease vary widely such that alterations in hormonal balance can result in children who are too fat, too thin, too short, or too tall. While the molecular explanations for states of excessive or insufficient hormone secretion constantly become more sophisticated with improvements in our understanding of the physiology and biochemistry, the clinical presentations of abnormal endocrine states remain constant. Recognition of the physical signs associated with these states is important as our ability to treat and correct these imbalances advances. The following descriptions will emphasize the physical signs associated with normal endocrine maturation and with states of hypo- and hyper-secretion of hormones.

THE ANTERIOR PITUITARY GLAND

The pituitary gland in humans contains anterior and posterior sections that have substantially different functions. In this chapter we will concentrate on the anterior section and on its relationship to the release of hormones in endocrine glands. The anterior pituitary contains cells that secrete three types of hormones: corticotropin-related peptide hormones, glycoprotein hormones, and somatomammotropins. These compounds have great biologic potency and, with the exception of prolactin, are regulated through closed feedback loops as well as through specific agonists and antagonists.

The **corticotropin-related peptide hormones** consist of adrenocorticotropic hormone (ACTH), α-melanocyte-stimulating hormone (α-MSH), and γ- and β-lipotropins (γ-LPH, β-LPH). These hormones are derived from a common precursor molecule, proopiomelanocortin, within whose amino-acid structure are contained their sequences. Within the subunit structure of β-LPH also are contained the important neuroendocrine molecules α-, β-, and γ-endorphin, and enkephalin. After posttranslational processing from this large precursor molecule, the secretion of ACTH is regulated by the level of corticotropin-releasing factor (CRF) in the pituitary portal plasma and by the level of plasma cortisol secreted from the adrenal gland, which then has a negative feedback effect on further secretion of ACTH (Fig. 9.1).

While the relationship between ACTH and cortisol secretion has been well studied, less is known about β-lipotropin secretion, along with secretion of its subunits α-, β-, and γ-endorphin, and about enkephalin and β-MSH secretion.

The **glycoprotein hormones** of the pituitary include follicle-stimulating hormone (FSH), luteinizing hormone (LH), and thyroid-stimulating hormone (TSH). Each of these hormones is composed of two dissimilar peptide subunits. The α chain is highly similar in structure among the three hormones. However, the β chain is unique and confers specificity from one hormone to another. These three hormones also contain significant amounts of carbohydrate and sialic acid residues along with their basic amino acid structures. As the corticotropin-related peptide hormones are stimulated by hypothalamic secretion, similarly, LH and FSH secretions are positively stimulated by gonadotropin releasing hormone (GnRH).

The primary action of FSH and LH is on the gonads. FSH directly stimulates gametogenesis in the testes and supports follicular development in the ovary. LH stimulates Leydig cell function of the testes, producing testosterone, and acts to promote luteinization of the ovaries (Fig. 9.2). The negative feedback effect of sex steroids on LH and FSH production is dramatically emphasized in the postmenopausal woman or in the young girl with Turner syndrome in whom marked elevations of these hormones occur.

TSH stimulates many aspects of thyroid function. These aspects include increasing the size of thyroid cells and also the vascularity of the gland. Specific increases in the size of follicular epithelial cells and in the amount of colloid may easily be determined. Moreover, TSH increases radioactive iodide uptake, thyroglobulin synthesis, and thyroxine and triiodothyronine release from the thyroid gland. Basic alterations in thyroid cell biochemistry also may occur following TSH administration. The rate of TSH secretion appears to be determined by the level of circulating thyroid hormone as well as by the hypothalamic hormone, thyrotropin-releasing hormone (TRH). However, negative feedback of TSH secretion by circulating thyroid hormone occurs mainly at the pituitary level (Fig. 9.3).

The somatomammotropin hormones, **prolactin** (PRL) and

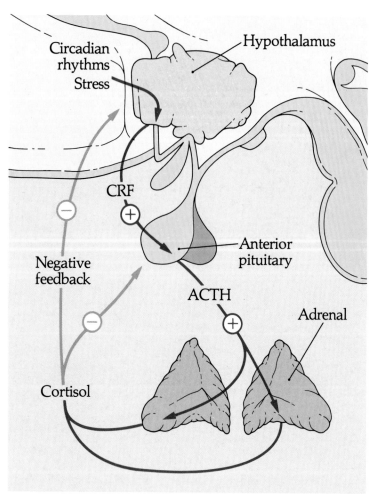

FIG. 9.1 Feedback regulation of adrenocorticotropic hormone (ACTH) at the level of the hypothalamus, pituitary, and adrenal glands.

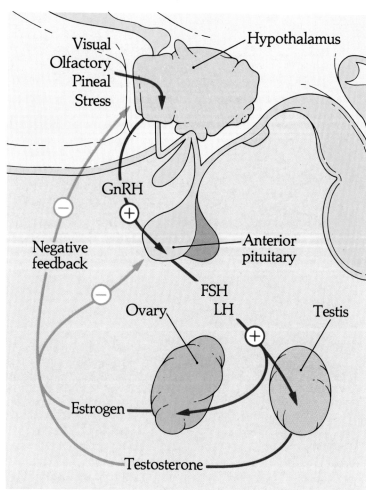

FIG. 9.2 Feedback regulation of luteinizing hormone (LH) and follicle-stimulating hormone (FSH) at the level of the hypothalamus, pituitary, and gonads.

growth hormone (GH), have similar chemical structures as well as some overlap of their biologic activity. The amino acid sequences of both contain two or three disulfide bridges.

PRL acts directly on its target organs and does not require an intermediary secondary endocrine gland. PRL's only major function in humans is the initiation and maintenance of lactation. In contrast to the other anterior pituitary hormones, prolactin appears to be under tonic stimulation. Chronic inhibition through hypothalamic secretory mechanisms appears to be the major regulator of unrestrained prolactin secretion. Dopaminergic pathways and dopamine have potent prolactin inhibitory properties and, in fact, dopamine appears to fit many criteria for the physiologic prolactin inhibiting factor.

GH modulates complex metabolic processes. Although the molecular basis of GH action continues to remain obscure, its obvious effects can be seen in hypopituitary children in whom it has been used for treatment. GH stimulates an increase in lean body mass as well as a marked increase in the size of the heart, pancreas, liver, and kidneys. It also has positive effects on carbohydrate, fat and protein metabolism, and causes a decrease in body fat. GH inhibits carbohydrate uptake by muscle. This diabetogenic effect of GH action has been well demonstrated and is a known complication of GH hypersecretion. On the other hand, hypoglycemia is seen in patients who are GH deficient.

GH appears to mediate some of its effects on bone and linear

growth via the somatomedins. These peptides have some structural similarity to proinsulin. Somatomedin C appears to mediate sulfate and phosphate incorporation into cartilage. Somatomedin C is identical to the peptide originally called insulin-like growth factor I (IGF I). GH is regulated on chronic and acute levels through a variety of mechanisms. A rapid fall in plasma glucose concentration may elicit a brisk rise in GH secretion. However, hypoglycemia of slow onset may not activate GH secretion. Neural factors such as sleep, stress, and α-adrenergic agonists may result in augmentation of GH secretion. Glucagon and vasopressin appear to cause hormonal augmentation of GH secretion. A fall in plasma somatomedin also may result in GH elevations. Recently, the hypothalamic GH releasing factor (GHRF) has been identified and appears to be an important physiologic stimulant of GH secretion, just as the hypothalamic peptide somatostatin appears to be important in the inhibition of GH secretion (Fig. 9.4).

The anterior pituitary, with its diverse cell types and hormonal secretory patterns, controls many important biologic processes. Anterior pituitary hormone deficiencies cause subsequent deficiencies in the output of secondary endocrine glands. Consequently, specific aspects of growth and development are consistently disturbed by oversecretion or undersecretion of the pituitary. Particular alterations in physical appearance should alert physicians to an abnormality in the anterior pituitary, and to subsequent secondary deficiencies (e.g., in the thyroid or adrenals).

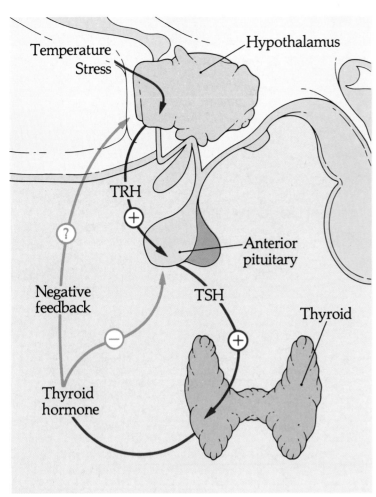

FIG. 9.3 Feedback regulation of thyroid-stimulating hormone (TSH) at the level of the hypothalamus, pituitary, and thyroid gland.

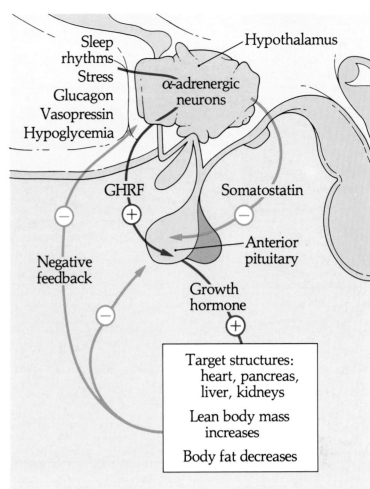

FIG. 9.4 Feedback regulation of growth hormone (GH) at the level of the hypothalamus, pituitary, and target organs.

SPECIFIC HORMONAL IMBALANCES
Growth Hormone Deficiency

The phenotypic features of a child with GH deficiency are most striking. GH deficiency tends to be recognized by the characteristic features of abnormal body proportion and increased adiposity around the trunk and extremities. As seen in Figure 9.5, GH-deficient children have delicate features, and, in males with this disorder, the genitalia frequently are small. Children with hypopituitarism tend to have high-pitched voices compared with other children of the same age.

Children with a variety of midline defects have a higher incidence of hypopituitarism when compared with normal children. The child seen in Figure 9.6 has a single central maxillary incisor—an example of a midline abnormality consistently associated with GH deficiency. Other physical findings suggestive of pituitary endocrine abnormalities include the syndrome of septo-optic dysplasia with pale optic discs (Fig. 9.7), and children with cleft lip and cleft palate. These embryologic defects, presenting in infancy, also may be associated with significant risks of hypoglycemia. Recurrent protracted hypoglycemia may be an early presentation of hypopituitarism. The hypoglycemia is effectively treated with GH replacement therapy.

Normal growth occurs at a varying rate, through the process. of normal development. Moreover, wide variability

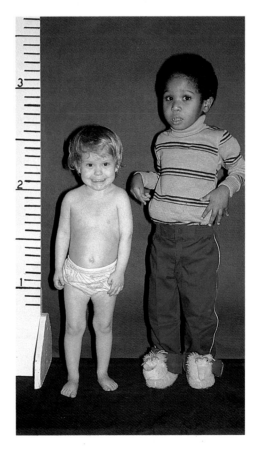

FIG. 9.5 The normal 3½-year-old boy is in the 50th percentile for height. The short 3-year-old girl exhibits the characteristic "Kewpie" doll appearance, suggesting a diagnosis of GH deficiency.

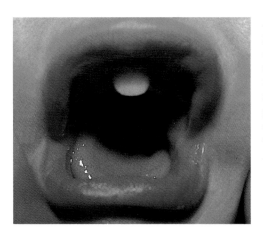

FIG. 9.6 The presence of a single central maxillary incisor should alert the clinician to investigate the possibility of GH deficiency. (Courtesy of Dr. P. Lee)

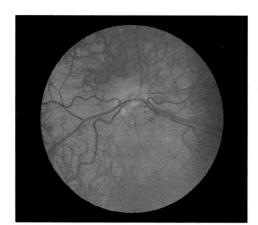

FIG. 9.7 Pale optic discs, suggesting optic atrophy, often are seen with septo-optic dysplasia. This finding also suggests pituitary endocrine deficiencies ranging from isolated GH deficiency to panhypopituitarism. (Courtesy of Dr. D. Hiles)

exists in growth rates between individual children at different ages. Incremental growth rate is one of the most important elements in assessing whether a child has a pathologic abnormality of growth. As seen in Figure 9.8, the growth velocity curve may be calculated as the first derivative of the linear growth curve. This manipulation graphically illustrates the wide variability in growth rates at different ages. The curve also illustrates that in the first 2 to 3 years of life growth is constantly decelerating. During the latency years, a long period of constant growth occurs and is followed by a sharp acceleration in growth velocity during adolescence. This sharp increase in growth velocity is the harbinger of puberty. The growth velocity of adolescence also is the only time during which the rapid growth of the infant is recapitulated.

It is important to remember that of those children with short stature and normal body proportions who are brought to their pediatrician for evaluation, only a few will have growth failure of an endocrine origin. In fact, the vast majority of short children who have organic illness suffer from major systemic diseases of cardiac, pulmonary, gastrointestinal, or renal origin. The most common etiology of short stature in children is short parents. The genetic potential of a child is heavily determined by the growth achieved by both parents and by their relatives, and this information should be part of a careful history taken in evaluating short children. Genetic syndromes (such as Turner syndrome or Down syndrome) provide examples of cases in which chromosomal abnormalities limit physical growth. Congenital disorders of bone mineralization and bone growth, such as the chondrodystrophies, also represent an important cause of short stature. An aggressive endocrine investigation should be undertaken to ascertain the presence or absence of hypopituitarism and GH deficiency only after these other diseases have been eliminated from consideration.

While deficiencies of other anterior pituitary hormones, such as TSH or ACTH, may result in secondary hypothyroid and hypoadrenal states, these states tend to be milder than those of primary hypothyroidism or Addison's disease and hence their clinical signs are not as striking. The most striking feature of the panhypopituitary patient remains that of growth retardation.

Thyroid Gland Disorders

The thyroid gland is situated in the neck or, rarely, at the base of the tongue or in the mediastinum. Both overactivity and underactivity of the thyroid gland may be associated with goiter; however, the signs of hyperthyroidism and hypothyroidism are dramatically different. Examination of the thyroid gland is an important step in the evaluation of a suspected abnormality in thyroid hormone release.

As seen in Figure 9.9, the thyroid gland usually can best be palpated with the examiner behind the patient. After identification of the cricothyroid cartilage, the second and third fingers are moved laterally along the trachea just medial to the sternocleidomastoid muscles. Two distinct lobes are palpable, the right lobe usually greater in size than the left lobe. With goiter present, these lobes may be quite easily identified. The texture of the gland will vary in hyperthyroidism and hypothyroidism; the former usually being soft and fleshy, and the latter usually firm or bosselated. Since the thyroid is directly supported by the trachea, having the patient swallow several mouthfuls of water will elevate and depress a palpable gland along with the trachea during the swallowing motion.

Most physicians are familiar with the symptoms associated with hyperthyroidism, or Graves' disease. An acceleration in basal metabolism with concomitant tachycardia, weight loss, heat intolerance, and nervousness are characteristic. Exophthalmus, a characteristic eye finding of Graves' disease, usually is less dramatic in children than in adults, but the appearance of proptosis can easily be appreciated (Fig. 9.10). The hyperthyroid gland can become quite large, as much as 3 to 4 times normal size, and it is quite warm during palpation. A bruit often may be heard over a hyperthyroid gland.

Either congenital or acquired hypothyroidism may also produce goiter. Goiter in an infant with congenital hypothyroidism is suggestive of an enzymatic defect in thyroid hormone biosynthesis. To demonstrate goiter in a newborn infant, the examiner's hand is placed gently under the back and shoulder blades of the infant, and the infant's trunk is raised from the bed (Fig. 9.11). As the head falls backward, the neck is elevated and a goiter, if present, will be displayed

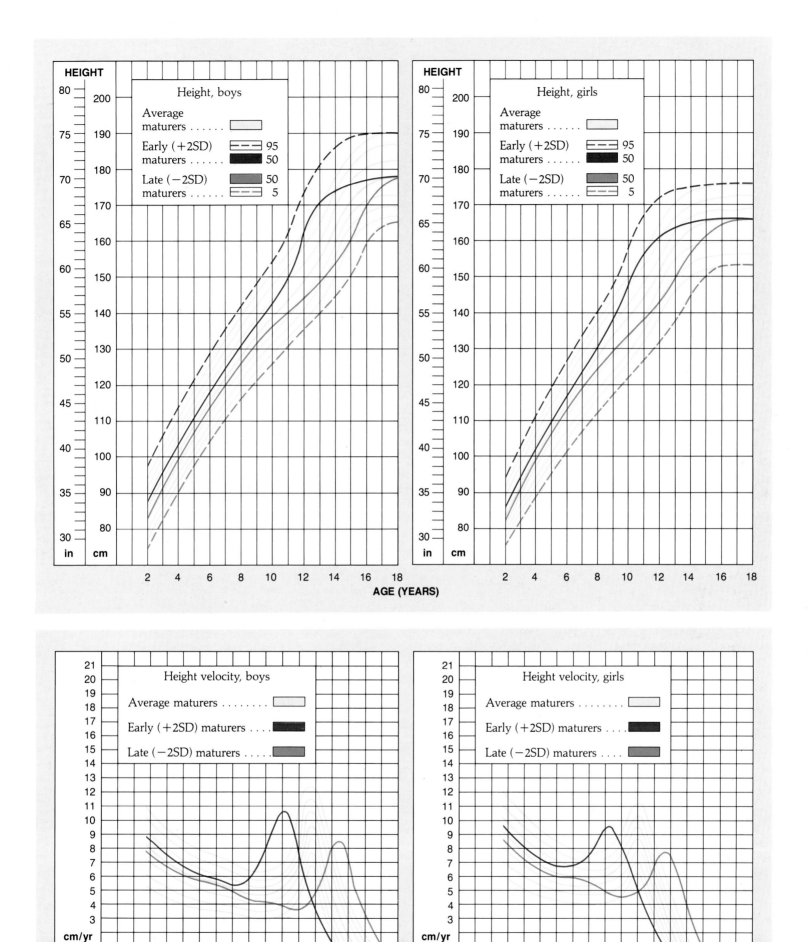

FIG. 9.8 Linear growth and growth velocity curves for boys and girls. (Adapted from Tanner JM, Davies PSW: Clinical longitudinal standards for height and height velocity for North American children. J Pediatr 107:317–329, 1985)

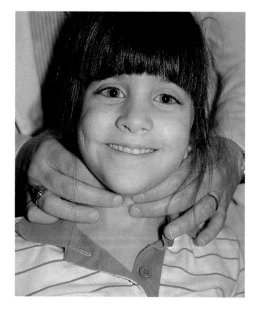

FIG. 9.9 Correct palpation of the thyroid gland is performed from behind the child.

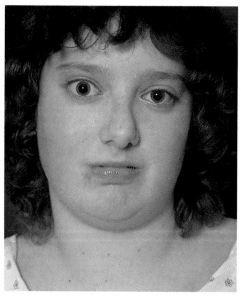

FIG. 9.10 These patients with Graves' disease illustrate both thyromegaly and

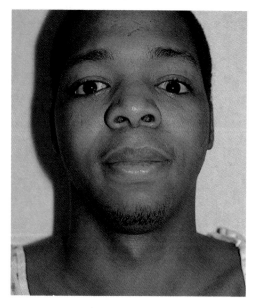

significant proptosis or ophthalmopathy.

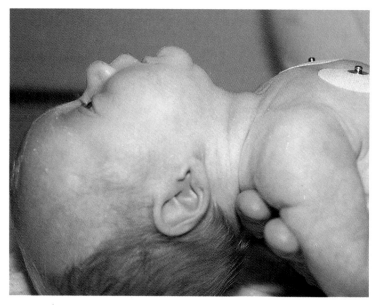

FIG. 9.11 Examination of the neonatal thyroid gland may be effectively performed by elevating the infant's trunk and allowing the head to drop back gently, as shown.

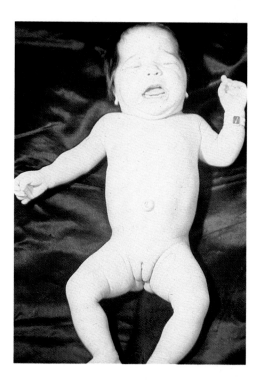

FIG. 9.12 A child with cretinism. (Courtesy of Dr. T.P. Foley, Jr.)

prominently. Because of neonatal thyroid screening, the coarse features of the congenital hypothyroid baby referred to as a cretin (Fig. 9.12), hopefully are now a thing of the past. However, the broad nasal bridge, thick lips, and dull appearance characteristic of a cretin were seen regularly in endocrine clinics and pediatric offices not long ago because of the difficulty of making this diagnosis in early life. It is now clear that all of these physical findings may be absent or too subtle to diagnose with certainty. This uncertainty, in combination with the success of early treatment of congenital hypothyroidism, mandates continued neonatal thyroid screening.

Acquired hypothyroidism, most frequently caused by Hashimoto's thyroiditis, may also present in a subtle fashion. The most dramatic expression of acquired hypothyroidism may be a sharp deceleration in growth, as seen in the growth curve shown in Figure 9.13. Following institution of thyroid hormone therapy, rapid catch-up growth occurs, returning the child to normal growth percentiles. Despite the subtlety of these clinical findings, the astute clinician will still take note of the dry skin, constipation, hair loss, depressed or delayed relaxation phase of deep tendon reflexes, and weakness of the child with acquired hypothyroidism.

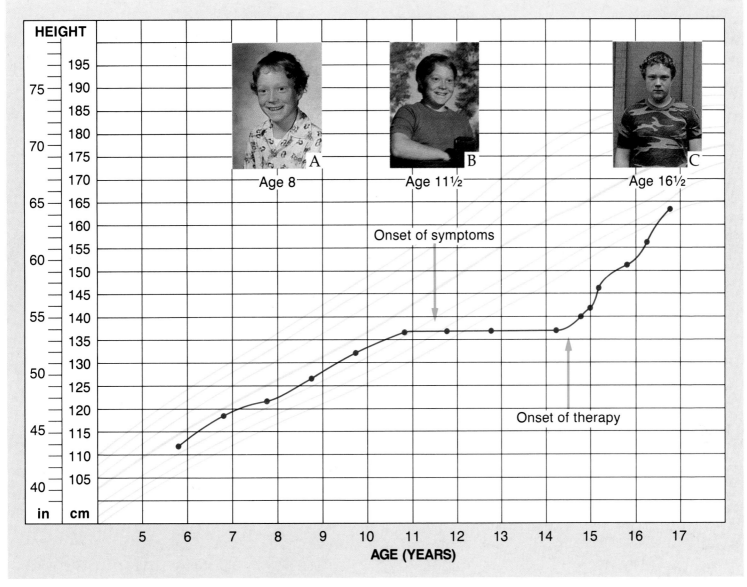

FIG. 9.13 The growth curve of this child with acquired hypothyroidism shows marked growth deceleration. Following thyroid replacement, significant catch-up growth occurs. The inserted photographs illustrate (**A**) the child prior to the onset of acquired hypothyroidism, (**B**) the change in body habitus associated with acquired hypothyroidism, and (**C**) resolution following thyroid replacement at the indicated times.

Parathyroid Gland Dysfunction

Dysfunction of the parathyroid glands usually does not present a unique phenotype. Chvostek's sign (distortion of the face when the seventh nerve is stimulated with a reflex hammer) or Trousseau's sign (cramping of the hand when a blood pressure cuff is elevated significantly above the systolic blood pressure) may be the only significant sign seen in an individual with hypocalcemia. However, Albright's hereditary osteodystrophy, one specific form of hypoparathyroidism, is associated with a very characteristic phenotype. These patients may have a round facies, short stature, obesity, skin hyperpigmentation with irregular margins, and a short thick neck (Fig. 9.14A). Shortening of the metacarpals and metatarsals is seen most commonly in the fourth digit, and less commonly in the other digits (Figs. 9.14B and C). These patients may have decreased intelligence as well as subcutaneous calcification, may present with hypocalcemia and hyperphosphatemia, and characteristically have reduced phosphaturia when given exogenous parathyroid hormone. This disorder is hereditary and is passed with an inheritance suggestive of an X-linked dominant gene. Albright's hereditary osteodystrophy should be suspected in a short child who is having difficulty with hypocalcemia and whose history reveals similarly affected family members.

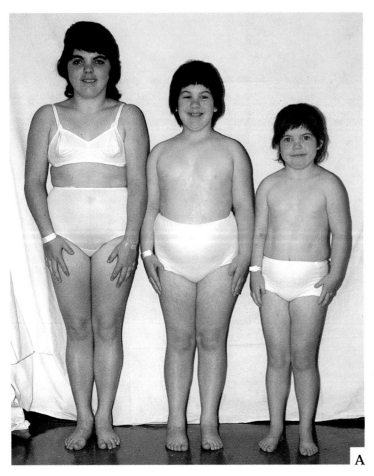

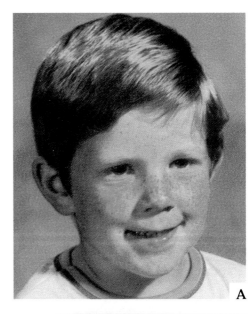

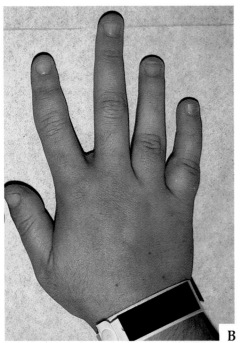

FIG. 9.14 **A**, Sisters with Albright's hereditary osteodystrophy (pseudohypoparathyroidism). **B**, The short fourth metacarpal may easily be appreciated in this photograph. **C**, Radiograph of the hand illustrates the short fourth metacarpal seen in pseudohypoparathyroidism as well as in other syndromes such as Turner syndrome. This child also has a short third and a short fourth metacarpal, as well. (**A** and **B** courtesy of Dr. J. Parks, **C** courtesy of Dr. J. Medina)

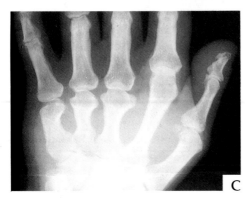

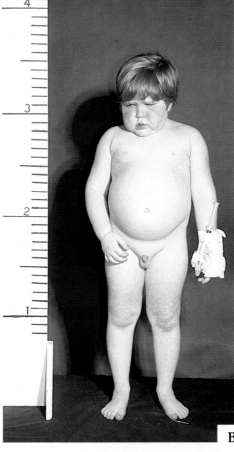

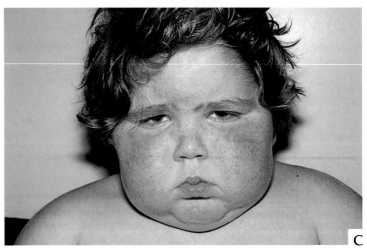

FIG. 9.15 Cushing syndrome. These photographs show how dramatic the changes associated with Cushing syndrome are, and how rapidly they can occur. **A**, Patient prior to the onset of Cushing syndrome. **B**, Patient 4 months after **A** was taken. Note the centripetal obesity of the trunk compared with the extremities after the onset of Cushing syndrome. **C**, Moon facies is clearly demonstrated and should raise the diagnostic index of Cushing syndrome. In diagnosing Cushing syndrome equally important to the physical manifestations shown here is the presence of growth failure.

THE DIFFERENTIAL DIAGNOSIS OF CUSHING SYNDROME AS INTERPRETED FROM THE DEXAMETHASONE SUPPRESSION TEST

	Normal	Adrenal Tumor	Pituitary Hypersecretion
	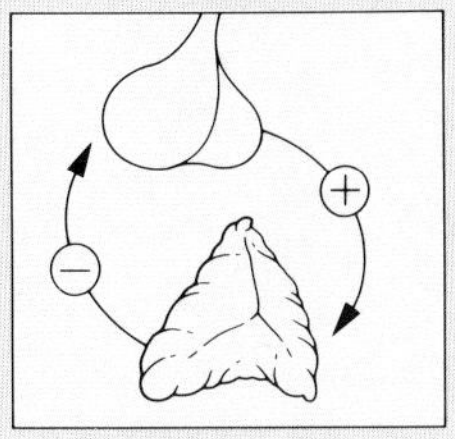	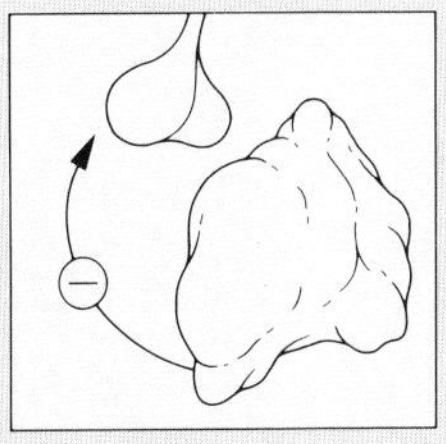	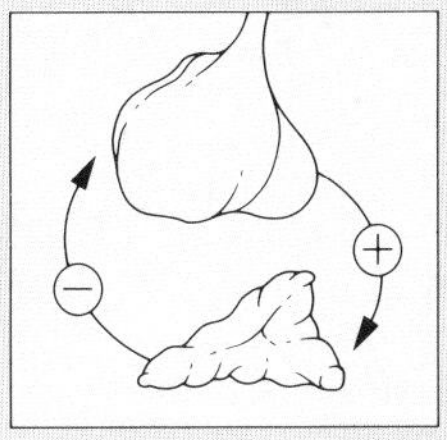
Plasma cortisol diurnal rhythm	10–25 µg% rhythmic	High no rhythm	High no rhythm
Plasma ACTH	Normal	Low	High
Plasma ACTH after adrenalectomy, on normal cortisol replacement	Normal	Low	High
Plasma glucocorticoid response to ACTH	3–5 fold rise	+, 0	+
Urinary glucocorticoid response to metyrapone	2–4 fold rise	0	+
Plasma glucocorticoid response to dexamethasone	Supressed	No fall	Partial fall

FIG. 9.16 The differential diagnosis of Cushing syndrome as interpreted from the dexamethasone suppression test. (Adapted from Williams RH: Textbook of Endocrinology, 6th ed. Saunders, Philadelphia, 1981, p.272)

Adrenal Gland Dysfunction

Hyperfunction or hypofunction of the adrenal glands results in some of the most dramatic physical alterations of any endocrinologic disorder. Cushing syndrome, the phenotype resulting from excess glucocorticoid action, is seen in endogenous as well as in exogenous steroid exposure. Rounded facies, plethora, and a central obesity are characteristic of Cushing syndrome (Fig. 9.15). The so-called Buffalo hump behind the neck has been described frequently. These children often may show centripetal obesity. Because of their excessive metabolism, muscle weakness and muscle wasting occur, resulting in comparatively thin extremities (see Fig. 9.15 B). These children frequently are irritable and quite miserable. The skin is usually thinned and easily bruised. Hypertension and, ultimately, loss of bone mineral and osteoporosis occur with long-standing glucocorticoid exposure.

Endogenous Cushing syndrome may be caused by adrenal tumors, pituitary adenoma, or ectopic ACTH production.

The high- and low-dose dexamethasone suppression test remains the most important diagnostic study for differentiating between the etiologies of Cushing syndrome. The development of effective ACTH assays and of urinary free-cortisol measurement has added new diagnostic power to this classic study. Following two days of baseline studies, dexamethasone is administered in a "low dose" of 0.005 to 0.006 mg/kg, or 0.25 mg, every 6 hours for three days in the older child or adult. Following the low-dose administration, a "high dose" of 0.02 to 0.025 mg/kg, or 2 mg, every 6 hours is administered for the last three days of the tests. The differential findings in the specific etiology of Cushing syndrome are listed in Figure 9.16. Improvement in surgical technique has been responsible for an improved outcome in the treatment of pituitary Cushing syndrome. Medical therapy for adrenal tumors or to supress pituitary ACTH production is still inadequate.

In striking contrast to the obesity seen with glucocorticoid excess, patients with Addison's disease (glucocorticoid and

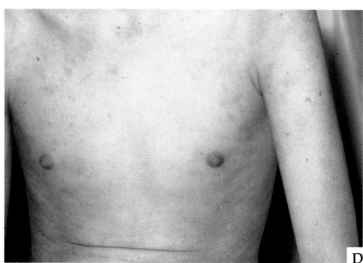

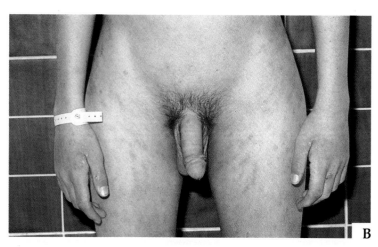

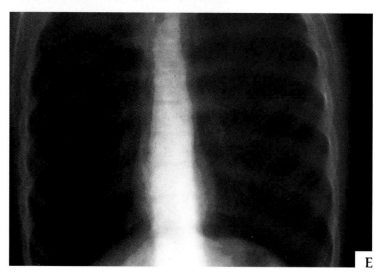

FIG. 9.17 **A**, This patient shows the thin habitus and ill appearance characteristic of Addison's disease. **B–D**, Hyperpigmentation may be marked. **E**, Microcardia is characteristically seen on chest radiograph. (**A** through **D** courtesy of Dr. M. New, **E** courtesy of Dr. J. Medina)

mineralocorticoid deficiency) present with a thin body habitus and wasting of subcutaneous tissue (Fig. 9.17A). There is little change seen in overall growth rate. Frequently a striking hyperpigmentation or bronzing of the skin occurs, with emphasis of this pigmentary change in flexor creases and in scars, and over the areolae of the nipples (Fig. 9.17B through D). Vitiligo may occur as well. Frequently patients may be confused and weak. In far-advanced Addison's disease vascular collapse is common. The decreased circulating plasma volume is reflected by the thinned narrow heart shadow seen on a chest radiograph (Fig. 9.17E). If untreated, patients with

Addison's disease gradually weaken and die. However, replacement of glucocorticoid with cortisol, and of mineralocorticoid with a compound such as 9 - α - fludrocortisone (Florinef) allows the patient with Addison's disease to lead a normal life. Tuberculosis was formerly the most common cause of Addison's disease. Autoimmune destruction of the adrenal gland has now replaced tuberculosis as the most common cause of Addison's disease. The clinical manifestations of Addison's disease are less fully expressed in individuals who have either isolated ACTH deficiencies or hypothalamic alterations in corticotropin-releasing factor kinetics.

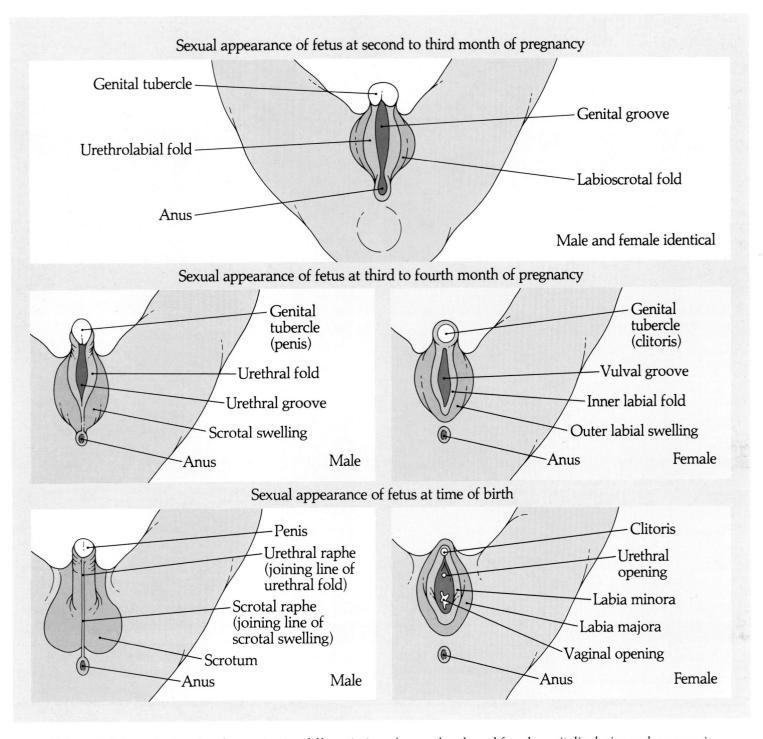

FIG. 9.18 Schematic drawing demonstrating differentiation of normal male and female genitalia during embryogenesis.

SEXUAL MATURATION

Anomalies of Early Sexual Development

Sexual maturation begins in fetal life. With normal progression, a normal internal and external male or female genital anatomy is formed (Fig. 9.18). If normal progression of sexual development fails, however, children may be born with ambiguous genitalia (Fig. 9.19), which presents a difficult and urgent diagnostic problem for the obstetric/pediatric team. Children with ambiguous genitalia must be evaluated with urgency and a diagnosis determined as quickly as possible. This provides the basis for an appropriate recommendation to parents regarding the sex of rearing, and also for the rapid and appropriate institution of therapy in cases where medical intervention is necessary.

The classification of anomalous sexual development can be based on gonadal development. Some disorders of gonadal differentiation (such as Klinefelter syndrome, Turner syndrome, and their variants) may not necessarily present with anomalous external genitalia. True hermaphroditism, while rare, frequently may present with ambiguous genitalia at birth. Female pseudohermaphrodites (genotype, XX) are those individuals who have ovaries, although they present with ambiguous external genitalia. The most common cause of female pseudohermaphroditism is virilizing adrenal hyperplasia. However any androgen or synthetic progestin transferred from the maternal circulation, either exogenously administered to the mother or endogenously produced by the mother, may result in virilization of the fetal genitalia.

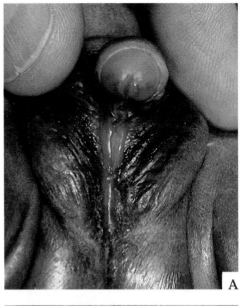
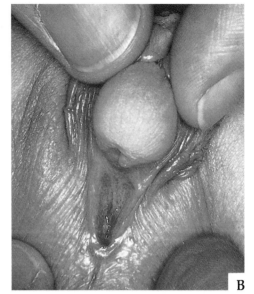
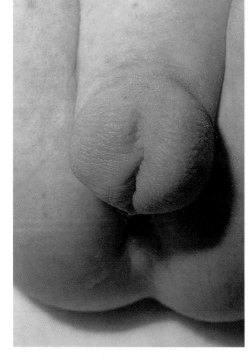

FIG. 9.20 Agenesis of the phallus.
(Courtesy of Dr. D. Becker)

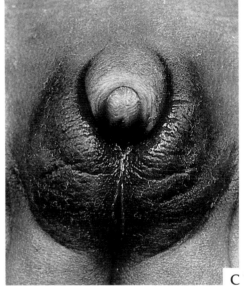
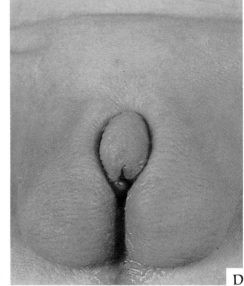

FIG. 9.19 Examples of ambiguous genitalia. These cases include (**A**) a true hermaphrodite, and (**B–D**) congenital virilizing adrenal hyperplasia. (**B** through **D** courtesy of Dr. D. Becker)

Teratogenic factors also may have an effect on the development of the external genitalia. These factors are constantly being elucidated as new drugs are introduced into the environment. Male pseudohermaphroditism is the term applied to individuals (genotype, XY) who have testes and ambiguous external genitalia. The etiologies of male pseudohermaphroditism are multiple and complex, and reflect the complex biosynthetic and hormonal processes required to induce normal development of the male external genitalia. Testicular unresponsiveness to either human chorionic gonadotropin (HCG) or LH is an early developmental error that will affect external genital development. Inborn errors of testosterone biosynthesis at both adrenal and testicular levels also will interfere with external genital development, since the development of external genitalia in the male is induced by the effects of both testosterone and dihydrotestosterone. A deficiency in the hormone may induce these abnormalities, or a defect in the hormone receptor may affect development, with inadequate recognition of androgenic hormones resulting in feminization of normal males. This is seen in its most dramatic form in the syndrome of testicular feminization, where the genitalia show no ambiguity, although the gonads are testes, and the individual's karyotype is XY. Karyotypic abnormalities, especially variants of the mixed or XY gonadal dysgenesis syndrome, also may be associated with ambiguous genitalia. Rare cases of ambiguous genitalia are unclassifiable and the mechanisms associated with these disorders remain to be elucidated.

It is important to remember that some children born with anatomic variants such as agenesis of the phallus (Fig. 9.20) may have neither a karyotypic nor a biochemical defect, but rather, a simple developmental anomaly. These also may outlie the classification of ambiguous genitalia described above. Regardless, any child seen at birth with ambiguous genitalia should not receive a sex assignment until such time as the appropriate sex of rearing may be properly assessed and assigned. An appropriate sex assignment must be based on the following considerations: potential for mature sexual function, potential fertility, and the long-term psychological and intellectual impact on the child and family.

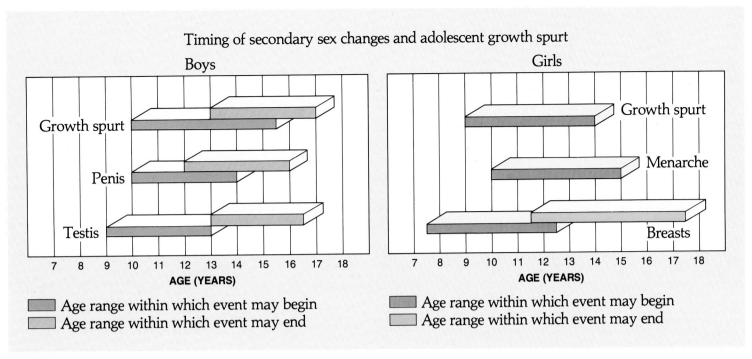

Timing of secondary sex changes and adolescent growth spurt

Boys

Girls

Age range within which event may begin
Age range within which event may end

FIG. 9.21 *Schematic representation of the onset of male and female puberty. (Adapted from Johnson TR, Moore WM, Jefferies JE: Children are Different: Development Physiology,* 2nd ed. *Ross Laboratories, Division of Abbott Laboratories, Columbus, OH, 1978, pp. 26–29)*

Development in Puberty

The pattern of timing of pubertal events for males and females is generally predictable (Fig. 9.21). However, for both males and females, the age of puberty varies in different regions of the world. In the United States, the onset of breast development and pubic hair growth occurs at approximately 10½ years of age, with menarche occurring at approximately 12½ years of age. However, considerable variations exist in these numbers for any individual patient.

THE TANNER STAGES

Because the onset and progression of puberty is so variable, Tanner has proposed a scale, now uniformly accepted, to describe the onset and progression of pubertal changes (Fig. 9.22). Males and females are rated on five-point scales. Males are rated for both genital development and pubic hair growth, while females are rated for breast development and also for pubic hair growth. The stages for male genital development are as follows (see Fig. 9.22A): STAGE I (Preadolescent). The testes, scrotal sac, and penis have a size and proportion similar to that seen in early childhood. STAGE II. There is enlargement of the scrotum and testes, and a change in the texture of the scrotal skin. The scrotal skin also may be reddened, a finding not obvious when viewed on a black and white photograph. STAGE III. Further growth of the penis has occurred, initially in length, although with some increase in circumference. There also is increased growth of the testes and scrotum. STAGE IV. The penis is significantly enlarged in length and circumference, with further development of the glans penis. The testes and scrotum continue to enlarge and there is distinct darkening of the scrotal skin. Again, this is difficult to evaluate on a black and white photograph. STAGE V. The genitalia are adult with regard to size and shape.

The stages in male pubic hair development are as follows (see Fig. 9.22B): STAGE I (Preadolescent). Vellous hair appears over the pubes with a degree of development similar to that over the abdominal wall. There is no androgen-sensitive pubic hair. STAGE II. There is sparse development of long pigmented downy hair, which is only slightly curled or may be straight. The hair is seen chiefly at the base of the penis. This stage may be difficult to evaluate on a photograph especially if the subject has fair hair. STAGE III. The pubic hair is considerably darker, coarser, and more curly. The distribution of hair has now spread over the junction of the pubes, and at this point the hair may be recognized easily on black and white photography. STAGE IV. The hair distribution is now adult in type but still is considerably less than that seen in adults. There is no spread to the medial surface of the thighs. STAGE V. Hair distribution is adult in quantity and type, and is described as an inverse triangle. There can be spread to the medial surface of the thighs.

In young women, the Tanner stages for breast development are as follows (see Fig. 9.22C): STAGE I (Preadolescent). Only the papilla is elevated above the level of the chest wall. STAGE II (Breast Budding). Elevation of the breasts and papillae may occur as small mounds along with some increased diameter of the areolae. STAGE III. The breasts and areolae continue to enlarge, although, they show no separation of contour. STAGE IV. The areolae and papillae elevate above the level of the breasts and form secondary mounds with further development of the overall breast tissue. STAGE V. Mature female breasts have developed. The papillae may extend slightly above the contour of the breast, due to recession of the areolae.

Pubic hair growth in females is staged as follows (see Fig. 9.22B): STAGE I (Preadolescent). Vellous hair develops over the pubes in a manner not greater than that over the anterior

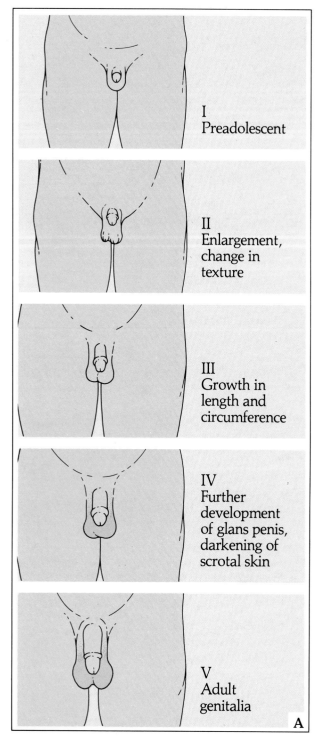

FIG. 9.22 Schematic drawings of male and female Tanner stages, showing (**A**) male genital development, (**B**) pubic hair development, and (**C**) breast development. (Adapted from Johnson TR, Moore WM, Jefferies JE: Children are Different:

abdominal wall. There is no sexual hair. STAGE II. Sparse, long pigmented downy hair, which is straight or only slightly curled, appears. These hairs are seen mainly along the labia. This stage is difficult to quantitate on black and white photography, particularly when pictures are obtained of fair-haired subjects. STAGE III. Considerably darker, coarser, and more curled sexual hair appears. The hair has now spread sparsely over the junction of the pubes. STAGE IV. The hair distribution is adult in type but decreased in total quantity. There is no spread to the medial surface of the thighs. STAGE V. Hair is adult in quantity and type, and appears in an inverse triangle of the classically feminine type. There is spread to the medial surface of the thighs but not above the base of the inverse triangle.

PRECOCIOUS PUBERTY

The Tanner classification has become an important instrument for communication among physicians, allowing a semiquantitative description of the pubertal progression of both boys and girls. However, variations in the timing and normal progression of puberty often are associated with specific pathologic entities. A diagnosis of precocious or early development may be made if sexual maturation begins under age 8 for girls and under age 9 for boys. In girls, the causes of isosexual precocity (development along lines of the same sex) are related to alterations in gonadal or central nervous system function. True precocious puberty follows an early onset of secretion of pulsatile LH and of FSH, and the subsequent re-

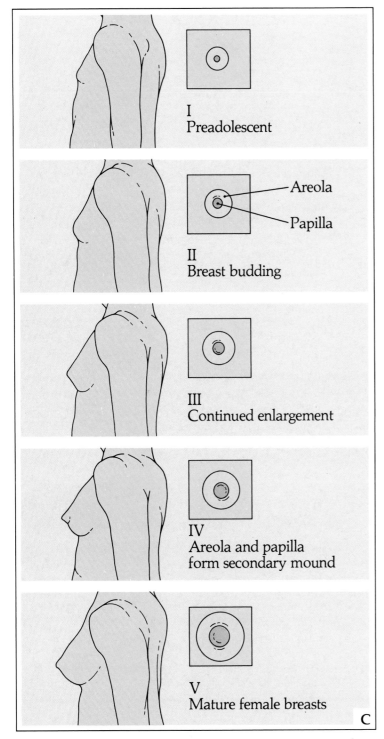

I
Preadolescent

II
Breast budding

Areola

Papilla

III
Continued enlargement

IV
Areola and papilla
form secondary mound

V
Mature female breasts

C

Development Physiology, 2nd ed. Ross Laboratories, Division of Abbott Laboratories, Columbus, OH, 1978, pp. 26–29)

sponse of the ovary. Estrogen-secreting tumors of the ovary, however, will suppress development of normal LH and FSH secretion. The McCune-Albright syndrome, polyostotic fibrous dysplasia with sexual precocity, has been associated with either central or peripheral etiologies for precocious puberty.

Isosexual precocity in young boys also may be caused by central nervous system abnormalities or by peripheral dysfunction. However, intracranial neoplasms are more commonly associated with precocious puberty in boys as compared with girls. Adrenal or testicular neoplasms in young boys are unusual but do occur. Late-onset congenital virilizing adrenal hyperplasia also may result in isosexual precocity in males.

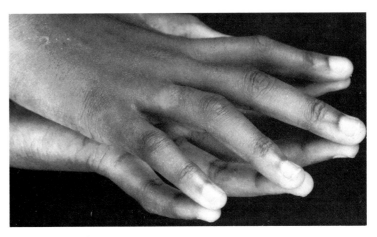

FIG. 9.23 Diabetic sclerodactyly is seen in this patient's inability to flatten the palms and fingers as he presses both hands together. (Courtesy of Dr. A. Rosenbloom)

INSULIN-DEPENDENT DISEASES
Diabetes Mellitus

Diabetes mellitus represents one of the most common of the chronic diseases seen by the endocrinologist. Prior to the institution of aggressive insulin therapy, children with diabetes mellitus and short stature were seen frequently in endocrine clinics and represented instances of the Mauriac syndrome. This syndrome is characterized by poorly controlled diabetes, short stature, hepatomegaly, and sexual infantilism. This is now a very rare occurrence. In a carefully treated child with type I or insulin-dependent diabetes mellitus, growth rate should be indistinguishable from that of a normal child. However, one physical finding still frequently seen in diabetic patients is that of limited joint mobility. Figure 9.23 shows the inability of a diabetic child to flatten the palms because of waxy thickened skin in the areas of the proximal and distal interphalangeal joints. Although this phenomenon is not as yet completely understood, it has been associated with poor diabetic control. The development of specific skin lesions such as necrobiosis lipoidica diabeticorum also may be associated with diabetes. Figure 9.24 shows such a lipid-filled skin lesion, which may occasionally be seen in a child with type I diabetes.

Hypoglycemia

Specific syndromes associated with hypoglycemia may be diagnosed at first glance during the patient's examination. The most striking of these is Beckwith-Wiedemann syndrome (Fig. 9.25), associated with macrosomia, macroglossia, omphaloceles, hemihypertrophy, and embryonal tumors. The hypoglycemia has been attributed to hyperinsulinism. These individuals may require aggressive treatment with diazoxide or in fact may come to partial or complete pancreatectomy because of the severity of the hypoglycemia.

Another rare cause of hypoglycemia, which may be quickly diagnosed, is leprechaunism. A small wizened infant presenting with severe recurrent hypoglycemia can readily be diagnosed as having leprechaunism. The etiology of the hypoglycemia seems to be that of hyperinsulinism and an abnormal cellular responsiveness to insulin's action. In this case however, the hyperinsulinism seems to be a state associated with an unusual response to insulin with hypoglycemia, as opposed to simple hyperinsulinism.

SUMMARY

As seen in the above illustrations, endocrine imbalances may result in dramatic alterations in a child's phenotype. These alterations should be readily recognized, and thus direct the diagnostic approach. Careful attention to the appearance of children requiring evaluation by a physician should allow early diagnosis of endocrine disorders, resulting in prompt therapeutic intervention and in restoration of the child's appearance and overall state of well-being.

BIBLIOGRAPHY

Bacon GE, Spencer ML, Hopwood NJ, and Kelch RP: A Practical Approach to Pediatric Endocrinology, 2nd ed. Year Book, Chicago, 1982.

Frasier SD: Pediatric Endocrinology. Grune & Stratton, Orlando, Florida, 1980.

Hung W, August GP, Glasgow AM: Pediatric Endocrinology. Medical Examination, Hyde Park, New York, 1983.

Kaplan SA: Clinical Pediatric and Adolescent Endocrinology. W. B. Saunders, Philadelphia, 1982.

Williams RH: Textbook of Endocrinology. W. B. Saunders, Philadelphia, 1981.

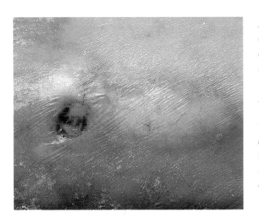

FIG. 9.24 Necrobiosis lipoidica diabeticorum is characterized by the presense of yellow waxy skin lesions that exhibit reddened components. Small areas of ulceration also may be seen. (Courtesy of Dr. B. Cohen)

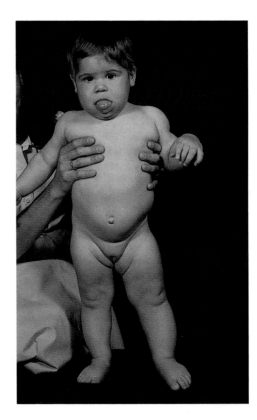

FIG. 9.25 Beckwith-Wiedimann syndrome. Note hemihypertrophy on the left side, along with the prominence of the tongue. (Courtesy of Dr. D. Becker)

PEDIATRIC NUTRITION AND GASTROENTEROLOGY

J. Carlton Gartner Jr., M.D.

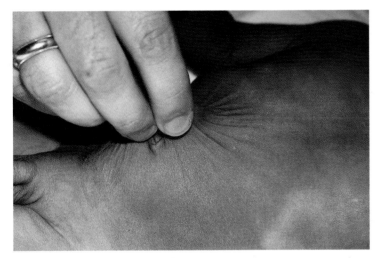 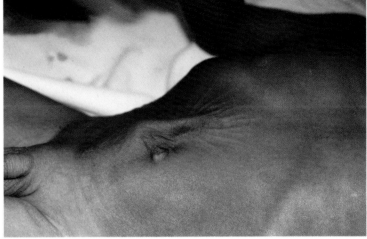

FIG. 10.1 Dehydration. In this patient with severe dehydration (left), skin turgor is poor indicating decreased extracellular volume. Skin remains tented after release and retracts quite slowly (right).

Nutrition and gastroenterology are areas closely related to the daily activities of most pediatricians. As a world health problem, the cycle of diarrhea, poor nutrition, and consequent absorptive disorders causes untold harm. This chapter will initially deal with nutritional assessment and malnutrition in children and then with some rarer nutritional deficiencies which may be diagnosed by careful examination and limited laboratory testing. This will supplement material already available in standard textbooks. The gastroenterology section will feature the conditions which may be diagnosed on clinical grounds, including cystic fibrosis, and will include several hepatic disorders based on our extensive experience as a transplant center.

NUTRITION

Nutritional awareness is mandatory for child health workers, given the importance of growth and development during infancy and childhood. Each pediatric visit, whether for routine care or serious illness, should include at least a basic nutritional assessment. This may include dietary, clinical, anthropometric, and detailed laboratory data. In a well child this process involves only a brief dietary history (adequate formula in sufficient quantity) and a plot of height, weight, and head circumference on standard curves. The ill child may require more careful assessment to clarify acute and/or chronic malnutrition in order to plan effective therapy.

Clinical Observations of Malnutrition

Clinical signs of chronic malnutrition are relatively easy for most observers to recognize. However, a cycle of recurrent gastrointestinal disturbances is the most common prodrome to undernutrition. Dehydration must be recognized early (dry mucous membranes, oliguria) before more serious complications ensue (depressed fontanelle, sunken eyes, diminished skin turgor) (Fig. 10.1). Rapid treatment and follow-up of nutritional depletion may interrupt the vicious cycle of malnutrition. Perhaps the major advance in world

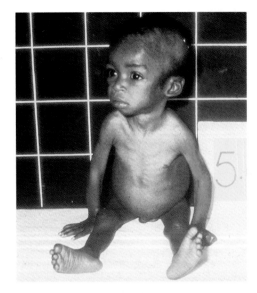

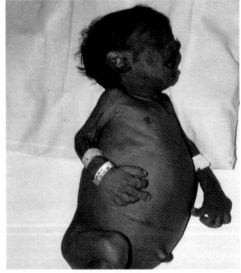

FIG. 10.2 *Marasmus. Note profound wasting and sparse hair* (left), *producing a characteristic simian appearance* (right).

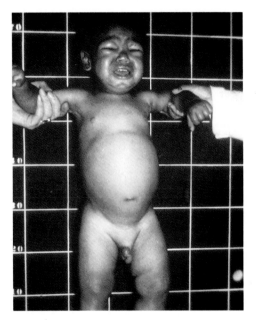

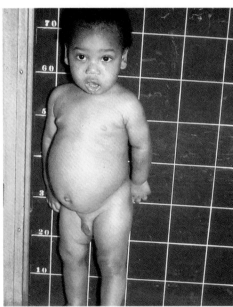

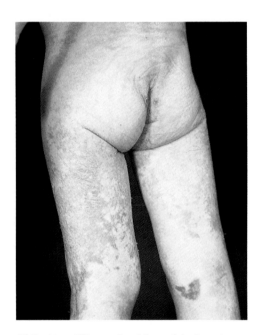

FIG. 10.3 Kwashiorkor. (Left) *This patient has a typical "sugar baby" appearance with generalized edema. Note the periorbital and limb edema.*

(Right) *The same patient after nutritional repletion. He has lost the edema, but retains the protuberant abdomen of malnutrition.*

FIG. 10.4 *The rash of kwashiorkor is scaly, erythematous, and may weep, especially in edematous areas.*

health in recent years is the use of oral rehydration solutions (ORS) to effectively treat gastroenteritis. Numerous studies have shown the advantages of this inexpensive, readily available mixture which does require potable water and appropriate dilution.

Clinical descriptions of malnutrition differentiate between marasmus (caloric deficiency with wasting of tissue) and kwashiorkor (protein deficiency with edema). More recently it has become evident that these conditions often overlap and have a similar pathogenesis. For both conditions, physical signs and descriptions are helpful in patient evaluation and treatment. Malnourished children are often apathetic and have decreased physical activity. Marasmus is characterized by a marked weight-for-height reduction with emaciation, loss of subcutaneous fat, lusterless and sparse hair, and poor nail growth, producing a rather simian appearance (Fig. 10.2).

A classic kwashiorkor patient looks well-nourished ("sugar babies") without wasting. The initial "moon face" of kwashiorkor is often mistaken for good nutrition. In fact the child is often edematous, which becomes striking after nutritional repletion (Fig. 10.3). These children usually suffer acute protein deficiency in addition to preexisting caloric deprivation. Skin changes in kwashiorkor include hyper- and hypopigmentation with a scaly, weeping dermatitis which may ulcerate and desquamate (Fig. 10.4). The rash is often more prominent in skin areas which are chronically irritated (groin in infants and areas of peripheral edema). It resembles pellagra but is seen in areas other than those exposed to sunlight.

Anthropometric Measurements and Laboratory Tests

After the initial clinical exam of the malnourished patient is completed, anthropometric measurements should be made. These enable large groups of children to be followed sequentially, and aid in distinguishing between acute and chronic malnutrition and assessing the effects of protein or total calories. Using standard curves such as 1976 National Center

GRADING OF NUTRITIONAL STATUS

Grade	Height for Age	Weight for Height
I	<95%	<90%
II	<90%	<80%
III	<85%	<70%

FIG. 10.5 Grading of nutritional status.

ANTHROPOMETRIC ASSESSMENT OF NUTRITIONAL STATUS

Measurement	Deficiency	Indicated Deficiency
Weight for age	<90% of standard	Protein–Calorie
Height for age	<95%	Protein–Calorie
Weight for height	<90%	Protein–Calorie
Triceps skinfold	<5%	Calorie
Midarm muscle circumference	<5%	Protein

FIG. 10.6 Anthropometric assessment of nutritional status.

for Health Statistics charts, height-for-age deficit [actual height divided by expected height-for-age (50th percentile) × 100] and weight-for-height deficit [actual weight divided by expected weight-for-height (50th percentile) × 100] may be calculated. Diminished height for age most commonly reflects chronic undernutrition, while low weight for height may indicate more acute malnutrition. Grading of nutritional status is done using these two parameters (Fig. 10.5). In addition, measurements of triceps skinfold thickness and midarm muscle circumference aid in further delineating protein and calorie deficits (Fig. 10.6).

Laboratory testing can be helpful in some malnourished children. Not only is the degree of chronicity of the insult confirmed, but certain specific deficiencies may be uncovered. Unfortunately, an inexpensive laboratory test for early malnutrition is not yet available. Amino acid nomograms may aid early diagnosis but are expensive and require a sophisticated laboratory. Decreases in body proteins are helpful but reflect the time for normal body catabolism. Consequently, retinol binding protein ($t_{1/2}$ 12 hours) and transferrin ($t_{1/2}$ 9 days) indicate more current nutritional status than the standard albumin ($t_{1/2}$ 20–24 days). An additional aid in assessing lean body mass is a comparison of 24-hour creatinine excretion to standard norms for height (creatinine height index).

As infection is a major cause of morbidity and mortality in the malnourished patient, a basic immunologic assessment is indicated. Total lymphocyte counts and skin tests are a minimal baseline, as the major effects are in the T-lymphocyte system.

NUTRITIONAL DEFICIENCIES WITH CHARACTERISTIC PHYSICAL SIGNS

Vitamin/Mineral	Signs/Symptoms
Calcium, phosphorus, vitamin D	Rickets/osteomalacia
Vitamin A	Night blindness, xerophthalmia, Bitot's spots, follicular hyperkeratosis
Vitamin C	Scurvy: bone lesions, bleeding
Vitamin E	Hemolytic anemia, peripheral neuropathy
Vitamin K	Petechiae, ecchymoses
Thiamine B_1	Beriberi: heart failure, increased intracranial pressure
Niacin	Pellagra: dermatitis (sun-exposed areas)
Riboflavin B_2	Angular stomatitis, cheilosis
B_6	Anemia, dermatitis, neuropathy
B_{12}	Anemia, neuropathy
Folate	Anemia
Iron	Anemia, koilonychia
Biotin	Rash, hair loss
Essential fatty acids	Rash, coagulopathy
Zinc	Rash (acrodermatitis), growth failure, delayed sexual development, ageusia
Copper	Bone changes, hypopigmentation, anemia, neutropenia
Selenium	Heart failure

FIG. 10.7 Nutritional deficiencies with characteristic physical signs.

Therapy

After clinical, anthropometric, and laboratory assessments are completed, decisions about aggressive nutritional repletion or mere maintenance therapy can be made. Obviously patients with hypoproteinemia and major changes in weight for height will need more vigorous therapy. In this country we have the advantage of many modified and elemental formulas for children with acute or chronic digestive disturbances. As malnutrition has profound effects on intestinal absorption, several of these formulas may be invaluable. It is important to know the specific content of each product used. High osmolar formulas are often not tolerated, especially by the compromised small-bowel mucosa. Occasionally parenteral nutrition may be lifesaving in these children.

Prior to initiating nutritional therapy (or after a period of hyperalimentation) it is helpful to look for specific vitamin, mineral, and trace element deficiencies. The more common and previously well-described deficiencies are listed in Figure 10.7. It is often difficult to assign individual findings, such as

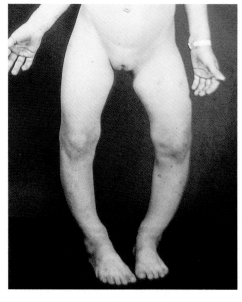

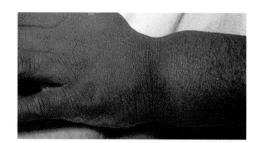

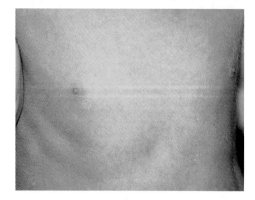

FIG. 10.9 Infantile rickets marked by widened wrists (top) and enlargement of the costochondral junction ("beading") (bottom). The latter occurred as the result of a rapid growth spurt following liver transplantation.

FIG. 10.8 Hypophosphatemic ricket marked by the obvious bowing.

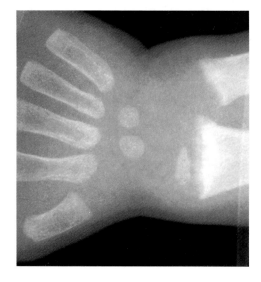

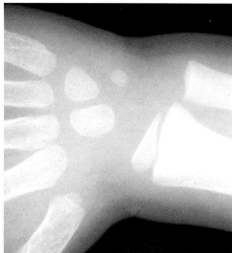

FIG. 10.10 Radiograph of the wrist in a patient with rickets (left) shows irregularity and widening of the epiphyses in the distal radius and ulna. With appropriate therapy (right), remineralization and healing occurs.

angular stomatitis, to specific deficiencies in a child with chronic, severe malnutrition. Several deficiencies, often seen in a hospital population, will be discussed below.

Rickets (or osteomalacia in nongrowing bone) from vitamin D deficiency remains a world health problem. However, the increased survival of tiny premature infants has led to biochemical rickets from calcium or phosphorus deficiency. Increased supplements of both of these minerals leads to reversal of the changes. The resurgence of breast feeding, especially in dark-skinned or vegetarian populations, has produced clinical rickets. It should be noted that disorders of two other organ systems—liver and kidney—may produce clinical or biochemical osteomalacia. Poor bile flow and consequent malabsorption is the primary etiology in hepatobiliary disorders. Additionally, end-stage renal disease with failure of renal hydroxylation of vitamin D₃ or renal tubular wasting of phosphorus may cause poor bone matrix formation.

In all of the above conditions which cause osteomalacia, the physical changes are similar: poor growth, curvature of weight-bearing bones (Fig. 10.8), widening of epiphyses, and costochondral beading (Fig. 10.9). Softening of the skull

(craniotabes) is seen in infants. With appropriate vitamin and mineral supplementation, radiographic healing occurs followed by bony remodeling (Fig. 10.10).

Deficiencies of other fat-soluble vitamins (E, K, A) may occur as well. Clinical vitamin E deficiency can progress from absence of peripheral deep-tendon reflexes to marked ataxia. Vitamin K deficiency, seen in patients with long-standing steatorrhea or liver disease, causes prolongation of the prothrombin time and can be associated clinically with easy bleeding and bruising. Vitamin A deficiency causes follicular hyperkeratosis, xerophthalmia, night blindness, and unusual shiny gray, triangular lesions on the conjunctivae (Bitot's spots).

Parenteral nutrition has been lifesaving, especially for neonates with major intestinal disorders complicated by malnutrition. Unfortunately, as trial-and-error methods were used in early hyperalimentation, numerous deficiencies were uncovered during prolonged periods of alimentation. Examples of this include fatty acid deficiency with the typical scaly dermatitis, and zinc deficiency with alopecia, diarrhea, and acrodermatitis; these conditions are now rare. Prior to reformulation of our own hyperalimentation mixture several

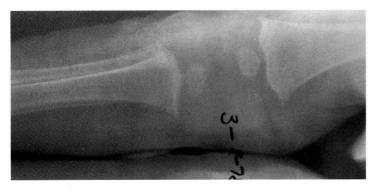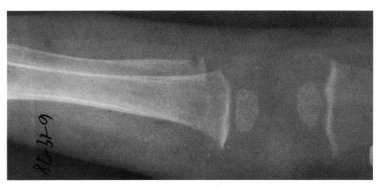

FIG. 10.11 Radiograph of a child with copper deficiency (left) reveals irregular epiphyses with spur formation, cloaking of metaphyses, periosteal new bone formation, and osteoporosis.

After 3 months of intravenous copper (right), the child demonstrates healing of the metaphyses.

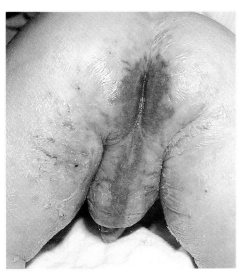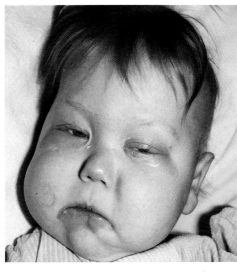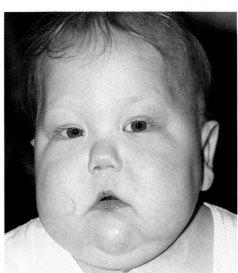

FIG. 10.12 Biotin deficiency. (Top) This child on chronic hyperalimentation developed dermatitis in perianal, perioral, and lid areas along with some thinning of hair. (Bottom) The rash has cleared dramatically after 4 days of biotin.

years ago, other unusual problems were uncovered. A child on hyperalimentation for 6 months developed irritability, bone pain, and decreased hair pigmentation. Anemia and progressive neutropenia ensued, and a skeletal survey as well as copper and ceruloplasmin determinations confirmed copper deficiency. Bone changes included osteoporosis, metaphyseal spurs, and periosteal new bone formation. Hematologic and then bone changes reversed with copper administration (Fig. 10.11). Another patient with short-gut syndrome on home hyperalimentation developed a peculiar weeping dermatitis in the perioral, perianal, and lid areas

along with lethargy and malaise. Changes reversed in only 4 days when intravenous biotin was added (Fig. 10.12).

Conclusion

Careful nutritional assessment followed by detailed clinical examination can uncover specific nutritional deficiencies as well as delineate the severity and chronicity of malnutrition. These facts will then allow a more specific plan of nutritional repletion to be formulated using a combination of parenteral and enteral routes.

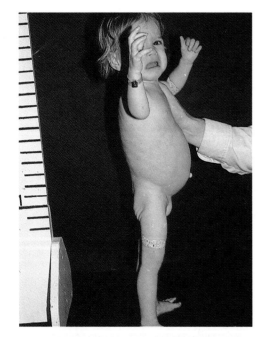
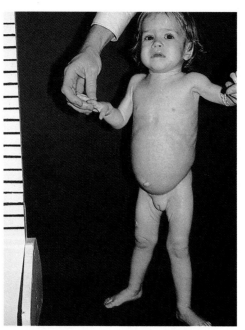
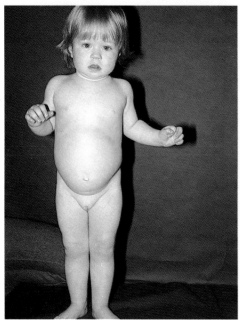
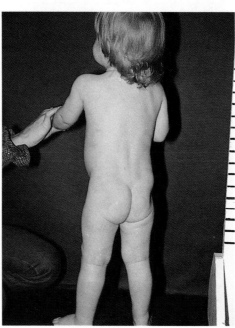

FIG. 10.13 Celiac disease. (Top) This child had a potbelly, vomiting, and weight loss as her major symptoms and was originally thought to have psychosocial failure to thrive. When celiac disease was suspected, the child was placed on a gluten-free diet. Note the protruding abdomen and wasted buttocks. (Bottom) After 10 weeks on the diet the improvement is obvious.

GASTROENTEROLOGY

Disturbances of gastrointestinal function are common in pediatric practice, perhaps second only to respiratory symptoms as a reason for office visits. However, clues to specific disorders are uncommon. This section will emphasize the major symptoms which bring patients with GI disease to medical attention and define entities which may be diagnosed by examination. Later in this section we will also discuss cystic fibrosis and liver disorders.

Malnutrition

As discussed earlier, malnutrition is a common sign in all GI diseases and generally does not aid specific diagnosis. Most clinicians, however, suspect celiac disease when they see a child with "potbelly" and wasted extremities and buttocks. A gluten-free diet is prescribed, and the results are quite rapid and dramatic (Fig. 10.13). As this is a lifelong condition, careful confirmation by repeated small intestinal biopsies is indicated.

Vomiting

Recurrent vomiting is a frequent symptom in childhood, most commonly associated with diarrhea (gastroenteritis).

PYLORIC STENOSIS
Early onset, a forceful projectile quality, continued hunger, and associated constipation are characteristic of hypertrophic pyloric stenosis. Giant gastric peristaltic waves and the typical firm pyloric olive are noted on examination (Fig. 10.14). In questionable cases, radiographs may be confirmatory by demonstrating a stringlike pyloric channel (Fig. 10.15). Abdominal ultrasonography can also demonstrate the pyloric tumor.

REFLUX
Gastroesophageal reflux is a common and usually self-limited condition beginning in early infancy. Many of these children "spit up" frequently in small amounts, both immediately and for hours after feedings. The problem usually lessens and gradually disappears by 1 year of age. Compli-

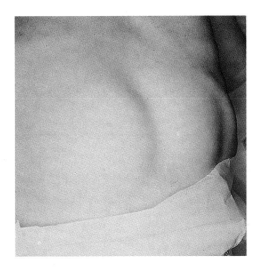

FIG. 10.14 Pyloric stenosis. The giant gastric waves are best seen just after a feeding.

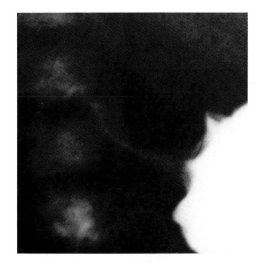

FIG. 10.15 This typical barium study in a patient with pyloric stenosis demonstrates a "stringlike" pyloric channel.

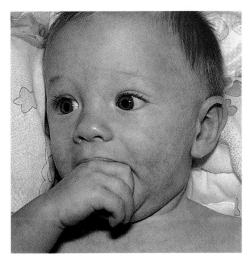

FIG. 10.16 Rumination. Note hand in mouth used to stimulate regurgitation and reswallowing.

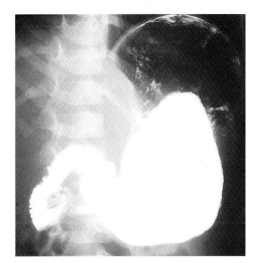

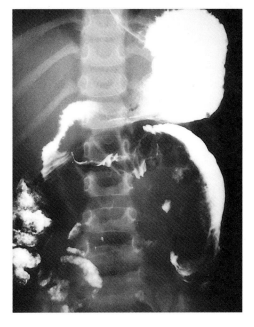

FIG. 10.17 Upper GI series demonstrates poor flow through the duodenum (top), and mass effect of the hematoma displacing other loops of bowel (bottom).

cated reflux—failure to grow, aspiration, esophagitis, hemorrhage, apnea—is less frequent. Clinical diagnosis is sufficient in mild cases, but more persistent or difficult problems may require further diagnostic testing. Barium swallow is helpful but diagnostic of abnormality in only 50 percent of the cases. Twenty-four hour (or shorter) esophageal pH-probe measurements, esophagoscopy and/or biopsy, aspiration nuclear scans, and esophageal manometric studies may all be necessary before arriving at a final assessment. Occasionally, peculiar posturing movements of the head and neck (as in Sandifer syndrome) are a clue to the problem. Additionally, psychophysiologic factors may predominate in the rumination syndrome. In late stages these children regurgitate constantly and swallow in a self-stimulating fashion (Fig. 10.16).

Therapy in mild cases involves more frequent and thickened feedings in an upright position—sitting and leaning forward rather than in a burp chair. Bethanechol chloride or metoclopramide hydrochloride may be of additional benefit. Persistent complicated reflux requires surgery, usually a Nissen-type fundoplication.

TRAUMA

No discussion of pediatric differential diagnosis is complete without a mention of trauma or child abuse. The GI tract may figure in subtle forms of abuse: chronic diarrhea from laxative abuse and feigned bleeding episodes are reported (Münchausen syndrome by proxy). Likewise, vomiting may be induced by occult trauma or abuse. Blunt injury to the abdomen, such as that from a bicycle handlebar, may produce an intramural duodenal hematoma with partial or complete obstruction and a fullness or mass on radiographic abdominal examination (Fig. 10.17). Resolution usually takes place slowly, and parenteral nutrition may be required for a period of time. As with other suspicious injuries, skeletal survey and detailed family evaluation are mandatory if the trauma is not explained by an obvious accident.

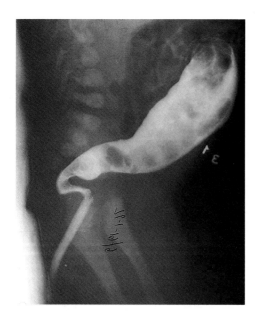

FIG. 10.18 The tapered transition zone to a normal-caliber colon is characteristic of Hirschsprung's disease.

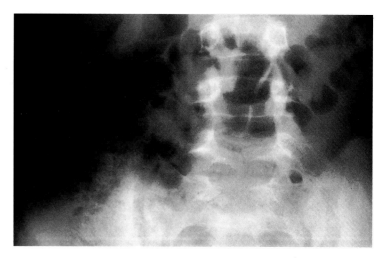

FIG. 10.19 An appendiceal fecalith can be seen in the right lower quadrant in this child with surgically proven acute appendicitis.

Constipation

Chronic constipation is usually seen on a functional basis and is often related historically to problems at the time of toilet training. Overflow incontinence (encopresis) may result and is usually manageable by a period of catharsis and bowel "retraining" in preschool or younger school-age children. Occasionally, major psychopathology is uncovered, especially in the older child, and appropriate intervention is necessary. Bladder dysfunction with recurrent urinary tract infections may be associated with major long-standing constipation.

Examination of the child with constipation usually reveals palpable stool in the descending colon and rectum. If the history dates to early infancy and obstipation is present as well, one should consider Hirschsprung's disease. Barium enema radiographic studies are usually diagnostic (Fig. 10.18), though rectal biopsy for ganglion cells and special stains are necessary for confirmation. In older children, rectal manometric studies may be helpful in separating organic from functional disorders.

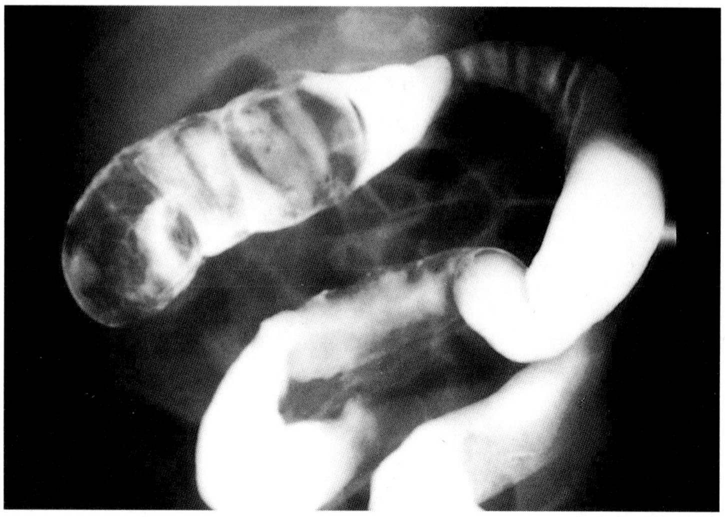

FIG. 10.20 Intussusception. Barium outlines the intussuscepted segment. Unfortunately, this lesion required laparotomy as reduction did not occur during the barium enema.

Abdominal Pain

Recurrent abdominal pain (RAP), often vague and nonspecific, is found in as many as 25 percent of school-age children. Despite careful evaluation, a precise etiology is seldom determined. In one long-term follow-up study at the Mayo Clinic, the only condition which appeared to be missed, though rarely, was regional enteritis. Unfortunately, 20 percent of RAP children are subjected to laparotomy.

Acute appendicitis may not have the classic sequence in pediatric patients, and suspicion must be high in any acute illness. All too often perforation has occurred prior to the diagnosis, and an appendiceal fecalith may be a good though infrequent clue (Fig. 10.19).

Less than one-third of patients with intussusception will have the classic triad: colicky pain, currant jelly stools, and an abdominal mass (Fig. 10.20). Neurologic symptoms such as lethargy or seizure are occasional clues to the diagnosis. Reduction by barium enema simplifies management of this disorder in most instances.

Hemorrhage

The etiology of GI hemorrhage usually requires detailed endoscopic and X-ray examination. In younger infants, the diagnosis may remain unclear in over 50 percent with a benign outlook. Portal hypertension, often of extrahepatic origin, is suggested by splenomegaly which may only become evident when volume status has been normalized after a recent hemorrhage. Other clues of chronic liver disease or colitis may be helpful. Perioral melanotic spots (Peutz-Jeghers syndrome; see Fig. 15.63) and other manifestations of intestinal polyposis syndromes (such as Gardner syndrome) can be detected by examination.

Diarrhea

Diarrhea is a symptom with many etiologies. Watery small-bowel diarrhea seldom yields a specific clue on examination.

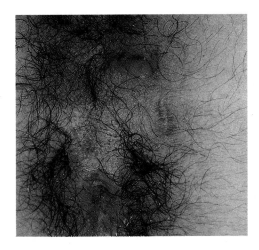
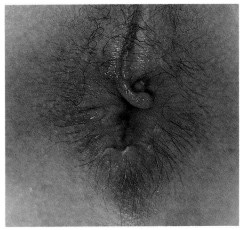

FIG. 10.21 (Left) *In this patient with Crohn's disease, the slightly raised, erythematous lesion eventually drained and represented a fistulous opening. Note a scar from previous incision and drainage (right). Perianal skintags are common in Crohn's disease and a good clue to diagnosis.*

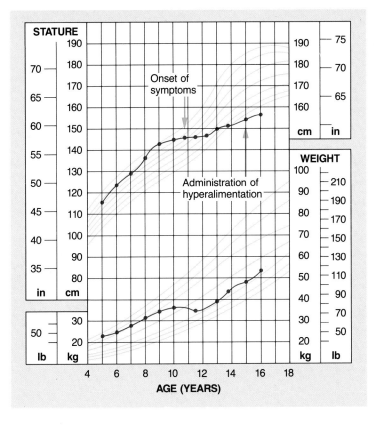

FIG. 10.22 *Crohn's disease. This growth curve demonstrates a falloff prior to onset of disease symptoms and continued poor growth through many exacerbations requiring steroid therapy. Home hyperalimentation has maintained weight gain.*

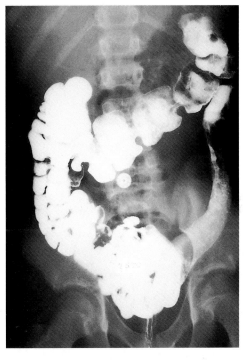

FIG. 10.23 *X-ray findings in Crohn's disease. Segmental narrowing of the left colon.*

INFLAMMATORY BOWEL DISEASE

Crampy abdominal pain with mucus and blood suggests large-bowel involvement, and numerous clues may suggest chronic inflammatory bowel diseases such as Crohn's disease or ulcerative colitis. While clinical distinctions are at times blurred in these latter disorders, severe perianal disease with fistulas and fissures along with perianal skintags is more common in Crohn's disease (Fig. 10.21). Additionally, poor growth prior to major GI symptoms is often a clue to Crohn's disease (Fig. 10.22). Rectal disease is characteristic of ulcerative colitis, perianal disease less common. Histologically, Crohn's disease is characterized by transmural inflammation with granuloma formation and skip areas. This deep inflammatory process accounts for the tendency to form fistulas and abscesses. Crypt abscesses are often seen in ulcerative colitis and help distinguish this disorder from many other causes of acute colitis. Radiographically, Crohn's disease may involve the entire bowel, with segmental narrowing, skip areas, and fistula formation (Fig. 10.23). Ulcerative colitis is a mucosal inflammation confined only to the large bowel (Fig. 10.24).

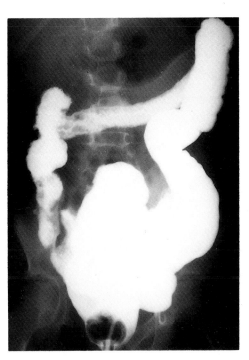

FIG. 10.24 *X-ray findings in ulcerative colitis. There is narrowing and loss of haustral markings, especially in the transverse colon. Mucosal irregularities are prominent in the right colon.*

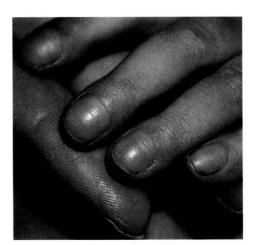

FIG. 10.25 *Osteoarthropathy (clubbing). Note thickening and loss of the angle at the nail bed.*

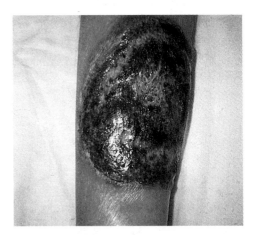

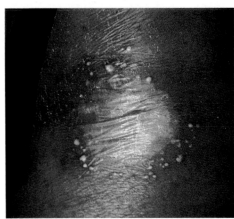

FIG. 10.26 *Pyoderma gangrenosum associated with inflammatory bowel disease (top). Initial papulopustules (bottom) coalesce to form a deep necrotic lesion.*

PRESENTATIONS OF CYSTIC FIBROSIS

General
    Failure to thrive
    Salty taste

GI/Nutritional
    Meconium ileus
    Foul-smelling stools, bloating, abdominal pain
    Rectal prolapse
    Intestinal impaction and obstruction
    Pancreatitis, acute and chronic
    Hypoproteinemia and edema
    Neonatal hyperbilirubinemia
    Cholelithiasis, cholecystitis
    Cirrhosis/portal hypertension
    Fat-soluble vitamin deficiency (E, K, A, D)

Metabolic
    Hyponatremic dehydration
    Heat stroke
    Metabolic alkalosis
    Diabetes mellitus

Respiratory
    Clubbing
    Asthma
    Chronic obstructive pulmonary disease
    Recurrent pulmonary infiltrates
    Chronic cough/sputum
    Barrel chest
    Hemoptysis
    Pneumothorax
    Cor pulmonale
    Nasal polyps

Other
    Infertility (males)

FIG. 10.27 *Presentations of cystic fibrosis.*

Osteoarthropathy, or clubbing in its mildest form, is seen not only in many conditions in which there is overt cardiopulmonary disease such as cyanotic heart disease or lung disease but also in gastrointestinal diseases (especially Crohn's) and liver disorders. Pathogenetic mechanisms are not clear, but shunting from right to left via pulmonary or abdominal vessels is a possibility. Earliest signs of osteoarthropathy are softening and loss of a normal angle at the base of the nail (Fig. 10.25).

Many rashes accompany inflammatory bowel disease, including erythema nodosum, erythema multiforme, papulonecrotic lesions, and ulcerative erythematous plaques. Perhaps the most characteristic rash is pyoderma gangrenosum. Initial lesions are papular, then become bullous, and finally deeply ulcerated and necrotic. The most frequent locations are the cheeks, thighs, feet, hands, legs, and inguinal regions (Fig. 10.26).

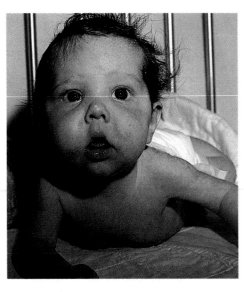

FIG. 10.28 *Cystic fibrosis. This patient was not gaining sufficient weight from breast feeding and was switched to soy formula. He became edematous, especially in the facial area.*

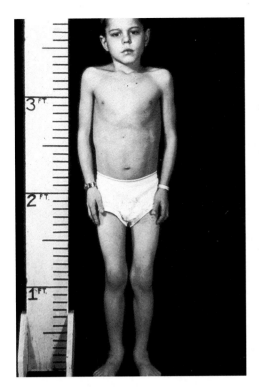
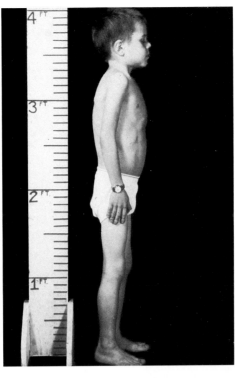

FIG. 10.29 Cystic fibrosis. This child presented with chronic cough. Note an increased AP chest diameter and overall poor nutrition as well as clubbing.

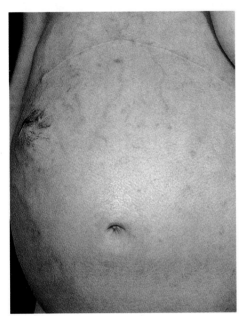

FIG. 10.30 Chronic liver disease/portal hypertension. This child had biliary atresia with good bile flow following a portoenterostomy procedure. Cirrhosis developed late, with physical signs of prominent abdominal veins and ascites.

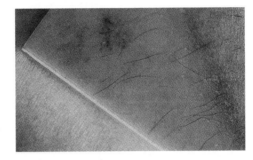

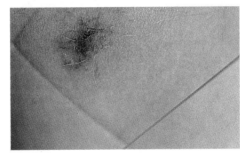

FIG. 10.31 Spider nevus. The vascular lesion blanches with compression by a glass slide (top), but reappears when pressure is released (bottom).

Cystic Fibrosis

Cystic fibrosis is the most common inherited lethal disorder in whites, with predominantly pulmonary and GI manifestations (Fig. 10.27). Clues to the diagnosis of cystic fibrosis are myriad and involve multiple systems. Few clinicians would fail to think of the diagnosis with meconium ileus, chronic cough, failure to thrive, and malabsorptive stools, so a few less common presentations were selected for discussion here.

Edema in an infant who is breast-fed or on soy formula and consuming adequate calories should strongly suggest cystic fibrosis (Fig. 10.28). As noted in the section on kwashiorkor, these infants often appear well-fed but quite thin after fluid is diuresed. The older child with asthma or recurrent bronchitis should be examined closely for signs of chronic lung disease. Subtle increases in AP chest diameter, clubbing, and rather poor general nutrition make a sweat test mandatory (Fig. 10.29).

Chronic Liver Disease

Children with chronic liver disease and cirrhosis have many clinical features in common. The liver is usually firm, often irregular and enlarged, though in late stages it may decrease in size. Splenomegaly follows portal hypertension. Portosystemic venous anastomoses lead to the development of dilated vessels in the abdominal wall (caput medusae) and gastrointestinal tract (varices, hemorrhoids) (Fig. 10.30). Ascitic fluid may form, and when in sufficient quantity, flank dullness and fluid wave may be elicited. Ultrasonography may detect even smaller amounts of free fluid. Spider nevi, dilated vascular channels which disappear with pressure, are seen in normal adolescents but should suggest chronic liver disease if other historical or examination clues are present (Fig. 10.31).

A large number of patients with intrahepatic biliary atresia (IBA) with narrow but patent extrahepatic ducts have been evaluated for possible liver transplantation. Unfortunately,

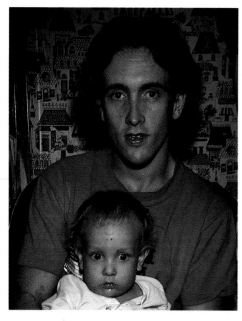

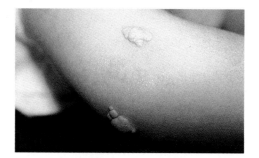

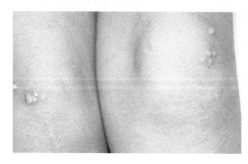

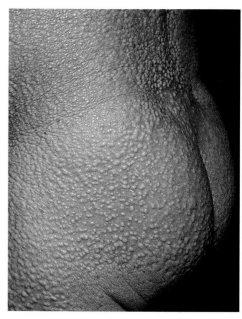

FIG. 10.32 Alagille syndrome. The child has intrahepatic biliary hypoplasia, butterfly vertebrae, and mild pulmonic stenosis. The father does not have liver disease but does have moderate pulmonic stenosis and poor growth. Note the narrow, thin face and pointed chin of both father and child.

FIG. 10.33 Xanthomas in chronic liver disease. Characteristic areas in the early stages of disease are "pressure points"

such as elbows and knees; later, xanthomas may become generalized.

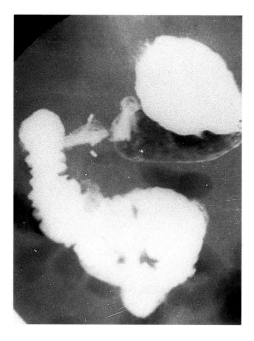

FIG. 10.34 Malrotation in biliary atresia. The duodenal "C" loop is not closed and is displaced to the right.

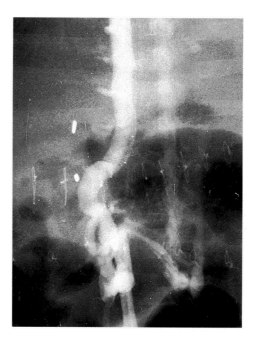

FIG. 10.35 Vascular anomaly in biliary atresia. The inferior vena cava is interrupted and continues as an azygous vein.

these patients are often subjected to portoenterostomy procedures which may actually do harm by increasing the incidence of cholangitis. Many IBA patients show features of arteriohepatic dysplasia (Alagille syndrome), a condition probably inherited as a dominant trait. Features include triangular face, deep-set eyes, prominent nose, poor growth, cardiac murmur, usually pulmonic stenosis, butterfly vertebrae, and persistence of posterior embryotoxon seen by slit-lamp examination of the eye (Fig. 10.32). Many individuals have only a few features of the disorder; prognosis

is variable. These patients often suffer from xanthoma formation and severe pruritus which may occasionally be features of other chronic liver diseases (Fig. 10.33).

Extrahepatic biliary atresia (EBA), with an incidence of 0.65 in 10,000 live births, is the most common cause of end-stage pediatric liver disease. Approximately 350 children per year are born with this condition in the United States. EBA may be associated with abnormalities of other organ systems, situs inversus viscerum, and polysplenia with or without congenital heart disease. Additionally, GI tract

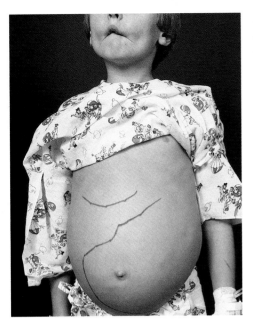

FIG. 10.36 Congenital hepatic fibrosis. This clinically well child had hematemesis and hypersplenism with normal liver function studies. Note massive splenic size and large left lobe of liver. Portosystemic shunting was effective therapy.

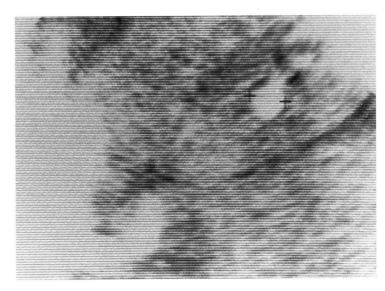

FIG. 10.37 Ultrasonogram of the kidney in a patient with congenital hepatic fibrosis reveals a cystic structure.

anomalies such as malrotation (Fig. 10.34) and vascular anomalies (Fig. 10.35) may complicate surgery and later attempts at transplantation.

Finally, one chronic hepatic disorder can usually be recognized by examination alone. The healthy-appearing child with massive splenomegaly and a large, firm left lobe of the liver with no stigmata of chronic liver disease except GI hemorrhage almost certainly has congenital hepatic fibrosis (Fig. 10.36). It should be remembered that these children may be part of the spectrum of polycystic kidney disease in childhood, and renal function studies are warranted (Fig. 10.37). Therapy for this condition may include shunting procedures for portal hypertension, as liver function may remain normal indefinitely.

BIBLIOGRAPHY

Ament M: Inflammatory disease of the colon: Ulcerative colitis and Crohn's colitis. J Pediatr 86:322–334, 1975.

Chase HP, Long MA, Lavin MH: Cystic fibrosis and malnutrition. J Pediatr 95:337–347, 1979.

Shaw JCC: Trace metals in the fetus and young infant. II. Copper, manganese, selenium, and chromium. Am J Dis Child 134:74–81, 1980.

Suskind RM (ed.):Textbook of Pediatric Nutrition. Raven Press, New York, 1981.

Suskind RM, Varma RN: Assessment of nutritional status of children. Pediatr Rev 5:195–202, 1984.

PEDIATRIC HEMATOLOGY

J. Jeffrey Malatack, M.D.
Julie Blatt, M.D.
Lila Penchansky, M.D.

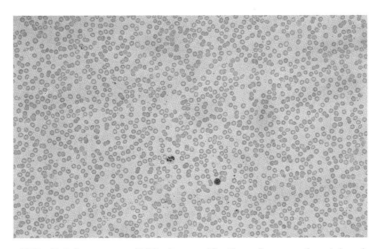

FIG. 11.1 *Low power (100×) magnification of a normal peripheral blood smear.*

INTRODUCTION

The tools of the clinical pediatric hematologist have evolved over recent years, as techniques previously limited to research and laboratory settings have moved into the realm of normal investigation and therapeutics. Despite such advances, however, the core of hematologic diagnosis continues to reside in a thorough medical history and physical examination and in evaluation of the patient's peripheral blood smear, CBC, reticulocyte count, and occasionally, a bone marrow examination. It is these same time-honored investigations that have allowed for the systematic ordering of diagnoses—first, with regard to the cell line involved, next, with regard to the nature of that involvement, and, finally, with regard to the very cause of that involvement itself.

This chapter will highlight common hematologic conditions as well as rarer entities for which the peripheral blood smear is an important diagnostic tool. Conversely, because bone marrow aspiration is not a technique used routinely by most pediatricians and because it is not needed to investigate the majority of common pediatric hematologic problems, we have not included an exhaustive review of marrow morphology.

THE RED BLOOD CELL

The red blood cell (RBC), or corpuscle, is the most ubiquitous of the blood's cellular components. Its primary function is to mediate the exchange of respiratory gases (oxygen and carbon dioxide) between the lungs and body tissues. Collectively this is accomplished by the presence of a critical red cell mass, which is under close homeostatic control. The homeostasis is maintained by alterations in red cell production under the stimulus of tissue hypoxia. Singularly, the red cell accomplishes its function by the critical biochemical features of its oxygen-carrying intracellular components and by the peculiar physical properties of the red cell itself.

The Peripheral Blood Smear

The red cell can be investigated along with other cellular elements by scrutiny of the peripheral blood smear. Such scrutiny has two functions. First, it provides confirmation of the values given on the standard Coulter counter printout. For example, on the Coulter counter, falsely elevated white blood cell (WBC) counts may result from the presence of nucleated

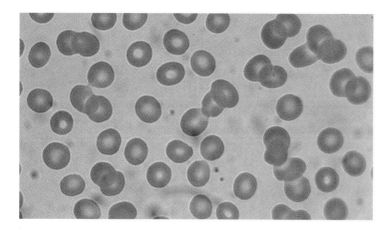

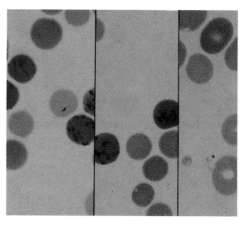

FIG. 11.3 Reticulo-cyte-stained periph-eral blood as seen in a patient with (left) a high reticulocyte count, (center) a normal reticulocyte count, and (right) a low reticulocyte count.

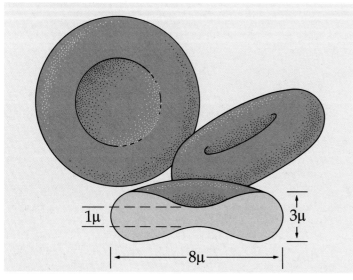

FIG. 11.2 (Top) High-power (400×) magnification of a normal pe-ripheral blood smear. (Bottom) Schematic drawing of a red blood cell (RBC) in two views to demonstrate features of the normal bicon-cave disc.

HEMOGLOBIN (Hgb) AND MEAN CORPUSCULAR VOLUME (MCV) VALUES AT VARIOUS AGES

Age	Hemoglobin (g/d1)	MCV (fl)
Birth (cord blood)	16.5	108
1 to 3 days (capillary)	18.5	108
1 week	17.5	107
2 weeks	16.5	105
1 month	14.0	104
2 months	11.5	96
3 to 6 months	11.5	91
0.5 to 2 years	12.0	78
2 to 6 years	12.5	81
6 to 12 years	13.5	86
12 to 18 years—female	14.0	90
male	14.5	88
18 to 49 years—female	14.0	90
male	15.5	90

FIG. 11.4 Hemoglobin (Hgb) and mean corpuscular volume (MCV) values at various ages. (Adapted from Dallman PR, in Rudolph A (ed): Pediatrics, 16th ed. Appleton-Century-Crofts, Inc., New York, 1977, p. 1111)

RBCs (see Fig. 11.9). In addition, the presence of red cell fragments may result in falsely elevated platelet counts. Sec-ondly, review of the peripheral smear also provides infor-mation regarding the differential WBC count as well as on red cell, white cell, and platelet morphology.

A systematic approach to looking at the smear can max-imize the amount of information extracted. The slide first is scanned under low power and an area is chosen, such that the red cells are just barely touching (Fig. 11.1). Areas in which the red cells are too dense or too sparse are fraught with artifact. Under low power, both mononuclear and polymorphonuclear cells are visible. By using the high-dry or oil lens, normal red cell morphology is revealed in which the normal biconcave disc is seen, wherein an area of central pallor is surrounded by an otherwise homogeneous red circle (Fig. 11.2). Beyond the newborn period, the RBC is about the size of the nucleus of the small lymphocyte. Next, a white cell differential count can be done and the morphology of the cells examined. Finally, platelets should be scrutinized for number (each platelet/high-dry field represents approxi-mately 10,000 platelets per mm³). Furthermore, it should be noted that a blood smear made from anticoagulated blood may have artifact such as vacuolation of the WBCs. Also platelets, which should clump on smears obtained by finger stick, may not form clumps if blood has been collected in anticoagulant.

Red Cell Production

Red cell production usually occurs in the bone marrow but under conditions of disease it also can occur in extramedullary locations such as the spleen. For the first 48 hours after it has joined the peripheral circulation, the newly formed red cell, or reticulocyte, has a number of unique characteristics, one of which is its ability to be stained with supravital stains. This allows for easy identification of its presence in the peri-pheral circulation. In the normal setting, the reticulocyte count is a reflection of the replacement of senescent red cells. Since the red cell life span is approximately 120 days, every day 0.8 percent of the red cell mass must be replaced by retic-ulocytes. Since reticulocytes maintain their staining charac-teristics up to 48 hours, the normal reticulocyte count at any given time is approximately 1.6 percent (0.8 to 2.4 percent).

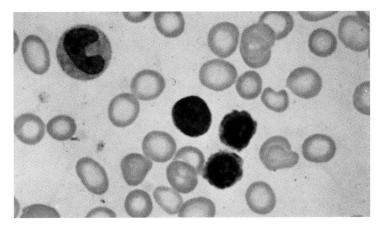

FIG. 11.5 *Microcytic hypochromic anemia of iron deficiency anemia. This 16-month-old patient has a history of excessive milk intake. Note the marked central pallor of the RBC with a small rim of hemoglobin, as well as its small size in comparison to that of the adjacent small lymphocyte nucleus.*

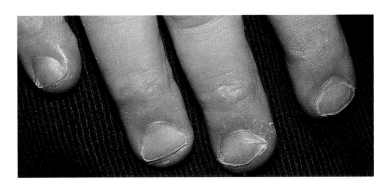

FIG. 11.6 *Spooning of fingernails in child with iron deficiency anemia.*

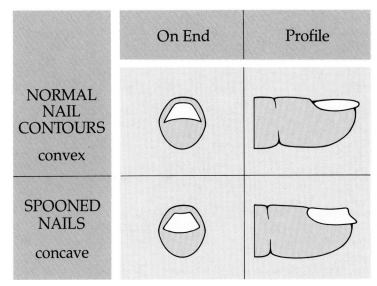

FIG. 11.7 *Schematic diagram to show that spooning occurs in both a mediolateral as well as in a proximodistal direction.*

(This figure is 1 to 2 percent higher in the adult menstruating female.) Increased reticulocyte counts are a reflection of increased red cell loss (through hemolysis or hemorrhage) while decreased reticulocyte counts are indicative of decreased red cell production.

Either of the above pictures can result in a decrease in RBC mass beyond a critical level, leading to anemia. Anemia may be an isolated finding or it may be a part of the spectrum of pancytopenia, in which WBCs and platelets also are affected (see below). When associated with decreased RBC production, anemia is characterized by an inappropriately low reticulocyte count, whereas most often, when anemia is associated with increased red cell destruction, the reticulocyte count is elevated (Fig. 11.3).

Normal values for RBC number and volume are age and sex related and are listed in Figure 11.4. Specifically, the mechanisms by which anemia occurs include:

1. Decreased production of RBCs by the bone marrow
2. Increased destruction, either of mature red cells peripherally or of their precursors while they are still in the bone marrow ("ineffective erythropoiesis")
3. Hemorrhage

The causes of anemia by any of these mechanisms are numerous. Anemias due to decreased red cell production include the microcytic anemias, pure red cell aplasia, and megaloblastic anemia. Anemias that are characterized by increased destruction, with no evidence of blood loss or of ineffective erythropoiesis (hemolytic anemias), include red cell membrane defects, intracellular RBC defects, and extra RBC factors causing hemolysis.

Anemias Due to Decreased Red Cell Production

MICROCYTIC ANEMIAS

The most common result of isolated failure of RBC production is the microcytic/hypochromic anemias. Normally, genetic control of the size of the red cell versus the volume of its intracellular contents is maintained in a presumed attempt to keep the physical properties of the red cell nearly constant. Any process that decreases hemoglobin production without affecting red cell precursors themselves leads to a hypochromic (hemoglobinized rim of the red cell less than two-thirds of the entire cell diameter) microcytic (small compared with the nuclei of the neighboring small lymphocyte) anemia.

Iron Deficiency Anemia

Iron deficiency anemia is the most common of the pediatric microcytic/hypochromic anemias. It occurs in infants whose rapidly increasing red cell mass is not paralleled by their dietary iron intake. This lack of iron leads to failure of hemoglobin production, and hence, to the formation of microcytic cells. Since the normal full-term infant has adequate iron reserves to accommodate the increasing red cell mass through the first 5 months of life, iron deficiency usually is seen in the second half of the first year of life, and iron deficiency anemia is seen most often at approximately 1 to 1½ years of age.

Figure 11.5 shows the peripheral blood of a 16-month-old child who has been fed large amounts of whole cow's milk from 3 months of age. The RBCs are microcytic and hypochromic. The platelets are characteristically increased in number (not shown), although they may be normal or even decreased. In severe iron deficiency anemia, anisocytosis (varied RBC size) and poikilocytosis (varied RBC shape) may be noted, as well as nonspecific morphologic abnormalities such as the presence of ovalocytes or basophilic stippling.

The child with iron deficiency anemia may be asymptomatic despite significant degrees of anemia. However when symptoms are present, irritability is the primary finding. Children also have been shown to demonstrate decreases in Bayley IQ scores, as well as a peculiar physical finding of "spooning" of the fingernails and toenails (koilonychia) (Figs. 11.6 and 11.7).

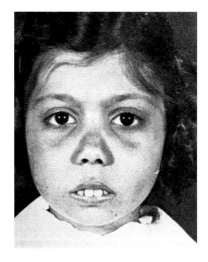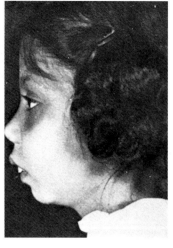

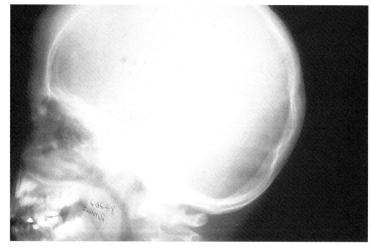

FIG. 11.8 (Left and Center) *Maxillary hyperplasia due to increased marrow space in child with thalassemia major.* (Right) *Skull* radiograph of the same patient demonstrates an increased marrow cavity of the skull and facial bones.

FIG. 11.9 *Peripheral blood smear of child with thalassemia major. Note the microcytic hypochromic anemia and prominent nucleated red cells surrounding the polymorphonuclear cells and lymphocytes.*

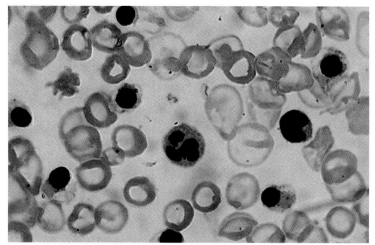

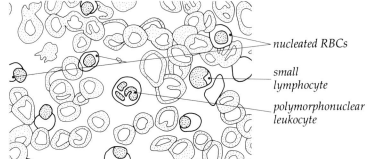

nucleated RBCs

small
lymphocyte

polymorphonuclear
leukocyte

Thalassemia

The thalassemias are the second most common cause of microcytic hypochromic anemia in the pediatric patient, and they result from ineffective erythropoiesis due to an imbalance between alpha and beta globin chain synthesis. In the homozygous form of this disease (thalassemia major, or Cooley's anemia), increased marrow activity results in expanded medullary spaces producing characteristic bony hyperplasia with physical and radiologic correlations (see Fig. 11.8). Untreated children with Cooley's anemia have chronic anemia with marked hepatosplenomegaly, scleral icterus, listlessness, and eventual overt cardiac failure. In addition, malocclusion may occur with malar hypertrophy. The clinical picture of Cooley's anemia should not be confused with that of iron deficiency anemia. Thalassemia major displays a characteristic abnormal smear with microcytes, target cells, basophilic stippling, and often, large numbers of nucleated RBCs (Fig. 11.9).

Beta thalassemia trait (thalassemia minor) is a common cause of mild to moderate anemia in blacks and in people of Mediterranean origin. Alpha thalassemia trait (another form of thalassemia minor most common in Asians) may be clinically indistinguishable from iron deficiency anemia. As a rule, for a given level of hemoglobin, the mean corpuscular volume (MCV), a measure of the red cell size, will be lower in thalassemia trait than in iron deficiency. However, in practice, a battery of laboratory tests including a hemoglobin electrophoresis and a therapeutic trial of iron may be needed to distinguish among thalassemia trait, iron deficiency, and other causes of microcytic anemia.

Lead Poisoning

Lead intoxication also leads to a microcytic anemia. However, nonhematologic manifestations of lead intoxication, particularly neurological complications, often dominate the picture. The spectrum of clinical presentation of lead intoxication ranges from acute encephalopathy with rapid progression to coma and death at one end, to vague symptoms including abdominal pain, vomiting, malaise, and behavior changes at the other end. Significant radiographic changes also are seen in lead intoxication (Figs. 11.10 through 11.12). Lead intoxication occurs due to excessive environmental lead intake. Both aerosolized and oral lead-containing environmental contaminants are major sources of lead intoxication. Pica associated with flaking lead paint represents neither the only nor the prevailing cause of lead intoxication although clearly it is a common mechanism of poisoning. The finger sucking behavior of children in homes where lead paint has become an intimate part of house dust is perhaps a more important source of environmental lead.

Hematologic abnormalities of lead intoxication are a direct result of the effects of lead on enzymes involved in heme pro-

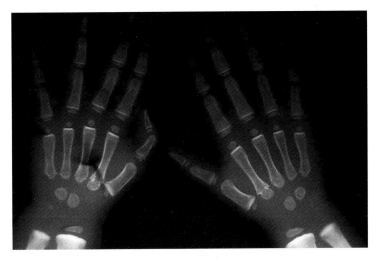

FIG. 11.10 Hand radiograph of child with lead intoxication reveals marked linear increases in the density of the metaphyses. These should not be confused with the growth arrest lines seen following a variety of illnesses.

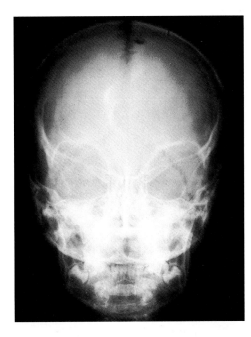

FIG. 11.11 Skull film of patient with lead intoxication, with encephalopathy. Note the split sutures indicative of increased intracranial pressure.

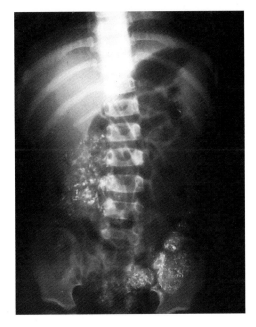

FIG. 11.12 Abdominal radiograph of a child with a history of pica and lead intoxication reveals radio-dense lead-containing paint chips scattered throughout the colon.

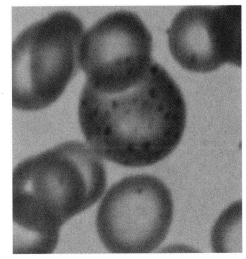

FIG. 11.13 Microcytic hypochromic anemia due to lead intoxication. Note prominent basophilic stippling. This finding is not specific for lead intoxication and may be seen in thalassemia and, though rarely, in iron deficiency.

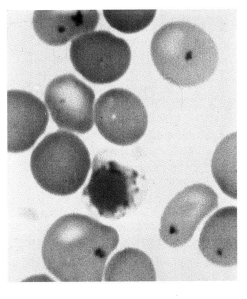

FIG. 11.14 Ringed sideroblast (iron-containing normoblast) on iron stain of the bone marrow. They are present in patients with sideroblastic anemia.

duction. Lead inhibits this enzyme system, causing failure of the placement of iron into the protoporphyrin ring. Thus, despite the presence of normal intracellular iron, the iron is unable to be incorporated into heme and, hence, hemoglobin production fails. This leads to a microcytic hypochromic anemia. Basophilic stippling, a second hematologic manifestation of lead intoxication, occurs as a result of inhibition of yet another enzyme. Nucleotide chains, normally removed from the RBC after its nucleus has been extruded, persist because of inhibition of this second enzyme. These remnants stain blue and cause stippling of the red cell (Fig. 11.13).

Sideroblastic and Other Anemias

The sideroblastic anemias are characterized by the presence of a minor or major population of hypochromic microcytic cells in the peripheral blood and of the ringed sideroblast in the bone marrow (Fig. 11.14). The sideroblastic anemias either are hereditary or acquired. The hereditary form is due to a deficiency of an enzyme or of enzyme activity required for hemoglobin production. The acquired forms may be secondary to drugs or toxins (lead being the most important of those in childhood), malignancy, inflammatory endocrine disease, or idiopathic disease. Copper deficiency and chronic disease, although generally resulting in normocytic anemia, occasionally may cause a microcytic picture.

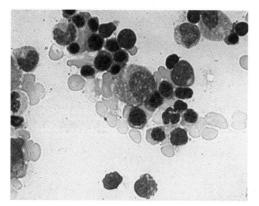
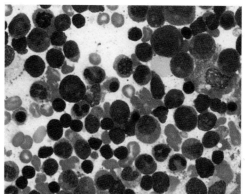

FIG. 11.15 (Left) *Normal bone marrow aspirate with plentiful erythroblasts (small cells approximately the size of a RBC with round very darkly staining nuclei and dark blue cytoplasm). (Right) Bone marrow aspirate of patient with Blackfan-Diamond syndrome. Note the clear decrease of erythroblasts.*

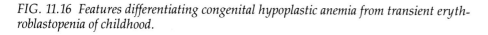

FEATURES DIFFERENTIATING CONGENITAL HYPOPLASTIC ANEMIA FROM TRANSIENT ERYTHROBLASTOPENIA OF CHILDHOOD

| | Disease | |
RBC Characteristic	Congenital Hypoplastic Anemia	Transient Erythroblastopenia of Childhood
Hemoglobin (Hgb)	Increased fetal Hgb	Normal fetal Hgb
Cellular antigen	i	I
MCV	Increased	Normal
RBC enzyme activity	Normal or high	Low

FIG. 11.16 *Features differentiating congenital hypoplastic anemia from transient erythroblastopenia of childhood.*

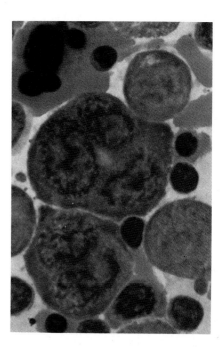

FIG. 11.17 *Congenital dyserythropoietic anemia type III. Note the centrally located gigantoblast.*

PURE RED CELL APLASIA

Pure red cell aplasia or hypoplasia refers to conditions in which red cell production fails to keep pace with normal red cell destruction, thus leading to anemia. Characteristically other cellular elements are unaffected. A congenital form of red cell aplasia/hypoplasia (variously referred to as congenital hypoplastic anemia, chronic idiopathic erythroblastopenia, chronic congenital aregenerative anemia, erythropoiesis imperfecta, or Blackfan-Diamond syndrome) is characterized by the onset of anemia by 6 months of age with a low absolute reticulocyte count. Approximately 25 percent of patients have minor congenital anomalies, including thumb anomalies as well as those found in the Turner syndrome phenotype. While a percentage of these patients go into spontaneous remission, others may remit many years following onset of the disease once they are placed on corticosteroid therapy. Still other patients do not improve and remain transfusion-dependent for the rest of their lives. The etiology of this disease remains unknown, although a defect in the erythroid stem cell may be a factor. The peripheral blood smear reveals macrocytic normochromic red cells. Examination of the bone marrow reveals erythroblastopenia (Fig. 11.15).

Pure red cell aplasia also may be an acquired disease, with drugs, toxins, and viral infections having been implicated as possible causes. Acquired pure red cell aplasia occurs more frequently in adults than in children, and in adult patients frequently is associated with thymoma and also is suspected to be on an autoimmune basis. Rarely does autoimmunity appear to be etiologic in childhood pure red cell aplasia, and thymoma is almost nonexistent. While drugs (particularly chloramphenicol) have been responsible for a significant percentage of cases of pure red cell aplasia in children, transient erythroblastopenia of childhood (TEC) is by far the most frequent cause of acquired childhood pure red cell aplasia.

TEC generally occurs from 1 to 4 years of age and appears 2 weeks to 2 months following a respiratory or gastrointestinal viral illness. The major differential diagnostic consideration for TEC is congenital hypoplastic anemia. The two diseases can be distinguished by their red cell characteristics. TEC cells, prior to recovery, have normal red cell characteristics while those of congenital hypoplastic anemia have fetal characteristics (Fig. 11.16).

While the peripheral blood smear from a patient with RBC aplasia often is nonspecific (although it may show atypical lymphocytes as vestiges of a residual viral infection), the bone marrow aspirate rarely may be more specific. It may show the vacuolated erythroblasts of chloramphenicol effect or the multinucleated giant cell indicative of the rare congenital dyserythropoietic anemia (Fig. 11.17).

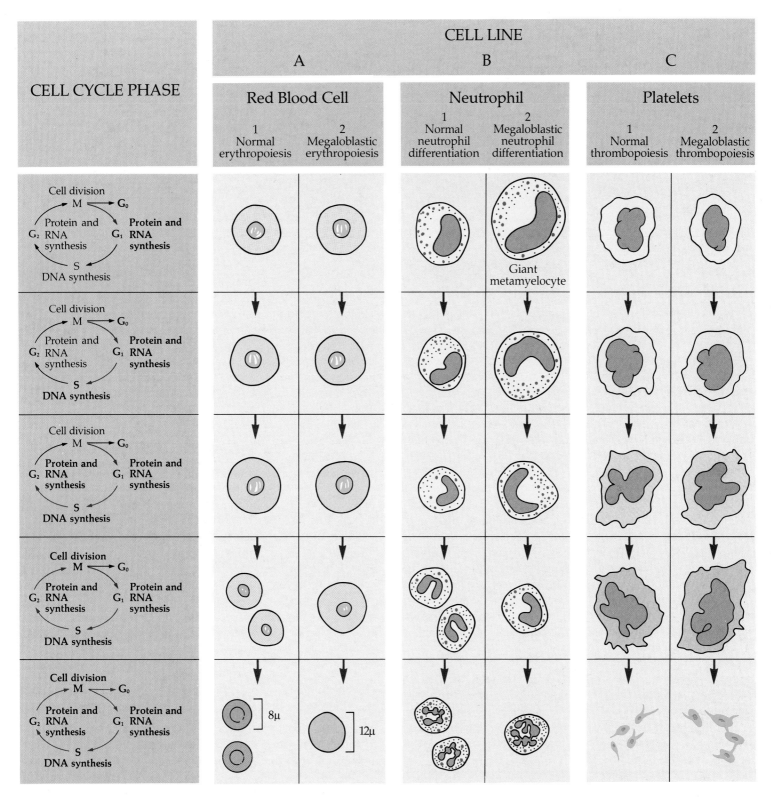

FIG. 11.18 Schematic comparison of normal cellular maturation and megaloblastic differentiation of three cell lines. The cell cycle phase is identified to the left of the figure. Note that megaloblastic cells fail to undergo DNA replication and cellular division at S and M phases respectively, leading to large red cells, hypersegmented polys, and large bizarrely shaped platelets.

MEGALOBLASTIC ANEMIAS

The megaloblastic anemias are another group of conditions characterized by failure of adequate red cell production. Although the etiology of the megaloblastic anemias varies, common morphologic abnormalities of the erythropoietic cells exist. The hallmark is the megaloblast, a marrow cell with a nucleated red cell, a lacy chromatin pattern, and a dyssynchrony of maturation between cytoplasm and nucleus. The morphologic alterations are a direct result of decreased nucleoprotein (DNA) synthesis compared with cytoplasmic protein synthesis, and they stem from a relative decrease in the factors needed in DNA replication, namely, folate or cobalamin (B_{12}).

While red cells primarily are affected in megaloblastic anemia, all of the actively dividing marrow cells fail to have normal DNA duplication and hence will become involved in the pathologic process. This leads to a decrease in all of the cellular elements.

Figure 11.18 depicts the alterations that occur in marrow production, due to inadequate DNA replication as seen in

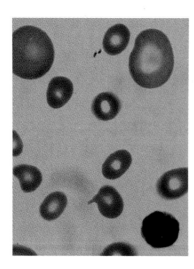

FIG. 11.19 Peripheral blood smear of patient with megaloblastic anemia. Note the enlarged red cell (macrocyte) at the upper left. It is much larger than the normal small lymphocyte in the same field.

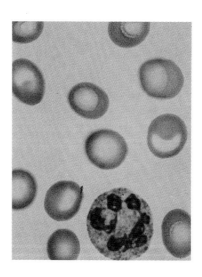

FIG. 11.20 A hypersegmented polymorphonuclear leukocyte in patient with phenytoin-induced folate deficiency.

megaloblastic anemia. The normal cell proceeds through the cell cycle with progressive condensation of the nucleus and nuclear chromatin, and with a progressive increase in the relative amount of cytoplasm. Progressive acidophilic staining of the cytoplasmic contents occurs as the cell becomes mature. The final cell division leads directly to the normal peripheral red cell. In megaloblastic anemia failure of DNA replication in the S phase of the cell cycle leads to a failure in the final cell division at M phase, resulting in a larger than normal red cell in the peripheral circulation—a macrocyte (Fig. 11.19).

Neutrophils also can be affected by a decrease in available DNA precursors. In fact an increase in nuclear lobulations is one of the earliest indications of megaloblastic neutrophil differentiation (Fig. 11.20). Figure 11.18 also shows normal neutrophil differentiation, in which a marrow metamyelocyte undergoes its final cell division leading ultimately to the presence of two mature neutrophils in the peripheral circulation. Figure 11.18 (B2) shows the giant metamyelocyte that is a bone marrow hallmark of megaloblastic neutrophil differentiation. Failure of DNA replication leads to failure of final cell division and, in some yet unknown fashion, to an increase in nuclear lobulations. As DNA precursor deficiency becomes more severe, not only are neutrophil nuclei altered, but also the white blood cell count in general becomes depressed.

Finally, thrombopoiesis can be altered by megaloblastic changes. Normal platelet differentiation occurs in a way that differs from that of the classic cell cycle. DNA replication occurs repeatedly in the megakaryocyte nucleus such that its ploidy is variable. The megakaryocyte nucleus then segments. This segmentation, however, does not occur in a one to one ratio to the cell's ploidy. Figure 11.18 reveals that with normal platelet maturation, dividing membranes develop in the megakaryocytic cytoplasm after DNA synthesis ceases. These divided segments of cytoplasm then break to form peripheral platelets.

Megaloblastic differentiation, by way of contrast, ultimately leads to bizarre-shaped and excessively sized platelets, presumably because the megakaryocyte never reaches its ploidy potential. With megaloblastic anemia the platelet number can be decreased and the platelet size and shape altered.

The etiology of the megaloblastic anemias is varied and, while it includes dietary folate or B₁₂ deficiency, in the Western world it is more likely to be malabsorption, drug-induced (notably phenytoin and methotrexate) or a number of inherited metabolic abnormalities. Pernicious anemia, which is due to the absence or deficiency of intrinsic factor required for vitamin B₁₂ absorption, has the peculiar physical finding of a smooth tongue. Patients also can suffer ataxia and paresthesias.

The Hemolytic Anemias

Anemias characterized by active hematopoiesis and premature destruction of the red blood cell without any blood loss or evidence of ineffective erythropoiesis collectively are called the hemolytic anemias. Patients with hemolytic anemia suffer from fatigue, pallor, and hyperdynamic cardiovascular states, and they frequently display jaundice. If the anemia has persisted for at least several days, the reticulocyte count is elevated and evidence of hemolysis (including increased carboxyhemoglobin, LDH, and decreased haptoglobin) is found. Because hemolytic anemias may be episodic, these characteristics may not be present at all times.

Differential diagnosis of hemolytic anemias rests largely on the recognition of specific morphologic abnormalities as listed in Figure 11.21.

MEMBRANE DEFECTS
Hereditary Spherocytosis

The most common cause of hemolytic anemia in the Caucasian population is hereditary spherocytosis (HS), a red cell membrane defect that leads to a characteristic peripheral blood smear. HS is transmitted most frequently as an autosomal dominant trait and is named for the peculiar appearance of its RBCs in the peripheral blood smear. The red cell membrane defect, which appears to be due to inherent membrane instability, leads to loss of membrane. Membrane repairs occur, which decrease the normal surface to volume ratio thereby leading away from the biconcave disc and toward a spherical shape (Fig. 11.22). The direct consequence of this new morphology is a less deformable cell. The inability of this new cell to deform leads to RBC destruction in the spleen. Consequently, the characteristic smear of HS may become more dramatic following splenectomy, when spherocytes are less prone to destruction (Fig. 11.23). Spherocytes also can be seen in immune-mediated (usually Coombs-positive) hemolytic anemias, which themselves can

CLASSIFICATION OF COMMON RED CELL HEMOLYTIC DISORDERS BY PREDOMINANT MORPHOLOGY*

Spherocytes
  Hereditary spherocytosis
  ABO incompatibility in neonates†
  Immunohemolytic anemias with IgG- or C3-coated
    red cells†
  Hemolytic transfusion reactions†
  Severe burns, other red cell thermal injuries

Bizarre Poikilocytes
  Red cell fragmentation syndromes (microangiopathic
    and macroangiopathic hemolytic anemias)
  Hereditary elliptocytosis in neonates

Elliptocytes
  Hereditary elliptocytosis
  Thalassemias
  (Other hypochromic-microcytic anemias)
  (Megaloblastic anemias)

Spiculated or Crenated Red Cells
  Acute hepatic necrosis (spur cell anemia)
  Uremia
  Abetalipoproteinemia

Prominent Basophilic Stippling
  Thalassemias
  Unstable hemoglobins
  Lead poisoning‡

Irreversibly Sickled Cells
  Sickle cell anemia
  Symptomatic sickle syndromes

Intraerythrocytic Parasites
  Malaria
  Babesiosis
  Bartonellosis

Target Cells
  Hemoglobins S, C, D, and E
  Hereditary xerocytosis
  Thalassemias
  (Other hypochromic-microcytic anemias)
  (Obstructive liver disease)
  (Postsplenectomy)

Nonspecific or Normal Morphology
  Embden-Meyerhof pathway defects
  HMP shunt defects
  Adenosine deaminase hyperactivity with low
    red cell ATP
  Unstable hemoglobins
  Paroxysmal nocturnal hemoglobinuria
  Dyserythropoietic anemias
  Copper toxicity (Wilson's disease)
  Erythropoietic porphyria
  Vitamin E deficiency
  Hypersplenism

*Nonhemolytic disorders of similar morphology are enclosed in parentheses for reference.
†Usually associated with positive Coombs test.
‡Disease sometimes associated with this morphology.

FIG. 11.21 Classification of common red cell hemolytic disorders by predominant morphology. (Adapted from Nathan DG, Oski FA (eds): Hematology of Infancy and Childhood, 2nd ed. W B Saunders Co, Philadelphia, 1981, p. 483, with permission)

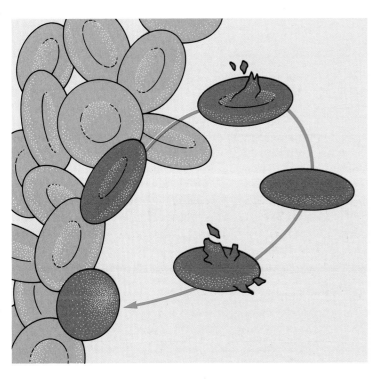

FIG. 11.22 Schematic drawing shows a developing spherocyte due to the process of repeated membrane fragmentation, loss, and repair.

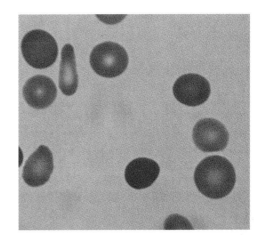

FIG. 11.23 Peripheral blood smear of patient who underwent splenectomy for hereditary spherocytosis (HS). Note the presence of small perfectly round cells without an area of central pallor. The MCHC may be normal but often is increased in patients with HS. Reticulocytosis also may be prominent.

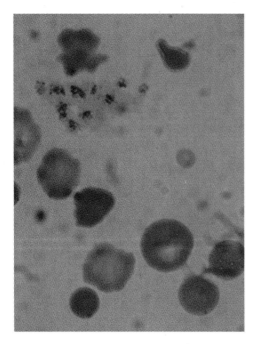

FIG. 11.24 Coombs-positive hemolytic anemia. Note spherocytes and a large RBC with polychromasia indicating the presence of regenerative anemia.

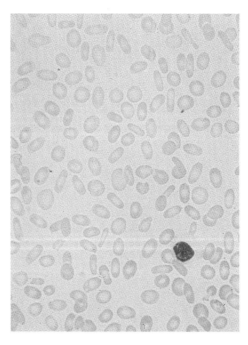

FIG. 11.25 Peripheral blood obtained incidentally from a 3-year-old child with elliptocytosis. Over 90 percent of the cells are elliptocytes. The child had a history of neonatal jaundice, but had been well before and has been well since.

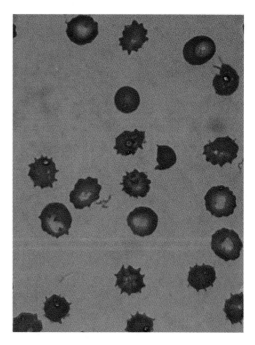

FIG. 11.26 Spiculated cells seen in a patient suffering from acute hepatic necrosis. The associated hemolytic anemia—spur cell anemia—was severe.

be triggered from a variety of disorders such as ABO incompatibility or postviral Coombs-positive warm-agglutinin-mediated hemolytic anemias (Fig. 11.24). Rh disease of the newborn however is a notable exception, as spherocytes characteristically are absent. As with all hemolytic anemias, Rh incompatibility and hemolysis are accompanied by a brisk compensatory reticulocytosis that on Wright's stain of the peripheral blood is seen as polychromasia.

Elliptocytosis

Another membrane defect that is morphologically distinct from HS is hereditary elliptocytosis (see Fig. 11.25). The pathophysiology of red cell destruction in hereditary elliptocytosis is probably very similar to that of HS. Also, like HS, hereditary elliptocytosis appears to be transmitted as an autosomal dominant trait. In most instances hereditary elliptocytosis is a mild well-compensated hemolytic anemia that is clinically insignificant unless splenic hypertrophy develops due to another disease process. Elliptocyte forms, less extensive than those seen in Figure 11.25, also are seen in a number of other anemias including thalassemia minor and iron deficiency anemia.

Other membrane abnormalities lead to still other morphologic defects, although they are mentioned here only in passing as their rarity precludes a more lengthy discussion.

Acanthocytic/Echinocytic Anemias

A number of hemolytic anemias are characterized by spiculated red cells referred to as acanthocytes or echinocytes. Abetalipoproteinemia is one disorder in which a red cell membrane defect leads to acanthocyte formation. Patients develop a progressive ataxia, retinitis pigmentosa, fat malabsorption, and the absence of chylomicrons, VLDLs, and LDLs. In addition roughly 50 to 90 percent of their red cells

are acanthocytes, which develop as a direct result of the alterations of serum lipids. Altered membrane lipid composition changes the fluidity of the RBC membrane, which leads to the acanthocytic form. Because of fat-soluble vitamin malabsorption in acanthocytosis, the red cells also are vitamin E deficient. However, despite altered membrane fluidity and vitamin E deficiency, hemolysis in abetalipoproteinemia is mild.

Spur cell anemia is another disease characterized by acanthocytes. However, the hemolysis in this disorder, unlike that of abetalipoproteinemia, may be brisk. Spur cell anemia develops in the setting of hepatic decompensation from a variety of causes. This leads to an alteration in the serum lipid profile, which leads to altered membrane fluidity and finally to hemolysis (Fig. 11.26). Spiculated cells, however, also can be seen in a large number of other conditions (see Fig. 11.21).

Target Cells

Target cells are produced in a variety of conditions and for the most part represent an increased ratio of red cell membrane to intracellular contents. Consequently any process that increases membrane surface area or decreases its intracellular contents can cause target formation. Liver disease (particularly obstructive hepatopathy with its secondary alteration of serum lipids and membrane lipid loading) is a well-known cause of targeting. Splenectomy, with its subsequent decrease in red cell molding, also leads to target formation. In addition, processes causing a decrease in hemoglobin production, as previously discussed (i.e., thalassemia, iron deficiency anemia) also can lead to targeting. Finally targets, or more correctly, pseudotargets, are formed when hemoglobin aggregates in the red cell center (see section on hemoglobinopathies).

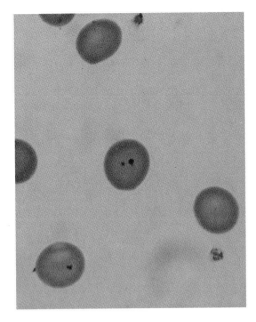

FIG. 11.27 "Heinz body prep" of 2-week-old infant with brisk hemolytic anemia. Note the dark-staining material in two of the red cells.

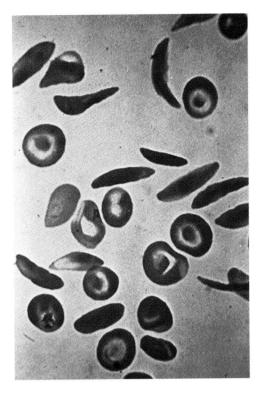

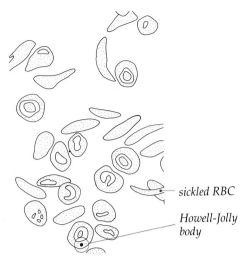

FIG. 11.28 Peripheral blood smear of a black child with HgbSS disease. Note the prominent targets and sickle cells, and the Howell-Jolly body.

sickled RBC

Howell-Jolly body

INTRACELLULAR RED BLOOD CELL DEFECTS
Hemoglobinopathies

The hemoglobinopathies often result in characteristic and even diagnostic peripheral blood smears. They can be responsible for hemolysis due to unstable hemoglobin variants or to altered (decreased) hemoglobin solubility.

Unstable Hemoglobins. Unstable hemoglobins, unlike most hemolytic hemoglobinopathies, rarely have a characteristic morphology although basophilic stippling and Heinz bodies may be noted on special staining of peripheral blood (Fig. 11.27). The Heinz bodies represent globin aggregates that have precipitated intracellularly. Red cells in Heinz body anemias usually are normocytic but they may be hypochromic as a result of splenic "pitting" of precipitated hemoglobin. Because precipitated hemoglobin may be mistaken for reticulin, reticulocyte counts may be spuriously high. Methylene blue staining of red cells after they have incubated for a few hours may demonstrate characteristic Heinz bodies. Hemolysis may be mild (Hgb Köln) or brisk (Hgb Bristol), or it may be induced by drugs such as sulfonamides (Hgb Zurich).

Sickle Cell Disease. Of the hemoglobinopathies that have altered hemoglobulin solubility, none are as well known or as ubiquitous as sickle cell anemia. Alterations of the amino acid sequence in the beta chain of the hemoglobin molecule lead to cross-linking of these beta chains when hemoglobin is in the deoxygenated state. It is this cross-linkage that ultimately leads to decreased hemoglobin solubility and to the sickling of the red cell (Fig. 11.28). The sickled red cell in any of the sickle cell anemias (SS, SC, S-thal) has lost its ability to distort its shape to navigate the microcirculation thereby leading to a log-jam phenomenon. It is this log-jamming, in combination with decreased red cell survival, that leads to the multiple clinical manifestations of sickle cell disease. These include the "painful" crisis (infarction secondary to log-jamming of the microcirculation), sequestration crisis, and aplastic crisis (usually a postviral decrease in red cell production in the face of shortened red cell survival). In contrast, however, the in-

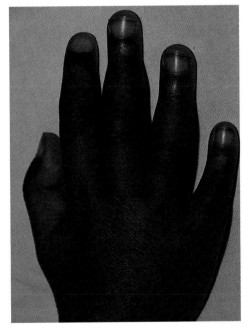

FIG. 11.29 Dactylitis (hand-foot syndrome) in a 3-year-old girl with sickle cell disease. This syndrome, which primarily affects toddlers, is seen less frequently in older children after the bone marrow of the small bones of the hands loses hematopoietic activity.

crease in susceptibility to certain infections with encapsulated bacteria, most frequently the pneumococcus, cannot be explained simply by the log-jam phenomenon.

While intravascular sickling in children with hemoglobinopathies can occur anywhere in the body, characteristically it occurs in the small vessels. In toddlers often the phalanges can be involved, leading to dactylitis (Fig. 11.29).

Hemoglobin C Disease. This hemoglobinopathy (HgbCC) also alters hemoglobin solubility but less significantly than does HgbS. Vaso-occlusive phenomena in this disease are rare but can occur. More frequently HgbC is a problem when it is paired in a double heterozygous state with HgbS. These patients have a form of sickle cell anemia (HgbSC) albeit somewhat less severe than that of HgbSS. The peripheral blood smear of homozygous C disease reveals targets. Unlike target cells in general, however, the targeting in C disease is not due to alterations in the cell membrane/cell

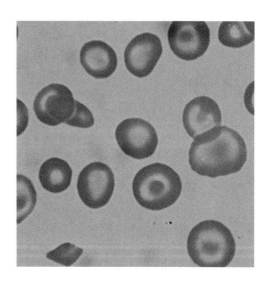

FIG. 11.30 Peripheral smear of SC disease with target cells. Sickled cells are less frequent in this disease than in SS disease.

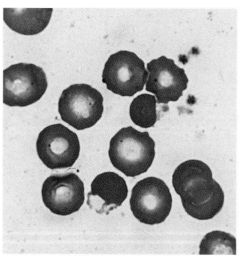

FIG. 11.31 Peripheral smear of patient with G6PD deficiency in the midst of a hemolytic episode. Note blister cells with hemoglobin condensed in the remaining (nonblistered) portion of the cell.

LIST OF DRUGS USUALLY ASSOCIATED WITH CLINICALLY SIGNIFICANT HEMOLYSIS IN G6PD DEFICIENCY

Antimalarials	Sulfa Drugs
Pamaquine	Salicylazosulfapyridine
Pentaquine	N-Acetylsulfanilamide
Primaquine	Sulfapyridine
Quinocide	Sulfamethoxypyridazine
	Thiazolsulfone

Antipyretics/Analgesics	Miscellaneous
Acetanilid	Fava beans
Aminopyrine	Nalidixic acid
Antipyrine	Naphthalene
	Phenylhydrazine
	Toluidine blue
	Acetylphenylhydrazine

FIG. 11.32 List of drugs usually associated with clinically significant hemolysis in G6PD deficiency.

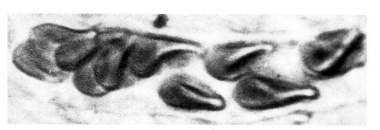

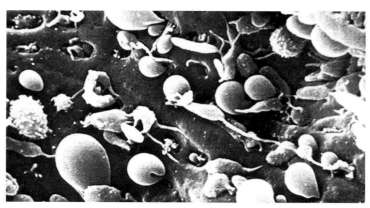

FIG. 11.33 (Top) RBC fluidity is demonstrated as cells move in a laminar fashion through a 12-micron vessel. (Bottom) RBCs being deformed as they traverse the microcirculation of the splenic sinusoids. (Top figure from Skalak R, Branemark PI: Deformation of red blood cells in capillaries. Science 164:717-719, May 9, 1969, Copyright 1969 by the AAAS, with permission; bottom figure from Zucker-Franklin D, Greanes MF, Grossi CE, Marmont AM: Atlas of Blood Cells, Edi. Ermes, Milan, Italy, 1981, with permission)

content ratio but rather to the aggregation of C hemoglobin in the red cell center, leading to a target appearance (Fig. 11.30).

Red Blood Cell Enzyme Abnormalities
Abnormalities in RBC enzymes are yet another intracellular cause of hemolysis. The most frequent of the enzyme defects leading to hemolysis are glucose-6-phosphate dehydrogenase (G6PD) deficiency (Fig. 11.31) and pyruvate kinase deficiency. The RBC morphology of these disorders often is normal or nonspecific.

Over 75 variants of G6PD have been identified in which enzyme activity may be elevated or severely deficient. Clinical syndromes may vary as well, with the degree of hemolysis paralleling the level of G6PD activity. Severely deficient patients may have chronic ongoing hemolysis. Other patients may have hemolysis induced by certain drugs that are known to generate free radicals and peroxides unable to be detoxified by the patient deficient in G6PD. The action of these compounds on sulfhydryl groups in the membrane and on hemoglobin and cytoplasmic proteins is what leads to hemolysis. Listed in Figure 11.32 are some of the drugs associated with clinically significant hemolysis in patients with G6PD deficiency.

Pyruvate kinase (PK) deficiency is the second most common type of glycolytic enzyme deficiency in the RBC. It remains, however, a far second to G6PD, with approximately 500,000 cases of G6PD deficiency occurring worldwide for every single case of PK deficiency. Like G6PD deficiency, wide clinical variability exists with PK deficiency. Mild fully compensated hemolytic anemia may occur, as well as severe neonatal hemolysis and hyperbilirubinemia. Hemoglobins range from 6 to 10 g per dl with normochromic but macrocytic indices. The reticulocyte count may range from 5 percent up to 90 percent in the splenectomized patient. Peripheral blood smears demonstrate poikilocytosis with teardrops, echinocytes, and polychromatophilia. Splenectomy may ameliorate or eliminate the need for repeated transfusions.

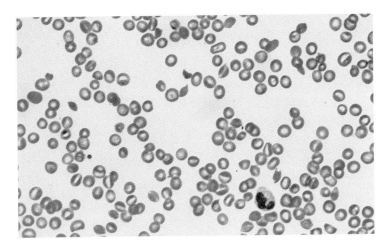

FIG. 11.34 *Peripheral blood smear of a child with disseminated intravascular coagulation (DIC) secondary to meningococcemia. Note RBC fragments and decreased platelets.*

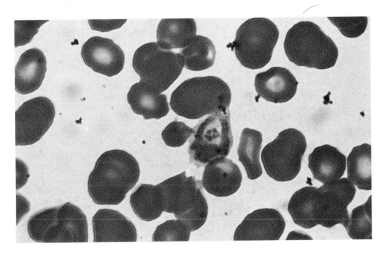

FIG. 11.35 *A peripheral blood smear prepared by the so-called "thick prep" method. Plasmodia vivax malaria are seen intracellularly in the RBC in the center of the smear.*

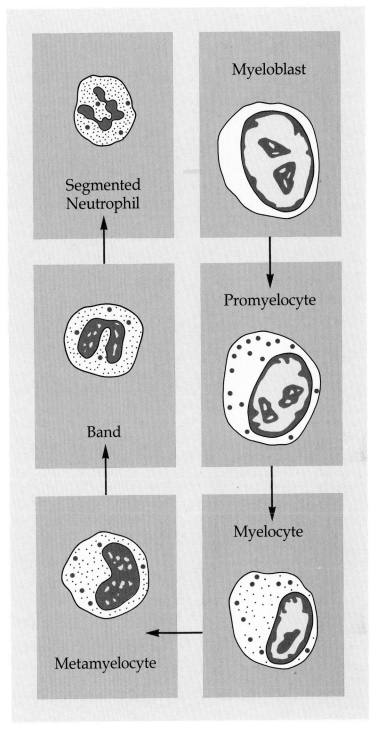

FIG. 11.36 *Schematic diagram of normal myeloid maturation.*

EXTRA RED BLOOD CELL FACTORS CAUSING HEMOLYSIS

The biconcave disc structure of the RBC, as well as its deformability, enhances blood flow through both the macrocirculation and microcirculation (Fig. 11.33). However, significant RBC fragmentation may occur in the microcirculation and is characteristic of the microangiopathic syndrome, disseminated intravascular coagulation (DIC) (Fig. 11.34). In DIC, the production of fibrin leads to its deposition in capillaries. Red cells become shorn as they transit these fibrin networks, resulting in the "microangiopathic smear." The presence of such a smear, with numerous RBC fragments, is helpful but not necessary for a diagnosis of DIC. The list of causes of DIC is long, although overwhelming bacterial infection is by far the most frequent cause of DIC in children.

Malaria, a worldwide cause of hemolysis, may be diagnosed by modification of the peripheral blood smear. A thick smear enhances finding the plasmodium organism (Fig. 11.35).

WHITE BLOOD CELLS

Examination of the peripheral smear together with the Coulter counter printout provides information about both quantitative and morphologic abnormalities of white cells. In general, however, the smear is not predictive of functional abnormalities, which may be present even when the smear is normal.

Although early myeloid precursor cells usually are present only in the bone marrow, in certain clinical situations they may be present in the peripheral blood as well. Their recognition, therefore, is important and is schematized in Figure 11.36. Immature lymphoid cells also may be found in the peripheral blood and are described below.

	12 months	4 years	10 years	21 years
Leukocytes, Total	11.4(6.0–17.5)	9.1(5.5–15.5)	8.1(4.5–13.5)	7.4(4.5–11.0)
Neutrophils, Total	3.5(1.5–8.5) (31%)	3.8(1.5–8.5) (42%)	4.4(1.8–8.0) (54%)	4.4(1.8–7.7) (59%)
Neutrophils, Band Forms	0.35 (3.1%)	0.27(0–1.0) (3.0%)	0.24(0–1.0) (3.0%)	0.22(0–0.7) (3.0%)
Neutrophils, Segmented	3.2 (28%)	3.5(1.5–7.5) (39%)	4.2(1.8–7.0) (51%)	4.2(1.8–7.0) (56%)
Eosinophils	0.30(0.05–0.70) (2.6%)	0.25(0.02–0.65) (2.8%)	0.20(0–0.60) (2.4%)	0.20(0–0.45) (2.7%)
Basophils	0.05(0–10) (0.4%)	0.05(0–0.20) (0.6%)	0.04(0–0.20) (0.5%)	0.04(0–0.20) (0.5%)
Lymphocytes	7.0(4.0–10.5) (61%)	4.5(2.0–8.0) (50%)	3.1(1.5–6.5) (38%)	2.5(1.0–4.8) (34%)
Monocytes	0.55(0.05–1.1) (4.8%)	0.45(0–0.8) (5.0%)	0.35(0–0.8) (4.3%)	0.30(0–0.8) (4.0%)

*Values are expressed as cells $\times 10^3/\mu l$. Mean values are given; ranges are in parentheses. Percent is for mean values.

FIG. 11.37 Normal leukocyte and differential counts. (From Altman PL, Dittmer DS (eds): Blood and Other Body Fluids, Federation of American Societies for Experimental Biology, Washington, DC, 1961, with permission)

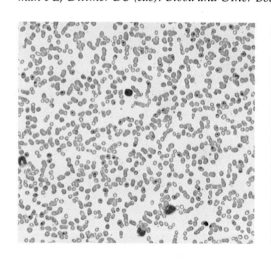
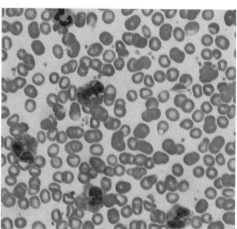

FIG. 11.38 (Left) Monocytosis in a child recovering from chemotherapy-related neutropenia. (Right) Eosinophilia with an increase in white blood cell count. This patient suffered from a parasitic infection that triggered the increase in eosinophils.

Quantitative Abnormalities of White Cells

Normal values for total white cell number and differential counts are age-related as seen in Figure 11.37. Black individuals may have lower granulocyte counts than Caucasians of the same age.

Both leukocytosis and leukopenia are common pediatric hematology problems. Increases in WBC number—lymphocytosis, neutrophilia or granulocytosis, monocytosis, eosinophilia (Fig. 11.38) or basophilia—can be seen, as well as decreases in specific types of WBCs. Numerous disorders can cause an increase in the number of immature white cell elements.

LEUKEMOID REACTION

Figure 11.39 shows a leukemoid reaction, which is characterized by a high white cell count (usually greater than 50,000/mm³) with an increase in the number of immature myeloid cells ("shift to the left"). There are many etiologies for leukemoid reactions, including Down syndrome and sepsis. Leukemoid reactions must be distinguished from leukemia (discussed below). Another differential diagnostic consideration is that of leukoerythroblastosis, in which increased numbers of immature granulocytes are accompanied on smear by nucleated red cells and red cell fragments, teardrops, target cells, and large platelets. This morphologic picture, in turn, has a long list of causes, which includes the

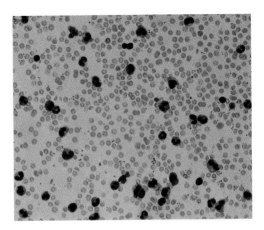

FIG. 11.39 Leuke-moid reaction in a patient with pneumococcal sepsis. A·higher magnification would reveal toxic granulations and Döhle bodies (see Fig. 11.54) in the polymorphonuclear leukocytes.

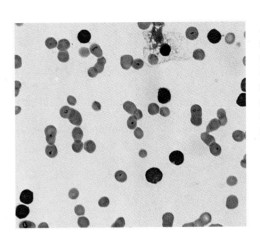

FIG. 11.40 Peripheral blood smear of a child with acute lymphocytic leukemia (ALL). Note the decreased platelets on the smear and the absence of normal WBCs.

MORPHOLOGIC CRITERIA FOR "LYMPHOBLASTIC" LEUKEMIC CELLS

Cytologic Features	L1	L2	L3
Cell size	Small cells predominate	Large; heterogeneous in size	Large and homogeneous
Nuclear chromatin	Homogeneous in any one case	Variable; heterogeneous in any one case	Finely stippled and homogeneous
Nuclear shape	Regular; occasional clefting or indentation	Irregular; clefting and indentation common	Regular; oval to round
Nucleoli	Not visible or small and inconspicuous	One or more present; often large	Prominent; one or more vesicular
Amount of cytoplasm	Scanty	Variable; often moderately abundant	Moderately abundant
Basophilia of cytoplasm	Slight or moderate; rarely intense	Variable; deep in some	Very deep
Cytoplasmic vacuolation	Variable	Variable	Often prominent

FIG. 11.41 Morphologic criteria for "lymphoblastic" leukemic cells.

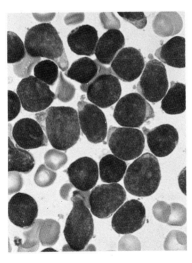

FIG. 11.42 Bone marrow aspirate from the child with ALL whose peripheral blood is shown in Figure 11.40. Note the monotonous pattern of the blastic cells (L1).

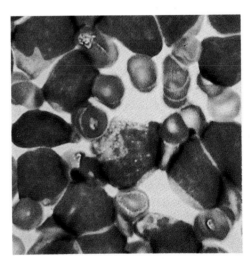

FIG. 11.43 L2 lymphoblasts in another patient with ALL. These lymphoblasts are larger and more heterogeneous in appearance than the L1 lymphoblasts and the nuclear to cytoplasm ratio is lower than that for L1 lymphoblasts. The nucleoli are prominent.

spectrum of myeloproliferative disorders ranging from myelofibrosis to chronic myelogenous leukemia, polycythemia vera, or essential thrombocythemia.

LEUKEMIA

Perhaps the most worrisome reason for an increase in immature white cells is leukemia. Childhood leukemias also may present as isolated or combined cytopenias with or without the presence of "blasts" on smear. Figure 11.40 shows the peripheral blood from a typical child with acute lymphoblastic or lymphocytic leukemia (ALL). The smear demonstrates thrombocytopenia, neutrophils appear to be decreased, and there are cells with the characteristics of lymphoblasts (Fig. 11.41). These cells are seen more clearly on bone marrow aspirate (Fig. 11.42). Alternatively, lymphoblasts may be the L2 variety (Fig. 11.43). Rarely, L3 or Bur-

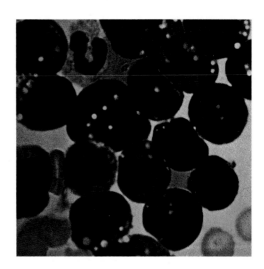

FIG. 11.44 L3 lymphoblasts represent the third morphologic presentation of ALL. These lymphoblasts are large deeply staining cells that often are vacuolated.

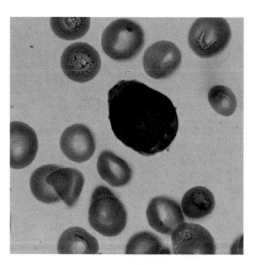

FIG. 11.45 A lymphoblast in the peripheral blood of a young infant with an overwhelming viral infection. This patient was also thrombocytopenic.

MORPHOLOGIC CRITERIA FOR "MYELOID" LEUKEMIC CELLS*

Myeloid Leukemias	
M1	Myeloblastic leukemia— no maturation
M2	Myeloblastic leukemia— with maturation
M3	Promyelocytic leukemia
M4	Myelomonocytic leukemia
M5	Monocytic leukemia
M6	Erythroleukemia
M7	Megakaryoblastic leukemia

*According to the standard French-American-British (F.A.B.) method of classification.

FIG. 11.46 Morphologic criteria for "myeloid" leukemic cells.

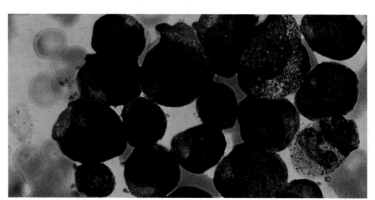

FIG. 11.47 Peripheral blood smear shows an Auer rod (red barlike figure in the cytoplasm) in a myeloblast of a patient with acute nonlymphocytic leukemia (ANLL).

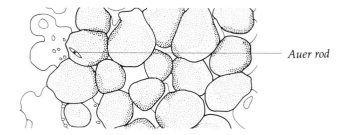

— Auer rod

kitt's type lymphoblasts (Fig. 11.44) will be seen and can be readily identified by the use of immunocytochemical markers. In diagnosing leukemia it is important to remember that:

1. A normal peripheral blood smear does not rule out the possibility of acute leukemia.
2. The presence of blasts in the peripheral blood does not confirm a diagnosis of leukemia.

This is particularly true in infants and younger children in whom the release of young cells from the bone marrow into the peripheral blood may occur in response to a range of problems including infection (Fig. 11.45).

In acute nonlymphoblastic leukemia (ANLL), the "blasts" belong to the myeloid or monocyte series and fall into one of six morphologic categories designated M1 to M6, (Fig. 11.46). A recent addition to this classification schema is M7, or megakaryoblastic leukemia, a nonlymphoid leukemia derived from platelet precursors. Although the presence of Auer rods is helpful in distinguishing ANLL from ALL (Fig. 11.47), the peripheral smear alone may not be sufficient for

distinguishing between these two forms of leukemia.

Figure 11.48 shows the peripheral blood of a child with the uncommon entity of adult type (Philadelphia-chromosome-positive) chronic myelogenous (granulocytic) leukemia (CML) in the chronic phase. This phase is characterized by a dramatic increase in white cell number, which usually exceeds 100,000/mm³. Mature granulocytes, band forms, and metamyelocytes predominate, although less mature myeloid cells, including an occasional myeloblast, may be seen. Eosinophilia, basophilia, and thrombocytosis also may be present, as well as nucleated red cells. Children with CML inevitably progress to a "blast crisis" (Fig. 11.49), which can have the morphologic appearance of either ALL or ANLL. Another form of the disease, juvenile (Philadelphia-chromosome-negative) CML, may present with morphologic findings similar to those of adult CML. However, the leukocytosis in juvenile CML tends to be less dramatic than in adult CML and there may be an increase of monocytoid cells. Anemia and thrombocytopenia are more profound than in adult CML.

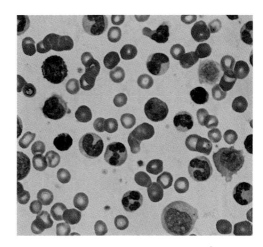

FIG. 11.48 CML in the chronic phase. Note the presence of all stages of myeloid maturation.

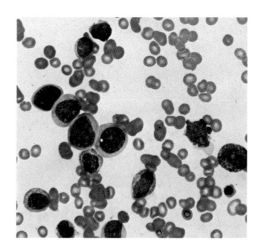

FIG. 11.49 Large numbers of blasts are seen in the peripheral blood of a CML patient in "blast crisis."

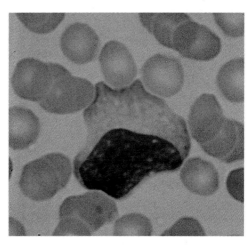

FIG. 11.50 An atypical lymphocyte from patient with infectious mononucleosis. The nucleus is large and the cytoplasm is abundant. Note that where the lymphocyte cytoplasm abuts a red cell, the lymphocyte deforms around it.

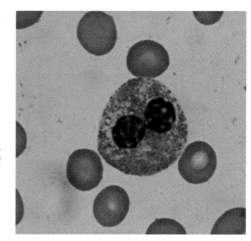

FIG. 11.51 Pelger-Huët anomaly. Note the uniform bilobed nucleus of the granulocyte.

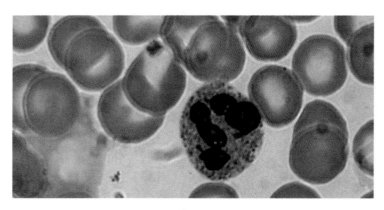

FIG. 11.52 Nuclear appendages, which can be seen normally in female polymorphonuclear leukocytes. An increase in appendages is seen in trisomy 13–15.

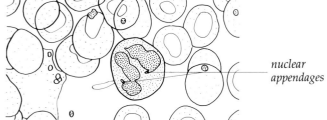

nuclear appendages

Morphologic Abnormalities of White Cells

ATYPICAL LYMPHOCYTES

Probably the most commonly seen morphologic abnormality of white cells is the atypical lymphocyte (Fig. 11.50). This is a large cell with an irregular plasma membrane, which often "hugs" adjacent red cells. Its nucleus also is large, and nucleoli may be visible. The abundant cytoplasm typically is basophilic and may contain vacuoles and azurophilic granules. Morphologic subtypes of atypical lymphocytes may occur but clinically, their recognition is of little use. Although infectious mononucleosis comes to mind when atypical lymphocytes are seen, these lymphocytes are not specific and may be present in many other situations, most notably in almost any viral illness. Immature lymphocytes, intermediate in maturity between lymphoblasts and mature lymphocytes, should be distinguished from atypical lymphocytes, although the two cell types are associated with overlapping differential diagnoses.

NEUTROPHIL ABNORMALITIES

Occasionally, mature neutrophils may be large in members of a given family, the so-called hereditary giant neutrophils. In addition, neutrophils or other polymorphs may be of normal size but have hereditary or acquired hypersegmentation or reduced numbers of nuclear segments, as in the Pelger-Huët anomaly (Fig. 11.51). Increased numbers of nuclear appendages also may occur (Fig. 11.52), such as may be seen in the neutrophils of patients with trisomy 13-15. These however may be difficult to distinguish from normal neutrophil "drumsticks," which are nuclear appendages that occur in 2 to 10 percent of the neutrophils of normal females.

Vacuoles can occur in any white cell for a variety of reasons, including artifact from anticoagulant, infections, or storage diseases. Certain types of inclusions, such as those seen in Gaucher's disease, are limited to bone marrow histiocytes and therefore are not detected on examination of the peripheral smear.

Toxic granulations, prominent azurophilic granules, are

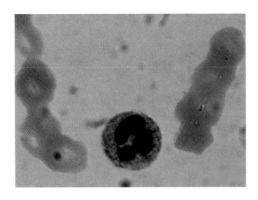

FIG. 11.53 Toxic granulations and a Döhle body are found in child with sepsis. The Döhle body appears as a gray-blue staining area, which in this cell is located at the inferior border of the cell.

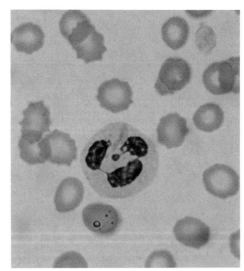

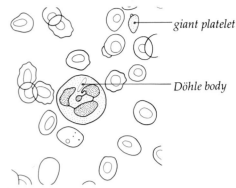

FIG. 11.54 The May-Hegglin anomaly showing a Döhle body in the white cell, and giant platelets that may be decreased in number.

— giant platelet

— Döhle body

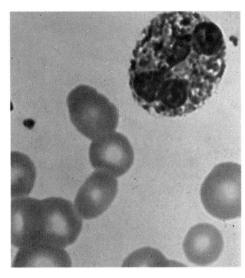

FIG. 11.55 Polymorphonuclear leukocytes with prominent granules characterize Alder-Reilly bodies as seen in Hurler's disease.

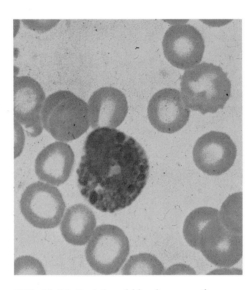

FIG. 11.56 Peripheral blood smear of a child with Chédiak-Higashi syndrome. (Courtesy of Dr. William Zinkham)

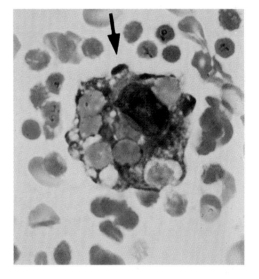

FIG. 11.57 Prominent erythrophagocytosis in which numerous RBCs are engulfed by white cell cytoplasm.

another common type of white cell inclusion. They are nonspecific but can be seen in both viral and bacterial infections (Fig. 11.53). Toxic granulations are to be distinguished from the hereditary dense granulation that can be present in the neutrophils of rare normal individuals. Döhle bodies, pale blue inclusions that usually are located peripherally in the cytoplasm of neutrophils, may coexist with toxic granulations. Together with giant platelets, Döhle bodies are seen in patients with the dominantly inherited May-Hegglin anomaly (Fig. 11.54).

Alder-Reilly bodies, or Reilly bodies, are prominent granules that are metachromatic when stained with toluidine blue, and which can be present in any of the white cells of patients with Hurler's disease for which they are virtually pathognomonic (Fig. 11.55). Coarse azurophilic neutrophilic granules that resemble Alder-Reilly bodies but are not metachromatic have been reported in Batten's disease. Likewise, large greenish-brown neutrophil inclusions are characteristic of the rare patient with Chédiak-Higashi syndrome (Fig. 11.56). Such granules may appear in eosinophils and basophils, as well.

White cells also may acquire inclusions by engulfing particles from their surroundings. Erythrophagocytosis (Fig. 11.57) is a nonspecific finding that presumably is immune-

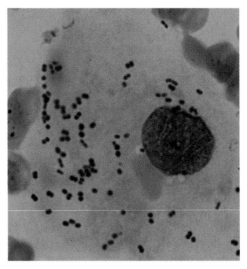

FIG. 11.58 Intracellular bacteria on Wright's stain of a buffy coat smear from a neutropenic patient. Note the numerous darkly stained bacteria in the cytoplasm.

mediated and is seen in viral infections and primary diseases of the reticuloendothelial system. LE cells of systemic lupus erythematosis are a diagnostically useful example of cellular phagocytosis although in general they are not seen on routine peripheral blood smears. Figure 11.58 shows a buffy coat preparation from a patient with suspected sepsis, demonstrating intracellular bacteria.

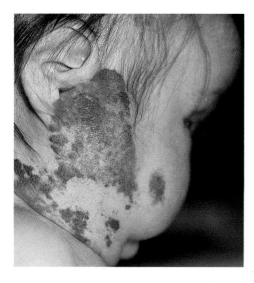

FIG. 11.59 Hemangioma of child with Kasabach-Merritt syndrome.

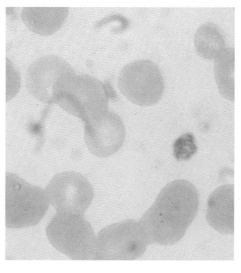

FIG. 11.60 Megathrombocyte in the peripheral blood of a patient with idiopathic thrombocytopenia purpura (ITP).

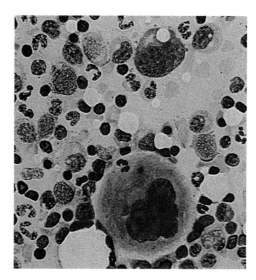

FIG. 11.61 High-power view of a megakaryocyte in the bone marrow of a patient with ITP.

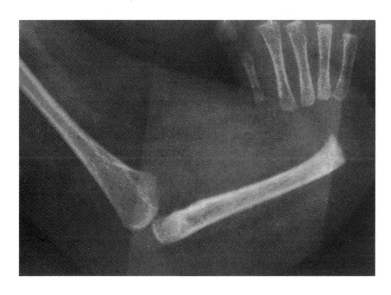

FIG. 11.62 Radiograph of the right arm of a child with thrombocytopenia-absent radius (TAR) syndrome. This patient had absent radii bilaterally.

PLATELETS

As with white cells, the CBC and smear generally are not useful for evaluating the functional abnormalities of platelets. Such abnormalities may be drug-related (e.g., aspirin) or inherited (e.g., von Willebrand's disease) and may require specific laboratory confirmation, which will not be discussed here. On the other hand, the diagnosis of quantitative and morphologic abnormalities of platelets, which may go hand in hand, is easily approached by examination of the smear. Platelets can be roughly quantified from the smear. A normal platelet count at any age is 150,000/mm³ to 450,000/mm³, although, clinically, thrombocytopenia may be inapparent until the platelet count gets well below 100,000/mm³.

As with the other hematopoietic cell lines, isolated thrombocytopenia may result either from decreased production or from increased destruction. The etiologies for the latter are numerous and include the idiopathic or immune thrombocytopenias, hypersplenism, and DIC. Figure 11.59 shows a patient with a large strawberry and cavernous hemangioma who had a platelet count of 3,000/mm³ as the result of consumption within the hemangioma (Kasabach-Merritt syndrome). Characteristically, in patients with in-

creased peripheral destruction, the platelets although decreased in number are large in size ("megathrombocytes") (Fig. 11.60). Although in some instances of increased destruction these diagnoses are clinically obvious or can be confirmed by laboratory tests (such as the measurement of antiplatelet antibodies or a DIC screen), often the diagnosis is made by ruling out causes of decreased platelet production by doing a bone marrow aspirate. In cases of increased destruction the bone marrow aspirate is notable because of the presence of normal or increased numbers of megakaryocytes (Fig. 11.61) and the absence of infiltrative processes such as leukemia. Large platelets are not always associated with thrombocytopenia and may be associated with functional abnormalities, as in the rare patient with Bernard-Soulier disease. On the other hand, patients with isolated thrombocytopenia on the basis of failure of production will have decreased or absent megakaryocyte precursors. Differentiation of the several causes of this finding, such as the thrombocytopenia-absent radius (TAR) syndrome and amegakaryocytic thrombocytopenia, may rest on clinical findings (Fig. 11.62). In some patients, such as those with Wiskott-Aldrich syndrome, abnormally small platelets are found that also may be decreased in number as a result of both failure of production and increased destruction.

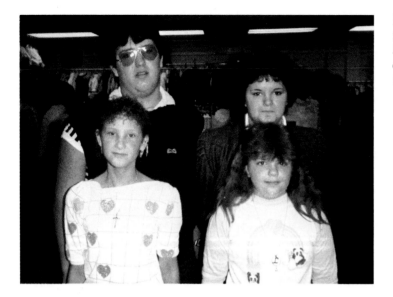

FIG. 11.63 A patient with Fanconi's anemia (shortly after bone marrow transplantation) and her three siblings. The patient (front left) presented with a hemoglobin of 3.5 g %, short stature, and increased skin pigmentation. Note the patient's diminutive size with respect to her more robust siblings.

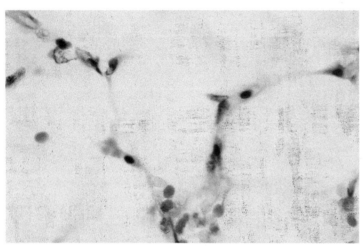

FIG. 11.64 Bone marrow biopsy of patient with acquired aplastic anemia. Stomal marrow cells are present with virtually no hematopoietic cells.

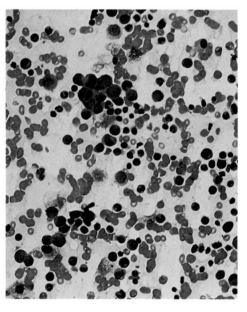

FIG. 11.65 Pseudorosettes (clumps of tumor cells) are particularly characteristic of a neuroblastoma metastasized to the bone marrow.

PANCYTOPENIA

Pancytopenia refers to a reduction in all three formed elements of the blood. In an analogous manner to anemia, pancytopenia is not a single disease entity but rather may result from a number of disease processes. Pancytopenia may occur due to bone marrow failure or to extramedullary cellular destruction (as seen in autoimmune disease, particularly SLE), or as a combination of depressed marrow function and increased cellular destruction. When pancytopenia is due to destruction of the formed elements of the blood, invariably there is another underlying disease. On the other hand, the pancytopenia due to bone marrow failure can be divided into genetically predisposed (constitutional) marrow failure syndromes, acquired marrow failure syndromes, and marrow replacement.

The most frequent of the constitutional marrow failure syndromes is Fanconi's anemia. Fanconi's anemia is a familial disorder marked by the association of pancytopenia and marrow hypoplasia with a variable constellation of congenital anomalies of the skin, skeleton, central nervous system, and genitourinary tract (Fig. 11.63). Fragility of the chromosomes further characterizes this syndrome, and it occurs even in the absence of physical anomalies. Patients can present with anemia very early in life but generally de-velop signs of marrow failure in midchildhood. The abnormal chromosomes are the most characteristic laboratory finding and chromosome breaks, gaps, and rearrangements are common.

Acquired marrow failure syndromes (aplastic anemia) occur as a result of an insult to the bone marrow from a variety of sources including drugs, toxins, solvents and radiation, as well as autoimmune and postinfectious disorders. Nevertheless a full 50 percent of aplastic anemia cases have no apparent insulting agent and are idiopathic in origin.

The clinical course of aplastic anemia from any of these causes is that of inexorable bone marrow failure with anemia, thrombocytopenia and leukopenia, leading ultimately to death from bleeding or infection if spontaneous recovery or successful intervention fails to occur.

While the peripheral smear will reveal a paucity of platelets and WBCs with a low reticulocyte count and normochromic normocytic anemia, a marrow biopsy generally is needed to clarify the diagnosis (Fig. 11.64).

Marrow replacement, another cause of pancytopenia, occurs either with a hematopoietic malignancy such as leukemia (see Fig. 11.42) or from solid tumors invading the marrow (Fig. 11.65). Both a direct "crowding out" phenomenon and an alteration of the marrow "milieu" appear to contribute to marrow failure.

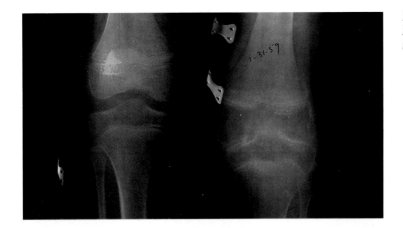

FIG. 11.66 Hemophiliac arthritis following recurrent hemarthroses. Note the widened joint space on the left knee as compared to that of the normal right knee.

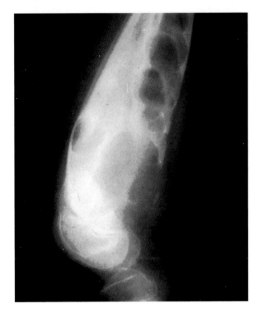
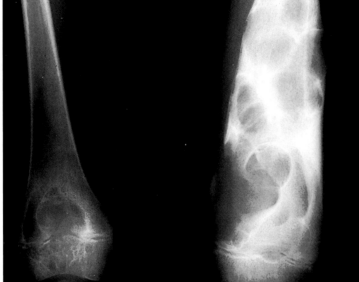

FIG. 11.67 (Left) Pseudotumor of the femur due to recurrent hemarthroses with subsequent bony destruction of the knee and adjacent bony structure. (Right) Note that the opposite knee also demonstrates early destructive changes in the distal femur and joint.

HEMOPHILIAS

Although several different types of hemophilia exist, hemophilia types A and B will serve as the prototypes for our discussion. All the hemophilias are caused by either a decrease or an absence of one of several vital coagulation factor activities. The factor may either fail to be synthesized or be synthesized in an altered form with less than adequate function.

Factor VIII deficiency hemophilia (type A, classical) is the most common form of this disease accounting for 85 percent of cases. Factor IX deficiency (type B, Christmas disease) accounts for nearly all of the remaining cases, with the exception of those rare patients who have other factor activity deficiencies. Because both hemophilia types A and B are transmitted in an X-linked recessive inheritance pattern, hemophilia is found to occur nearly always in males.

The hemophilias may present with variable degrees of factor deficiency with commensurate degrees of clinical disease. Patients with mild hemophilia have factor activity between 5 to 30 percent and in general only suffer from coagulopathy if they undergo surgery or suffer major trauma. Patients with moderate hemophilia have a factor activity of 1 to 5 percent and suffer localized hemorrhage if significant trauma occurs. Finally and most frequently, patients with less than 1 percent of factor activity have spontaneous soft-tissue hemorrhage or bleeding associated with only minor trauma.

Patients with hemophilia may present with bleeding in the newborn period at the time of circumcision. Those infants who escape clinical problems at that time generally do not present until 12 to 18 months of age, when they have become more mobile and minor trauma from falls precipitates bleeding. Although the clinical manifestations of hemophilia can affect any organ, the musculoskeletal, central nervous, and urinary systems predominate. The most common of the clinical manifestations of hemophilia include hemarthroses, and soft-tissue bleeding with intramuscular hematomas. Secondary hemophiliac arthropathy also may occur, with knees, elbows, and ankles the most commonly involved joints. Recurrent untreated hemorrhages may lead to contractures (Fig. 11.66) and painful arthritis (Fig. 11.67). Finally, intramuscular bleeding can cause compartment syndromes with secondary peripheral nerve palsies.

BIBLIOGRAPHY

Miller DR, Pearson HA, Baehner RL, McMillan LW: Smith's Blood Diseases of Infancy and Childhood, 4th ed. C V Mosby Co, St. Louis, 1978.

Nathan DG, Oski FA: Hematology of Infancy and Childhood, 2nd ed. W B Saunders Co, Philadelphia, 1981.

Oski F, Naiman JL: Hematologic Problems of the Newborn, 3rd ed. W B Saunders Co, Philadelphia, 1982.

Wintrobe MM, et al: Clinical Hematology, 8th ed. Lea & Febiger, Philadelphia, 1981.

Zucker-Franklin D, Greanes MF, Grossi CE, Marmont AM: Atlas of Blood Cells, Edi. Ermes, Milan, Italy, 1981.

PEDIATRIC INFECTIOUS DISEASE

Holly W. Davis, M.D.

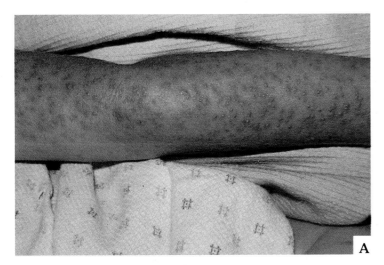

A

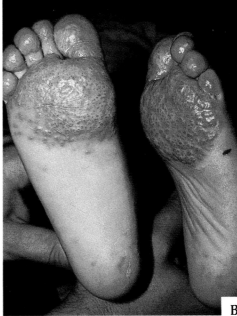

B

FIG. 12.1 Clustering of viral exanthematous lesions. In this child with underlying eczema and early varicella, the first crop of vesicles appeared in clusters at sites previously affected by eczema. **A**, The flexor surface of his arm is covered with numerous discrete lesions. **B**, Vesicles are confluent over the plantar surface of his toes and on the balls of his feet. (Courtesy of Dr. M. Sherlock)

In selecting infectious diseases for presentation in an atlas format, we have chosen to emphasize those disorders in which visual findings tend to be prominent, as well as those that either are common or are so potentially serious as to make early diagnosis important. Modes of presentation, patterns of clinical evolution, and spectrum of severity will be stressed. The following topics will be covered: infectious exanthems, mumps, bacterial skin and soft-tissue infections, infectious lymphadenitis, bacterial bone and joint infections, and congenital and perinatal infections.

INFECTIOUS EXANTHEMS

Exanthematous disorders are numerous, commonly encountered, and having many similarities often are a source of clinical confusion. In establishing a diagnosis the clinician should attend not only to the basic character of the exanthem but also to its mode of spread, its distribution, the evolution of lesions, and the constellation of associated symptoms. In some of these illnesses, the presence of characteristic oral enanthems can be helpful in establishing the diagnosis. It is also important to remember that the lesions of viral exanthems tend to appear first and to cluster most heavily at sites of prior skin irritation, such as the diaper area or sites of eczematous dermatitis (Fig. 12.1).

Viral Exanthems

Along with mumps three exanthems—measles or rubeola, rubella, and varicella—continue to be referred to as the usual childhood diseases. Measles and rubella were once so common and well described that their exanthems became paradigms, with the rashes of subsequently described disorders often being termed "rubeoliform" or "rubelliform," for example. As a result of immunization, however, measles and rubella are becoming relatively rare and now affect adolescents and young adults more often than young children. The current infrequency of these disorders in developed countries has created a situation in which younger practitioners are unfamiliar with them, and thus may be uncertain about diag-

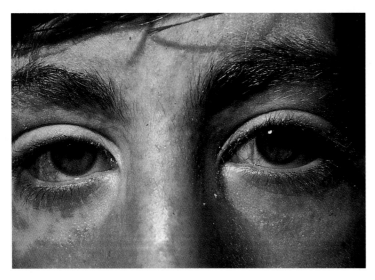

FIG. 12.2 Rubeola/measles. During and after the prodromal period, the conjunctivae are injected and produce a clear discharge. This is associated with marked photophobia. (Courtesy of Dr. M. Sherlock)

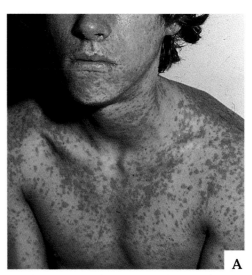

FIG. 12.4 **A**, The measles exanthem is a blotchy erythematous blanching maculopapular eruption that appears at the hairline and spreads cephalocaudally over 3 days (**B**) ultimately involving the palms and soles. With evolution lesions become confluent at proximal sites. (Courtesy of Dr. M. Sherlock)

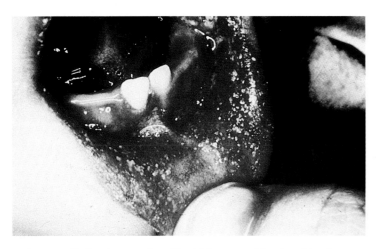

FIG. 12.3 Rubeola/measles. Koplik's spots, bluish-white dots surrounded by red halos, appear on the buccal and labial mucosae a day or two before the exanthem and begin to fade with onset of the rash. (Courtesy of Dr. S. L. Katz)

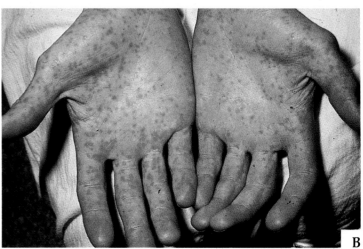

nosis. However, identification remains important because of contagion and potential complications. Accurate clinical diagnosis can be difficult in view of the fact that a multitude of other viruses, including adenoviruses, enteroviruses and the Epstein-Barr (EB) virus, can produce a variety of cutaneous exanthems, and that the clinical picture produced by a given pathogen can closely mimic that of others.

RUBEOLA (NINE-DAY OR RED MEASLES)
Measles is a highly contagious, moderate to severe acute illness with a typical prodrome and mode of evolution. Prodromal symptoms consist of fever, increasing malaise, dry cough, coryza, and conjunctivitis with clear discharge and marked photophobia (Fig. 12.2). One to two days after onset, a pathognomonic enanthem (Koplik's spots) appears on the buccal mucosa (Fig. 12.3). Lesions consist of tiny bluish white dots surrounded by red halos, which increase in number and then fade over a 2- to 3-day period. The exanthem is seen first on day 3 or 4, as prodromal symptoms and fever peak in severity. It is a blotchy, erythematous blanching maculopapular eruption that appears at the hairline and spreads

cephalocaudally over 3 days, ultimately involving the palms and soles (Fig. 12.4). Once generalized the rash becomes confluent over proximal areas but remains discrete distally. Older lesions tend to develop a rusty hue as a result of capillary leak and cease to blanch with pressure. Fading commences after 3 days with clearing 2 to 3 days later. Fine branny desquamation of the most severely involved areas may ensue. Generalized adenopathy may be present in moderate to severe cases.

During the acute phase of this illness, most patients appear to be quite ill systemically. They are lethargic, complain of moderate to severe malaise and anorexia, and prefer to be left alone to sleep in a darkened room.

The incubation period for measles is 9 to 10 days and patients are contagious from approximately 4 days before the appearance of rash until about 4 days after. The attack rate in exposed susceptible individuals is greater than 90 percent. Morbidity is rather high and mortality not uncommon, especially in third world countries. The peak season for measles is late winter through early spring. Potential complications (resulting either from extension of the primary infection or from secondary invasion by bacterial pathogens) include otitis media, pneumonia, obstructive laryngotracheitis, and acute encephalitis.

RUBELLA (GERMAN MEASLES)
While rubella has little or no prodrome in children, adolescents, like adults, may experience 1 to 5 days of low-grade

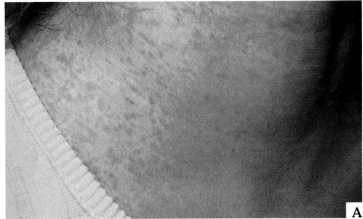

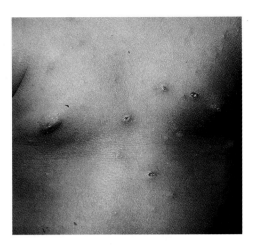

FIG. 12.6 Varicella/chickenpox. The characteristic finding of lesions in all stages of evolution is seen on the trunk of this child. Note the presence of papules, vesicles, umbilicated and scabbed lesions, all within a small geographic area.

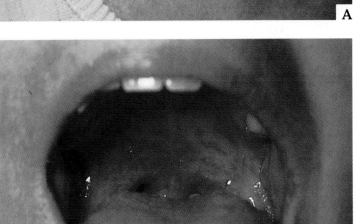

FIG. 12.5 Rubella/german measles. **A**, The exanthem of rubella usually consists of a fine pinkish-red maculopapular eruption that appears first at the hairline and rapidly spreads cephalocaudally. Lesions tend to remain discrete. **B**, The presence of red palatal lesions (Forscheimer spots), seen in some patients on day 1 of the rash, and occipital and posterior cervical adenopathy are suggestive findings of rubella. (Courtesy of Dr. M. Sherlock)

fever, mild malaise, adenopathy, headache, sore throat, and coryza. Fever, if present at all in young children, is low grade and rarely lasts more than a day. The exanthem is a discrete pinkish-red fine maculopapular eruption, which, like measles, typically begins on the face and spreads cephalocaudally (Fig. 12.5A). Generalization occurs within 24 hours, whereupon fading begins, with clearing complete by 72 hours. Forscheimer spots, an enanthem consisting of small reddish spots on the soft palate, are seen in some patients on day 1 of the rash and can be helpful in differential diagnosis (Fig. 12.5B). Adenopathy, often generalized, is a common but not an invariable feature. Occipital, posterior cervical, and postauricular nodes tend to be those most prominently enlarged. Arthritis and arthralgias are frequent in adolescent and adult females, beginning on day 2 to 3 and typically lasting 5 to 10 days. Large or small joints may be affected.

Many patients infected with rubella do not manifest this typical picture. Up to 25 percent of infected individuals are asymptomatic yet are capable of transmitting the virus to others. In some the rash may last only 1 day and it may involve only the trunk; in others, the exanthem is absent and the patient will appear to have pharyngitis or an upper respiratory tract infection. Since a number of other viruses, including adenoviruses, coxsackie viruses and echoviruses, can produce a rubella-like picture, exact diagnosis requires serologic testing. Such testing is important if the patient is pregnant or has been in contact with a pregnant woman, or if arthritis is a prominent feature simulating the picture of acute rheumatic fever or rheumatoid arthritis.

Peak incidence occurs in late winter and early spring, and patients are contagious from a few days prior to a few days after appearance of the exanthem. The incubation period ranges from 14 to 21 days. Complications are rare in childhood and include arthritis, purpura with or without thrombocytopenia, and mild encephalitis. The major complication results from spread of virus to susceptible pregnant women and their fetuses, resulting in congenital rubella syndrome (see section below on congenital infections). When such an exposure is thought to have occurred, acute and convalescent titers should be obtained from the index patient, and the pregnant woman should be tested for hemagglutination inhibition antibody. If this is positive, immunity can be assumed; if it is negative, she should be retested in 2 weeks. If antibody is detected in the second specimen, infection has occurred and the fetus is at risk.

VARICELLA (CHICKENPOX)

Varicella in the normal host is a relatively benign albeit highly contagious illness caused by the varicella-zoster virus. A brief prodrome of low-grade fever, upper respiratory tract symptoms, and mild malaise may occur, and if present is followed rapidly by the appearance of a pruritic exanthem. Lesions appear in crops and evolve rapidly over several hours. Most patients will have three crops although some may have only one and others may have as many as five. Initial crops involve the trunk and scalp, while subsequent crops are distributed more peripherally; thus, the mode of spread is centrifugal. The presence of scalp lesions with the initial crop often is helpful in diagnosing the patient who presents early in the course of the disease. Lesions begin as tiny erythematous papules that rapidly enlarge to form thin-walled superficial central vesicles surrounded by red halos. Vesicular fluid changes promptly from clear to cloudy; then drying begins, resulting in an umbilicated appearance. As surrounding erythema fades a central crust or scab is formed which sloughs after several days. A hallmark of this exanthem is the finding of lesions in all stages of evolution within a relatively small geographic area of skin (Fig. 12.6). Generally all scabs have sloughed in 10 to 14 days. Scarring does not occur unless lesions become secondarily infected.

An enanthem is commonly seen and consists of thin-walled vesicles that rapidly rupture to form shallow ulcers.

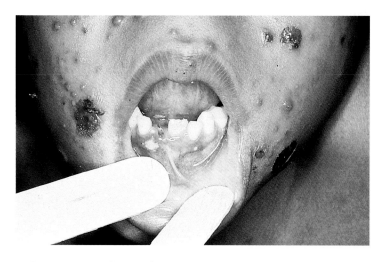

FIG. 12.7 Varicella/chickenpox. On mucosal surfaces, thin-walled vesicles may form which rapidly rupture forming painful shallow ulcers. (Courtesy of Dr. E. Wald)

Any mucosal surface may be affected (Fig. 12.7). While skin lesions are pruritic, those present on oral, rectal or vaginal mucosal surfaces, or those involving the external auditory canal or tympanic membrane, can be very painful necessitating analgesia. Systemic symptoms generally are mild, although low-grade to moderate fever may be present during the first few days. In most cases pruritus is the child's major complaint. In adolescents however, as in adults, the illness is more likely to be severe with prominent systemic symptoms and with more extensive exanthematous involvement.

Varicella occurs year round, with peak periods in late autumn and in late winter through early spring. The period of communicability begins 1 to 2 days before the appearance of lesions and lasts until all lesions have crusted over. The incubation period ranges from 10 to 21 days, with very high secondary attack rates in susceptible individuals. The most common complication in normal hosts is that of secondary bacterial infection of excoriated skin lesions. Such infection can range from impetiginization to cellulitis. Other complications, though rare, include pneumonia, hepatitis, and encephalitis. The onset of these complications typically is heralded by a secondary fever spike concurrent with an increase in general systemic symptoms. With encephalitis an altered level of consciousness will be apparent along with other signs of neurologic dysfunction. Reye's syndrome, an encephalopathy of unclear etiology, is now a well-recognized complication that can occur as a child is recovering from acute varicella. Repetitive pernicious vomiting is followed by an altered level of consciousness in which periods of lethargy alternate with periods of delirium or combativeness.

In the immunocompromised or immunosuppressed host with deficient cellular immunity, varicella is an extremely severe and often fatal disease with CNS, pulmonary, and generalized visceral involvement. Skin lesions often are hemorrhagic and tend to remain vesicular for a prolonged period of time (Fig. 12.8). In the potentially compromised host who has not had varicella previously (including those on short-course high-dose steroids), parents must be forewarned of these dangers and thereby instructed to notify their physician immediately of any suspicion of exposure. This enables the administration of zoster immune globulin or zoster immune plasma within 72 hours of exposure, thus reducing the severity of illness.

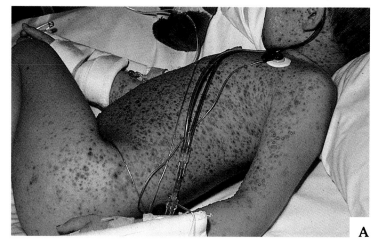

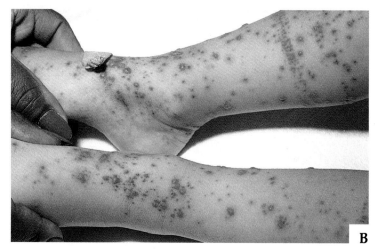

FIG. 12.8 Disseminated hemorrhagic varicella. **A**, In the immunocompromised child skin lesions tend to be hemorrhagic and nearly confluent. **B**, Lesions also evolve more slowly than usual, remaining vesicular for a prolonged period.

ADENOVIRUS INFECTIONS
There are approximately 30 distinct types of adenovirus capable of producing a variety of clinical illnesses including conjunctivitis, upper respiratory tract infections and pharyngitis, croup, bronchitis, bronchiolitis and pneumonia (occasionally fulminant), gastroenteritis, myocarditis, nephritis, cystitis, and encephalitis. An exanthem occasionally accompanies other symptoms, and a variety of rashes have been described. The eruption may consist of discrete nonspecific blanching maculopapular lesions or it may be morbilliform, rubelliform, rubeoliform, or on occasion petechial. Typically it is generalized when first noted. The most readily identifiable clinical constellation consists of conjunctivitis, rhinitis, pharyngitis and a discrete blanching maculopapular rash (Fig. 12.9). Anterior cervical and preauricular lymphadenopathy, low-grade fever, and malaise are common associated findings. The peak season for adenovirus infections in temperate climates is late winter through early summer and patients are maximally contagious during the first few days of illness. The incubation period ranges from 6 to 9 days.

COXSACKIE HAND-FOOT-AND-MOUTH DISEASE
Of the enteroviruses coxsackie group A16 produces the most easily recognizable exanthem, known as "hand-foot-and-

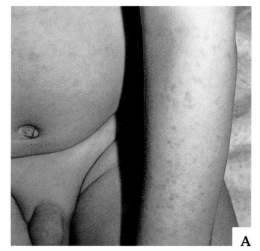
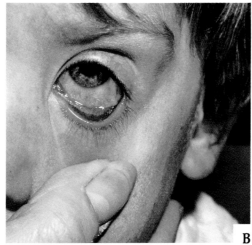

FIG. 12.9 Adenovirus. **A**, This discrete erythematous blanching maculopapular rash was generalized when first noted, and occurred in association with pharyngitis and (**B**) nonpurulent conjunctivitis. (Courtesy of Dr. M. Sherlock)

A

B

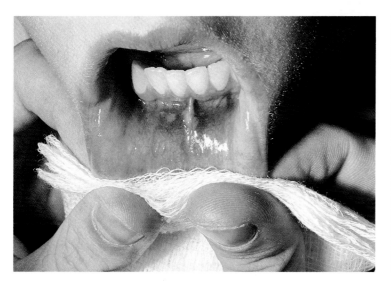

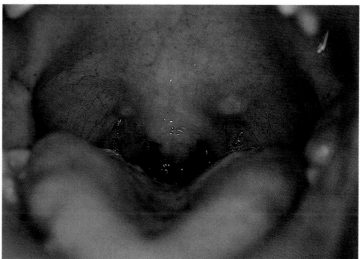

FIG. 12.10 Coxsackie hand-foot-and-mouth disease. The enanthem of this disorder is characterized by lesions consisting of mildly painful, shallow yellow ulcers surrounded by red halos. These may be found on the labial or buccal mucosa, the tongue, soft palate, uvula, and anterior tonsillar pillars. When oral lesions occur in the absence of the exanthem, the disorder is called herpangina.

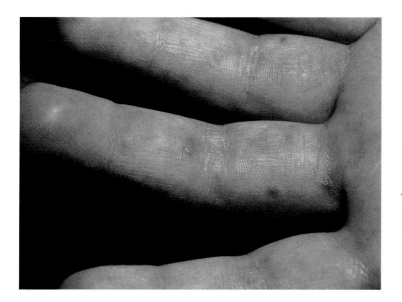

FIG. 12.11 The exanthem of coxsackie hand-foot-and-mouth disease involves the palmar, plantar and interdigital surfaces of the hands and feet, and consists of thick-walled gray vesicles on an erythematous base. (Courtesy of Dr. M. Sherlock)

mouth disease." Patients may have a brief prodrome consisting of low-grade fever, malaise, sore mouth and anorexia, during which time lesions are absent. Within 1 to 2 days oral lesions and, soon thereafter, skin lesions are noted in the typical case. The former consist of shallow yellow ulcers surrounded by red halos. They are found most frequently on the labial and buccal mucosal surfaces but also may affect the tongue, soft palate, uvula, and anterior tonsillar pillars (Fig. 12.10). These enanthematous lesions usually are only mildly painful. On occasion, when seen early in their evolution, small vesicles are noted on the palate or mucosal surfaces. The cutaneous lesions begin as erythematous macules on the palmar aspect of the hands and fingers, the plantar surface of the feet and toes, and the interdigital surfaces. They evolve rapidly to form small thick-walled gray vesicles on an erythematous base (Fig. 12.11), which may feel like slivers, be pruritic, or be asymptomatic. Over 90 percent of patients with this disease have oral lesions and about two-thirds have the exanthem. In those cases where cutaneous manifestations are absent, the process is called herpangina (caused by coxsackie and other enteroviruses) and may resemble early herpes gingivostomatitis. However coxsackie ulcers are less painful,

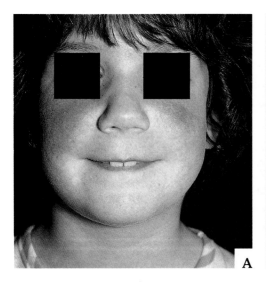
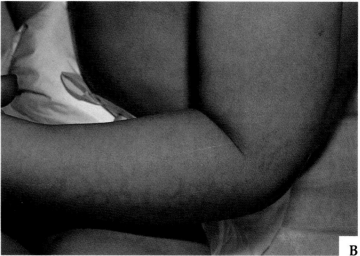

FIG. 12.12 Erythema infectiosum (fifth disease). **A**, On day 1, warm erythematous nontender circumscribed patches appear over the cheeks. These fade on the following day as (**B**) an erythematous lacy rash develops on the extensor surfaces of the extremities. (Courtesy of Dr. M. Sherlock)

less likely to involve gingival surfaces, and are not associated with the high fever and intense gingival erythema, edema, and bleeding typical of herpes.

Coxsackie hand-foot-and-mouth disease is highly contagious with an incubation period of approximately 2 to 6 days. Duration of symptoms ranges from 2 days to 1 week. The peak season is late summer through early fall.

Other enteroviral syndromes produced by the coxsackie group and by echoviruses include a mild nonspecific febrile illness with myalgias, headache, and abdominal pain; generalized exanthems that may be maculopapular, vesicular, or urticarial; encephalitis, acute cerebellar ataxia, and myelitis; pleurodynia; myocarditis; hemorrhagic conjunctivitis; and gastroenteritis.

ERYTHEMA INFECTIOSUM (FIFTH DISEASE)

Erythema infectiosum is a mildly contagious illness of preschool- and young school-age children that is thought to be of viral origin although, as yet, no specific organism has been isolated. The disorder is characterized primarily by its exanthem, as fever, constitutional, and other symptoms are unusual. Other symptoms when present may include headache, nausea, sore throat, myalgia, and arthralgias. The rash begins on the face, with large bright red erythematous patches appearing over both cheeks (Fig. 12.12A). These patches are warm but nontender, and have circumscribed borders that usually are macular but may be slightly raised. They are easily distinguished from those of cellulitis and erysipelas by their symmetry and lack of tenderness, and by the absence of high fever and toxicity. On the following day the facial lesions begin to fade and a symmetric, macular or slightly raised, lacy erythematous rash appears on the extensor surfaces of the extremities (Fig. 12.12B). The rash may spread over the next day or so to the flexor surfaces, buttocks, and trunk. Resolution occurs within 3 to 7 days of onset.

ROSEOLA INFANTUM (EXANTHEM SUBITUM)

Roseola infantum is a febrile illness that primarily affects young children between the ages of 6 and 36 months. It is thought to be of viral origin but as with fifth disease, no pathogen has as yet been identified. The clinical course begins abruptly with rapid temperature elevation, which occasionally precipitates a febrile seizure. Anorexia and irritability are the major associated symptoms. Examination reveals no source for the fever, which usually is higher than

39°C. Administration of an antipyretic produces only a transient decrease in temperature, which then rises rapidly to its former height. While most patients do not look toxic, many undergo a sepsis workup and lumbar puncture because of the combination of unexplained high fever and marked irritability. Fever persists for approximately 72 hours, whereupon the patient abruptly defervesces. In most cases an erythematous morbilliform exanthem appears simultaneously with defervescence, but in a small percentage of patients it develops 1 day before or after fever lysis. Lesions are discrete rose-pink macules or maculopapules that begin first on the trunk and then spread rapidly to the extremities, neck, and face (Fig. 12.13). They may last from several hours to a day or two before resolution.

While cases occur year round, roseola appears to be more common in late fall and early spring. Secondary cases are uncommon except in institutional settings. Duration of communicability is unclear, but the incubation period is thought to be 10 to 15 days.

MONONUCLEOSIS

The Epstein-Barr virus, in producing an infection that primarily involves the reticuloendothelial system, is recognized as the most common source of the mononucleosis syndrome, causing 90 percent or more of cases. Its peak season is mid to late winter, and its incubation period ranges from 14 to 50 days, although this tends to be shorter in young children. Transmission may occur by intimate mucosal contact via shared eating utensils, or by transfusion. The fact that in the young its incidence is highest in lower socioeconomic groups, while, in adolescence and early adulthood, it is seen more commonly in people of the middle and upper classes is perhaps in part attributable to the poorer hygienic conditions and practices found in lower socioeconomic circumstances and to the increase in intimate contact found in adolescence and young adulthood.

Although modes of presentation vary widely, two major clinical pictures of mononucleosis have come to be regarded as classic presentations: the first is that of pharyngeal glandular fever, consisting of fever, fatigue, malaise, pharyngitis, lymphadenopathy and atypical lymphocytosis, often accompanied by splenomegaly; the second is a typhoidal form, in which pharyngitis is absent and adenopathy is less prominent. The former has been reported to account for 80 percent of cases of EB virus mononucleosis, while the latter has been

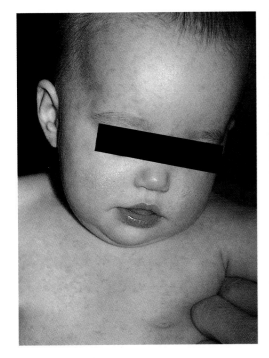
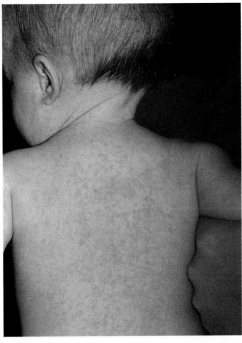

FIG. 12.13 *Roseola infantum/exanthem subitum. The exanthem of this disorder usually appears abruptly after 3 days of high fever and irritability. It is morbilliform in appearance and is comprised of discrete rose-pink macules. It may have become generalized when first noted, or centrifugal spread may be described.*

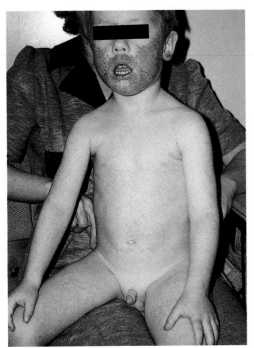
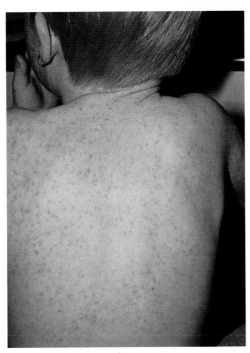

FIG. 12.14 *In this child with EB virus mononucleosis, a diffuse erythematous maculopapular rash was part of the clinical picture. Lesions on his face are hemorrhagic and confluent as a result of prior irritation. (He had practiced shaving two days before.) Note also the swelling in the region of the tonsillar node and the fact that the child is mouth breathing as a result of adenoidal hypertrophy. (Courtesy of Dr. M. Sherlock)*

held accountable for 20 percent. With the advent of definitive serologic tests however, it has become increasingly apparent that EB virus infection can result in a broad spectrum of clinical diseases with protean manifestations. Accurate clinical diagnosis is made even more difficult by the large number of differential diagnostic possibilities.

An exanthem is seen in as many as 15 percent of all patients with mononucleosis, although this percentage is greatly increased in patients for whom ampicillin has been prescribed for pharyngeal or respiratory symptoms. Usually an erythematous maculopapular rubelliform rash, the exanthem can be rubeoliform, scarlatiniform, urticarial, hemorrhagic, or even nodular in character (Fig. 12.14). In many cases the exanthem serves as the primary reason for seeking medical care, and in instances in which the overall clinical

picture is "atypical" it probably results in a significant number of misdiagnoses.

Clinical Features
of Classic Pharyngeal Glandular Fever

The classic pharyngeal glandular fever form of mononucleosis is encountered most commonly in the adolescent or young adult, although it also is seen occasionally in the preschool-age and school-age child. Onset usually is insidious, beginning with a prodrome, which may last from a few to several days, consisting of fatigue, malaise and anorexia, often in association with headache, sweats, and chills. Photophobia and edema of the eyelids and periorbital tissues may be noted in some patients during or shortly after this prodromal period. The acute phase usually is heralded by a

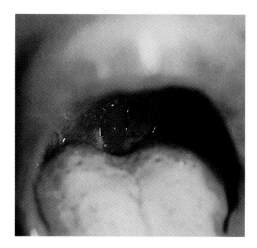

FIG. 12.15 EB virus mononucleosis. Severe pharyngotonsillitis is seen in this child whose tonsils are markedly enlarged and covered with a gray exudate. The uvula is erythematous and edematous. (Courtesy of Dr. M. Sherlock)

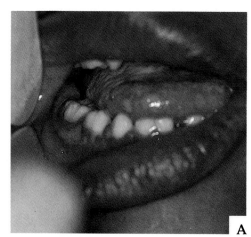

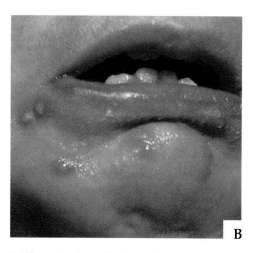

FIG. 12.16 Herpes simplex infections. **A,**Herpetic gingivostomatitis is characterized by discrete mucosal ulcerations and by gingival erythema, edema and friability in association with fever, dysphagia and cervical adenopathy.

B,These thick-walled vesicles on erythematous bases were noted in this child who had early findings of intraoral involvement, as well. (Courtesy of Dr. M. Sherlock)

further increase in temperature which may show wide daily fluctuations. Pharyngitis and cervical node enlargement then become apparent. The sore throat tends to increase in severity over several days before abating and may be associated with significant dysphagia. Tonsillar and adenoidal enlargement may range from mild to marked, and the tonsillar surface may vary in appearance from one of mild erythema to one of severe exudative inflammation with palatal and uvular edema (Fig. 12.15). Approximately one-third of patients have severe pharyngeal manifestations, and many of these also will have halitosis and palatal petechiae. The anterior cervical lymph nodes are routinely enlarged, and posterior cervical adenopathy is common. In classic cases diffuse adenopathy becomes apparent toward the end of the first week. Involved nodes are firm, discrete, and mildly to moderately tender. Approximately 50 percent of patients develop splenomegaly in the second to third week of illness, and as many as 30 to 40 percent have associated hepatic enlargement. The period of acute illness ranges in duration from 4 days to as long as 3 weeks.

Less Common Manifestations and Complications
A small percentage of patients develop less common manifestations or complications. These include pneumonitis with a pattern of a diffuse atypical pneumonia; hematologic abnormalities such as direct Coombs-positive hemolytic anemia and thrombocytopenia; icteric hepatitis; neurologic disorders such as acute cerebellar ataxia, encephalitis, aseptic meningitis, myelitis and radiculoneuritis; and, rarely, myocarditis and pericarditis. Neurologic and hepatic involvement occasionally can be fulminant, resulting in death. Other major complications include acute upper airway obstruction due to tonsillar and adenoidal hypertrophy, and splenic rupture, which may occur spontaneously or as a result of minor trauma, repeated palpation, or the increase in abdominal pressure associated with defecation.

Other Variations in Clinical Presentation and Course
While the classic cases of mononucleosis are not uncommon, there are many variations in presentation and clinical course, some of which are age related. Older patients, for example, may present with only a day or two of symptoms of acute illness and with no prodrome, yet on examination they may have marked adenopathy, splenomegaly, and severe pharyngotonsillar symptoms. The acute phase of the illness usually lasts a week or more, but in some cases improvement may be more rapid. Wide variations exist in the severity of systemic and focal symptoms.

In young children EB virus infection can present a particularly challenging diagnostic problem. Until recently the infection had been thought to be largely subclinical. It is now believed that more likely the process has not been accurately diagnosed, its manifestations being milder, less typical, and of shorter duration in this age group. Furthermore in children under 3 to 4 years of age, the most common diagnostic test, the Monospot, rarely is positive, necessitating the use of specific EB virus serological tests for confirmation. Many young children present with signs of a severe upper respiratory tract infection with fever, prominent cough, and rhinitis. Periorbital swelling, if present, can simulate one major mode of presentation of acute bacterial sinusitis. In many cases the general picture is one of prolonged pharyngotonsillitis (usually culture negative for group A streptococci), with or without rhinitis, and cough. Tonsillar exudates are common but by no means universal. The incidence of the exanthem is somewhat higher in preadolescent patients, approaching 35 percent in some series. If hepatosplenomegaly and/or prominent anterior and posterior cervical adenopathy is found along with one of the above clinical pictures, EB virus infection should be suspected. If these latter findings are absent, the diagnosis is unlikely to be considered, although definitive diagnosis is probably not as important in such mild cases.

While younger patients are somewhat less subject to the less usual manifestations and complications of mononucleosis, they are more vulnerable to acute upper airway obstruction as a result of tonsillar and adenoidal hypertrophy. Moreover, children under 5 years of age who develop significant tonsillar and adenoidal enlargement during the course of EB virus infection are more likely to have secondary otitis media, and may, subsequent to resolution of the acute process, become subject to recurrent bouts of otitis media, tonsillitis, and sinusitis as a result of persistent tonsillar and adenoidal hypertrophy.

Diagnostic Methods

A number of laboratory studies may be helpful in suggesting or confirming the diagnosis of infectious mononucleosis. A classic finding is that of lymphocytosis of 50 percent or more, with at least 10 percent atypical lymphocytes. These atypical lymphocytes will vary in appearance in contrast to the monotonous forms seen with leukemia. There is considerable variability, however, in the degree of lymphocytosis and in its timing. Fifty percent or more of patients will have mild elevations in liver enzymes early in the course of their illness. Most commonly diagnosis is confirmed by finding heterophil antibodies toward the end of the first week or at the beginning of the second week of illness (or earlier in cases where adenopathy and splenomegaly are present from the outset). Currently slide tests, of which the Monospot is best known, are the most prevalent method in use. With improvements in sensitivity, it has now become evident that 70 to 80 percent of children between the ages of 4 and 12 produce this heterophil antibody, although they do so in lesser amounts than adolescents, who have 80 to 90 percent positivity. In children under 2 years of age, this antibody is not detectable and, in children between ages 2 and 4, it may be found in approximately 30 percent of cases. A number of specific EB virus antibody titers also are available, but since they are expensive and require acute and convalescent titers their usefulness is limited to research, and to helping to confirm or disprove cases where there are severe, prolonged and/or or unusual manifestations, and a negative heterophil response.

Differential Diagnosis of Mononucleosis

The diagnosis of EB virus infection thus rests upon the combination of clinical picture and laboratory confirmation. In view of the multiple modes of presentation and in light of the wide variability in severity of illness, clinical manifestations and clinical course, there exists a wide range of differential diagnostic possibilities. Streptococcal pharyngotonsillitis, diphtheria, and sinusitis are major diagnostic considerations in the early phases of the pharyngeal glandular form of mononucleosis. In a small percentage of cases, patients with infectious mononucleosis may simultaneously have streptococcal pharyngitis although treatment with penicillin does not yield the expected clinical improvement. While rubella may produce anterior and posterior cervical adenopathy and an exanthem similar to that of mononucleosis, its milder course and the lack of tonsillitis and visceromegaly should help to distinguish it from mononucleosis. With rubeola the prodrome and mode of spread of the exanthem, along with the early presence of Koplik's spots, help in differentiation. Brucellosis and listeriosis, though relatively rare, also must be considered as differential diagnostic possibilities.

The typhoidal form of mononucleosis can present a major diagnostic challenge when there is no production of heterophil antibody. Cytomegalovirus infection, toxoplasmosis, postperfusion syndrome, and drug-induced mononucleosis caused by phenytoin, para-aminosalicylic acid, and diaminodiphenylsulfone are major differential diagnostic considerations. In patients with severe hepatic involvement, EB virus infection can simulate other forms of infectious hepatitis as well as leptospirosis. While the history and some aspects of the clinical picture may help in distinguishing one disease entity from another, specific serologic tests often are required. Moreover in patients with neurologic, pulmonary, hematologic and cardiac manifestations, a broad differential diagnosis must be considered.

HERPES SIMPLEX INFECTIONS

The herpes simplex viruses produce infections that primarily involve the skin and mucous membranes, although in neonates, in the immunocompromised host, or in a rare normal host, infection can result in disseminated disease and central nervous system involvement. The herpes simplex type 2 virus usually is manifest as a genital pathogen (see Chapter 16), although occasionally it is the source of oral lesions and is the usual agent associated with neonatal herpes (see section below on congenital infections). The herpes simplex type 1 virus is the more common pathogen and may produce a number of clinical pictures. The organism is ubiquitous, and infections are seen year round. Patients with primary infections may shed the virus in saliva, urine and stools, as well as from skin lesions. Intimate contact, shared eating utensils and respiratory droplets are major modes of spread, and infected adults, especially parents, are the most common source. The incubation period for herpes simplex type 1 ranges from 2 to 12 days with an average of 4 to 6 days. Over 90 percent of primary infections are subclinical or asymptomatic. Most patients with symptomatic primary infection are under 5 years of age and have an illness characterized by fever, malaise, localized vesicular lesions, and regional adenopathy. As is true of other herpes viruses, the herpes simplex type 1 virus appears to enter a latent or dormant stage in many patients, which later serves as a source of recurrence. With the herpes simplex virus local ganglia are thought to be the sites of residence.

Diagnosis of symptomatic herpes simplex infections often can be made on clinical grounds alone, particularly in cases of primary infection. When the diagnosis is in question, a Giemsa-stained smear of scrapings obtained from the base of a vesicle (see Chapter 16) usually will demonstrate ballooned epithelial cells with intranuclear inclusions and multinucleated giant cells when the lesion is herpetic. Viral cultures yield results in 24 to 72 hours. Acute and convalescent titers are less useful and are of no help during recurrences.

Herpetic Gingivostomatitis

Herpetic gingivostomatitis is one of the most common forms of primary symptomatic herpes simplex infection. Patients abruptly develop high fever, irritability, anorexia and mouth pain; infants and toddlers often drool copiously. The gingivae rapidly become intensely erythematous, edematous and friable and tend to bleed easily. Small yellow ulcerations with red halos are seen routinely on the buccal and labial mucosae, on the gingivae and tongue, and often on the palate and tonsillar pillars, as well (Fig. 12.16A). Within a short time yellowish-white debris builds up on mucosal surfaces and halitosis becomes prominent. Thick-walled vesiculopustular lesions also may develop on areas of perioral skin (Fig. 12.16B). The anterior cervical and tonsillar nodes are enlarged and tender. Symptoms range in duration from 5 to 14 days, but the virus may be shed for weeks following resolution, and the severity of illness may vary from mild to marked. Young children with prolonged high fever and intense pain may become dehydrated and ketotic and should be followed closely and hydrated as needed. The

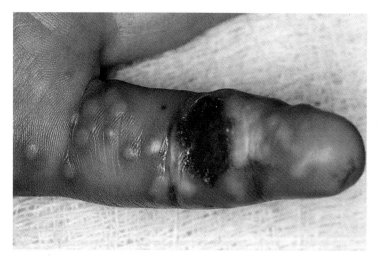

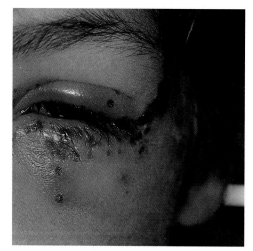

FIG. 12.18 Ocular herpes may be limited to involvement of the lids and periorbital skin but can spread to involve conjunctivae, cornea, and deeper structures with devastating results.

FIG. 12.17 Grouped thick-walled vesicles on an erythematous base which are painful and tend to coalesce, ulcerate, and then crust are the characteristic findings of an herpetic whitlow.

diffuseness of the ulcerations and mucosal inflammation, and the intense gingivitis help to distinguish this disorder from herpangina and exudative tonsillitis, as well as from other forms of gingivitis.

Primary Herpetic Skin Involvement
(Herpes Labialis and Herpetic Whitlow)

Patients with primary herpetic infections involving the skin present with fever, malaise, localized lesions, and regional adenopathy. Lesions consist of deep thick-walled painful vesicles on an erythematous base. They usually are grouped but may occur singly, and they evolve over several days becoming pustular, coalescing, ulcerating, and then crusting. Resolution occurs in 10 to 21 days. Lesions often develop as a result of direct inoculation of an area of traumatized skin, such as the site of an abrasion, burn, or small cut. While any portion of the skin may be involved, the lips (as in herpes labialis) and the fingers or thumbs (as in herpetic whitlow) are the most common sites of involvement (see Figs. 12.16B and 12.17 above). Children who suck their fingers or thumbs may develop hand lesions in concert with gingivostomatitis or herpes labialis. Adult health care workers, with no previous infection, may incur these lesions as a result of contact with infected patients. Wrestlers may develop lesions of the back, upper chest or any portion of the extremities, following a bout with an infected opponent. These lesions may simulate those of a bacterial infection, but the presence of thick-walled vesicles and the relative sparseness of bacteria on Gram stain should raise clinical suspicion of herpes, which can be confirmed by positive findings on Giemsa stain of scrapings from the base of a lesion.

Ocular Herpes

Rarely the periorbital area and eyelids are the site of primary herpetic infection or are inoculated by a child with oral disease. In such cases vesicular lesions involving the lids may be seen in isolation or in connection with conjunctival erythema and edema, and a purulent discharge (Fig. 12.18). Preauricular adenopathy is usual. Corneal clouding may be noted early on, and is associated with dendritic ulcerations visible on slit-lamp examination (see Chapter 17). While adenovirus and Newcastle virus also can produce severe

conjunctivitis with preauricular adenopathy, the presence of vesicular lid lesions usually seen in herpetic infection can help in making the differential diagnosis. Because of the risk of keratitis and iridocyclitis with permanent visual impairment, urgent ophthalmologic consultation is indicated whenever there is any suspicion of herpetic infection.

Eczema Herpeticum
(Kaposi's Varicelliform Eruption)

Patients with atopic eczema and other forms of chronic dermatitis are at risk for a particularly severe form of primary herpes simplex infection that is heralded by the abrupt onset of high fever, irritability, and discomfort. Lesions appear in crops and primarily involve areas of previously affected skin. Typically they evolve to form pustules, and then rupture and form crusts over the course of a few days. Not infrequently these lesions become hemorrhagic (Fig. 12.19). Multiple crops can appear over 7 to 10 days simulating varicella. However, the slower evolution of lesions, the tendency of such lesions to hemorrhage, their primary localization to eczematous areas, and the persistence of fever and systemic symptoms for as long as 1 week help to distinguish this disorder from varicella. Severity ranges from mild to fulminant, and is dependent in part on the extensiveness of the preceding dermatitis. When the area of involvement is large, fluid losses can be severe. There also is a significant risk of secondary bacterial infection. As many as 40 percent of cases are fatal.

Recurrent Herpes Simplex

As mentioned earlier, following primary infection the herpes simplex virus tends to incorporate itself into the genome of the ganglia that lie in the region of initial involvement such that reactivation of the latent virus results in localized recurrences at or near the site of previous infection. Fever, sunlight, local trauma, menses, and emotional stress are recognized triggers and, since the mouth is the major site of primary infection, labial and perioral lesions (cold sores) are seen most commonly. Many patients report a prodrome of localized burning along with stinging or itching, prior to the development of an area of edema, erythema, and tenderness over which grouped vesicles erupt. These vesicles contain

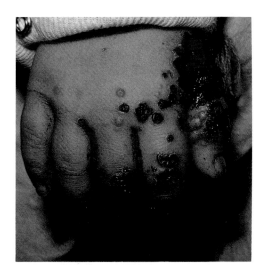

FIG. 12.19 Eczema herpeticum (Kaposi's varicelliform eruption). Primary herpes simplex infection in a child with underlying eczema produced crops of hemorrhagic vesiculopustular lesions limited to areas of preexisting dermatitis which then ruptured and crusted. (Courtesy of Dr. M. Sherlock)

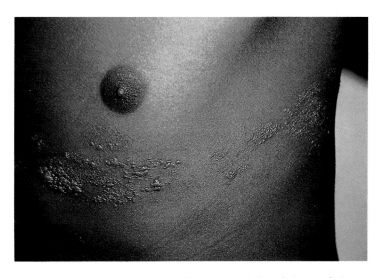

FIG. 12.20 Herpes zoster. The dermatomal distribution of these grouped vesicles is a hallmark of herpes zoster. The vesicles are rather thin-walled and coalescent, and they lie on an erythematous base. (Courtesy of Dr. M. Sherlock)

yellow serous fluid, and they often appear smaller and less thick-walled than primary lesions. After 2 to 3 days, the vesicular fluid becomes cloudy, and then crusts form. Although fever and systemic symptoms are absent, regional nodes may be enlarged and tender. The localization of the lesions to a small area helps to distinguish them from those of herpes zoster. Prodromal symptoms and discomfort help to distinguish recurrent herpes simplex from impetigo and from contact dermatitis.

HERPES ZOSTER (SHINGLES)

The varicella-zoster virus, like other herpesviruses, appears to take up permanent albeit generally quiescent residence in its host following initial infection, i.e., varicella. Generally the virus lies dormant in the genome of posterior nerve root cells, but it can reactivate though the pathogenesis of reactivation often is unclear. Mechanical and thermal trauma, infection, and debilitation all have been postulated as triggers. In the reactivated form, herpes zoster, lesions consist of grouped thin-walled vesicles on an erythematous base, which are distributed along the course of a spinal or sensory nerve root (Fig. 12.20). They evolve from macule, to papule, to vesicle, and then to a crusted stage over a few days. Hyperesthesia or nerve root pain may precede, accompany or follow the eruption, and has no correlation with severity of the rash. Pain, if present at all in pediatric patients, rarely is severe and generally is short lived, unless a cranial nerve dermatome is involved. Fever and constitutional symptoms may or may not be part of the picture, but regional adenopathy is common.

Thoracic dermatomes are involved in the majority of cases, and are followed in frequency by cervical, trigeminal, lumbar, and facial nerve regions. Cranial nerve involvement may produce a puzzling prodrome consisting of severe headache, facial pain or auricular pain with no evident cause, lasting up to several days prior to appearance of the eruption. Lesions appear unilaterally on the tonsillar pillars and uvula with involvement of the maxillary branch of the trigeminal nerve, on the buccal mucosa and palate with involvement of the mandibular division, and on the face, cornea, and tip of the nose with involvement of the ophthalmic branch (see Chapter 18). When the geniculate

ganglion is affected, vesicles are seen in the external auditory canal in concert with facial paralysis. Although varicella can be transmitted by patients with herpes zoster, contagion generally is less of a problem since most have lesions on areas that are covered by clothing and most do not have involvement of the oropharynx.

Bacterial Exanthems

STREPTOCOCCAL SCARLET FEVER

While most commonly associated with pharyngitis and impetigo, the group A β-hemolytic streptococci are frequently the cause of an illness that is characterized in part by a generalized exanthem commonly known as scarlet fever, or scarlatina. The exanthem is produced by an erythrogenic toxin excreted by the streptococcus. Streptococcal infections occur year round, although pharyngitis and scarlet fever have a peak incidence in winter and spring. Transmission requires close contact to enable the direct spread of large droplets, and those with nasal infection are particularly effective sources. Anal carriers as well as contaminated food sources also have been responsible for outbreaks. The incubation period for scarlet fever ranges from 12 hours to approximately 7 days. Patients are contagious during the period of the acute illness, and may transmit the organism during active subclinical infection, as well. An average of 50 percent of family members living with an index case will become secondarily infected, and up to half of these individuals will have subclinical disease.

Once a severe illness with high morbidity and mortality, scarlet fever has modified over the past several decades to become much milder. In the classic case, which is seen less than 10 percent of the time, the patient experiences an abrupt onset of fever, chills, malaise, headache, sore throat, and vomiting; abdominal pain may be a prominent complaint. Within 12 to 48 hours the exanthem appears and rapidly generalizes, usually beginning on the trunk and spreading peripherally, but sometimes spreading cephalocaudally. The face is flushed and smooth with perioral pallor. The remaining skin becomes diffusely erythematous and is covered by tiny pinhead-sized papules, giving the appearance of a sunburn with goose bumps. The texture is sandpapery on

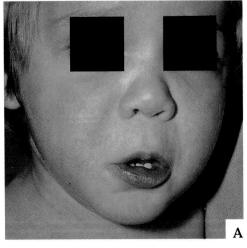

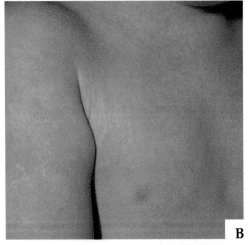

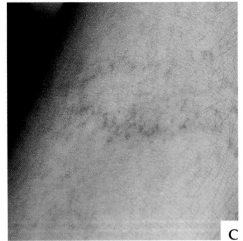

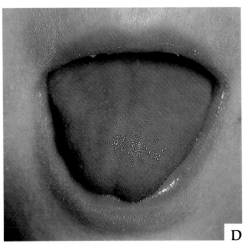

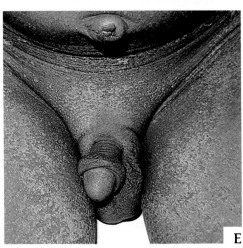

FIG. 12.21 *Streptococcal scarlet fever.* **A** *and* **B**, *In the classic case of this disease the exanthem is characterized by a flushed face, perioral pallor and a diffuse blanching erythematous rash that has a sandpapery consistency on palpation.* **C**, *Within 1 to 3 days of onset, Pastia's lines may be noted.* **D**, *The characteristic red strawberry tongue with glistening surface and prominent papillae is seen a few days after onset.* **E**, *Desquamation occurs in thin flakes as the acute phase of the illness resolves, and is proportional to the intensity of the exanthem.* (**A**, **B**, *and* **E** *courtesy of Dr. M. Sherlock*)

palpation and the erythema blanches with pressure (Fig. 12.21A and B). The skin may be pruritic, but it is not tender. Many patients also will have urticaria and dermatographism. In severe cases vesiculation may occur. Following generalization the rash becomes accentuated in skin folds or creases, and 1 to 3 days after its appearance petechiae may appear in a linear distribution along the creases, forming "Pastia's lines" (Fig. 12.21C). Examination of the oropharynx in the "textbook" case discloses large very erythematous and edematous tonsils which often are covered by exudate, along with palatal erythema and petechiae (see Chapter 20). The uvula may be erythematous and edematous as well. The tongue also shows characteristic findings. During the first two days it has a white coating through which erythematous and edematous papillae project, resulting in a "white strawberry tongue." Subsequently the white coat peels leaving a glistening red surface with prominent papillae, which is referred to as a "red strawberry tongue" (Fig. 12.21D). Tender cervical adenopathy is seen in 30 to 60 percent of cases. Without benefit of treatment the rash, fever, and pharyngitis resolve within 1 week; with treatment improvement is relatively rapid. Desquamation occurs regardless of treatment and begins several days after onset, occurring in a cephalocaudal distribution (Fig. 12.21E). The skin is shed in fine thin flakes (in contrast to the thick flakes that characterize desquamation following staphylococcal exanthems), and the extent of this process is directly proportional to intensity of the exanthem.

Diagnosis is easy in the classic case, but in other cases wide spectrum in severity of disease and in its manifestations can result in confusion. Fever may be absent or low grade, and

malaise may be minimal. Pharyngitis may be mild (without exudate, petechiae, or marked erythema) or absent, even when the throat is the site of infection. In such cases tongue findings may be absent as well. When streptococcal skin or wound infections are the primary site of infection the oropharynx is normal. The appearance of the exanthem may vary as well. In some children it is patchy but continues to be most prominent near skin folds (Fig. 12.22). An occasional child may have diffuse petechiae. Still others may present with fever and/or nasopharyngitis and urticaria as their initial manifestations. In dark-skinned children erythema and perioral pallor may be difficult to appreciate and the papules may be larger thus producing a texture less like sandpaper.

Recognition followed by treatment with a 10-day course of penicillin or erythromycin is important not only to shorten the course of the illness but also to prevent rheumatic fever and pyogenic complications, the most common of which include adenitis, otitis, sinusitis, and peritonsillar and retropharyngeal abscesses. Poststreptococcal nephritis, however, is not prevented by antimicrobial therapy. Therefore in patients with fever or nasopharyngitis and urticaria and in children with scarlatiniform eruptions, a screening throat culture for group A streptococci should be obtained regardless of presence or absence of other symptoms.

STAPHYLOCOCCAL EXANTHEMS
Coagulase-positive staphylococci are ubiquitous organisms that are carried at any given time by approximately one-third of the population. While the hallmark of staphylococcal infection is the abscess, numerous forms of infection

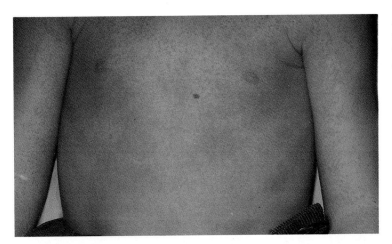

FIG. 12.22 There is a wide spectrum in severity and manifestations. In this child with streptococcal scarlet fever, the rash has a patchy distribution with accentuation in the axillae and other skin creases.

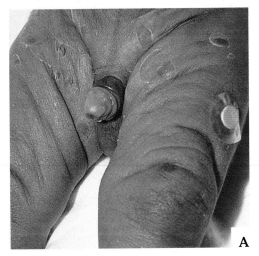

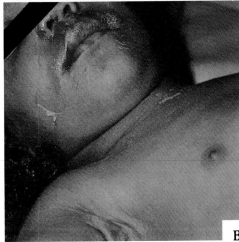

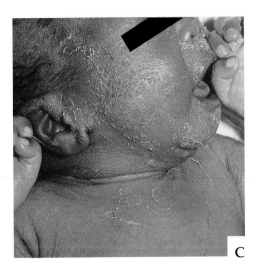

FIG. 12.23 Staphylococcal scalded skin syndrome. **A,** This infant shows evidence of epidermal separation and has numerous ruptured bullae over the inguinal region and thighs. **B,** In this older child, symptoms were mild and only the skin of the face, axillae, and perineum showed signs of epidermal separation. Note the evidence of a positive Nikolsky's sign on her upper lip and cheek, which resulted when she wiped her nose. **C,** A denuded area is evident on the upper chest and thick flakes have begun to form on the face. Culture of the purulent nasal discharge was positive for Staphylococcus aureus. *(Courtesy of Dr. M. Sherlock)*

are seen, and three distinct generalized exanthematous disorders have now been identified: staphylococcal scalded skin syndrome; staphylococcal scarlet fever; and toxic shock syndrome. In each case the organisms at the primary site of infection release exotoxins, which then produce the characteristic rash. Transmission may occur via direct contact with persons who are infected or who are carriers. Sites of carriage include the nose, skin, axilla, perineum, hair, and nails. Spread of infection also may occur via airborne particles or through contact with contaminated objects or food. Draining skin lesions, nasal discharge, and contaminated hands constitute particularly important sources of transmission. Traumatic or surgical wounds, burns, insect bites, areas of preexisting dermatitis, viral skin lesions, and prior viral respiratory tract infection all serve as major predisposing conditions.

Staphylococcal Scalded Skin Syndrome
A disorder seen most commonly in infants and young children, staphylococcal scalded skin syndrome is caused by phage group II coagulase-positive staphylococci. The primary infection usually is mild, with purulent nasopharyngitis, conjunctivitis, impetigo, and infections of the umbilicus and circumcision sites seen most commonly. Sepsis, pneumonia, or other severe invasive staphylococcal infections may precede onset of the exanthem though rarely.

The infecting organisms produce an epidermolytic exotoxin, which is spread hematogenously and which causes cleavage of the skin between the epidermis and the dermis. This process may begin within hours or days of the appearance of signs of the primary infection, and typically its onset is heralded by prodromal symptoms of fever and irritability, often accompanied by vomiting. These symptoms are followed by the abrupt development of a diffuse erythroderma that spreads rapidly from head to toe and simulates the appearance of a sunburn. In contrast to streptococcal scarlet fever, the involved skin is tender, even to light touch. Within 1 to 3 days thin-walled flaccid bullous lesions appear, which rupture soon after formation (Fig. 12.23A). Simultaneously larger portions of the epidermis begin to separate in sheets, and during this phase the placement of light lateral traction on the skin will cause the epidermis to pull away from the dermis leaving a raw weeping surface called Nikolsky's sign (Fig. 12.23B). Following exfoliation the surface gradually dries forming large thick flakes (Fig. 12.23C).

There is a broad spectrum of severity for this syndrome. In severe cases the patient appears toxic and miserable and sheds large portions of skin, resulting in significant fluid losses that may be accompanied by difficulties with temperature regulation. In mild cases (see Fig. 12.23B above)

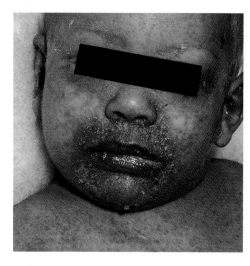

FIG. 12.24 Staphylococcal scarlet fever. Purulent conjunctivitis served as the primary source of infection in this child who presented with fever and a tender sandpapery scarlatiniform rash. This photo taken 2 days after onset shows the perioral cracking and thick flaking, which help distinguish this process from that due to streptococci.

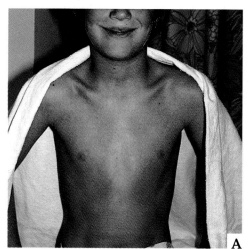

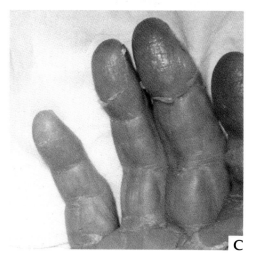

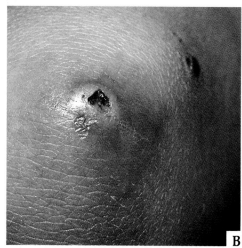

FIG. 12.25 Toxic shock syndrome. A, This young boy presented with diffuse erythema, fever, chills, myalgias, head- ache, vomiting, and orthostatic dizziness with mild widening of his pulse pressure. B, Examination disclosed an infected knee abrasion, which grew S. aureus. Though his illness was relatively mild, the association of gastrointestinal symptoms and orthostatic changes suggested TSS, which was confirmed by laboratory studies and by (C) subsequent desquamation. This begins periungually and the skin is shed on thick casts. (C, courtesy of Dr. G. Pazin)

toxicity may be absent and only localized areas of skin are denuded, with the face and perineum constituting the primary sites of shedding. The causative organism can be isolated from the site of primary infection, but it is absent at least initially from the bullae and from sites of skin separation.

Staphylococcal Scarlet Fever

Staphylococcal infection can result in an exanthem that initially is indistinguishable in appearance from that produced by Group A β-hemolytic streptococci. The illness is characterized by fever, irritability and moderate malaise, followed by the abrupt onset of a generalized erythematous rash often of sandpapery consistency with accentuation in the skin creases. In contrast to the exanthem seen in strep- tococcal scarlet fever, the involved skin usually is tender, the tongue is normal, and there is no palatal enanthem. Evo- lution of lesions also differs, as within 2 to 5 days the skin be- gins to crack and fissure, especially in the perioral and peri- orbital areas and in the skin creases (Fig. 12.24). It is then shed gradually in large thick flakes over 3 to 5 days. Local skin and wound infections are common antecedents and their presence often enables presumptive identification of staphylococci as causative agents early in the course of the disease. However, when nasopharyngitis is the source of pri- mary infection, the picture can be very difficult to distinguish from that of mild variants of the streptococcal infection, in which the strawberry tongue and palatal

petechiae often are absent. The same may be true when a local infection with lymphangitis is the source. In such cases the tendency for the staphylococcal rash to be tender may be the major clinical distinction, pending Gram stain and/or culture results. Unless the primary infection is severe enough to warrant parenteral treatment, oral antimicrobial therapy is sufficient.

Toxic Shock Syndrome

Toxic Shock Syndrome (TSS) is the third syndrome of staph- ylococcal origin to be characterized by a generalized exanthem. It is seen in children and adults who have localized infections caused by coagulase-positive staphylo- cocci of phage groups I or III, and in menstruating women and girls whose vagina and cervix are colonized with these organisms. In the latter subgroup of patients, there is a strong correlation with tampon use, suggesting that the impedence of normal menstrual flow and/or the presence of secondary abrasions may contribute to development of this syndrome. The fact that that cervical canal is open during menses also may be important, in allowing ascent of the organisms and in facilitating the more direct release of exo- toxin into the blood stream via contact with the denuded uterine lining. While infected menstruating patients may have a history of vaginal discharge (often purulent) or show signs of inflammatory vulvovaginitis, many do not. Patients in whom the site of primary infection is not gynecologic often on examination will be found to have an obvious primary focus of infection in the form of a skin lesion, an abscess, or purulent conjunctivitis (see Fig. 12.25B).

The clinical picture of TSS is characterized by a prodrome ranging from 1 to 7 days in duration and consisting of low-grade fever, malaise, myalgias, and vomiting. This is followed by an abrupt increase in fever, with chills and worsening myalgias, in association with nausea, vomiting, abdominal pain, headache, orthostatic dizziness, and weakness. Soon thereafter the patient's skin becomes diffusely erythematous, mimicking a sunburn and having an appearance very similar to that of staphylococcal scarlet fever (Figs. 12.25A and B). Conjunctivitis with photophobia as well as pain and erythema of the oropharyngeal mucosa commonly are associated. Many patients also have a strawberry tongue. Diarrhea, hypotension and oliguria often are prominent on the second day, sometimes followed by alterations in consciousness, and confusion. In severe cases findings of the adult respiratory distress syndrome may develop. Many patients have muscle tenderness and weakness as well as diffuse abdominal tenderness without peritoneal signs. A small proportion develop nonpitting edema of the face, hands, and feet. Over the ensuing few days, petechiae may appear on the skin, oral ulcers may be noted, and a secondary maculopapular rash may develop in some patients. Desquamation is routine and usually begins 1 week after onset. It is most prominent over the palms and soles and at the tips of the fingers and toes, where the skin is shed in casts (Fig. 12.25C).

Laboratory findings indicate multisystem involvement. Common hematologic findings include a leukocytosis with a left shift and relative lymphopenia, mild decreases in hematocrit, and decreased platelet counts. Hypoproteinemia, hypocalcemia, decreased creatinine clearance, elevated blood urea nitrogen, pyuria, proteinuria, impaired urinary concentrating ability, and sodium wasting also are frequent findings. Mild increases in serum bilirubin and hepatic enzymes reflect hepatic dysfunction, as does prolongation of the prothrombin time. Myoglobinuria may be encountered in a small proportion of patients. While sinus tachycardia is routine, arrhythmias are unusual. The clinical and laboratory findings suggest a process in which there is diffuse vascular leak with third-spacing of fluids, electrolytes, and protein. Secondary hypotension and hypoperfusion result in oliguria and azotemia, while the hepatic changes may be toxin related.

As recognition of TSS has increased, the existence of a wide spectrum of severity has become apparent. Mild cases closely mimic the picture of staphylococcal scarlet fever, and fever, chills, myalgias, headache, dizziness, and rash are routine. Headache usually is severe, and occasionally is accompanied by meningismus. Vomiting may be mild or pernicious, and diarrhea may vary widely from patient to patient, in frequency, duration, and character of stools although stools uniformly are found to contain increased numbers of leukocytes. Patients in whom gastrointestinal symptoms are mild tend to have much less evidence of fluid shifts and hypotension, and often escape problems of cardiovascular and renal dysfunction. Those with severe disease tend to require massive volume expansion and vasopressor therapy, and also are at risk for severe cardiovascular and renal compromise, with a significant potential for fatal outcome.

Antimicrobial therapy is important to eradicate the source of primary infection and thereby reduce the risk of recurrence. Prior to the recognition of coagulase-positive staphylococci as the causative agent of TSS, patients recovering from this illness were subject to multiple recurrences. This finding was particularly true for postmenarcheal females who often had repeated recurrences with menstrual periods. Treatment appears to reduce this risk markedly.

MENINGOCOCCAL EXANTHEMS

Neisseria meningitidis is capable of producing a number of clinical illnesses, two of which—acute meningococcemia, and meningococcosis or chronic meningococcemia—are characterized in part by a generalized exanthem. The organism is carried in the upper respiratory tract of humans who, though usually asymptomatic, nevertheless may transmit the organism via droplet spread of respiratory secretions. The majority of persons so exposed become carriers and produce antibodies but do not develop clinical disease. Clinical illness is most common in children under 5 years of age, with a peak incidence between 6 and 12 months of age. A secondary peak of lesser magnitude is seen in adolescence. Susceptibility to disease appears to be related to a lack of bactericidal antibody or to a failure to produce antibody in response to infection. It is still unclear as to whether or not antecedent viral respiratory infection is a predisposing factor. While meningococcal infection occurs year round, the peak season for these illnesses is late winter and early spring. Invasive disease occurs both endemically and epidemically. Persons who have intimate contact with infected patients, e.g., other members of the same household or persons in "closed communities" such as military barracks, dormitories or daycare centers, are at highest risk of becoming secondarily infected. The incubation period following exposure ranges from 1 to 10 days, with most clinical cases developing in less than 4 days. Secondary attack rates range from 0.3 to 10 percent and are highest during epidemic outbreaks. Any mucosal surface is subject to infection, which may remain localized or may serve as the source of more invasive disease.

Acute Meningococcemia

The two major invasive forms of meningococcal disease are meningitis and septicemia, which may occur singly or in combination. Patients usually experience a prodromal period ranging in length from a few hours to 5 days. During this phase symptoms of upper respiratory tract infection or nasopharyngitis are typical in association with fever. Patients also may have lethargy, headache, myalgias, arthralgias, and vomiting. Following this an abrupt change occurs, characterized by increased fever with chills (or occasionally hypothermia), worsening malaise, and lethargy. In the 90 percent for whom meningitis is the primary manifestation, vomiting, irritability (often with a high-pitched cry in infants), and meningismus are prominent. Delirium, combativeness, stupor, and seizures also may develop. While some of these patients also have meningococcemia, they are less likely to develop cutaneous manifestations. Endotoxic shock and disseminated intravascular coagulation (DIC) also are unusual, and mortality is relatively low.

In contrast approximately 10 percent of patients develop a picture of overwhelming sepsis with little or no evidence of meningitis. In these patients the abrupt change in clinical picture described above typically is associated with the development of a rash in association with manifestations of shock, including mottling, distal coolness with decreased capillary refill or cyanosis, and either widened pulse pressure or frank hypotension. Up to 85 percent of these patients will

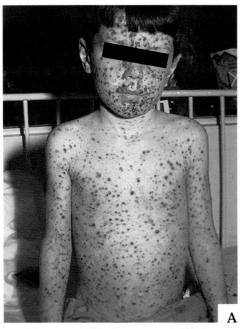

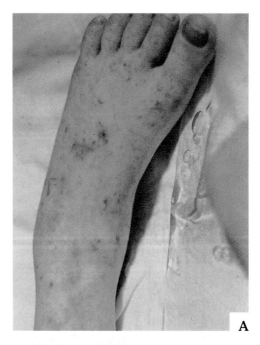

FIG. 12.26 Meningococcemia. **A**, This youngster manifests the generalized purpuric and petechial rash characteristic of acute meningococcemia. **B**, Petechiae are more apparent in this close-up of an infant. Gram stain of petechial scrapings may reveal organisms. **C**, Purpura may progress to form areas of frank cutaneous necrosis, especially in cases with DIC. (**B**, courtesy of Dr. M. Sherlock)

FIG. 12.27 Rocky Mountain spotted fever. **A**, The exanthem characteristic of this disease first appears distally on wrists, ankles, palms, and soles. It may be petechial from the outset or it may start as an erythematous, blanching macular or maculopapular eruption, which then becomes petechial as it spreads centripetally. **B**, In this child the rash has generalized. Both petechial and blanching erythematous lesions are present. (**A**, courtesy of Dr. E. Wald, **B**, courtesy of Dr. T. F. Sellers, Jr.)

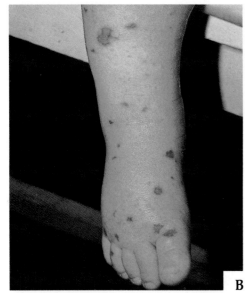

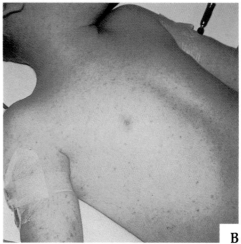

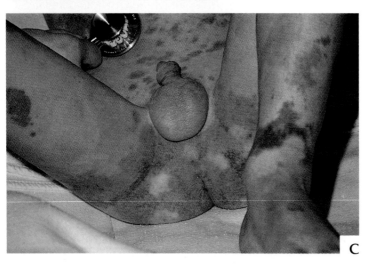

have cutaneous lesions involving the trunk and extremities. Such lesions may consist of tender pink macules; of petechiae, which often are palpably raised; and of purpura, which when present is most prominent on the extremities and may progress to form areas of frank necrosis (Fig. 12.26). The combination of purpura and shock is termed the "Waterhouse-Friderichsen" syndrome and has been associated in

some but not all instances with adrenal hemorrhage and secondary adrenal insufficiency. Evolution may be fulminant, resulting in prostration within a few hours, or it may be slower, occurring over a period lasting up to 24 hours. Patients with a short prodrome, fulminant progression and early appearance of purpuric lesions have a particularly poor prognosis. Over 60 percent of these have clinical evidence of hypotension and DIC on presentation, and approximately 50 percent have no leukocytosis, suggesting that their immune system has been overwhelmed. Only about 20 percent of these patients have meningitis. Mortality in these cases approaches 40 percent while only 3 percent of those with slower progression succumb. Most deaths occur within 24 hours of presentation and are the result of a combination of circulatory collapse and congestive heart failure due to endotoxic shock and myocarditis.

In many cases diagnosis can be suspected clinically and is confirmed by laboratory findings. Gram-stained smears of petechial lesions and of buffy coat preparations often will reveal gram-negative diplococci (see Chapter 11). Cultures of blood, CSF, and petechial lesions should be performed unless the severity of illness precludes lumbar puncture. Counterimmunoelectrophoresis of urine, CSF, or blood may provide rapid confirmation. Because of the potential for deterioration, aggressive empiric antimicrobial therapy and vigorous supportive measures should be instituted promptly whenever meningococcemia is suspected.

There are a number of differential diagnostic possibilities, which include other forms of bacterial sepsis, bacterial endocarditis, Rocky Mountain spotted fever, and various other disorders characterized by thrombocytopenia. Some forms of gram-negative septicemia initially may be clinically indistinguishable from meningococcal septicemia. Similarly *Haemophilus influenzae* type B septicemia as well as pneumococcal septicemia may be associated with the development of petechiae, though in these cases they are not palpable. The purpuric lesions of staphylococcal sepsis tend to become pustular early on, and the site of primary infection also helps distinguish this organism. Adenoviral and streptococcal infections may produce petechial rashes but usually they do not cause a septic picture. Other clinical characteristics help to distinguish patients with thrombocytopenia due to immune thrombocytopenic purpura, acute leukemia and mononucleosis, while the centripetal mode of spread of the petechial rash of Rocky Mountain spotted fever, and the initial distribution and subsequent mode of spread of Henoch-Schönlein purpura, help to distinguish these illnesses. Differentiation can be particularly difficult in the case of a child presenting with high fever with no source other than that of an upper respiratory tract infection, and a petechial rash. These findings may represent early nonfulminant meningococcemia, but they also can be the picture of viral illness or of another bacterial process; in such a case observation and/or presumptive therapy may be necessary.

Meningococcosis (Chronic Meningococcemia)

Meningococcosis, a disorder more indolent than acute meningococcemia, is defined as meningococcal sepsis with a fever of greater than 1 week's duration, without meningitis. The average length of symptoms prior to diagnosis is 6 to 8 weeks. In most cases symptoms are intermittent and in all cases they consist of fever and chills (without rigor), with an exanthem seen in nearly 95 percent of cases. The rash waxes and wanes, often in association with the fever. Lesions may consist of tender erythematous subcutaneous nodules, of erythematous macules and papules, or of petechiae, occurring singly or in combination. Urticarial lesions are seen occasionally. The feet, legs, upper arms, and trunk are the sites most commonly involved. Mild malaise and myalgias tend to accompany the fever, and headache and arthralgias also are common. In childhood cases swelling of hands, feet, knees and ankles may occur intermittently, without evidence of warmth or erythema; however when the legs are involved, the child may refuse to walk.

Diagnosis of meningococcosis can be difficult, since early blood cultures often are negative (although children are more likely than adults to have positive cultures) and skin lesions generally are negative for organisms, both on smear and culture. Throat culture usually is negative as well. Leukocytosis is seen with the fever. Sedimentation rate may be normal or elevated. Thrombocytopenia is seen occasionally. Close follow-up and monitoring of the clinical course, combined with repeated blood cultures, is the best way to confirm the diagnosis. Of the patients not diagnosed and treated, approximately one-third ultimately will develop severe localized infection (after an average of 10 weeks of illness) with meningitis, carditis, nephritis, and ocular infection occurring most commonly.

Miscellaneous Exanthems

ROCKY MOUNTAIN SPOTTED FEVER

Rocky Mountain spotted fever is an acute potentially severe exanthematous disease caused by the organism *Rickettsia rickettsii.* (A similar disorder occurs in South America and is termed "São Paulo disease.") These obligate intracellular parasites usually are transmitted to man via the bite of an infected tick, which injects organisms while it feeds on the host. Occasionally however inhalation of fomites is the route of acquisition. Once injected the organisms then multiply in the endothelium of small blood vessels, and are spread hematogenously resulting in a widespread vasculitis characterized by focal inflammation and thrombosis with secondary vascular leakage. Because ticks are active during warm months, the peak seasons for this disorder are spring and summer. The incubation period ranges from 2 to 14 days with an average of 4 to 8 days. Two-thirds of cases occur in children under 15 years of age. Yearly outbreaks tend to occur in very circumscribed geographic areas. Mortality is as high as 5 to 7 percent and often is due to a failure to diagnose and treat the condition in its early phase.

Onset may be acute or gradual and is characterized by nonspecific symptoms of which fever and headache are the most prominent. The fever may be constant or fluctuating while the headache, which may be frontal or generalized, typically is severe, unremitting, and unresponsive to analgesia. Headache may not be a major complaint in very young children, however. Other less constant symptoms include chills, anorexia, nausea and vomiting, sore throat, abdominal pain, diarrhea, arthralgias, and myalgias. Respiratory symptoms are uncommon. The spleen is enlarged in 30 to 50 percent of cases, but adenopathy is not prominent. The exanthem usually is noted on or about the third day of illness, but it may appear as late as the beginning of the second week.

In the majority of patients, the characteristic appearance and mode of spread of the exanthem is the most helpful clue to clinical diagnosis. The rash begins on wrists, ankles, palms and soles, usually appearing as an erythematous blanching fine macular or maculopapular eruption. It then spreads centripetally and becomes petechial (Fig. 12.27) although occasionally lesions are petechial from the outset. In some cases the eruption is not prominent and may even be transient, making diagnosis difficult. Lesions also can be difficult to appreciate in patients with dark skin. Conjunctival injection, with photophobia and petechial hemorrhages, often develops simultaneously with the rash. Firm nonpitting nondependent edema, beginning in the periorbital region and then generalizing, tends to develop a few days after the onset of symptoms. In some cases myalgias are severe and are accompanied by muscle tenderness particularly of the thighs and calves. In severe cases CNS symptoms develop with disease progression and range in severity from restlessness, irritability and anxiety to confusion, delirium, and coma. Meningismus may be noted on examination, with or without CSF abnormalities, e.g., lymphocytosis with mildly elevated protein levels and normal glucose. Seizures and signs of focal involvement, including cortical blindness and deafness, ataxia and spasticity, may supervene. Retinal hemorrhages, papilledema, and sixth nerve palsies ultimately may develop along with pathologic reflexes. Other features of advanced disease include ST-T segment changes on electrocardiography that are reflective of myocarditis; DIC with

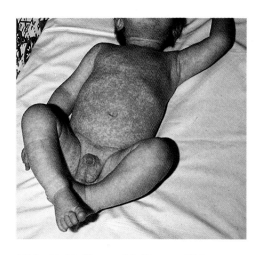

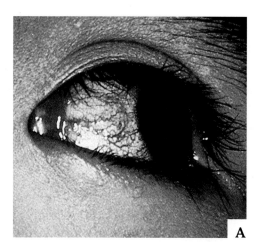

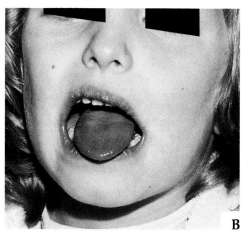

FIG. 12.28 Kawasaki disease. This toddler with Kawasaki disease has a generalized bright red morbilliform maculopapular exanthem, which is one of the more common forms of rash seen with this disorder. (Courtesy of Dr. W. Neches)

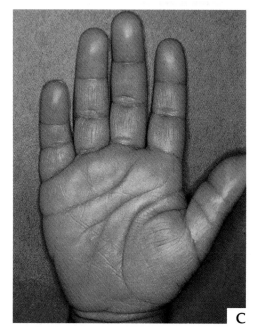

FIG. 12.29 Kawasaki disease. **A**, Non-purulent conjunctivitis, characterized by dilatation of the bulbar conjunctival vessels, and (**B**) labial erythema and a strawberry tongue also are common manifestations seen within a few days of onset of fever. **C**, Palmar erythema and indurated edema often are noted soon after the appearance of the rash; both were mild in this child. (Courtesy of Dr. W. Neches)

prolonged bleeding and the appearance of extensive areas of cutaneous hemorrhage and necrosis; renal failure; and cardiovascular collapse.

White blood cell counts are normal or low in the first few days, and then tend to rise. Thrombocytopenia is common. Other laboratory abnormalities include hyponatremia due to fluid shifts and renal losses; hypoproteinemia due to vascular and renal losses and hepatic dysfunction; elevated liver function tests; and hyperkalemia with increasing cell death.

Because there is no diagnostic test capable of providing prompt definitive results and because the early institution of antimicrobial treatment is crucial to a favorable outcome, the diagnosis of Rocky Mountain spotted fever must be made on clinical grounds and as early as possible. The diagnosis should be suspected in any child with fever, headache, toxicity and a centripetally spreading petechial rash, especially when the patient's history suggests or confirms an exposure to ticks. The *R. rickettsii* organisms are sensitive to both chloramphenicol and to tetracyclines, and recovery is usual if therapy is begun during the first week of illness. Sulfonamides are contraindicated. If treatment is delayed beyond the first week however, the outcome may be unfavorable despite antimicrobial therapy and vigorous supportive measures. Subsequent serologic confirmation may be made using the Weil-Felix test or complement fixation tests. Immunofluorescent examination of skin biopsy specimens obtained 4 to 8 days from onset can provide earlier confirmation but often this test is not readily available.

Rocky Mountain spotted fever usually can be distinguished from meningococcemia by virtue of the latter disorder's more rapid evolution, by the palpability of its petechiae, and by its positive Gram stain and culture results. The respiratory prodrome, the presence of Koplik's spots, and the different mode of exanthematous spread enable its distinction from rubeola, as does the milder symptomatology and shorter course of most enteroviral infections. The tick typhus fevers—variably named tick typhus, tick bite fever, and "fièvre boutonneuse"—produce milder disease and usually can be distinguished by the presence of a characteristic indurated skin lesion with a necrotic center at the site of the tick bite in association with regional adenopathy.

KAWASAKI DISEASE

Although the exact etiology of Kawasaki disease remains unknown, an as yet unidentified infectious agent is strongly suspected. While recognized worldwide Kawasaki disease is most prevalent among children of Japanese descent, suggesting an element of genetic susceptibility. Immunologic factors also are thought to play a role in its pathogenesis, particularly with respect to its vasculitic features. While the extensive work of Japanese and American investigators has clarified diagnostic criteria and has led to increased recognition of this disorder, previously termed infantile polyarteritis, there does appear to be an actual increase in its incidence. Cases have occurred individually and in epidemic clusters, with little seasonal prevalence except for slight

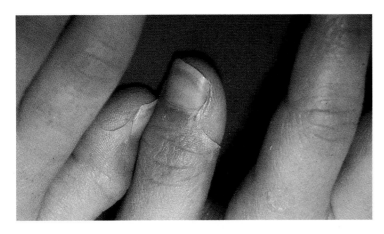

FIG. 12.30 Kawasaki disease. Early in the subacute phase desquamation occurs. This child shows early changes involving the tips and periungual portions of the fingers, a finding similar to that seen in TSS. (Courtesy of Dr. W. Neches)

increases in late spring and late fall. Neither person to person spread nor common source exposure has been confirmed, however. Eighty percent of cases occur in children under 4 years of age, with 50 percent occurring in children under age 2. It is found rarely in children over 8 years of age.

The clinical course of the disease is divided into three phases—an acute phase lasting approximately 10 days, a subacute phase lasting 2 to 3 weeks, and a convalescent phase lasting from a few weeks to several months. Diagnosis is based on the presence of five out of six major clinical criteria during the acute phase. These criteria include:

Fever of 5 or more days duration
Conjunctivitis
Oral inflammation
Extremity involvement
Rash
Adenopathy

Exclusion of other disorders is required as well.

The acute phase begins with the abrupt onset of high spiking fevers with multiple daily spikes. In the first week maximum daily temperatures range from 39° to 40° C. Thereafter peaks of 38° to 39° C occur for up to 2 weeks or longer. During this period the child is miserable, restless, and emotionally labile. An exanthem appears with the fever or soon thereafter. In all cases it is deep red and generalized in distribution, although it may be accentuated over the perineum and in intertriginous areas. It may take the form of a morbilliform maculopapular eruption, it may be pruritic and urticarial in appearance, or less commonly it may resemble the exanthems of erythema multiforme or of scarlet fever (Fig. 12.28). Facial swelling and pallor are common associated findings.

Within several days of onset of the fever and rash, a number of other manifestations may develop. These include:

1. A nonpurulent non-ulcerative conjunctivitis characterized by dilatation of bulbar conjunctival vessels (Fig. 12.29A)
2. Oral involvement characterized by erythema of the lips, which crack and bleed and become painful, diffuse nonpainful erythema of the oropharyngeal mucosa, and a strawberry tongue (Fig. 12.29B)
3. Intense erythema of the palms and soles associated with a variable degree of swelling that has a firm indurated quality and which may be accompanied by fusiform swelling of the fingers (Fig. 12.29C)

4. Cervical adenopathy seen in 50 to 70 percent of patients and usually consisting of unilateral firm nodal enlargement with overlying erythema.

Additional manifestations may include urethritis with pyuria (75 percent), arthralgias and arthritis (35 to 40 percent), diarrhea and abdominal pain (25 percent), aseptic meningitis (25 percent), hepatitis (10 percent), cholestatic jaundice and hydrops of the gallbladder (5 percent). During the acute phase polymorphonuclear leukocytosis is usual, and the sedimentation rate and C-reactive protein levels rise markedly.

The subacute phase begins about 10 days after onset as the fever and rash begin to moderate or subside. Arthritis and arthralgias are most likely to become manifest during the transition to this phase. Early in this period desquamation begins in the periungual area of the fingers, then spreading to the toes, and ultimately to the palms and soles, which are shed in casts (Fig. 12.30). During this stage findings of carditis, which becomes clinically apparent in approximately 20 percent of cases, are most likely to appear, although tachycardia and a gallop rhythm may have been noted during the acute phase and a few patients will have died early in the course of the disease as a result of fulminant pancarditis. Coronary artery vasculitis with aneurysmal dilatation is the most common pathologic finding. It is thought that all patients probably have some degree of coronary angiitis, but that in the majority of patients it is mild and remains subclinical. Patients who become symptomatic may develop signs of congestive heart failure, pericardial effusion, cardiac arrhythmias, mitral insufficiency, or myocardial infarction. The latter phenomenon due to coronary thrombosis is abetted by thrombocytosis, which peaks in the third week with platelet counts as high as 1.8 million. Most infarctions occur within 11 to 50 days from onset of symptoms and are the major source of the 0.5 to 2 percent incidence of mortality. Echocardiography has proven highly useful in detecting coronary artery aneurysms, even in patients without cardiac symptoms. Electrocardiographic monitoring detects arrhythmias, heart block and voltage changes suggestive of left ventricular hypertrophy in as many as 30 percent of patients, but it may be normal in patients with positive echocardiographic findings. In a few reported cases, aneurysmal dilatation of the brachial, iliac and cerebral arteries and of the abdominal aorta has become clinically evident, reflecting diffuse angiitis.

The convalescent phase begins in the fourth to fifth week and is defined as lasting until the sedimentation rate has returned to normal, some 6 to 10 weeks from onset. A number of cardiac deaths occur during this convalescent period. Coronary artery abnormalities as detected by serial echocardiography may persist for a year or more however, and there is increasing evidence of long-term cardiac sequelae.

Because there is no specific test for diagnosing Kawasaki disease, adherence to the strict diagnostic criteria listed above with elimination of other differential diagnostic possibilities is important in arriving at a diagnosis of this disorder. Differential diagnostic considerations include scarlet fever (both streptococcal and staphylococcal), staphylococcal scalded skin disease, TSS, leptospirosis, disseminated yersiniosis, Rocky Mountain spotted fever, rubeola, enteroviral infection, Reiter's disease, juvenile rheumatoid arthritis, and systemic lupus erythematosis. Cultures, serologic tests, patient age, and clinical course of disease will help in ruling out these other disorders.

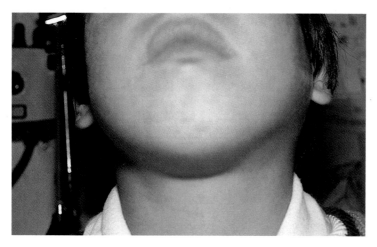

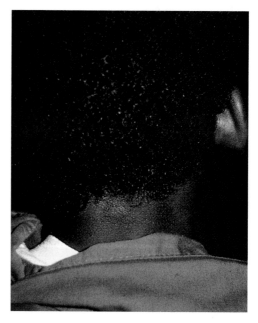

FIG. 12.32 Mumps. Postauricular swelling and secondary displacement of the auricle can be appreciated when the patient is viewed from behind. (Courtesy of Dr. M. Sherlock)

FIG. 12.31 Mumps. This young boy presented with unilateral parotid swelling, which was indurated and moderately tender. Visually it was appreciated best in this view, which reveals swelling anterior and inferior to his left ear.

MUMPS (EPIDEMIC PAROTITIS)

Mumps is an acute viral illness that preferentially involves neural and glandular tissues. While salivary glands, especially the parotid glands, are the most common sites of clinical involvement, the CNS may be affected as well as other glandular tissues in any combination. In as many as one-third of cases, infection is subclinical. Peak incidence is in late winter and spring. The incubation period is 16 to 18 days, with patients being contagious from 1 to 7 days prior to onset of clinical symptoms and for 5 to 9 days thereafter. Asymptomatic individuals also can transmit the virus.

Prodromal symptoms consist of fever, headache, malaise, and anorexia. In the typical case these symptoms are followed within 24 hours by the onset of an earache or face pain, which older children often can localize to the region of the pinna. Pain is aggravated by chewing and by stimulation of salivation (in particular, by sour foods). Parotid swelling generally becomes noticeable within the next 24 hours, increases gradually over the next few days and then abates over a similar period of time. Fever may persist for the duration of swelling but can disappear early in the course. On examination an area of tender indurated swelling, extending from the preauricular area through the subauricular space to the postauricular region, can be palpated (Fig. 12.31). With pronounced enlargement the pinna is pushed up and out (Fig. 12.32). The gland when palpated is discovered to be mild to moderately tender. The color of the overlying skin is normal. Intraoral examination may reveal erythema and edema of Stensen's duct. Bilateral involvement is usual although one gland will tend to enlarge before the other and up to 25 percent of symptomatic patients will have unilateral inflammation.

This "typical picture" is but one of many possible variants of clinical mumps. In some cases the parotid gland is spared and the submaxillary or sublingual salivary glands may be the primary site of involvement. In the former instance, indurated swelling is found below the mid-portion of the mandible; in the latter case bilateral submental swelling is seen externally with sublingual swelling noted intraorally. Preauricular swelling and induration, the Stensen's duct abnormality when present, and the absence of prominent overlying erythema help to distinguish parotid swelling from cervical adenitis involving the tonsillar node. In confusing cases and in cases where submaxillary or sublingual salivary glands are involved closely simulating adenopathy, the patient can be given lemon juice to sip or a lemon wedge to suck on. In patients with mumps this will result in a prompt increase in pain as it stimulates salivation, whereas no such change will be seen in patients with adenopathy. In cases of bacterial parotitis, the patient is likely to have high fever and to show signs of toxicity. The overlying skin is erythematous, with exquisite tenderness found on palpation. Inspection of Stensen's duct while the gland is massaged usually will show purulent drainage.

While it has been estimated that up to 75 percent of mumps patients may have CSF pleocytosis, symptomatic meningoencephalitis is seen only in about 10 percent of patients. CNS symptoms usually follow parotitis, but can develop prior to or even in the absence of salivary gland involvement. There is a wide spectrum in severity of these symptoms, ranging from isolated headache and malaise with fever to frank meningismus with nausea, vomiting, and severe alterations in sensorium. While permanent sequelae are rare, children recovering from severe mumps meningoencephalitis may not return to normal levels of school performance for up to 6 months or a year.

Orchitis is much less common in pediatric than in adult male patients in whom there is a 20 to 30 percent incidence. Orchitis usually follows salivary gland enlargement but may occur in its absence. Fever, chills, headache, nausea, vomiting, and lower abdominal pain are prominent and develop with the onset of painful generally unilateral testicular swelling. Epididymitis is an invariable accompaniment. Duration of this process ranges from 3 to 7 days. Oophoritis, seen in an occasional female patient, presents with a secondary temperature spike, nausea, vomiting, and severe lower abdominal pain and tenderness. Involvement may be unilateral or bilateral, and when unilateral and on the right side it may be indistinguishable from appendicitis. Pancreatitis is an uncommon though potentially severe manifestation. Patients tend to have sudden onset of excruciating boring epigastric pain in association with fever, chills, repetitive vomiting, weakness, and even prostration. This, too, tends to last for 3 to 7 days. Thyroiditis, mastitis, bartholinitis, and dacryocystitis have been reported in isolated cases, as well.

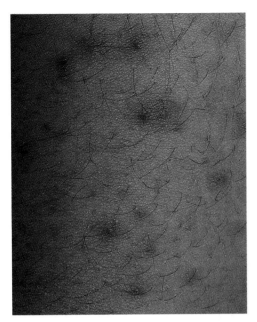

FIG. 12.33 Folliculitis. The extensor surfaces of the extremities and other hair-bearing areas are the most common sites of this superficial infection of hair follicles. Lesions begin as erythematous nodules at the base of a hair shaft and then evolve to form a central pustule with a thin red rim.

BACTERIAL SKIN AND SOFT-TISSUE INFECTIONS

Superficial bacterial skin infections occur with a relatively high frequency in childhood. In the majority of cases, the causative organisms are inoculated through a small wound such as a superficial cut, an abrasion, an insect bite, or a burn. Injection may occur at the time of the injury if the pathogen has colonized the site previously, or it may occur subsequently via scratching, touching, or contamination with dirt. The fact that young children, being active and impetuous, frequently incur minor injuries that produce breaks in skin continuity, and that they are less cognizant of keeping wounds clean and of washing their hands after sneezing, blowing or picking their noses, helps to explain their propensity to these infections. In some cases a preexisting dermatitis, by breaking down the skin barrier, sets the stage for secondary infection. The ever present risk of infection in these patients with preexisting dermatitis must be kept in mind, especially when steroids are being prescribed as therapy.

While most superficial infections are relatively minor in severity, diagnosis and proper treatment are important to reduce further spread of infection and to prevent its transmission to others. Deeper skin and soft-tissue infections, while less common, have the potential for considerably greater morbidity and even mortality. As with superficial lesions inoculation from without is the most common mode of acquisition with the organism simply having been injected more deeply. In a number of instances however, these infections represent metastatic foci of bacteremic spread.

Group A β-hemolytic streptococci and coagulase-positive staphylococci are the organisms most commonly responsible for these types of infections. Both organisms commonly reside in the nasopharynx, and staphylococci routinely colonize the skin, a phenomenon that is less likely though still possible with streptococci. Both organisms are transmitted readily by carriers or by persons with active nasopharyngeal or skin infections, with droplet, aerosol, and direct contact being the major modes of spread. Staphylococci are relatively resistant to heat and drying and can be transmitted via objects and fomites, as well. The fact that each pathogen produces relatively characteristic clinical features can help,

to some extent, in making clinical diagnoses. Staphylococci, for example, when injected below the epidermis are somewhat more likely to remain localized stimulating suppuration and tissue necrosis, whereas streptococcal infection tends to result in spread along tissue planes and through lymphatics, and thus, is more commonly associated with secondary cellulitis, lymphangitis, and regional adenopathy. It must be remembered, however, that other pathogens such as pseudomonas can mimic these clinical pictures and that staphylococcal infection can simulate some of the more typical findings of streptococcal infection. Additionally, in some cases infection is the result of action of multiple pathogens working in concert.

Folliculitis

Folliculitis is the term used to refer to superficial infection and/or irritation of hair follicles. The scalp, face, extensor surfaces of the extremities, and buttocks are the most common sites of involvement. Patients with dry atopic skin and keratosis pilaris (a condition in which follicles become blocked by keratin plugs) are particularly prone to this problem (see Chapter 8). Additional predisposing factors include seborrhea, excessive sweating, poor hygiene and topical application of or contact with oils, tars, and adhesives. In each of these situations, obstruction of follicles occurs setting the stage for inflammation and secondary infection. Following occlusion a superficial erythematous nodule develops around the hair. This nodule then evolves to form a thin-walled central pustule with a thin red rim (Fig. 12.33). The lesions may itch or burn mildly and subsequently may drain and crust. While healing of a given lesion occurs in 7 to 10 days without treatment, multiple crops may occur. With scratching the infection may be spread to other areas, and secondary impetiginous lesions may develop. Coagulase-positive staphylococci are the pathogens usually identified, although other skin colonizers may participate. Oral antimicrobial therapy directed at the staphylococcus and treatment of or avoidance of the predisposing condition are the measures indicated to clear the process.

On occasion the early lesions found in some forms of tinea capitis and tinea corporis may mimic folliculitis although itching usually is more prominent in these fungal infections and the surrounding rim of erythema tends to be wider. Tinea should be suspected especially when folliculitic lesions are localized to the hairline of the scalp. Older lesions, when present, may help in distinguishing between fungal and bacterial infections. Gram stains and KOH preparations and cultures are useful in evaluating questionable cases.

Impetigo

Impetigo is a superficial infection of the epidermis caused by streptococci, staphylococci, or both. Exposed portions of the body including the face, extremities, hands, and neck are the most common sites of involvement. Lesions are teeming with organisms and serve as a major source of transmission to others. In temperate climates the disorder has a peak season in summer and early fall because of increased exposure of greater areas of body surface to insect bites, injury, and colonization by pathogenic organisms. In warm climates impetigo is prevalent year round. Group A streptococci are believed to be the most common offending pathogens, being the sole organisms found in approximately 30 percent of

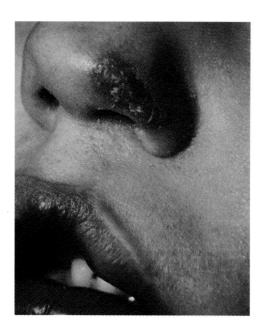

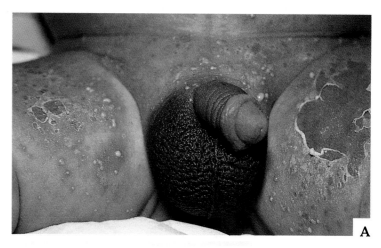

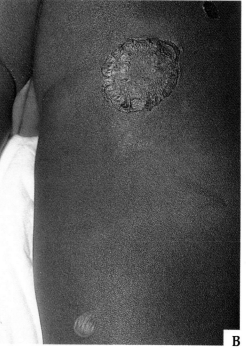

FIG. 12.34 Impetigo. This impetiginous lesion, caused by group A streptococci, has evolved from a papule to a vesicle that ruptured, producing this characteristic honey-colored crust. (Courtesy of Dr. M. Sherlock)

FIG. 12.35 Impetigo. This infant with staphylococcal diaper dermatitis (A) has multiple small thin-walled pustules that rupture rapidly and coalesce, leaving a shallow base and a superficial peeling rim. B, The various stages of bullous impetigo are evident in this child. An unruptured flaccid bulla is seen near an older lesion that has spread outward and crusted peripherally, and another that has just ruptured.

cases, and being isolated in combination with coagulase-positive staphylococci in about 60 percent of cases. In the latter group it is suspected that the staphylococci are secondary invaders. *Staphylococcus aureus* is the sole offender in about 10 percent of cases. Significant regional variations in the relative frequency of isolation of these pathogens do occur, however.

In patients without preexisting dermatitis, lesions tend to be localized, but when the child has an antecedent condition such as eczema, the infection can spread rapidly to involve extensive areas.

In cases due to Group A streptococci alone the lesion begins as a papule and evolves rapidly to form a small thin-walled vesicle with an erythematous halo. The initially serous vesicular fluid becomes cloudy and the vesicle ruptures, forming a superficial honey-colored crust (Fig. 12.34). If the crust is lifted, a shallow smooth weeping erythematous base is revealed. Secondary enlargement and tenderness of the regional lymph nodes is common. The initial macules of primary staphylococcal impetigo may evolve rapidly to form small thin-walled pustules or the larger flaccid bullae of bullous impetigo. The latter contain slightly cloudy fluid and often are a centimeter or more in diameter. In either case the pustules or bullae rupture rapidly leaving a shallow erythematous base surrounded by a superficial peeling rim (Fig. 12.35). In cases of more long-standing or combined infection, lesions may crust centrally and enlarge centrifugally. This may result in the formation of a superficial central scab surrounded by a bullous rim, or in evolution of a dried lesion with multiple concentric rings (Fig. 12.36). Lesions may coalesce over time and satellite lesions may form around larger primary lesions. Regardless of type, impetigo frequently is pruritic and thus the patient is stimulated to scratch, thereby spreading the infection to other sites or even inoculating the offending bacteria deeper into the skin.

The possible source of the causative organisms may be the patient's own skin or the nasopharynx or those of another infected person. In patients with facial and perinasal lesions, the nose and sinuses are the most likely sites of origin. Oral antimicrobial therapy is preferred for eradication and is particularly important when the source of infection is the nasopharynx, although topical antibacterial ointments may

serve to reduce the spread of infection to others in the child's environment. If the patient has a predisposing dermatosis, this too must be treated.

On occasion infection with other organisms can simulate the picture of impetiginous lesions. One form of tinea capitis produces lesions identical to those of streptococcal impetigo. Hence when small pustules and golden-crusted lesions are seen on the scalp or at the hairline, Gram stain and KOH preparations are indicated to ensure correct diagnosis. Candida can produce tiny pustules, which rupture and have a superficial peeling rim, at times simulating staphylococcal infection in the diaper area. However, with candidal diaper dermatitis, lesions usually are smaller, pustules are more evanescent, the inflammation is more diffuse and the erythema more intense than that seen with staphylococcal impetigo. In confusing cases a KOH preparation and/or Gram stain can be used to clarify the etiology.

Ecthyma

Ecthyma is an ulcerative skin infection that penetrates more deeply than impetigo, to involve the dermis. The disorder is most prevalent in tropical climates. Poor hygiene, insect bites, and trauma are the major predisposing factors, accounting for the fact that the lower extremities and the

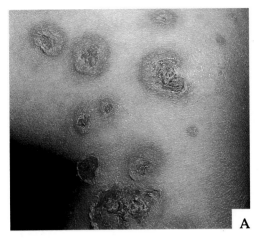

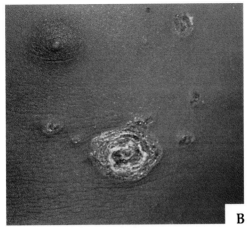

FIG. 12.36 Impetigo. In this child with staphylococcal impetigo (**A**) older lesions have central crusts with bullous rims that are spreading outward. The findings of long-standing impetigo are seen in this youngster (**B**) whose lesions are crusted in rings. Note also the smaller satellites surrounding the larger primary lesion. (**B**, courtesy of Dr. M. Sherlock)

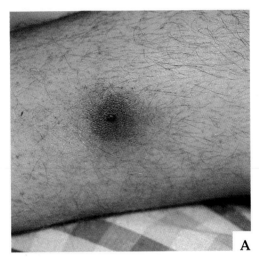

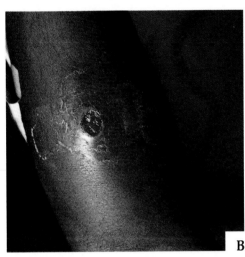

FIG. 12.37 Ecthyma. **A**, In focal ecthyma due to inoculation of group A streptococci, the lesion initially consists of a central vesicle or pustule (that rapidly crusts over) on a painful indurated erythematous base. With progression a deep widening ulcer forms, as seen in this child (**B**) following removal of the overlying crust. (Courtesy of Dr. E. Wald)

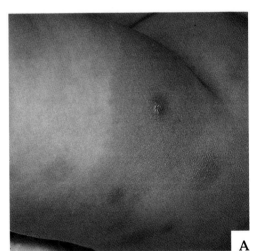

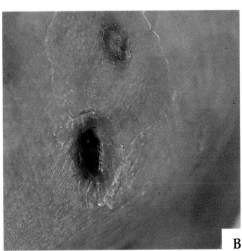

FIG. 12.38 Ecthyma. Pseudomonas septicemia may result in metastatic ecthymatous lesions that begin as pink macules and become hemorrhagic (**A**) and ultimately necrose centrally to form a black eschar (**B**). (Courtesy of Dr. E. Wald)

buttocks are the usual sites of involvement. Initially lesions may resemble impetigo consisting of a vesicle or a pustule on an erythematous base, which then ruptures and crusts over. In ecthyma however, the lesions are painful, and the crusts harder, thicker and more adherent than in impetigo, and the surrounding area of erythema is indurated. The ulcerative base beneath the crust gradually deepens and enlarges. Unroofing the crust uncovers a round deep punched-out ulcer with raised borders (Fig. 12.37). The size of the lesions ranges from ½ to 3 cm. Without treatment these lesions take weeks to heal, leaving a circumscribed scar.

In most cases ecthyma is the result of direct inoculation of organisms through the skin with group A β-hemolytic streptococci being the usual pathogen. On occasion staphylococci or pseudomonas may be causative; the latter organism, when infecting a small wound, is more likely to produce a central abscess that exudes a greenish or bluish purulent exudate when its crust is lifted. Pseudomonas septicemia also may result in metastatic ecthymatous lesions, which begin as pink macules and then evolve to hemorrhagic papules and then necrose centrally to leave a dark eschar on an erythematous base (Fig. 12.38). Subsequently ulceration occurs, along with deep necrosis. This metastatic form of ecthyma is distinguished easily from primary cases by virtue of the formation of multiple lesions and by the presence of systemic signs of sepsis.

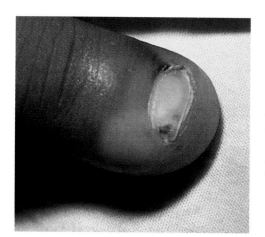

FIG. 12.39 Paronychia. Chewing on a hangnail predisposed this child to the development of a paronychia. Initially, erythema developed near the hangnail, and was followed rapidly by suppuration.

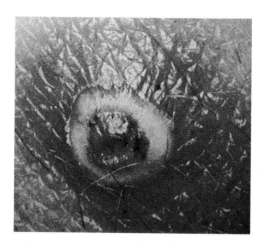

FIG. 12.40 Furuncle. In this well-developed furuncle, the abscess has burrowed to the surface and the skin has thinned centrally and begun to necrose. There is a wide surrounding rim of erythema and induration. (Courtesy of Dr. B. Cohen)

Abscesses of the Skin and Soft Tissues

Abscesses are localized collections of purulent material, which are buried in a tissue, an organ, or in a confined space. They result from the deep seeding of pyogenic organisms, which, in the case of abscesses involving the skin and its appendages, usually are coagulase-positive staphylococci. As the area of inflammation expands outward, central necrosis occurs and the process tends to produce an increase in pressure with resultant burrowing toward the surface or along tissue planes, resulting in further local tissue destruction. Drainage is essential for healing, as the abscess contents provoke a continuing inflammatory response, and antimicrobials are unable to penetrate to the necrotic center of the lesion. Abscesses of the skin and soft tissues are categorized in part according to the site of involvement and in part according to the structure involved. The types most commonly encountered in childhood will be discussed below.

PARONYCHIA (PERIUNGUAL ABSCESS)

A paronychia is a relatively superficial abscess that develops under the cuticle or along the nail fold of a finger or a toe. Staphylococci and occasionally streptococci gain access through a traumatized hangnail, or through lesions created by clipping a cuticle or by chewing on the fingers. Occasionally an ingrown toe nail is the predisposing condition, and in such cases the nail, which usually was cut improperly, grows laterally into the nail fold, lacerating the soft tissue and setting the stage for infection. In typical cases erythema, pain and tenderness develop at the site of injury, and are followed rapidly by suppuration (Fig. 12.39). The infection then advances from the portal of entry around the nail fold and if treatment is delayed, it can burrow beneath the base of the nail creating a subungual abscess. Occasionally secondary lymphangitis may develop. Drainage is accomplished readily by undermining the involved portion of the cuticle and nail fold with a scalpel blade. Unless secondary complications have developed, subsequent soaking usually is sufficient for healing.

ABSCESSES OF SKIN APPENDAGES
Furuncle

A furuncle or boil is a perifollicular dermal abscess that is usually caused by coagulase-positive staphylococci, perhaps in concert with other skin flora. It may be the result of extension of a superficial folliculitis or of direct inoculation via minor trauma. Hairy areas subject to friction and/or maceration are particularly vulnerable. Skin contact with oc-clusive agents such as oils, tars, and adhesives is another common predisposing factor. Older children and adolescents have a much higher incidence than do younger children.

The lesion begins as a small dermal nodule around a hair follicle, which initially may produce a sensation of mild discomfort and itching. As it gradually increases in size, pain worsens and is aggravated by touching and motion of the involved area. With expansion the overlying skin becomes reddened, central necrosis begins to occur, and with increased inflammation and pressure the infection begins to burrow and seek egress. In the case of most furuncles, the abscess burrows toward the surface of the skin, which becomes thinned and shiny as the abscess becomes fluctuant (Fig. 12.40). Application of warm compresses can hasten this process. At this point incision and drainage is indicated. Without intervention spontaneous drainage of bloody purulent material ultimately occurs in most cases, and the patient experiences prompt relief of pain. In areas such as the nape of the neck or the upper back, where the overlying skin is thick enough to resist external pointing, the process may take a path of lesser resistance, burrowing outward from the center through the subcutaneous tissues and along fascial planes. If this process is not interrupted by early surgical intervention, the result is the gradual formation of a *carbuncle* which consists of an extremely painful exquisitely tender multilocular mass of interconnected dermal and subcutaneous abscesses, with multiple points of partial drainage at the skin surface. Carbuncle formation often is accompanied by fever, chills and increasing malaise, and there is a significant risk of secondary bacteremia. Even with treatment, sloughing and extensive scarring tend to result.

Hidradenitis Suppurativa

In hidradenitis suppurativa an apocrine gland is the site of infection and abscess formation. Hence, localization in these cases is limited to the axillae, perineum and areolae, and the disorder is not seen until the onset of puberty. Occlusion, maceration and poor hygiene are major predisposing factors, fostering inflammation of the gland with resultant obstruction and providing a favorable environment for multiplication of staphylococci. As the inflammatory process expands, the gland ultimately ruptures and an abscess forms. In contrast to the perifollicular furuncle, this infection is deeper and slower to localize and suppurate. It begins as a firm mildly tender nodule that enlarges very gradually, becoming increasingly uncomfortable and ever more tender to the touch. Recurrences are considerably more common with this disorder than is the case with furuncles.

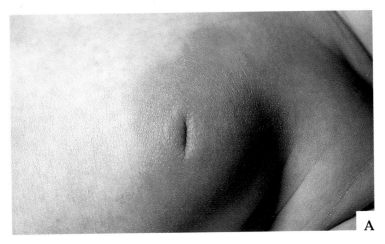

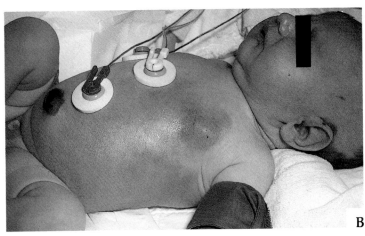

FIG. 12.41 Breast abscess. **A**, The typical manifestations of a breast abscess were seen in this neonate—swelling, induration, tenderness, warmth, and erythema. With compression, pus could be expressed from the nipple. **B**, This unfortunate infant was not brought to the hospital until subcutaneous rupture and extensive cellulitic spread had occurred. She was febrile, toxic, irritable, and listless on presentation.

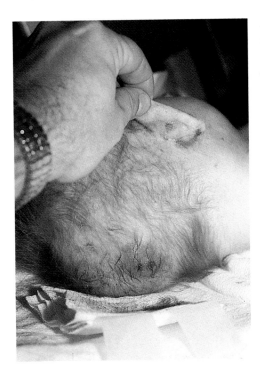

FIG. 12.42 Scalp abscess. Several days after discharge from the newborn nursery this infant presented with two scalp abscesses and an impetiginous lesion behind the right ear. The surface of the larger abscess is marked by two puncture wounds, which were the site of placement of monitor leads during labor. (Courtesy of Dr. B. Zitelli)

ABSCESSES OF SPECIAL SITES

The breasts, scalp, and perianal areas are three specific sites of abscess formation of particular importance in pediatrics. Breast and scalp abscesses are discussed below. Perirectal abscesses are described in Chapter 15.

Breast Abscess

Breast abscesses occur with a small but significant frequency in pediatric patients with incidence peaks in the neonatal and pubertal age groups. Newborns greater than 31 weeks gestation at delivery have the highest incidence, due in part to physiologic hypertrophy of breast tissue as a result of stimulation by maternal hormones. Colonization of the skin and/or of the nasopharynx with virulent organisms (*S. aureus* or coliforms) during delivery or in the nursery is another important predisposing factor. Up to 25 percent of affected infants have overt staphylococcal diaper dermatitis at the time of presentation. Minor local trauma also is thought to be a predisposing factor. The majority of cases occur during the second or third week following delivery, but infection may occur as late as 8 weeks of age. The problem first manifests as swelling and tenderness of the affected breast. Unilateral involvement is the rule. With time local warmth and overlying erythema become evident, and it may become possible to express a purulent discharge from the nipple (Fig. 12.41A). Axillary adenopathy may be present as well. Only 25 percent of infants have low-grade temperature, and other systemic symptoms are uncommon unless treatment is delayed. Depending on the time of presentation, a firm tender nonfluctuant nodule may be found on palpation, or the mass clearly may be fluctuant, indicating suppuration and necrosis. In the former instance parenteral antibiotic therapy and close monitoring for progression to fluctuance are indicated. In the latter instance prompt surgical incision and drainage are required. Broad-spectrum coverage should be provided pending culture results. Commonly recovered organisms include *S. aureus*, *Escherichia coli*, salmonella species, *Streptococcus agalactiae*, *Proteus mirabilis*, and mixed flora. Delay in diagnosis and institution of treatment may result in subcutaneous rupture and cellulitic spread with secondary bacteremia (Fig. 12.41B). Delay in surgical drainage of fluctuant lesions also can result in permanent loss of breast tissue, which in females can produce a cosmetically deforming breast asymmetry that is first noted at puberty.

Breast abscesses may be seen again following puberty. Minor trauma, cutaneous infections, epidermal cysts, and duct blockages appear to be the common antecedent conditions. The clinical picture is similar to that seen in infants. Coagulase-positive staphylococci are the usual offending organisms.

Scalp Abscess

As is the case with breast abscesses, pyogenic infections of the scalp are particularly common in the neonatal period. Trauma is the predominant predisposing factor, and in neonates these abscesses commonly develop at the site of insertion of scalp leads for fetal monitoring during labor. Affected infants occasionally are found to have staphylococcal diaper dermatitis, as well. In the majority of cases, the infection is localized and consists of a tender nodule with overlying erythema (Fig. 12.42). The nodule commonly is fluctuant at

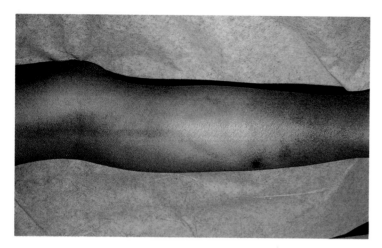

FIG. 12.43 Lymphangitis. An insect bite was the source of inoculation of group A streptococci in this child who subsequently developed secondary cellulitis and lymphangitis. The erythematous streaks coursing up the leg were tender and slightly indurated.

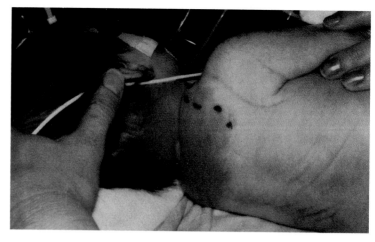

FIG. 12.44 Erysipelas. A 6-week-old infant presented with fever, lethargy, irritability, and hypotension in association with erysipelas. The purplish-red lesion was raised, indurated, and tender. The border, though irregular, was sharply demarcated from the adjacent skin. The involved skin appeared edematous and had a "peau d'orange" quality. Cultures of blood and tissue aspirate grew group A streptococci.

the time of presentation enabling prompt incision and drainage. Staphylococci and coliforms are the major pathogens recovered. Because of the neonate's immunologic immaturity, antimicrobial therapy also is recommended and in most cases can be administered orally. On rare occasions infection is extensive and takes the form of a necrotizing fasciitis (see below). In these patients and in the rare infant with a localized abscess and systemic symptoms, parenteral broad-spectrum antibiotic treatment (pending culture results) is indicated in addition to incision, drainage, and debridement.

When scalp abscesses are encountered in older children, care should be taken to determine the responsible pathogen. While staphylococci may be the source, invasive fungi are more likely to be the responsible organisms. These fungi produce a thick-walled boggy multilocular abscess termed a "kerion" (see Chapter 8). Gram stain and KOH preparations of purulent contents and of pulled hairs are important, for while incision and drainage is the treatment of choice for abscesses of bacterial origin, oral antifungal and steroid therapy are indicated for the kerion.

Lymphangitis

Inflammation of lymphatic channels is actually a secondary manifestation of infection at a distal site. The phenomenon is the result of invasion of lymphatic vessels by pathogenic organisms, which then spread along these channels toward regional lymph nodes. Group A β-hemolytic streptococci, by virtue of elaborating fibrinolysins and hyaluronidases, are the most common source of lymphangitis, although wounds infected by staphylococci and pseudomonas also may result in overt lymphangitis. Clinically tender, erythematous, and irregular linear streaks are seen extending from the primary site toward the draining regional nodes (Fig. 12.43). The primary site may be an infected wound or an area of cellulitis. Systemic symptoms consisting of fever, chills, and malaise are often but not invariably present. Without appropriate antimicrobial therapy, cellulitis may develop or extend and necrosis and ulceration may occur with attendant risk of bacteremia. Culture and Gram stain

of material from the primary site will aid in selection of antimicrobials; however, presumptive initial therapy is necessary pending culture results.

Erysipelas

Group A β-hemolytic streptococci are the source of this unusual distinctive infection involving a localized area of the dermis and superficial lymphatics. The causative organisms usually are found in the upper respiratory tracts of afflicted patients and are inoculated through a break in the skin that may elude detection on presentation. Hematogenous seeding has been postulated in some cases, however. Systemic symptoms are prominent and precede appearance of the characteristic skin lesion. The onset is abrupt and is heralded by fever and chills often in association with nausea, vomiting, and headache. This prodrome is followed by the appearance of an intensely painful skin lesion that consists of a circumscribed raised plaque that is a deep purplish-red in color (Fig. 12.44). The raised border, although irregular, is well demarcated and spreads centrifugally. Red lymphatic streaks may advance ahead of it toward the regional nodes. On close inspection the skin is seen to be edematous and may have a thickened "peau d'orange" character. On palpation it is indurated, hot, and exquisitely tender. With evolution small surface blebs containing yellow fluid may form. The malar portion of the face is the site most commonly involved, with the trunk, neck, and extremities being less frequent areas of localization. Patients may become bacteremic, developing metastatic foci of infection. Infants are at particular risk for systemic spread. The clinical picture of erysipelas is so characteristic that streptococcal infection can be presumed and parenteral antimicrobial treatment initiated. Cultures of tissue aspirate from the advancing border of the lesion and of the nose and throat typically are positive for group A streptococci, as are blood cultures in septic patients.

Cellulitis

Cellulitis is an infection of bacterial origin in which subcutaneous loose connective tissue is the primary site of in-

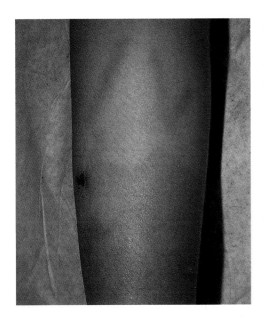

FIG. 12.45 Wound-related cellulitis. The infected mosquito bite that served as the source of cellulitis in this child can be seen on the left. The area of erythema was indurated and exquisitely tender. Note how the borders fade gradually into the adjacent normal skin.

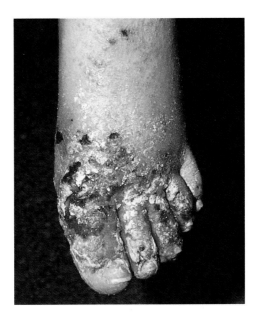

FIG. 12.46 This patient with wound-related cellulitis had been on topical steroid therapy for contact dermatitis for about 48 hours when he experienced explosive onset of swelling, redness, and pain. Impetiginous changes are apparent, as well. (Courtesy of Dr. M. Sherlock)

flammation. With progression the process extends centrifugally through the subcutaneous tissue and also may ascend to involve the lower dermis. Although cellulitis may develop anywhere on the body, it occurs most commonly on the extremities and face. There are three major modes of origin:

1. Extension from a wound
2. Hematogenous seeding
3. Extension from a deeper infection

Clinically cellulitis is characterized by painful tender indurated subcutaneous swelling. The overlying skin is smooth, warm, often shiny, and usually erythematous (see Fig. 12.45). Occasionally it has a violaceous hue. In contrast to erysipelas, the margins or borders of both the edema and erythema are indistinct, fading imperceptibly into the surrounding tissues. Prior to therapy rapid extension is the rule. Systemic symptoms are common, particularly when infection is due to hematogenous spread or to extension from deeper sites. In such cases fever, chills, malaise, and headache are typical. When hematogenous seeding is the source, toxicity may be marked.

WOUND-RELATED CELLULITIS
Extension of infection from an external wound such as a puncture, laceration, abrasion or insect bite is perhaps the most common source of cellulitis, particularly in school-age children and in adolescents. Mild local erythema immediately surrounding a wound, an impetiginous lesion or a pustule may have been noted, prior to the abrupt onset of increased pain and the rapid evolution of subcutaneous inflammation that herald the development of cellulitis. In the majority of cases, the primary lesion is readily identifiable at the time of presentation (Fig. 12.45) but in some instances it may no longer be detectable. Occasionally secondary infection of a preexisting dermatitis may result in a cellulitis that spreads with frightening speed (Fig. 12.46). Group A streptococci and coagulase-positive staphylococci are the organisms recovered most commonly in these circumstances. Pseudomonas and mixed flora may be responsible for cellulitis occurring secondary to puncture wounds of the foot. While rapid peripheral spread, overt lymphangitis and regional adenitis are regarded as highly characteristic of streptococcal infection, this same picture may be seen with cellulitis due to any

of these wound-related pathogens. Fever and other systemic symptoms may be present with this form of cellulitis, but they are more likely to occur with cellulitis due to hematogenous seeding or to extension of inflammation from deeper structures.

Hands, feet, and extremities are the most common sites of wound-related cellulitis. This necessitates close assessment and monitoring for further spread and for secondary neurovascular compromise. Inward spread to tendon sheaths of a hand or a foot can have disastrous consequences; hence, cellulitis involving these structures must be treated aggressively, and clinical status must be monitored very closely. When an extremity is encircled by cellulitis, swelling and increased pressure can result in extensive damage distally if the area is not surgically decompressed. Gram stain and culture of material obtained from the primary wound and/or from tissue aspirate from the center and margin of the inflamed area may be helpful in identifying the specific pathogen. Successful aspiration necessitates the use of a large syringe to provide high-pressure suction and may require prior injection of nonbacteriostatic saline. Blood cultures should be obtained in all patients with systemic symptoms. Prompt treatment is essential to prevent further spread and complications. Antimicrobial therapy often has to be selected empirically, pending culture results. Coverage for penicillinase-producing staphylococci is essential.

Major differential diagnostic considerations include angioedema due to insect bites and delayed hypersensitivity reactions to hymenoptera stings. The former is pruritic, nontender and often has an identifiable central punctum, while the latter is pruritic, and mildly painful and tender. Both are unassociated with systemic symptoms or with adenopathy or lymphangitis. The history, lack of erythema, presence of ecchymotic discoloration and absence of systemic symptoms all help to distinguish swelling due to trauma.

HEMATOGENOUS CELLULITIS
Hematogenous seeding is another common source of cellulitis, particularly in infants and young children. While young infants may present with sudden onset of sepsis followed soon thereafter by the appearance of cellulitis, older infants, toddlers and preschool-age children commonly have antecedent upper respiratory tract symptoms. This

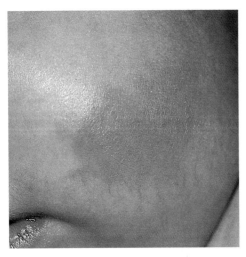

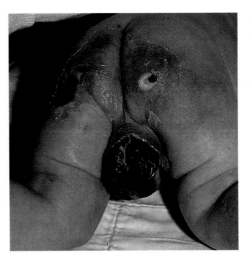

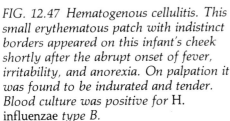

FIG. 12.47 Hematogenous cellulitis. This small erythematous patch with indistinct borders appeared on this infant's cheek shortly after the abrupt onset of fever, irritability, and anorexia. On palpation it was found to be indurated and tender. Blood culture was positive for H. influenzae type B.

FIG. 12.48 Necrotizing fasciitis. The extent of cellulitis and tissue necrosis are visibly evident in this child who is recovering from necrotizing fasciitis due to group A streptococci. On presentation he was thought to have cellulitis but was more ill systemically and appeared much more uncomfortable than would be expected. Furthermore, on presentation the area of induration extended well beyond the overlying erythema. (Courtesy of Dr. M. Sherlock)

prodrome is followed by the sudden development of a high fever that begins nearly simultaneously with the appearance of a nondescript area of swelling. Often this swelling is localized in the periorbital region (see Chapter 20), but at times may be located over a cheek or over the neck or an upper extremity. The overlying skin rapidly becomes pink, red, or violaceous as the area of edema spreads in extent. Irritability, anorexia and signs of toxicity become increasingly marked, in most cases prompting presentation for medical care within 24 hours. H. influenzae type B is a particularly likely source of this picture, but it is by no means the only organism to produce cellulitis in this age group or in these anatomical regions. Streptococcus pneumoniae, as well as group B streptococci (in infants under 3 months of age) can produce an identical picture. However Haemophilus influenzae type B does appear to be the sole pathogen responsible for cellulitis of the cheek, also termed "buccal cellulitis." In this form of cellulitis, a type limited exclusively to infants, the swelling and erythema are located over the midcheek near the mandibular ramus (Fig. 12.47). Ipsilateral otitis and localized erythema of the underlying buccal mucosa are common associated findings. The systemic symptomatology and exquisite tenderness help to distinguish it from "popsicle panniculitis," which results from cold injury. The latter is characterized by formation of a mildly tender, discrete indurated disc-shaped subcutaneous mass located at the angle of the mouth, with reddish-purple discoloration of the overlying skin. Systemic symptoms, induration, and tenderness also help to distinguish hematogenous cellulitis at other sites from sympathetic swelling and from angioedema due to insect bites.

The severity of illness and the inevitability of bacteremia with its attendant risks warrant expeditious evaluation and treatment. Blood cultures are positive in a very high percentage of patients and may be supplemented by culture of tissue aspirates from the area of cellulitis. Counterimmunoelectrophoresis also may be helpful. High-dose antimicrobial therapy should be administered parenterally, and selected to ensure coverage for β-lactamase-producing haemophilus.

CELLULITIS DUE TO EXTENSION OF INFECTION FROM DEEPER STRUCTURES

Though less common than the other forms, cellulitis may result from extension of infection and inflammation, from deeper structures toward the skin surface. This possibility necessitates paying close attention to examination of underlying structures in evaluating any patient with evidence of cellulitis. Dental abscesses (see Chapter 18) and acute sinusitis (see Chapter 20) may underlie facial cellulitis. Osteomyelitis may produce secondary cellulitic changes of overlying soft tissues, especially following subperiosteal extension (see below). Suppurative lymphadenitis and subcutaneous rupture of skin, scalp, and breast abscesses are other common sources (see Fig. 12.41B). Fever, toxicity, and other systemic symptoms are not unusual with this form of cellulitis. Antecedent history along with findings on careful examination usually will result in identification of this type of cellulitis and in recognition of the primary source.

Necrotizing Fasciitis

Variously termed necrotizing fasciitis or cellulitis, synergistic cellulitis or gangrene, necrotizing erysipelas and streptococcal gangrene, this dreaded disorder is a severe deep necrotizing soft-tissue infection, which at a minimum involves subcutaneous tissues and fascial sheaths and often extends to underlying muscle. This process spreads relentlessly along fascial planes producing edema, vascular thrombosis, and ever-widening necrosis resulting in extensive soft-tissue destruction. Deep surgical and traumatic wounds are major predisposing factors, although injection sites, cutaneous ulcers, and abscesses may serve as the initiating condition. Diabetics with vascular disease have an especially increased risk. The extremities, perineum, buttocks, trunk, and abdominal wall are the most common sites of involvement. Causative organisms include Group A β-hemolytic streptococci, *S. aureus*, *Pseudomonas aeruginosa*, *E. coli*, and mixtures of aerobes and anaerobes, and of anaerobes and facultative gram-negative rods.

Moderate to severe systemic symptoms are prominent clinically, and along with fever usually precede the appearance of cellulitic changes. The local area of inflammation initially may resemble ordinary cellulitis with nonraised indistinct margins, and localized subcutaneous edema with overlying erythema. However, on careful palpation, it often is possible to appreciate that the edema and induration may be palpably deeper and often are noted to be far more extensive than the overlying erythema. Pain is remarkably severe early on and the lesion is exquisitely tender. With progression the overlying skin itself may become edematous simulating erysipelas. Later its color changes, from that of red or purple to a patchy gray-blue, and surface bullae, often filled with hemorrhagic fluid, may appear. At this point numbness and decreased sensitivity to pain may be noted centrally. With further evolution central necrosis or cutaneous gangrene supervenes (Fig. 12.48). When anaerobes are involved crepitance may become evident clinically or subcutaneous emphysema may be visible on radiography. As the localized process evolves, systemic symptoms increase. Signs of poor perfusion, pallor, and mottling often are accompanied by grunting respirations and by alterations in level of consciousness including disorientation, obtundation, and seizures. This picture may culminate in frank prostration, often in association with generalized edema. Common laboratory findings in advanced cases include anemia due to hemolysis and marrow suppression, proteinuria, hypoproteinemia, hypocalcemia due to saponification of necrotic fat, and hyponatremia. Blood and wound cultures are routinely positive. Mortality ranges from 8 to 70 percent depending on the series, and morbidity and disfigurement are high in survivors. Delays in diagnosis and inadequate surgical debridement are major factors in cases with poor outcome.

Early recognition is crucial to ensure appropriate intervention and to improve prognosis. This can be particularly difficult in cases resembling ordinary cellulitis that initially improve on antimicrobial therapy before worsening. Necrotizing fasciitis should be suspected in any patient with cellulitis (particularly around a deep wound) who has unusually severe pain and systemic symptoms that are out of proportion to local findings. This can enable exploration before advanced skin changes and loss of sensation appear, signaling that necrosis already is extensive. If such changes are present, this process must be presumed. In early cases examination of frozen sections of biopsy material may confirm the diagnosis. Incision and passage of a probe also can be helpful. If the probe passes easily along fascial planes, the diagnosis is confirmed. Control necessitates wide exci-

sion with extensive exposure and debridement of all necrotic tissues, in combination with broad-spectrum antimicrobial therapy (guided in part by Gram-stain results pending cultures). Aggressive supportive measures are important, as well.

INFECTIOUS LYMPHADENITIS

Lymph nodes respond to both systemic and local infections with increased cellular multiplication and activity, clinically manifest as enlargement and tenderness. When enlargement and degree of inflammation are mild, this often is called "reactive adenopathy." Nodes usually are 2 cm or less in diameter, and they are discrete, slightly firm or rubbery in consistency, and mobile. Discomfort and tenderness are mild. However when enlargement is marked and inflammation is pronounced, the phenomenon is termed "adenitis." In the latter cases nodes usually exceed 2 to 3 cm in diameter, and overlying soft tissues may become edematous making it difficult to distinguish exact margins. With progression the overlying skin often becomes erythematous and may become adherent, reducing mobility. Discomfort and tenderness are usually but not always marked. Depending on the causative organism, suppuration may occur. Adenopathy may be generalized or regional, but adenitis tends to be localized to a single node. Whereas adenitis is invariably of infectious etiology, adenopathy may be a feature of collagen vascular disease or it may be of neoplastic origin. Malignant nodes usually are very firm or hard, but occasionally they are rubbery in consistency. They also may be discrete but not infrequently they are matted and often appear fixed or poorly mobile. Tenderness is unusual. Depending on the type of malignancy, the adenopathy may be isolated to one region, or it may be generalized and associated with hepatosplenomegaly and with such systemic symptoms as anorexia, fatigue, weight loss, night sweats, and bone pain. Many of the infectious diseases associated with generalized or cervical adenopathy have been discussed earlier in this chapter. Figure 12.49 presents in tabular form some of the distinguishing features of the adenopathy characteristic of these disorders. Neoplastic disorders are discussed in Chapter 11.

In this section we will concentrate on the manifestations and causes of focal lymphadenitis. Almost any organism capable of infecting tissue can produce adenitis, hence the number of potential pathogens is large. Assessment is facilitated by knowledge of patterns of lymphatic drainage, of the differential diagnostic possibilities of an inflammatory mass in a given region, and of the differential clinical characteristics of adenitis produced by individual organisms. By definition infection of a lymph node is a secondary phenomenon occurring as a result of drainage through lymphatic vessels to a regional node. Identification of the primary source, when possible, is important in narrowing the list of potential causative organisms. In many instances close examination of those areas whose lymphatics drain to the affected region will reveal the source. However it is not uncommon for the primary site to have healed by the time adenitis becomes clinically manifest. In these cases careful history taking concerning prior distal wounds or inflammation, as well as about any possible environmental exposures, may disclose the probable pathogen. This can be particularly important in cases caused by organisms not readily grown on culture, and for those cases in which prior administration of antibiotics has suppressed the causative organism resulting in negative cultures.

Disorder	Site of Adenopathy	Character of Nodes	Other Features	Laboratory Findings
EB virus mononucleosis	Anterior and posterior cervical, or generalized	Soft to firm, discrete, mildly to moderately tender	Pharyngitis; splenomegaly (50%); rash (15%); fever, malaise, fatigue	Atypical lymphocytosis; +Monospot (80%>4 yrs); + EB virus titers; may have abnormal LFTs
Cytomegalovirus infection	Generalized or cervical	Soft to firm, discrete, mildly tender	Fever, malaise, fatigue; occasionally hepatosplenomegaly	Atypical lymphocytosis; abnormal LFTs; urine + for inclusions and + for CMV on culture; + CMV titers
Toxoplasmosis	Generalized or cervical	Smooth, firm, mildly tender	Myalgias, fatigue, coryza; occasionally splenomegaly and maculopapular rash	Atypical lymphocytosis (frequent); + toxoplasma titers
Brucellosis	Generalized or cervical and axillary	Discrete, may be mildly tender or nontender	History of contact with sick farm animal or ingestion of raw milk; afternoon fever and chills; sweats, malaise, headache and backache, arthralgia; splenomegaly; lasts weeks and may become chronic with metastatic abscesses	Normal or decreased WBC with lymphocytosis; +cultures and serologic tests
Rubella	Anterior and posterior cervical	Soft to mildly firm, discrete, mildly tender or nontender	Fine discrete maculopapular rash; Forscheimer spots on palate	+Rubella titer
Streptococcal pharyngitis	Anterior cervical	Soft to mildly firm, discrete, tender	Pharyngitis or nasopharyngitis; headache, malaise; abdominal pain; may have palatal petechiae and/or scarlatiniform rash	+Throat culture for group A β-hemolytic streptococcus
Herpes simplex	Anterior cervical and submandibular	Soft to mildly firm, discrete, mobile, tender	Gingival erythema and edema with discrete mucosal ulcers; high fever	+Viral culture (diagnosis usually made on clinical grounds)
Coxsackievirus herpangina	Anterior cervical	Soft to mildly firm, discrete, mobile, slightly tender	Discrete ulcers on labial mucosa, gingiva, tongue, and tonsillar pillars; may have vesicles on palms and soles	+Viral culture (diagnosis usually made on clinical grounds)
Adenovirus	Anterior cervical and pre-auricular	Soft to mildly firm, discrete, mobile, mildly tender	Nonspecific pharyngeal inflammation, occasionally with exudate; may have conjunctivitis	+Viral culture

FIG. 12.49 Common infectious causes of generalized or prominent cervical adenopathy.

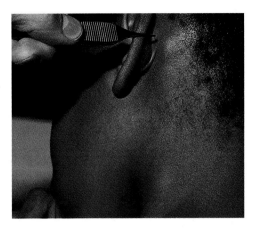

FIG. 12.51 Acute lymphadenitis. This child presented with folliculitic and crusted scalp lesions and a tender 1½-cm postauricular node with overlying erythema. The initial suspicion of bacterial infection was not confirmed. KOH preparation and fungal culture identified tinea capitis as the primary process.

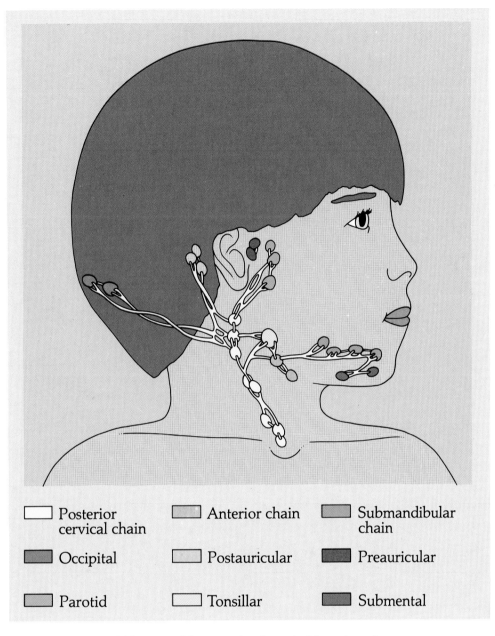

Posterior cervical chain	Anterior chain	Submandibular chain
Occipital	Postauricular	Preauricular
Parotid	Tonsillar	Submental

FIG. 12.50 The superficial cervical lymph nodes.

The Superficial Regional Lymph Nodes

THE CERVICAL LYMPH NODES

The cervical nodes, being numerous and draining multiple structures, are particularly common sites of acute adenitis (Fig. 12.50). In addition to infections of the upper respiratory tract, those of the skin of the face, the scalp, conjunctivae, teeth, gingivae, ears, and neck all may serve as primary sites of infection. Nasal and oropharyngeal infections drain to the tonsillar and anterior cervical nodes. Superficial facial infections and facial cellulitis may drain to the anterior cervical chain or to the preauricular or submental nodes, depending on location. The occipital, posterior cervical, preauricular, and postauricular nodes receive lymphatic drainage from nearby portions of the scalp, and thus may become inflamed and enlarged in connection with secondary infection of seborrhea, impetigo, wound infections, tinea capitis or head lice infestation (Fig. 12.51). Conjunctival infections may result in adenitis of the preauricular node. The dentition, gingivae and tongue are drained by lymphatics coursing to the submental and submandibular nodes, which can be secon-

darily involved in cases of dental abscess, gingivitis, and stomatitis. Infections of the external auditory canal and of the auricle may drain to the preauricular or postauricular nodes, while those involving the neck may affect the anterior or posterior cervical chain, depending on location.

While the number of potential causative organisms is high, an individual pathogen often can be implicated by careful history taking and physical examination. Differentiation also must be made from other masses that may be present in the cervical region, many of which are congenital and subject to secondary infection, simulating adenitis. A number of these and their clinical characteristics are enumerated in Figure 12.52.

THE AXILLARY AND EPITROCHLEAR LYMPH NODES

Over a dozen nodes occupy the axilla. Those in the anterior pectoral portion drain the breast and chest wall, those in the lateral or mid-portion receive drainage from the hand and arm, and those in the posterior subscapular region drain portions of the back. The epitrochlear node receives lymphatic vessels from the fingers, hand and skin of the forearm, but it is a much less common site of adenitis than are the axil-

DIFFERENTIAL DIAGNOSIS OF CERVICAL ADENOPATHY/ADENITIS

Type of Mass	Usual Site	Character	Time of Appearance
Lymphangioma	Preauricular, submental, submandibular, supraclavicular	Soft, compressible; transilluminates; margins often indistinct; may increase in size with crying or straining; nontender unless infected	Birth to 2 years
Hemangioma	Preauricular, post-auricular, may occur along or under sternocleidomastoid	Soft, compressible; margins often indistinct; increases in size with crying, straining, and dependency; nontender unless infected	Birth to 1 year; gradually enlarges during first year, then regresses
Branchial cleft cyst	Preauricular, at mandibular angle, along anterior border of sternocleido-mastoid, suprasternal	Discrete; usually has overlying or nearby pore or fistula, which may retract with swallowing; nontender unless infected	Present at birth; often not noticed until infection produces enlargement, pain, and overlying erythema with or without drainage
Thyroglossal duct cyst	Midline, often at level of hyoid or just below	Discrete; usually has overlying pore or fistula; moves with tongue movement	Present at birth; often not noticed until infection produces enlargement, pain and overlying erythema, with or without drainage
Dermoid cyst	Midline, often submental or suprasternal	Discrete, smooth; doughy or rubbery; nontender; does not retract with swallowing	Infancy/childhood
Laryngocele	Just lateral to midline along anterior border of sternocleidomastoid	Soft, compressible, may gurgle on compression; increases in size with straining or crying; nontender unless infected; may have associated stridor or hoarseness; may have air fluid level on X-ray	Infancy/childhood
Esophageal diverticulum	Paratracheal, usually on the left	Soft, compressible; increases in size with crying or straining; nontender; may have history of dysphagia and/or aspiration	Infancy/childhood
Sialadenitis	Preauricular extending under and behind ear, submandibular, submental	Firm; mildly tender when viral; exquisitely tender when suppurative, with pus exuding from orifice; pain increased with eating, especially lemons; elevated serum or urine amylase	Any age
Teratoma	Midline or paramedian	Solitary; firm with irregular border; rapid increase in size; may have calcifications on X-ray	Infancy/childhood

FIG. 12.52 Differential diagnosis of cervical adenopathy/adenitis.

lary nodes. Wound and skin infections, cellulitis, and herpes zoster are major sources of axillary adenitis in childhood.

THE INGUINAL LYMPH NODES

The inguinal nodes are divided into two groups by Poupart's ligament, with those above the ligament being termed inguinal nodes and those below it termed femoral. The inguinal group receives lymphatics from the external genitalia, anus, umbilicus, lower abdomen and back, buttocks and upper thigh, and also may drain the lower leg. Thus, in addition to wound and skin infections, perianal, intra-ab-

DIFFERENTIAL DIAGNOSIS OF CERVICAL ADENOPATHY/ADENITIS

Type of Mass	Usual Site	Character	Time of Appearance
Thyroid goiter	Isthmus (midline), and lobes (paratracheal)	Diffuse enlargement; usually smooth contour and soft consistency, occasionally nodular; moves with swallowing	Occasionally neonatal (with maternal ingestion of iodides); childhood in endemic areas (iodine-deficient water); child-hood/adolescence in familial cases
Graves' disease	Isthmus (midline), and lobes (paratracheal)	Diffuse enlargement; smooth contour and soft consistency; moves with swallowing; associated signs of thyrotoxicosis and exophthalmos	Childhood/adolescence
Hashimoto's thyroiditis	Isthmus (midline) and lobes (paratracheal)	Diffuse enlargement; distinct contours; firm or rubbery; surface may be irregular; may have neck soreness and dysphagia; may have symptoms of mild hyperthyroidism	Childhood/adolescence
Thyroid carcinoma	Usually in lateral lobe or at junction of isthmus and lobe	Solitary mass; firm or hard and differs in consistency from rest of gland; may have associated adenopathy; may have past history of irradiation	Childhood/adolescence
Leukemia	Any cervical node or nodes	Firm to hard; often enlarges rapidly; may be fixed or matted; nontender; often other regions involved; often hepatosplenomegaly; may have fever, anorexia, weight loss, bone pain, pallor, petechiae	Any age
Non-Hodgkin's lymphoma	Spinal accessory, supraclavicular	Firm to hard; enlarges rapidly; may be fixed or matted; nontender; often other regions are involved; may have fever, anorexia, weight loss, bone and joint pain	5–15 years
Hodgkin's disease	Anterior or posterior cervical, preauricular, supraclavicular	Firm, occasionally rubbery; slow growing; may be mobile, fixed or matted; nontender; often otherwise asymptomatic; may have fever, malaise, weight loss, night sweats hepatosplenomegaly	Usually > 5 years
Rhabdomyo-sarcoma	Nasopharyngeal, parotid, anterior or posterior cervical	Primary nasopharyngeal: symptoms of enlarged adenoids; later serosan-guineous nasal discharge, weight loss, cranial nerve deficits, and secondary node enlargement. Primary parotid or cervical: hard, painless, nontender mass	Any age, but more common in early childhood

dominal, and genital infections may serve as sources of in-guinal adenitis. The femoral nodes primarily drain the foot and lower leg. The popliteal nodes receive drainage from the foot and lower leg, but like the epitrochlear nodes, they are unusual sites of adenitis.

Having discussed the general features of acute lympha-denitis in contrast to those of adenopathy, as well as the regions of involvement and their likely sources, we now can look at the characteristics of adenitis produced by the various causative organisms.

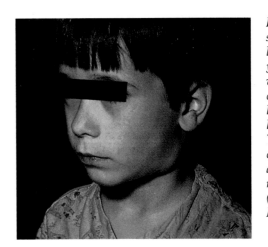

FIG. 12.53 Acute suppurative lymphadenitis. This youngster was seen within 24 hours of onset of painful enlargement of the left tonsillar node. There was mild overlying edema and the node was markedly tender. (Courtesy of Dr. M. Sherlock)

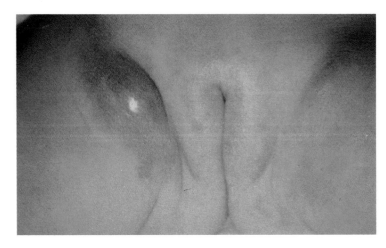

FIG. 12.54 Acute suppurative lymphadenitis. Increased pain and erythema, thinning of the overlying skin, and fluctuance on palpation signal that central necrosis has occurred. (Courtesy of Dr. M. Sherlock)

Acute Suppurative (Staphylococcal and Streptococcal) Lymphadenitis

Group A β-hemolytic streptococci and coagulase-positive staphylococci are responsible for the majority of cases of acute lymphadenitis, regardless of anatomical region. Together they account for up to 80 percent of cases of cervical adenitis alone. In recent years staphylococcal infections have surpassed in frequency those due to streptococci. Other than culture there is no way to distinguish between the two clinically, as the clinical picture for both consists of sudden painful and rapid enlargement usually of a single node. The involved node is firm and exquisitely tender, and may range in diameter from 2 to 6 cm (Fig. 12.53). Within 24 to 72 hours the overlying soft tissue becomes edematous and the skin, erythematous. As many as 50 percent of patients may be febrile and some appear toxic; bacteremia develops in a small percentage. Left untreated, suppuration occurs during the next several days, and is detectable as central fluctuance. Simultaneously, thinning of the overlying skin may be noted as the process points to the surface (Fig. 12.54). Occasionally the abscess may point inward rupturing into the soft tissues and dissecting along tissue planes with potentially catastrophic effects. Prompt institution of antimicrobial therapy can significantly alter this course. When high-dose oral therapy is started prior to development of overlying cellulitic changes, such changes may be prevented and enlargement halted and followed by regression. Even cases with swelling and erythema at the start of therapy may not progress to suppuration. Patients with high fever and toxicity require parenteral treatment, as do children who fail to improve on oral medication. Suppuration necessitates incision and drainage.

Cervical nodes, especially the tonsillar and anterior cervical, are the most common sites of adenitis due to streptococci or staphylococci. Patients usually are young children with a peak incidence between 1 and 4 years. Many have a history of antecedent rhinitis, often associated with impetiginization of the anterior nares and anterior cervical adenopathy. Cough, anorexia, vomiting, and fever also may be present. These findings may persist or they may clear prior to the onset of adenitis. In older children a recent episode of pharyngitis may be reported, and in a small percentage of these children, adenitis develops in association with a peritonsillar abscess (see Chapter 20). Secondarily infected dermatitis, insect bites, impetigo and wound infections may precede the onset of adenitis in other patients, in which case the node affected depends on the primary site. These infections as well as cellulitis are common antecedents of axillary and inguinal adenitis due to these organisms. Primary sources may be evident at the time adenitis develops, but often they have healed. It is also important to remember that invasive forms of tinea capitis may closely mimic streptococcal and staphylococcal infection, both in appearance of the primary lesion and in the character of the secondary adenitis, although progression to suppuration is unusual. Adenitis due to *Pasteurella multocida* may be clinically indistinguishable, but rarely is associated with systemic symptoms. Furthermore, a history of an antecedent cat or dog bite is common with adenitis due to this organism.

Adenitis Due to Other Bacterial Respiratory Pathogens

On occasion adenitis may be due to infection with *H. influenzae* or with *S. pneumoniae*. In the vast majority of cases nodal inflammation appears in concert with periorbital or buccal cellulitis and is associated with fever and toxicity. Bacteremia is usual. Because patients with these infections receive prompt parenteral therapy, suppuration is rare and regression generally is prompt.

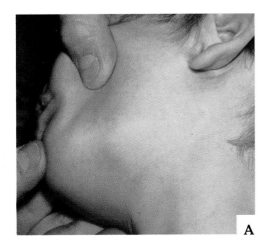 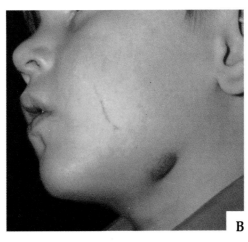 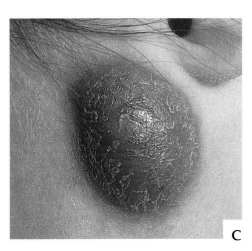

FIG. 12.55 Mycobacterial adenitis. **A,** Early in the course of adenitis due to M. tuberculosis *or atypical mycobacteria, enlargement of the node is gradual, ten-* derness is mild, and there is little or no sign of warmth or overlying inflammation. **B,** After a few to several weeks the overlying skin becomes thickened, tense, discolored, and adherent to the node. **C,** This node was fluctuant, indicating suppuration. (Courtesy of Dr. M. Sherlock)

Adenitis Due to Anaerobes and Mixed Flora

Clinically, this form of adenitis resembles that due to streptococci and staphylococci, although the involved node often is smaller and slower to suppurate. The vast majority of these cases are secondary to dental disease including dental abscesses, gingivitis, and stomatitis; as a result, the submental or submandibular nodes are more likely to be affected. On occasion the adenitis appears simultaneously with facial cellulitis stemming from a dental abscess (see Chapter 18).

Actinomycotic Adenitis

Dental disease is also the primary source of actinomycotic adenitis, which usually affects a submandibular node. Enlargement is gradual, and on palpation the node is firm and lumpy, has an irregular border and is mildly to moderately tender. Over time the center blackens and necroses, and a chronic draining sinus may form. Microscopic examination of the discharge discloses characteristic sulfur granules.

Mycobacterial Lymphadenitis

Although the incidence of tuberculosis has decreased markedly in developed countries, *Mycobacterium tuberculosis* and atypical mycobacteria (especially *Mycobacterium scrofulaceum*) continue to be important sources of lymphadenitis. Recognition of this form of lymphadenitis is important, as its management is considerably different from that of forms arising from other sources. Both typical and atypical organisms cause similar clinical findings. Nodal enlargement is gradual and persistent. The node is slightly to mildly tender and initially there is little or no sign of warmth or overlying inflammation (Fig. 12.55A). After a few to several weeks the node becomes adherent to the overlying skin, which itself becomes thickened and tense, and develops a reddish or reddish-purple discoloration (Figs. 12.55 B and C). Suppuration may occur several weeks to months after onset, and this may

result in rupture through the overlying skin with formation of a chronic draining sinus. The risk of chronic drainage is thought to be markedly increased if aspiration or incision and drainage are attempted. While local clinical findings are similar, there are historical and other differences that can help to distinguish tuberculous adenitis from atypical mycobacterial adenitis.

TUBERCULOUS LYMPHADENITIS

Children with tuberculosis may be of any age and frequently have a positive history of exposure to another infected individual. In the United States they are more likely to be black and to live in cities. Posterior cervical and supraclavicular nodes are the most common sites involved, and in a small percentage of cases adenitis is bilateral. Generalized adenopathy may be noted in as many as 20 percent of patients. Up to 50 percent have systemic symptoms that may include fever, cough, night sweats, anorexia, and malaise. Chest radiographs reveal positive findings suggestive of tuberculosis in 75 percent of cases; the sedimentation rate exceeds 30 in up to 80 percent; and the PPD is positive with more than 10 mm of induration. Treatment of tuberculous adenitis is pharmacologic, with excision reserved for cases with chronic drainage.

ADENITIS DUE TO ATYPICAL MYCOBACTERIA

Patients with atypical mycobacterial adenitis usually are under 4 years of age and are unlikely to have a history of exposure to tuberculosis. In the United States they tend to be Caucasian and from rural areas. A submandibular, preauricular, anterior cervical, inguinal, or epitrochlear node may be the site of involvement. Bilateral adenitis and generalized adenopathy do not occur and systemic symptoms are rare. Chest radiographs rarely are abnormal; only one-third have elevated sedimentation rates; and the PPD is positive with induration ranging from 5 to 10 mm. Atypical mycobacteria typically are resistant to multiple drugs, hence excisional biopsy generally is the treatment of choice. Spontaneous regression can occur, however, making observation a reasonable course if suppuration and/or drainage have not occurred.

Adenitis Associated With Animal or Vector Contact

In a number of children, acute local lymphadenitis is the result of inoculation of a pathogen via an animal scratch or bite, via the bite of an insect vector transmitting a pathogen from an animal host, or by contact with a contaminated animal carcass. In some of these disorders, systemic symptoms are very prominent; in others the local adenitis is the primary manifestation.

PASTEURELLA MULTOCIDA ADENITIS
Suppurative adenitis due to *P. multocida* may occur in patients who develop local infection at the site of a scratch or bite inflicted by a dog or cat. Soon after the manifestations of local infection appear at the primary site, a regional node enlarges and becomes tender. Overlying swelling and redness are common and suppuration may occur early. This picture is clinically indistinguishable from adenitis due to streptococci or staphylococci, but often *P. multocida* infection can be suspected by history. Axillary and inguinal nodes are the most common sites of involvement. Systemic symptoms are unusual.

CAT SCRATCH DISEASE
Adenitis is a primary feature of cat scratch disease, which is thought to be due to an as yet unidentified pleomorphic bacillus that is seen in Warthin-Starry stained sections of biopsied nodes. Low-grade fever may occur in about 25 percent of affected patients. Ninety percent have a history of either an antecedent cat scratch or of contact with cats or kittens. While inoculation via a cat scratch is the most common means of infection, splinters, puncture wounds, and dog scratches also have been implicated. Incidence is highest in fall and winter in temperate climates, with cases occurring with equal frequency year round in tropical areas. Most patients are in the 5 to 14 year age range, but family clusters that include younger children and adults have been reported. Onset of symptoms begins 3 to 30 days following inoculation, with 7 to 12 days being the most common time. A red papule or series of papules is commonly noted at the site of inoculation. Shortly thereafter one or more regional nodes enlarge, becoming mildly painful and tender. Involved nodes are firm, and overlying warmth and mild redness may develop within a few days of enlargement. In order of frequency, axillary, cervical, submandibular, preauricular, epitrochlear, and inguinal nodes have been reported as sites of involvement. In cases involving a preauricular node, associated conjunctivitis is common suggesting conjunctival inoculation as the source. Discomfort generally subsides in 4 to 6 weeks, but the node may remain enlarged or may fluctuate in size for months. Suppuration occurs in about one-third of patients.

As skin test materials generally are unavailable and as methods of culturing the organism are still in the process of being developed, diagnosis is made primarily on the basis of history, clinical picture and course, and/or pathologic findings on excisional biopsy. When infection is suspected expectant follow-up is recommended. If suppuration occurs aspiration is believed by most authorities to be preferable to incision and drainage because of concerns that the latter procedure may lead to prolonged drainage and scarring. In protracted or atypical cases excisional biopsy is suggested.

TULAREMIA
Francisella tularensis may produce an illness in which adenitis is prominent in concert with systemic symptoms. Rabbits, hares, muskrats, and voles serve as endemic sources of this pathogen. Children may acquire the glandular or ulceroglandular form of the disease by handling or skinning dead animals (often encountered on hunting trips or hikes), following an animal bite (especially that of a cat who hunts rabbits), or occasionally from the bite of an insect vector (mosquito, mite, or tick). The incubation period for this illness ranges from 1 to 21 days with an average of 3 to 4 days. Onset generally is abrupt and is characterized by moderate to high fever, chills, headache, myalgias, vomiting, and possibly photophobia. Within 2 days of onset of systemic symptoms, axillary, epitrochlear or inguinal adenitis is noted, and soon thereafter a painful papule appears distal to the involved node at the site of inoculation. This papule ruptures within 1 to 2 days, forming a central ulcer with a raised edge. The involved node is firm and tender and may be associated with overlying erythema. Generalized adenopathy and hepatosplenomegaly may be noted in some cases, and in the second week of illness a blotchy erythematous maculopapular rash (or occasionally a vesicular, pustular or nodose exanthem) may appear. Without treatment fever may persist for 2 to 3 weeks, and the ulcer may take as long as a month to heal. The diagnosis is suggested by history, clinical picture and course, and is confirmed by serologic tests. Streptomycin is the treatment of choice.

BUBONIC PLAGUE
Now rare in developed countries, this infection continues to appear sporadically in people who live or hunt in areas in which infection is endemic in the wild rodent population. Its usual means of transmission is via flea bite, but on occasion inoculation occurs through a break in the skin as a result of handling an infected carcass. Thus inguinal and axillary nodes are the most common sites of bubo formation. The incubation period ranges from several hours to 10 days and is terminated by the abrupt onset of high fever, chills, malaise, weakness, and headache. Pain in the area of a regional node precedes rapid nodal enlargement. The node is fixed, firm, and exquisitely tender with overlying edema. Purplish discoloration is common. The inoculation site may appear normal, or it may be manifest as a skin abscess. Rapid progression of systemic symptoms occurs, with the patient appearing toxic and apprehensive, and often manifesting delirium and signs of neurologic dysfunction. DIC and septic shock may supervene if treatment is not instituted promptly. When infection is suspected the node should be aspirated for culture, blood cultures should be obtained, and broad-spectrum parenteral therapy instituted.

General Approach to Diagnosis of Lymphadenitis

Because of the wide range of pathogens that may produce lymphadenitis, meticulous care must be taken in the process of clinical assessment. The history should include questions concerning antecedent and current signs and symptoms, which may include prior wounds such as cuts, bites, punctures, splinters, or scratches distal to the inflamed node. Exposure to other ill persons or to animals, as well as recent travel, should be determined. Questions also must be asked about the presence or absence of systemic symptoms and their course, and about the rapidity of evolution of the adenitis itself. History of past problems and medication intake are important as well. Physical examination must include precise measurement of size of the inflamed node, in addition to inspection of overlying soft tissue and palpation to determine contour, consistency, and degree of tenderness. The region drained by the involved node must then be inspected for clues as to the probable primary source of infection. Finally close attention should be paid to the child's general status and to other portions of the reticuloendothelial system, e.g., to other nodal regions as well as to the liver and spleen.

With the above information the specific pathogen may be evident on clinical grounds alone or the differential diagnostic possibilities may be considerably narrowed, enabling confirmation by a minimum of laboratory tests. Close follow-up is important for all children treated as outpatients, to monitor their clinical course and response to therapy.

BACTERIAL BONE AND JOINT INFECTIONS

Osteomyelitis

The anatomy and physiology of growing bone places children at particular risk for bacterial infection, and in fact 85 percent of cases of osteomyelitis occur in children under 16 years of age. The highest incidence occurs in infancy with a secondary peak between 8 to 12 years, in most series. During infancy males and females are affected with equal frequency but thereafter, males predominate in a ratio of 2–3 to 1. The advent of antimicrobial therapy and advances in diagnostic techniques have significantly altered the course and outcome. Mortality has fallen from 25 percent in the pre-antibiotic era, to 1 to 2 percent; morbidity has dropped from 50 percent to less than 15 percent.

S. aureus and β-hemolytic streptococci are the most commonly identified pathogens in all age groups. *H. influenzae* type B and *S. pneumoniae* also are important causes in children under 2 years of age. *Staphylococcus epidermidis*, combined infections, and gram-negative organisms account for a smaller percentage of cases. Salmonella is of particular importance in children with sickle hemoglobinopathies, and pseudomonas often is isolated in cases resulting from puncture wounds to the foot. Despite cultures, in 15 to 20 percent of cases no causative organism is identified, often as a result of suppression by prior antibiotic therapy. Once bacteria have become established within bone, they stimulate an inflammatory response with formation of exudate. As this collects local pressure increases, promoting extension outward and causing further vascular stasis and thrombophlebitis. The resultant ischemia causes local bone necrosis. With further progression dead bone can form a sequestrum surrounded by purulent material, which becomes inaccessible to antimicrobial penetration.

An appreciation of the anatomic and physiologic features of bone in general and of growing bone in particular is essential to an understanding of the pathophysiology of osteomyelitis in childhood. Nutrient vessels enter the diaphysis from the periosteum and extend to the metaphysis (or, in flat and irregular bones, to the area adjacent to the epiphysis) where terminal arterioles form loops and empty into larger sinusoidal veins. This area is one of sluggish somewhat turbulent blood flow, which is prone to thrombosis and which serves as an ideal site for bacterial deposition in the face of bacteremia. Furthermore, being devoid of phagocytic macrophages, the sinusoidal veins lack a major line of defense against bacteria. In infants under 8 to 12 months of age, a number of additional factors facilitate the rapid extension of infection, once it is present. As the epiphyseal plate has not fully formed, the nutrient arterioles penetrate into the epiphysis; hence rupture of infection into the adjacent joint is common. The cortex of the infant's metaphysis is thin and the trabeculae are fewer in number, facilitating penetration outward to a more loosely attached periosteum, as well as extension toward the diaphysis. Thus infants are far more likely to have extensive involvement, even with early diagnosis. Once the epiphyseal growth plate has formed, it serves as a relatively effective barrier to joint extension, substantially reducing the frequency of secondary septic arthritis, although sympathetic joint effusions are not uncommon. Exceptions to this are cases of hematogenous osteomyelitis involving the proximal metaphysis of the humerus or femur and of the distal fibula, where the synovium of the adjacent joint inserts so as to include the metaphysis within the joint.

Based on the mode of acquisition, osteomyelitis has been classified into three major categories. Hematogenous spread accounts for over 50 percent of cases in childhood. Areas of rich blood supply and sluggish flow are most vulnerable to bacterial seeding, hence the metaphyseal portions of long bones and the subepiphyseal portions of flat and irregular bones are the usual sites of involvement in this category. In many cases of hematogenous osteomyelitis, prior respiratory and skin infections appear to be the original source of infection and bacterial seeding. Children with sickle hemoglobinopathies are particularly vulnerable to hematogenous osteomyelitis as a result of their vulnerability to bacteremia and sepsis and because of their predisposition to sludging and infarction. Spread from a contiguous focus of infection accounts for most of the remaining cases of osteomyelitis in childhood. Infections of fracture sites, surgical wounds, and puncture wounds, or extension of infection from an adjacent cellulitis or abscess serves as the predisposing condition, with localization dependent on the original site of injury or infection. While important in adults peripheral vascular disease is rarely a predisposing condition in childhood. When such cases are seen, the patient usually is an adolescent with long-standing diabetes mellitus, and the small bones of the hands or feet are the most common sites of involvement. In all three categories of osteomyelitis, trauma appears to be a significant predisposing factor, perhaps by virtue of producing local small-vessel occlusion with secondary stasis, anoxia, and necrosis.

In addition to categorization by mode of spread or acquisition, osteomyelitis is further subdivided into acute, subacute, and chronic forms according to duration of symptoms. Of these the acute form is by far the most common. The major clinical findings in each form consist of localized bone pain, which typically is constant, severe, and exacerbated by movement. The overlying soft tissues may be warm, swollen and occasionally erythematous, but in contrast to the findings in cellulitis, they generally are not indurated. Spasm of overlying muscles is often intense adding to discomfort, and the adjacent joint may be held in

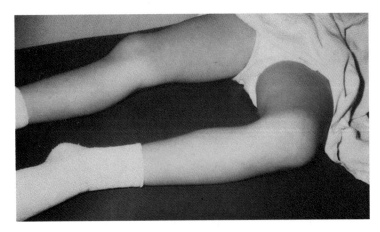

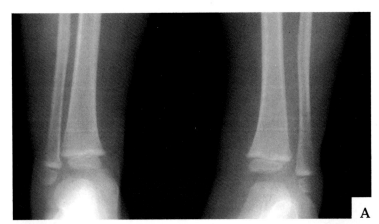

FIG. 12.56 Osteomyelitis. Fever, hip and thigh pain, and a refusal to walk were the chief complaints of this 5-year-old child with osteomyelitis of the proximal femur. On inspection she lay quite still, holding the left leg externally rotated and flexed at the hip and knee. This same position also is adopted by children with acute arthritis of the hip.

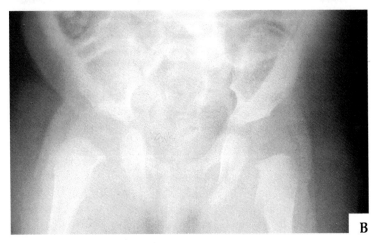

FIG. 12.57 Radiographic findings of acute osteomyelitis. Radiographic changes lag behind the clinical in osteomyelitis. **A**, The first noticeable change, about 3 days after onset, is deep soft-tissue swelling, seen here adjacent to the metaphysis of the distal tibia on the left. **B**, In this neonate a radiolucency is evident in the proximal metaphysis of the right femur, which also is displaced upward and laterally. On aspiration of the hip, purulent fluid was obtained confirming the suspicion of rupture of the infection into the hip and of secondary septic arthritis. (**A** courtesy of Dr. J. Ledesma-Medina, **B** courtesy of Dr. R. Dominguez)

flexion. Beyond these common features there is a wide range of clinical pictures. Appreciation of this spectrum is important to ensure early diagnosis, thus resulting in a more favorable outcome.

ACUTE OSTEOMYELITIS
Acute Hematogenous Osteomyelitis

In the acute hematogenous form of osteomyelitis, the mode of presentation and clinical findings are significantly age dependent, although most patients present within 1 week of onset of symptoms. Infants under 6 months of age often have no systemic signs of infection. However, a small percentage may have low-grade fever, and a few may present with a frankly septic picture. Early on, irritability and anorexia are the major manifestations. Within a few days evidence of pain on movement and/or of decreased use of a limb may be noted (pseudoparalysis). At this time or soon after, localized soft-tissue swelling may be noted. This often extends rapidly to involve the entire extremity, reflecting rapid spread of infection in the underlying bone. For the same reason tenderness also is diffuse. Furthermore multiple bones may be involved. Careful attention must be given to joint examination because of the high risk of early joint extension and secondary septic arthritis.

In children 8 months to 2 years of age, fever and signs of toxicity are common although not universal. History and/or persistent signs of antecedent upper respiratory tract or skin infection are present in over 50 percent of cases. In many cases systemic symptoms consist primarily of fever and irritability in association with a refusal to walk, a limp, or decreased use of an extremity. A small percentage present with more severe systemic symptoms that may include chills, lethargy, irritability, anorexia, vomiting, and dehydration. At this age children often are unable or unwilling to point to the site of discomfort, but on observation may be found to avoid moving the involved extremity or to hold a particular joint in flexion *consistently*. Soft-tissue swelling and warmth may be noted overlying a metaphysis, but this often is subtle or absent in early cases, and it is undetectable in cases where the proximal femur is involved. Comparative circumferential

measurements of suspected areas, and painstaking care in first eliciting the child's cooperation, and then in palpating for evidence of muscle spasm and/or point tenderness are well worth the effort when osteomyelitis is suspected. Even then, focal tenderness may be difficult to detect early in the course.

Children over 2 years of age with acute osteomyelitis are usually febrile but rarely toxic. They are more likely to complain of and point to a specific site of pain, and point tenderness generally is easy to elicit unless presentation is very early. Older patients describe the pain as deep, intense, and constant. Signs of adjacent joint flexion and of nearby muscle spasm are common (Fig. 12.56) but, again, overlying soft-tissue swelling may be subtle. Unless a sympathetic effusion has developed, the adjacent joint may be passively moved through its full range of motion, although this will exacerbate the pain.

When bones other than the long tubular bones of the extremities are the site of infection, the clinical picture can be especially confusing. Osteomyelitis of the pelvic bones can mimic numerous other conditions. While fever and an abnormal gait are the most common presenting complaints,

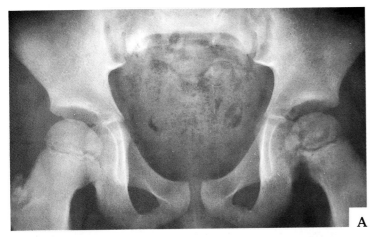

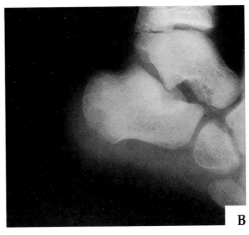

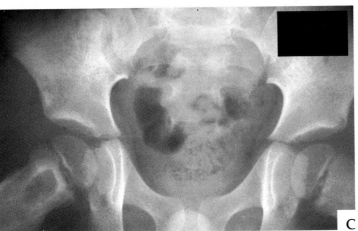

Fig. 12.58 Radiographic findings of acute osteomyelitis. **A,** The epiphysis and proximal metaphysis of the left femur have a moth-eaten appearance in this older child. **B,** Deep and superficial soft-tissue swelling overlie the radiolucent lesion of the calcaneus in this boy who developed pseudomonas osteomyelitis following a puncture wound of the heel. **C,** The late changes of a lytic lesion with sclerotic margins are seen in the right femoral metaphysis of this child who was completing his course of therapy. (**A** and **C** courtesy of Dr. R. Dominguez, **B** courtesy of Dr. E. Wald)

lower abdominal and groin pain, hip and/or buttock pain, sciatica, and thigh pain (with swelling) each have been prominent early complaints in individual patients. Often the initial clinical picture is more suggestive of appendicitis, pelvic abscess, or of infection of the hip or femur than of pelvic osteomyelitis. Diagnosis necessitates a high level of suspicion and great care in examination. In patients presenting with abdominal complaints, the lack of rebound tenderness, the lesser prominence of gastrointestinal symptoms, the onset of pain in the lower abdomen rather than in the periumbilical region, and normal findings on rectal examination can help to distinguish the process from that of acute appendicitis. Furthermore, while the majority of patients have pain on hip motion in one or more planes, range of motion either is normal or only slightly limited, and with careful examination point tenderness usually can be detected.

Acute Osteomyelitis Due to Contiguous Spread

Acute osteomyelitis as a result of contiguous spread of infection must be suspected in those patients with prior puncture wounds, deep lacerations, surgical incisions, fractures, abscesses, or cellulitis who experience a sudden onset of increased pain at the wound site. This pain is perceived as deep, severe and constant, and is aggravated by movement. In these cases soft-tissue cellulitis is a common associated finding and fever is usual. Often when extension of primary soft-tissue infection is the source, the patient may have worsened clinically after a period of improvement on antimicrobial therapy or may have failed to show the expected response to therapy.

Diagnostic Methods in Acute Osteomyelitis

Short of definitive cultures standard radiographic and laboratory studies are of somewhat limited use in the diagnosis of acute osteomyelitis. The sedimentation rate is elevated in the vast majority of cases and exceeds 40 in about 80 percent. This finding is helpful primarily in confirming that an inflammatory process is the source of symptoms. White blood cell counts, while usually elevated with a left shift in differential, may be normal in as many as 50 percent of cases and thus are less useful. Radiographic changes lag behind the clinical process and can be subtle. The first noticeable change, which is seen about 3 days after onset of symptoms, is the presence of deep soft-tissue swelling displacing fat lines adjacent to a metaphysis (Fig. 12.57A). In ensuing days the swelling increases to obliterate fascial planes, and then extends to involve subcutaneous tissues. These soft-tissue changes can be very difficult to appreciate when osteomyelitis involves bones of the trunk or pelvis; however, in cases of pelvic osteomyelitis, clouding of the obturator foramen, distortion of the fascial planes around the adjacent hip, or even displacement of the bladder may be detectable. When a sympathetic joint effusion is present or when rupture into the adjacent joint has resulted in secondary septic arthritis, joint-space widening and/or bony displacement may be evident (Fig. 12.57B). Bony changes are not visible radiographically until 7 to 10 days after onset in untreated patients. These changes consist of periosteal elevation followed by focal evidence of bony lysis, and subsequently, by sclerosis or new bone formation at the margins of the lytic lesion (Fig. 12.58). Early diagnosis and treatment may prevent bony radiographic changes completely.

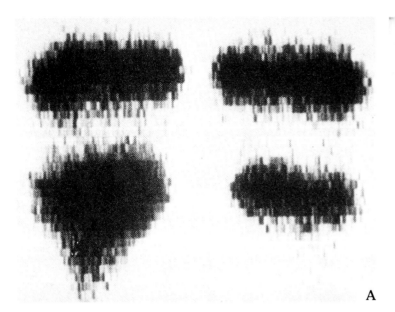
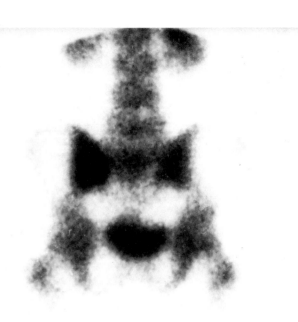

A   B

FIG. 12.59 Technetium scan findings in acute osteomyelitis.
A, *In this radionuclide scan, selectively increased uptake is seen in the proximal right tibial metaphysis. The uptake in the epiphyses is normal reflecting active bone growth.* **B**, *This youngster presented with a puzzling picture of abdominal pain* *suggestive of an acute abdomen. A bone scan was obtained after other studies were unrevealing. The increased uptake in the right sacroiliac area helped to identify osteomyelitis as the source of symptoms. (Courtesy of Dr. E. Wald)*

Technetium scanning has provided a better means of early identification and localization of sites of acute osteomyelitis. It can be positive as early as 24 to 48 hours after onset of symptoms revealing discrete areas of increased uptake (Fig. 12.59A). The procedure has been particularly useful as a diagnostic adjunct in cases of pelvic and vertebral osteomyelitis in which the mode of presentation has simulated the clinical picture of another condition (Fig. 12.59B). It also can be helpful in distinguishing osteomyelitis from cellulitis, septic arthritis, and acute bony infarcts. With cellulitis, intense deep soft-tissue uptake is seen with faint diffuse uptake in underlying bone; in septic arthritis the scan may be normal, or when accompanied by overlying cellulitis, it may show increased periarticular soft-tissue uptake; in early infarcts, uptake is decreased. Scans also are helpful in delineating additional areas of involvement in the small percentage of cases with multiple sites. Standard radiographs remain important, however, in identifying fractures and malignancies, which may simulate the appearance of osteomyelitis on bone scan. Bone scans have the additional limitation of an occasional false-negative reading, possibly due to local ischemia. When clinical suspicion remains high, a repeat technetium scan or a gallium scan (which identifies purulent exudate) should be considered or aspiration should be performed.

Vigorous attempts must be made to isolate the causative organism to optimize therapy on the basis of known sensitivities and a determination of bactericidal levels. Aspiration of the site of maximal tenderness or maximal uptake as revealed by bone scan can be very useful in that it provides material for Gram stain and culture. In cases where purulent material is obtained, operative drainage should be considered strongly. Even in the absence of exudate, flushing the aspirating needle with culture media often will enable isolation of the causative organism. Blood cultures are positive in over 50 percent of cases of acute hematogenous osteomyelitis and should be drawn in all suspected cases.

Complications of osteomyelitis include secondary septic arthritis with resultant joint damage, epiphyseal injury with long-term morbidity from impaired bone growth, progression to chronic osteomyelitis (now seen in less than 4 percent of cases), and rarely pathologic fractures. The rate of complications is highest in young infants who often have extensive bony involvement and secondary septic arthritis by the time the diagnosis is made. Care in clinical assessment and aggressive attempts to confirm the diagnosis of acute osteomyelitis as early as possible are as important to ensuring good outcome and minimizing complications as are adequate antimicrobial therapy and recognition of the need for surgical intervention where appropriate. Close collaboration between pediatrician and orthopedic surgeon is essential in order to optimize decisions regarding the route and duration of pharmacotherapy, and the need for and timing of surgical intervention when indicated.

SUBACUTE OSTEOMYELITIS

Approximately 10 percent of cases of hematogenous osteomyelitis have an insidious onset and a subacute course often characterized by mild to moderate local pain in an extremity, with or without swelling. Fever is unusual and other systemic symptoms are absent. Typically the patient has had symptoms for a few to several weeks prior to presentation. In some instances this subacute course appears to be related to partial suppression of the infection by antibiotics that have been administered for infection at another site (such as for otitis media, tonsillitis, or impetigo). In these patients pain may improve during the period of antimicrobial therapy only to worsen once they stop taking the medication. In other cases in which antibiotics have not been prescribed, reduced bacterial virulence is postulated. On examination local tenderness is evident and overlying soft-tissue swelling may be noted. By the time diagnosis is made, multiple sites are involved in as many as 20 percent of patients. However secondary sites may not be symptomatic.

While white blood cell counts usually are normal, the sedimentation rate is elevated in most (but not all) patients. Blood cultures rarely are positive. Radiographs may show one of several possible findings. In children presenting within

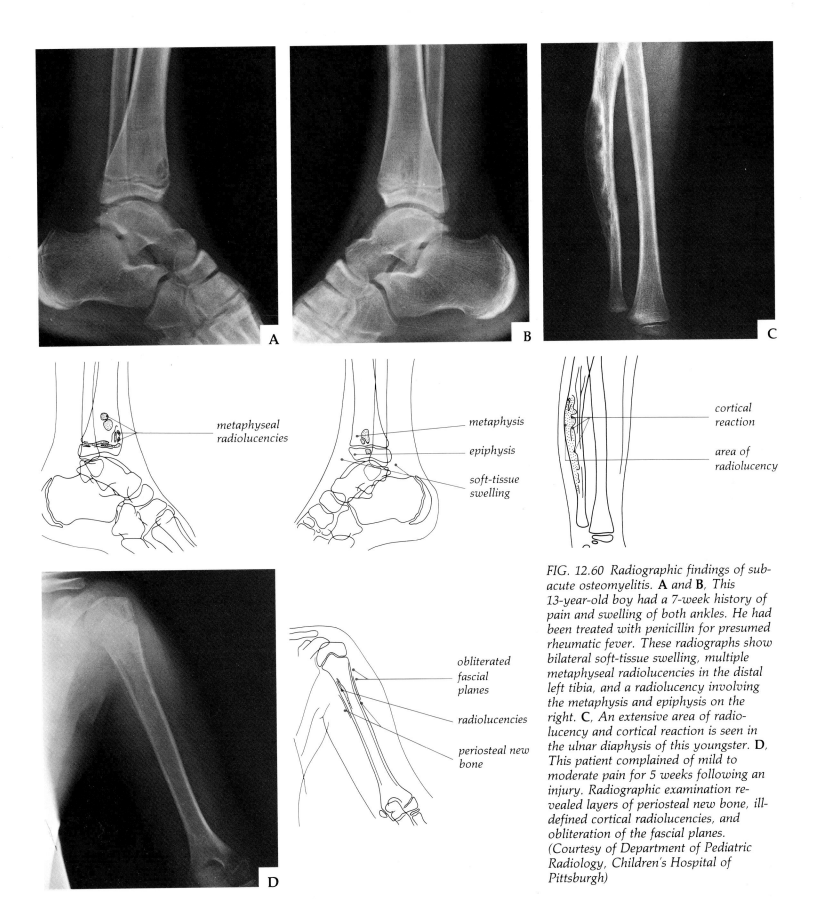

FIG. 12.60 Radiographic findings of subacute osteomyelitis. **A** and **B**, This 13-year-old boy had a 7-week history of pain and swelling of both ankles. He had been treated with penicillin for presumed rheumatic fever. These radiographs show bilateral soft-tissue swelling, multiple metaphyseal radiolucencies in the distal left tibia, and a radiolucency involving the metaphysis and epiphysis on the right. **C**, An extensive area of radiolucency and cortical reaction is seen in the ulnar diaphysis of this youngster. **D**, This patient complained of mild to moderate pain for 5 weeks following an injury. Radiographic examination revealed layers of periosteal new bone, ill-defined cortical radiolucencies, and obliteration of the fascial planes. (Courtesy of Department of Pediatric Radiology, Children's Hospital of Pittsburgh)

a few weeks of onset who have taken antibiotics, radiographic findings may simulate the deep soft-tissue swelling characteristic of early acute osteomyelitis. Other configurations include an isolated metaphyseal radiolucency surrounded by reactive bone (Brodie's abscess); a metaphyseal radiolucency with loss or disruption of cortical bone simulating a tumor; excessive cortical reaction in the diaphysis simulating an osteoid osteoma; or multiple layers of subperiosteal new bone overlying the diaphysis, at times mimicking the appearance of Ewing's sarcoma (Fig. 12.60). While a bone scan is not of great use in distinguishing subacute osteomyelitis from a primary bone tumor, it can be very helpful in revealing other sites of involvement. Because the long course, clinical picture and radiographic findings of this infection often are indistinguishable from those of a neoplastic process, biopsy generally is required to establish the diagno-

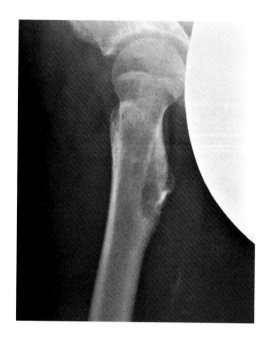

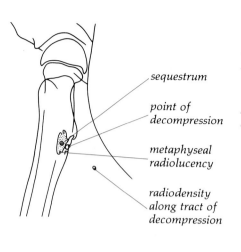

FIG. 12.61 Chronic osteomyelitis. Inadequate initial treatment resulted in progression to chronic osteomyelitis in this child. In this radiograph, taken 6 months after onset of symptoms, a radio-dense sequestrum is seen within the metaphyseal radiolucency. The process also had begun to decompress into the soft tissues of the thigh. (Courtesy of Department of Pediatric Radiology, Children's Hospital of Pittsburgh)

sequestrum

point of decompression

metaphyseal radiolucency

radiodensity along tract of decompression

sis and to isolate the causative organism. In the vast majority of cases, a coagulase-positive staphylococcus is found. Surgical curettage, immobilization, and antimicrobials are the mainstays of treatment.

CHRONIC OSTEOMYELITIS

With the advent of antimicrobial therapy and improvements in diagnostic techniques, chronic osteomyelitis has become a relatively rare entity in countries where there is ready access to medical care. Delay in diagnosis, inadequate antimicrobial and/or surgical therapy, and unusually resistant organisms are the major factors associated with this outcome. Pathophysiologically, extensive necrosis, sequestrum formation as a result of bone death, and decompression via fistulization through the overlying soft tissues are characteristic (Fig. 12.61). Patients continue to be troubled by local pain of varying severity and by chronic draining sinuses. Aggressive surgical curettage and long-term antimicrobial therapy are required to achieve resolution, but, despite this, permanent functional disability and deformity are not uncommon once osteomyelitis has progressed to a chronic phase.

JUVENILE DISCITIS AND VERTEBRAL OSTEOMYELITIS

Inflammation of an intervertebral disc space in childhood is a puzzling disorder, both in terms of the elucidation of its exact pathophysiology and in terms of its mode of presentation. Prior to the third decade of life, vascular channels penetrate through the vertebral end plates and communicate with the intervertebral disc. Thus it is thought that hematogenously spread organisms are more likely to alight in the disc space of children and adolescents, whereas thereafter they may lodge in vascular arcades adjacent to the subchondral plate of the vertebra itself. This factor has been used to explain the higher frequency of discitis in childhood and the relative infrequency of acute vertebral osteomyelitis prior to adulthood. However, differences in clinical picture, the lower frequency of isolation of pathogens, and evidence that immobilization alone is effective in treating discitis, while antimicrobial therapy is required in vertebral osteomyelitis have led to speculation that disc-space inflammation may be due to a low-grade viral or bacterial infection.

Known predisposing conditions in adults include urinary tract infections, pelvic inflammatory disease and bowel and urinary tract surgery, while in children they include upper respiratory tract infection, gastroenteritis, and genitourinary infection. The importance of antecedent trauma is unclear. Hematogenous spread may occur through the valveless veins of Batson's plexus or via the vertebral branches of the posterior spinal arteries. In both discitis and vertebral osteomyelitis, coagulase-positive staphylococci are the organisms most commonly isolated, followed by streptococci, gram-negative enteric pathogens, and corynebacteria. The lumbar spine and the lower thoracic spine are the most common sites of involvement for both entities.

The clinical picture of discitis, which is seen predominantly in children under age 4, is dominated by pain and progressive limp. Often the pain is perceived as focal back pain of progressively worsening severity. In a few instances it may be perceived as primarily worse in the flank, abdomen, or hip. It is constant, may be aggravated by sitting, standing, or movement, and typically it is worse at night. Children who are too young to describe their pain may present with a picture of irritability and the refusal to walk or even sit. In some cases increased irritability has been noted during diaper changes. Adoption of an abnormal posture is a frequent finding. Most commonly this posture is one of exaggerated lumbar lordosis, but in some cases the lumbar spine may be held stiff and straight. Toddlers may assume a knee-chest position. Fever often is present during the first week or two of symptoms, but it may be absent and often is low grade. Other systemic symptoms are unusual. Occasionally abdominal distension is prominent, raising suspicion of intra-abdominal pathology.

Failure to remember that vertebrospinal pathology may result in a limp or refusal to walk, and thus failure to carefully examine the backs of such patients, often results in long delays in diagnosis. Such examination when done may reveal paravertebral muscle spasm with guarding and exquisite focal tenderness, although in some cases tenderness may be vague or absent. Resistance to flexion and extension of the spine is common, and in the young may simulate meningismus. Pain on straight-leg raising and hip motion also may be encountered.

RELATIVE FREQUENCY OF PATHOGENS IN SEPTIC ARTHRITIS ACCORDING TO AGE

Neonate	1 Month–2 Years	2–5 Years	>5 Years
S. aureus	H. influenzae type B	S. aureus	S. aureus
Group B streptococci	Group A streptococci	Group A streptococci	Group A streptococci
Gram-negative enteric pathogens	S. pneumoniae	H. influenzae type B	Neisseria gonorrhoeae
	N. meningitidis	N. meningitidis	P. aeruginosa
	P. aeruginosa	S. pneumoniae	
	Salmonella species		

FIG. 12.62 Relative frequency of pathogens in septic arthritis according to age.

The sedimentation rate is elevated unless symptoms have been present for many months, but white blood cell counts are elevated only during the first few weeks. Specific radiographic changes do not appear until 2 to 6 weeks after onset, at which point disc-space narrowing becomes evident. In ensuing weeks irregularities of the adjacent vertebral end plates become apparent. The loss of normal lumbar lordosis or the presence of local scoliosis may be noted early on. A technetium scan can reveal focal increased uptake as early as 1 week after onset of symptoms. Culture of biopsy specimens of the disc space, when obtained early in the course, may yield an offending organism but commonly are negative after a few weeks of symptoms. Blood cultures rarely are positive. The majority of patients improve symptomatically with immobilization alone, and the process appears to resolve after several weeks of casting.

The clinical picture of adult vertebral osteomyelitis, seen sometimes in adolescents, usually is one of insidious onset of gradually progressive back pain that is constant, aggravated by movement, and resistant to analgesics. Fever is absent or low grade. Occasionally the onset is acute with fever and generalized systemic symptoms accompanying the abrupt appearance of pain. In the rare cases reported in young children, onset usually has been acute and the clinical picture dominated by abdominal and/or flank pain, with associated tenderness and often guarding. In some patients paraspinous or spinous process tenderness, back stiffness, and pain on leg motion or lower extremity weakness also may be noted. Laboratory findings are similar to those of children with discitis, with the exception that blood cultures obtained in the acute phase generally are positive. Early radiographic findings also are similar, but following the appearance of disc-space narrowing, frank destructive lesions of the vertebral body are seen. Cultures of operative biopsy specimens usually are positive for S. aureus. Antimicrobial therapy is necessary to achieve clinical resolution, and surgical debridement is more likely to be required.

Septic Arthritis

Bacterial invasion of the synovial membrane with resultant septic arthritis is a condition with a high potential for long-term morbidity. Release of lysosomal enzymes by attracted leukocytes, abscess formation, formation of granulation tissue, and ischemia resulting from increased intra-articular pressure act in concert to damage the articular surface and to promote synovial fibrosis and bony ankylosis. Early diagnosis and treatment are essential to prevent or at least to minimize the extent of irreversible damage. This however is hindered in many cases by overlap, in both clinical picture and laboratory findings, with viral and other forms of acute arthritis.

Septic arthritis is a disorder primarily of young children with two-thirds to three-fourths of cases occurring in patients under 5 years of age. Males are affected twice as often as females. Ninety percent of cases are the result of hematogenous seeding in the course of bacteremia, and while in most cases the affected joint becomes the primary site of localization it is not uncommon for septic arthritis to develop in a child with bacterial meningitis or pneumonia, often becoming manifest early in the course of treatment. As many as 40 percent of patients have a history and/or signs of an antecedent upper respiratory tract infection at the time of diagnosis. This is especially common in cases caused by H. influenzae type B. Streptococcal skin and soft-tissue infections may antedate septic arthritis due to this pathogen. In older children or in adolescents, gonococcal urethritis, vaginitis, and/or cervicitis assumes importance as an antecedent to hematogenous seeding (see Chapter 16). Prior trauma also may predispose and is reported in a significant number of cases. In approximately 10 percent of patients, the septic arthritis is secondary to rupture of a primary osteomyelitis into the joint space. Direct penetrating injury accounts for a small percentage (see Chapter 19).

Bacterial pathogens are isolated in 65 to 75 percent of cases, either from synovial fluid culture, blood culture, or both. The relative frequency of pathogens varies considerably with patient age, as shown in Figure 12.62. Children with sickle hemoglobinopathies are particularly vulnerable to salmonella septic arthritis. Failure to isolate an organism can be explained in some instances by suppression due to prior antibiotic administration, while in other cases it is unclear as to whether the synovium is involved and synovial fluid is spared, whether synovial fluid may impede growth,

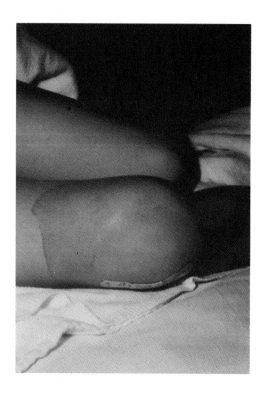

FIG. 12.63 Septic arthritis. This 8-year-old boy awoke suddenly at 3 AM with severe knee pain. By 8 AM he was noted to be febrile and had marked swelling and extreme limitation of movement. There was no overlying erythema. Examination of joint fluid revealed gram-positive cocci in chains, with a white blood cell count of 24,000. Cultures were positive for group A streptococci.

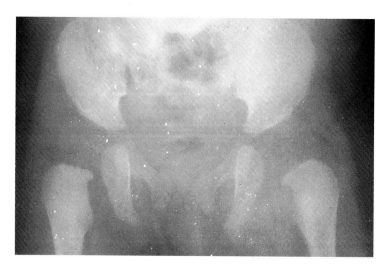

FIG. 12.64 Radiographic findings of septic arthritis. While radiographs may be normal early on, in most cases joint-space widening can be detected. In this infant who presented with fever, toxicity and refusal to move the left leg, capsular swelling and displacement of the proximal femur are readily apparent. (Courtesy of Dr. R. Dominguez)

or whether in some instances the arthritis reflects the actions of bacterial toxins rather than of the organisms themselves.

The knee, hip, elbow and ankle are the joints most commonly affected. The wrist and shoulder are involved less often, with other joints being rare sites of septic arthritis. In over 90 percent of cases, only a single joint is affected. *Neisseria gonorrhoeae* is the organism most commonly associated with multiple joint involvement, but other pathogens may be responsible, particularly coagulase-positive staphylococci and also *H. influenzae* type B. The hip and shoulder joints when involved are particularly prone to damage. Being somewhat hidden, clinical signs may be subtle and thus diagnosis often is delayed. Further, as the synovium inserts distal to the epiphysis of the proximal humerus and femur, compromise of the blood supply to the epiphysis is more likely to occur as a result of increased intra-articular pressure.

The typical clinical picture of hematogenous septic arthritis is one of a young child who presents with moderate to high fever that often is accompanied by signs of toxicity, in association with severe localized joint pain, overlying swelling, and marked limitation in range of motion. The fever may be quite acute in onset or it may have been present for a few days, but presentation tends to occur soon after the onset of joint symptoms. Variations in this picture depend in part on the age of the patient, the joint involved, the causative organism, and the duration of symptoms. Infants and toddlers cannot describe focal pain and thus they tend to present with fever and irritability, the latter of which is aggravated by movement. Refusal to bear weight or decreased use of an extremity may or may not have been noted by the family. When a knee, ankle, wrist, or elbow is involved, local swelling and warmth usually are evident (Fig. 12.63). However with early presentation, swelling may be subtle and high fever may make differential warmth hard to distinguish. Surface erythema often is absent. When a hip is involved, swelling and warmth are not evident externally and pain may be referred to the knee or thigh. Often the position adopted by the patient is the best diagnostic clue. To minimize intra-articular pressure and pain, the child prefers to lie still with the knee and hip flexed and with the hip externally rotated (see Fig. 12.56). In cases of septic arthritis of the shoulder, subtle swelling may or may not be evident but the shoulders may not be held at the same level and the arm on the involved side will be held against the chest to splint the joint.

Septic arthritis of the sacroiliac joint, which accounts for about 1 percent of cases, can present a particularly confusing picture often mimicking hip or intra-abdominal disease. Only one-third of patients have an acute presentation, the remainder having a subacute course. Buttock pain, limp, and fever are the most common presenting complaints. Unilateral radicular pain may be described by as many as one-third of patients. Findings of lower abdominal and rectal tenderness in association with normal hip motion may fool the examiner who fails to recognize that leg and buttock pain necessitate meticulous examination of the lower back. Such an exam will reveal tenderness over the involved sacroiliac joint, and pelvic compression will replicate the pain as will hyperextension of the ipsilateral hip, with the patient supine and dangling his leg over the edge of the table.

Limitation of joint motion and evidence of pain on motion are perhaps the most valuable clinical clues to the diagnosis of septic arthritis. Limitation usually is severe unless presentation is very early, and motion obviously provokes marked discomfort. In young patients with fever and decreased use of an extremity but without clear-cut swelling, localization often is possible if, after careful inspection and palpation for bony tenderness, each joint is gently moved while the examiner carefully guards the other joints, without touching them. Diagnosis can be particularly difficult in neonates and very young infants, who may be afebrile and often will have no systemic symptoms. In such cases decreased use of an extremity often is the earliest clue. Pain on motion usually is evident, however, even before the appearance of localized swelling.

When septic arthritis is the result of rupture of a focus of osteomyelitis into a joint, distinction between the two processes can be very difficult to establish clinically. Focal pain generally is of longer duration, but as most cases occur in infants under 8 months this clue often is unavailable. In older children the hip, shoulder, and ankle are the major sites of this secondary form of septic arthritis. These children usually will have a history of prolonged focal pain, antedating a brief period of respite, followed by the sudden return of pain that is markedly aggravated by joint motion. In the days following a penetrating joint injury, a sudden increase in pain and swelling should lead to immediate suspicion of secondary septic arthritis.

Because of the high cost of delays in diagnosis in terms of morbidity, any child with fever, acute onset of pain, and limited motion of a joint should be presumed to have septic arthritis until proven otherwise. These findings should prompt expeditious diagnostic investigation. Plain radiographs with comparison views should be obtained without delay and inspected carefully for even subtle signs of joint-space widening or capsular distention, although in early cases findings may be normal. When the hip is the suspected site of pathology, lateral and upward displacement of the femoral head may be noted along with displacement of the gluteal fat lines (Fig. 12.64). A bone scan is perhaps the best method of evaluating the child with suspected septic arthritis of the sacroiliac joint. Arthrocentesis should be considered early, as examination of joint fluid is the study most likely to yield definitive results. A heparinized syringe should be used to prevent spontaneous clotting. Positive findings on Gram stain are particularly helpful; cultures are positive in 60 percent or more of cases. Pleocytosis is common with two-thirds of patients having more than 50,000 white blood cells. It is crucial to remember, however, that there is considerable overlap with nonbacterial arthritis in cell counts, differential counts, and protein and glucose levels found on examination of synovial fluid. Thus septic arthritis cannot be ruled out when these values are within the normal range. Peripheral white blood cell counts and sedimentation rate may add suggestive evidence, but again there is overlap with viral arthritis. As many as 20 percent of patients have white blood cell counts under 10,000, although most have a significant left shift. The sedimentation rate may be markedly elevated, but it is under 40 in as many as 45 percent of cases. Blood cultures are positive in up to 40 percent of patients. Counterimmunoelectrophoresis studies may be helpful in identifying the responsible pathogen before culture results are available and in cases where cultures prove negative. Bone scans are useful in identifying patients with underlying osteomyelitis.

Diagnosis thus is dependent on assessment of the assembled data including clinical course, physical findings, and results of multiple laboratory studies. Even with a negative Gram stain, empiric antimicrobial therapy selected to cover the most likely pathogens (see Fig. 12.62) should be started, pending cultures, for cases in which septic arthritis is deemed likely on the basis of other available findings. As is true of osteomyelitis, collaboration between pediatric and orthopedic colleagues is essential, for drainage of infected material is essential to good outcome.

Any disorder associated with acute arthritis must be considered as part of the differential diagnosis. In some instances the clinical picture of an obvious viral or vasculitic syndrome enables differentiation. The polymigratory picture of acute rheumatic fever and the much less acute onset of juvenile rheumatoid arthritis help to distinguish these conditions.

Adenopathy, visceromegaly, anemia, and radiographic changes help distinguish malignant joint infiltration.

CONGENITAL AND PERINATAL INFECTIONS

A number of pathogens that produce relatively mild or even subclinical disease in children and adults can cause severe disease with devastating sequelae, when infection is acquired prenatally or perinatally. Toxoplasmosis, rubella, cytomegalic inclusion disease, herpes simplex infection (the TORCH diseases), and congenital syphilis are well-known sources of pathology. In addition sepsis, meningitis, pneumonia, and other infections due to numerous perinatally acquired bacterial pathogens are the cause of significant neonatal morbidity and mortality, especially in infants born prematurely. Because of the breadth of this subject and because of limitations of space, we have elected to limit discussion to three disorders that tend to produce distinctive physical findings.

Congenital Toxoplasmosis

Toxoplasma gondii is an intracellular protozoan that is acquired primarily from consumption of infected raw or undercooked meat, or via ingestion or inhalation of oocysts excreted in cat feces. Occasionally transmission occurs via transfusion or organ transplantation. While most cases of postnatal infection are thought to be subclinical, a mononucleosis-like syndrome and cervical adenopathy have been identified as clinical features, and it may well be that in many cases the clinical picture simulates a viral illness and thus the true cause goes unrecognized.

Prenatally acquired infection has the potential for serious harm to the developing fetus. It is estimated that in the United States 1–2 per 1000 live-born infants have congenitally acquired toxoplasmosis. Maternal infection during pregnancy results in fetal infection less than 50 percent of the time, however. Risk of transmission to the fetus increases as gestation advances, but the severity of fetal injury is greater the earlier the infection occurs during pregnancy. Major sites of involvement are the CNS, retina, choroid, and muscles. As a result of these factors 70 percent of congenitally infected infants appear normal at birth, about 10 to 20 percent are overtly symptomatic, and approximately 10 percent have detectable chorioretinitis without other abnormalities (see Chapter 17). Infected infants without signs of disease and those with mild chorioretinitis alone are at risk for progressive ocular and on occasion CNS involvement if not diagnosed and treated. In many instances, however, the diagnosis is not suspected until signs of visual impairment, strabismus, or developmental delay prompt careful ophthalmologic and neurologic assessment.

In severely infected infants, the clinical picture may closely simulate that of other congenital infections, especially cytomegalovirus. These infants tend to be small for gestational age, may be microcephalic or hydrocephalic, develop early onset jaundice, have hepatosplenomegaly and diffuse adenopathy, and often are covered with petechial and purpuric lesions or with a generalized maculopapular rash. Seizures are common in these infants as is a CSF pleocytosis with increased protein and xanthochromia. Skull radiographs may reveal diffuse cortical calcifications in contrast to the periventricular pattern seen with cytomegalic inclusion disease (Fig. 12.65). Interstitial pneumonitis and myocarditis may be

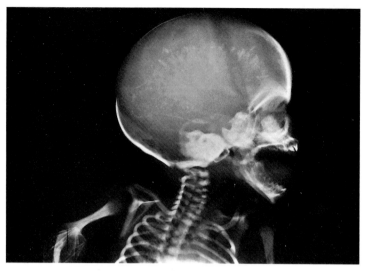

FIG. 12.65 Congenital toxoplasmosis. Microcephaly, ventricular dilatation, and cerebral calcifications were prominent findings in this infant with severe congenital toxoplasmosis. (Courtesy of Department of Pediatric Radiology, Children's Hospital of Pittsburgh)

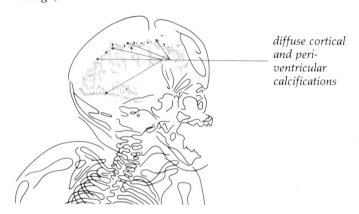

diffuse cortical and peri-ventricular calcifications

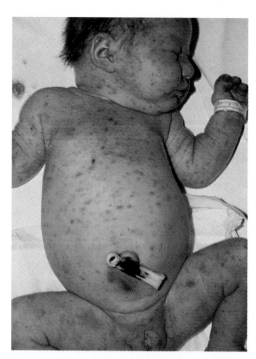

FIG. 12.66 Congenital rubella. This newborn had the full-blown picture of the "expanded rubella syndrome," including a generalized blueberry muffin rash, diffuse petechiae, hepatosplenomegaly, early onset of jaundice and neurologic depression. (Courtesy of Dr. M. Sherlock)

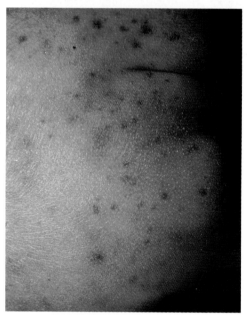

prominent features as well. These infants have a high risk of severe neurodevelopmental sequelae, if they survive. Other infants may appear normal initially but may rapidly develop signs of neonatal myocarditis with minimal CNS manifestations, although they too may have cerebral calcifications, as may infants with apparently isolated chorioretinitis.

Diagnosis is best confirmed by IgM fluorescent antibody testing or, in cases presenting with ocular findings later in infancy, by the Sabin-Feldman dye test. Treatment with pyrimethamine and triple sulfa or sulfadiazine for a 4-week course appears to interrupt the infection and prevent the progression of ocular and CNS injury.

Congenital Rubella

Despite its usually mild manifestations when acquired postnatally, prenatal infection with rubella virus is far from being a benign process. Intrauterine death, variable constellations of congenital anomalies, and severe perinatal illness may result. The mother may or may not have symptomatic illness. In the viremic phase the virus is transmitted to the placenta, and thence in most instances to the fetus. If the fetus becomes infected, mitotic activity is reduced and focal cytolysis and vascular injury occur, resulting in congenital malformations. The earlier in gestation the infection occurs, the greater the potential for injury. Of fetuses infected during the first 8 weeks, 39 percent will spontaneously abort or be stillborn, 25 percent will have gross anomalies noted at birth, and 36 percent will appear normal. Ultimately 85 percent of all liveborn infants infected during the first 8 weeks will be found to have sequelae. Infections in the ensuing 12 weeks pose a gradually decreasing risk of anomalies, and those occurring thereafter do not cause defects. The most commonly encountered anomalies are central diffuse cataracts, congenital heart disease (patent ductus arteriosus, pulmonary artery stenosis, pulmonary valvular stenosis), and sensorineural deafness (usually bilateral, occasionally unilateral), seen singly or in combination.

There is thus a wide range of clinical manifestations. Some infants at risk are normal. Some appear normal at birth but later are found to have hearing loss. A number are small for gestational age and at birth have evidence of congenital heart disease and of ocular anomalies including microphthalmia, glaucoma, cataracts that may be central or diffuse, and pigmented retinopathy (see Chapter 17). While usually present at birth, ocular findings may be missed unless careful oph-

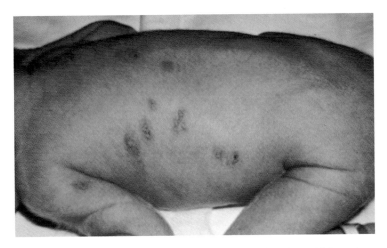

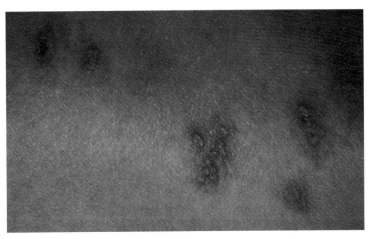

FIG. 12.67 Neonatal herpes simplex type 2 infection. Although normal at birth, this infant developed sudden onset of fever, lethargy, and decreased feeding at 6 days of age. On examination multiple grouped vesicular lesions were noted on the trunk and scalp. The liver and spleen were markedly enlarged and very firm. He had a fulminant course resembling that of septic shock, and died within 24 hours. (Courtesy of Dr. M. Sherlock).

thalmologic examination is performed. Many of these infants develop jaundice within 24 hours of delivery and have hepatosplenomegaly and diffuse adenopathy as well.

Ten to twenty percent of liveborn infants with congenital rubella manifest signs of severe disseminated infection at or shortly after delivery. In addition to early jaundice, hepatosplenomegaly and adenopathy, they often have signs of myocarditis with ischemic changes on electrocardiography, interstitial pneumonitis, thrombocytopenia with petechiae and purpura, and signs of CNS dysfunction that may range from lethargy and hypotonia to frank meningoencephalitis. Radiographs may reveal bony abnormalities consisting of metaphyseal lucencies and irregular epiphyseal mineralization. In some cases a rubelliform rash may be noted, or a characteristic raised bluish papular eruption, termed a "blueberry muffin rash," may be evident due to dermal erythropoiesis (Fig. 12.66). Most of these severely affected infants are microcephalic in addition to being small for gestational age. Survivors of this "expanded rubella syndrome" have a high likelihood of deafness and significant psychomotor retardation. In a small percentage of cases, delayed manifestations may surface. These include anemia toward the end of the first month, and at 3 to 4 months of age the insidious onset of interstitial pneumonitis and the appearance of a chronic generalized rubelliform exanthem. Still later immunodeficiency may be detected. Feeding difficulties, chronic diarrhea, and failure to thrive are common.

Infants with congenital rubella are chronically and persistently infected, and tend to shed live virus in urine, stools, and respiratory secretions for up to a year. Hence they should be isolated in hospitals and kept away from susceptible pregnant women when sent home. Diagnosis can be confirmed by viral culture and specific IgM titers.

Neonatal Herpes Simplex Infection

Infants born vaginally to mothers with genital herpes simplex type 2 are at significant risk for acquisition of infection. Typically the mother is asymptomatic and the infant appears totally normal at birth. Signs of infection may develop any time within the first 4 weeks, but usually they appear 4 to 8 days postpartum. Infection may be localized to the skin, eye, mouth or central nervous sytem, or it may be systemic. In the latter instance, onset begins with fever or subnormal temperature in association with lethargy, poor feeding, vomiting and jaundice. The liver and spleen are enlarged and often are remarkably firm. Respiratory distress supervenes, followed by a picture that is indistinguishable from that of septic shock with DIC. Approximately three-fourths of affected infants have typical herpetic skin or mucosal lesions (Fig. 12.67). The scalp and face are the sites most commonly involved. Occasionally lesions are limited to the conjunctiva or to the oral mucosa. In the absence of these lesions, accurate diagnosis is extremely difficult. Mortality is high, exceeding 50 percent, but has been reduced by early recognition and systemic antiviral therapy. Nevertheless, morbidity remains high in survivors. Infants with localized skin, eye, and/or oral involvement have a relatively good prognosis. Those with localized CNS disease have a better survival rate than those with systemic infection but they share severe morbidity.

Less frequently infections may occur prenatally as a result of ascent from the lower genital tract through ruptured membranes, or as a result of maternal viremia. With prenatal acquisition, the infant may die in utero or may be born with jaundice, skin lesions, and signs of systemic infection.

BIBLIOGRAPHY

Barton LL, Feigin RD: Childhood Cervical Lymphadenitis: A Reappraisal. J Pediatr 84: 846–852, 1974.

Cherry JD: Newer Viral Exanthems. Adv Pediatr 16: 233–286, 1969.

Chesney PJ, Davis JP, Purdy WK et al: Clinical Manifestations of Toxic Shock Syndrome. JAMA 246: 741–748, 1981.

Clain A: Demonstrations of Physical Signs in Clinical Surgery, 16th ed. John Wright-PSG, Littleton, Mass, 1980.

Committee on Infectious Diseases, American Academy of Pediatrics: Report of the Committee on Infectious Diseases—The 1982 Red Book, 19th ed. Am Acad Pediatr, Evanston, Illinois, 1982.

Dich, VQ, Nelson JD, Haltalin KC: Osteomyelitis in Infants and Children. Am J Dis Child 129: 1273–1278, 1975.

Feigin RD, Cherry JD: Textbook of Pediatric Infectious Disease. Saunders, Philadelphia, 1981.

Fleisher G, Ludwig S, Campos J: Cellulitis: Bacterial Etiology, Clinical Features and Laboratory Findings. J Pediatr 97: 591–593, 1980.

Hanshaw JB, Dudgeon JA: Viral Diseases of the Fetus and Newborn. Saunders, Philadelphia, 1978.

Krugman S, Katz SL: Infectious Diseases of Children, 7th ed. CV Mosby, St. Louis, 1981.

Lascari AD, Bapat VR: Syndrome of Infectious Mononucleosis. Clin Pediatr 9: 300–304, 1970.

Leibel RL, Fangman JJ, Ostrovsky MC: Chronic Meningococcemia in Childhood. Am J Dis Child 127: 94–98, 1974.

Mandell GL, Douglas RG Jr, Bennet JE: Principles and Practice of Infectious Diseases. Wiley, New York, 1979.

May M: Neck Masses in Children: Diagnosis and Treatment. Pediatr Ann 5: 517–535, 1976.

Melish ME, Hicks RV, Reddy V: Kawasaki Syndrome: An update. Hosp Pract 17: 99–106, 1982.

Melish ME, Hicks RM, Larson EJ: Mucocutaneous Lymph Node Syndrome in the United States. Am J Dis Child 130: 599–607, 1976.

Morrey BF, Bianco AJ, Rhodes KH: Septic Arthritis in Children. Pediatr Clin North Am 6: 923–934, 1975.

Nixon GW: Acute Hematogenous Osteomyelitis. Pediatr Ann 5: 65–81, 1976.

Rapkin RH, Bautista G: *Haemophilus influenzae* Cellulitis. Am J Dis Child 124: 540–542, 1972.

Season EH, Miller PR: Primary Subacute Pyogenic Osteomyelitis in Long Bones of Children. J Pediatr Surg 11: 347–353, 1976.

Sumaya CV: Infectious Mononucleosis in Children. Pediatr Update 1985, 13–31.

Toews WH, Bass JW: Skin Manifestations of Meningococcal Infection. Am J Dis Child 127: 173–176, 1974.

Tofte RW, Williams DN: Toxic Shock Syndrome, Evidence of a Broad Clinical Spectrum. JAMA 246: 2163–2167, 1981.

Wannamaker LW, Ferrieri P: Streptococcal Infections—Updated. DM, 1–40, Oct 1975.

Wilson HD, Haltalin KC: Acute Necrotizing Fasciitis in Childhood. Am J Dis Child 125: 591–595, 1973.

RENAL AND GENITOURINARY DISORDERS

Demetrius Ellis, M.D.
Ellis D. Avner, M.D.

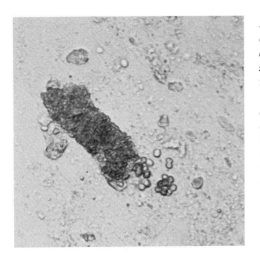

FIG. 13.1 Red blood cell cast from a patient with post-streptococcal glomerulonephritis. These casts are almost always associated with glomerulonephritis or vasculitis, and virtually exclude extra-renal disorders of bleeding.

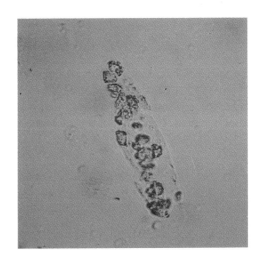

FIG. 13.2 White blood cell cast from a patient with chronic glomerulonephritis.

The manifestations of renal and genitourinary disorders range from readily apparent, gross structural abnormalities to subtle abnormalities of the urinary sediment. In this chapter we will utilize examples of physical findings, as well as characteristic urinary findings and radiographs, to demonstrate the broad spectrum of these disorders in the pediatric population.

GLOMERULAR DISORDERS

Acute Glomerulonephritis

Red blood cell casts (Fig. 13.1) were found in the urine of a 4-year-old male who presented with mild supraorbital edema, headache, and decreasing urine output during the preceding few days. The urine was described as being smokey or tea-colored. Medical history revealed that 2 weeks earlier the patient had suffered from a febrile illness with painful pharyngitis for which he sought no medical attention. Clinical examination revealed a blood pressure of 140/105 mmHg, mild periorbital edema, and tenderness on palpation of the kidneys. Laboratory studies were consistent with mild renal insufficiency. He also had a protein excretion of 2.1 g per 24 hours, a low plasma C3 complement level, and elevated

streptozyme and anti-DNAase B titers, evidence which strongly implicated a streptococcal infection in the pathogenesis of this child's glomerulonephritis. Complete, spontaneous recovery of all renal abnormalities occurred within 5 weeks with conservative management, although hematuria persisted for about 1 year.

Chronic Glomerulonephritis

White blood cell casts may be seen in the urine sediment of patients with acute or chronic glomerulonephritis, vasculitis, as well as pyelonephritis and other disorders resulting in tubulointerstitial nephritis. The cast shown in Figure 13.2 occurred in a child with systemic lupus erythematosus whose only presenting symptom was mild back pain. Urinalysis demonstrated 2+ protein, microhematuria, pyuria without bacteria, and red and white blood cell casts. Diagnosis was confirmed by immunologic studies including a low serum complement level, and positive titers of antinuclear antibody and antibodies to double-stranded DNA. Renal biopsy revealed diffuse proliferative glomerulonephritis. Note that formation of tubular casts is aided by diminished urine flow, high urinary solute concentration, and by the matrix of plasma- and tubule-derived protein in which cells become embedded.

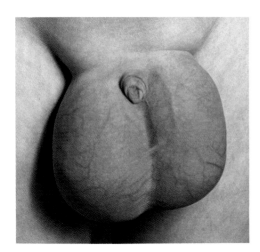

FIG. 13.3 Severe scrotal edema in a 6-year-old boy with nephrotic syndrome.

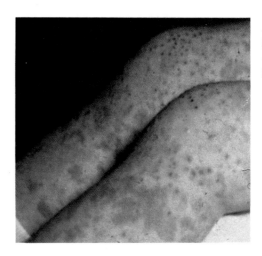

FIG. 13.4 Typical purpuric lesions of Henoch-Schönlein purpura.

Nephrotic Syndrome

Generalized edema and rapid weight gain are characteristic features of childhood nephrotic syndrome, with the former showing a predilection for the eyelids, pleural space, abdomen, scrotum, and legs (Fig. 13.3). Although edema per se usually provokes few complaints from most patients, it can at times be disfiguring, and produce skin induration and breakdown or interfere with respiratory, genitourinary, or gastrointestinal function. Symptoms may occasionally be confused with allergic edema. However, the findings of severe proteinuria, hypoalbuminemia, and hypercholesterolemia usually lead to correct diagnosis and treatment of nephrotic syndrome.

Henoch-Schönlein Purpura (Anaphylactoid Purpura)

Three weeks after an upper respiratory infection, a 2-year-old boy presented with generalized malaise, abdominal pain, periorbital edema, and difficulty walking "as if his legs were hurting." One day later, he developed an ecchymotic, purpuric rash (Fig. 13.4), the characteristic clinical manifestation of Henoch-Schönlein purpura. The rash was distributed over the extensor surfaces of the extremities and on the buttocks, but spared the trunk. Individual lesions faded over 1 week, but new lesions appeared or reoccurred over several weeks.

Some patients initially develop an urticarial-type eruption which subsequently becomes macular or maculopapular. Occasionally, younger patients develop an angioneurotic-like edema of the scalp, face, or dorsa of hands or feet. As was true in the aforementioned case, 90 percent of children with Henoch-Schönlein purpura have a prodrome consisting of an upper respiratory infection 1 to 3 weeks prior to the onset of symptoms, while 80 percent have gastrointestinal and/or arthritic symptoms. About half of the patients have renal involvement ranging from simple microhematuria and a variable degree of proteinuria to oliguria and renal failure. In contrast to adults, use of multiple medications is rarely related to the onset of this condition in children.

There are no distinct biochemical features of this condition. Some patients have leukocytosis and an elevated serum IgA level. Platelet counts and coagulation studies are normal. It is the skin rash which is essential for the diagnosis of Henoch-Schönlein purpura since the renal abnormalities may otherwise closely resemble another condition known as IgA nephropathy (Berger disease).

VESICOURETERAL REFLUX AND INFECTIONS

Vesicoureteral Reflux

Vesicoureteral reflux is a congenital condition in which the normal valve mechanism of the ureterovesical junction is impaired, leading to reflux of bladder urine into the ureter and/or kidneys. In a young child with urinary tract infection, such reflux of infected urine is a major risk factor for the development of pyelonephritis, renal scarring, and chronic renal damage.

The severity of vesicoureteral reflux is assessed by the findings on voiding cystourethrograms and classified according to the following international grading system (Fig. 13.5):

Grade I reflux—reflux into the ureter only (Fig. 13.6)

Grade II reflux—complete reflux into the ureter, pelvis, and calyces without any dilation of the structures (Fig. 13.7)

Grade III reflux—complete reflux with mild dilatation and/or tortuosity of the ureter, and mild dilatation of the renal pelvis but only slight blunting of the calyceal fornices (Fig. 13.8)

Grade IV reflux—complete reflux with moderate dilatation of the ureter, renal pelvis, and calyces; complete obliteration of the sharp angle of the fornices with maintenance of the papillary impressions of the calyces (Fig. 13.9)

Grade V reflux—gross dilatation and tortuosity of the ureter with gross dilatation of the renal pelvis and calyces; obliteration of the papillary impressions of the calyces (Fig. 13.10)

Grades I through III have a high rate of spontaneous resolution, and patients with such findings should be placed on suppressive antibiotic regimens to ensure maintenance of sterile bladder urine. Grades IV and V are generally associated with significant anatomic abnormalities of the ureteral orifice and require surgical correction.

Bacterial Cystitis

Young children presenting with an acute onset of fever, emesis, dysuria, suprapubic pain, and a urinary sediment such as that shown in Figure 13.11 should be suspected of having bacterial cystitis. Many more cells and bacteria may be seen when urine is examined after centrifuging at 3000 rpm for 5 minutes. By far the most common organism cultured from

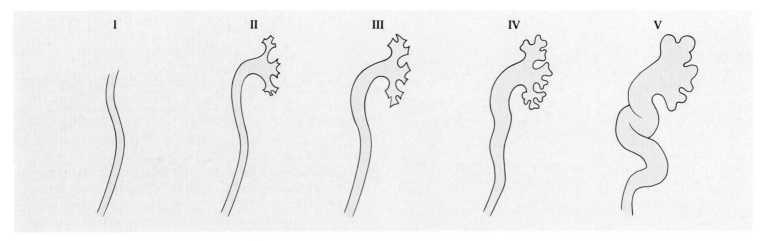

FIG. 13.5 Grades of vesicoureteral reflux, schematically presented.

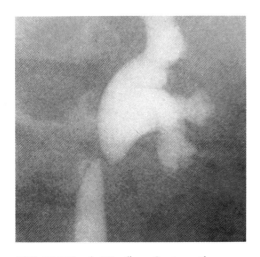

FIG. 13.6 Grade I reflux: Cystourethrogram shows reflux only into the ureter.

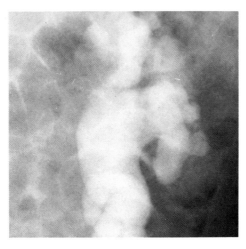

FIG. 13.7 Grade II reflux: Cystourethrogram shows complete reflux into the ureter, pelvis, and calyces; no dilatation.

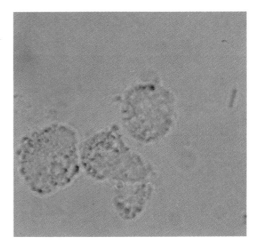

FIG. 13.8 Grade III reflux: Cystourethrogram shows complete reflux with mild dilatation of the ureter and renal pelvis, but only slight blunting of the calyces.

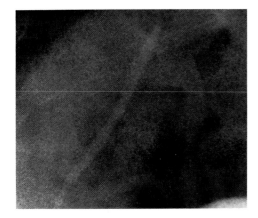

FIG. 13.9 Grade IV reflux: Cystourethrogram shows complete reflux with moderate dilatation of the ureter, pelvis, and calyces; complete obliteration of sharp angle of fornices.

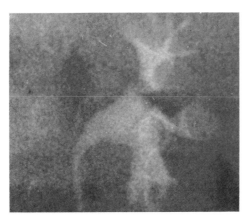

FIG. 13.10 Grade V reflux: Cystourethrogram shows gross dilatation of the ureter, pelvis, and calyces; obliteration of the papillary impressions of the calyces.

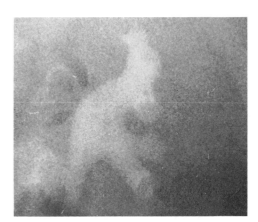

FIG. 13.11 High-power view of unspun urine shows several white blood cells and a rod-shaped organism, suggestive of bacterial cystitis.

patients with acute or chronic urinary tract infection is *Escherichia coli*, with Pseudomonas or Proteus species occasionally found, particularly in patients with abnormal genitourinary anatomy.

While the diagnosis of urinary tract infection is established by appropriate urine cultures. the site of infection may be unapparent when only presenting symptoms or urinalysis findings are considered. Evaluation with pyelography and micturition cystourethrography should be performed in all children under the age of 8 years following documentation of their first urinary tract infection. Such studies will usually define structural abnormalities leading to obstructive nephropathy or vesicoureteral reflux, and are essential in planning medical and surgical management of these patients.

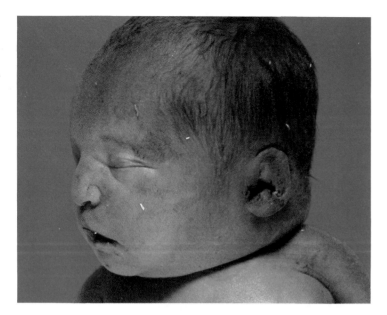

FIG. 13.12 Potter facies. This infant with bilateral multicystic dysplasia died at 12 hours of age with pulmonary insufficiency. The altered facies produced by the fetal compression syndrome of oligohydramnios includes small, posteriorly rotated ears, micrognathia, a beaked nose, and wide-set eyes. (Courtesy of Dr. MacPherson, Magee-Women's Hospital, Pittsburgh)

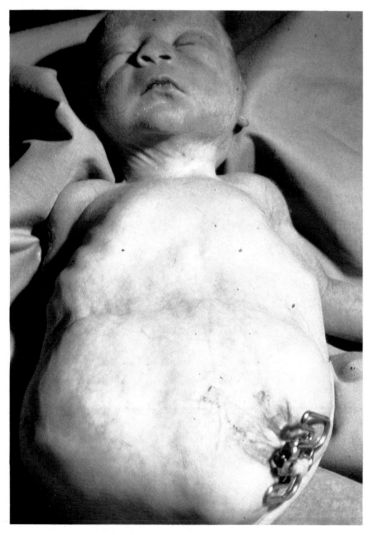

FIG. 13.13 Newborn with complete agenesis of the abdominal musculature. This patient had severe renal dysplasia and died soon after birth. The typical wrinkled skin of the abdominal wall ("prune belly") is not seen due to marked abdominal wall distention.

DEVELOPMENTAL ABNORMALITIES
Potter Syndrome

Oligohydramnios from any cause leads to a complex syndrome of fetal compression. Although chronic leakage of amniotic fluid may be responsible for oligohydramnios, it most commonly occurs secondary to decreased fetal urine formation because of renal agenesis or severe underlying renal structural disorders. The relative lack of amniotic fluid during fetal life leads to pulmonary hypoplasia and fetal compression, which consequently results in abnormal positioning of the hands and feet and the production of an altered facies characterized by abnormally small posteriorly rotated ears, a small chin, a beaked nose, and unusual facial creases (Fig. 13.12). Infants with Potter syndrome die of respiratory insufficiency secondary to the severe associated abnormalities of pulmonary development.

Prune-Belly Syndrome (Eagle-Barrett Syndrome)

This syndrome usually consists of the absence of abdominal musculature, renal and urinary tract abnormalities, and cryptorchidism (Fig. 13.13). Males are affected more severely and 20 times more frequently than females. Although, there is generally no ureteral obstruction, the ureters are dilated and tortuous, and 75 percent exhibit reflux. The bladder is enlarged despite low renal pelvic and intravesical pressures. Infection is quite common because of urinary stasis.

The major determinant of prognosis in these patients is the degree of associated renal dysplasia. Intestinal malrotation is a common associated abnormality; anomalies of the limbs and heart may occur but are uncommon. Infertility in males is universal even when it is possible to surgically place the testes into their normal intrascrotal position.

Extrophy of the Bladder

The embryology of this condition is poorly understood. It occurs more frequently in males, and although most cases are sporadic, it has occasionally occurred in siblings. Associated renal abnormalities are unusual but may include unilateral renal agenesis and horseshoe kidney. If the condition is not properly managed, infection and vesicoureteral reflux through incompetent ureteral orifices can lead to hydronephrosis, pyelonephritis, and eventually to renal failure. Moreover, even after primary closure, patients continue to be at risk for chronic cystitis and for tumor of the bladder (primarily adenocarcinoma). Other structural abnormalities frequently seen in association with bladder extrophy include abnormalities of the bony pelvis, epispadias, and other genital defects and anomalies of the alimentary tract (Fig. 13.14). Such a constellation of disfiguring and difficult problems makes bladder extrophy a most devastating abnormality of the genitourinary tract requiring a multidisciplinary treatment plan (surgical-medical-psychosocial).

Imperforate Anus

Because of common embryologic origins and the anatomic proximity of the genitourinary and lower gastrointestinal

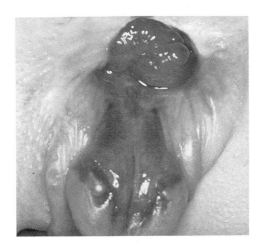

FIG. 13.14 Vesical extrophy. The penis is short, wide, and has prominent epispadias and absence of the corpus spongiosum.

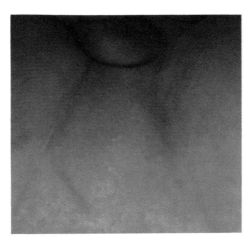

FIG. 13.15 Imperforate anus. This male newborn has an absent median raphe and anal atresia. On further study he was found to have agenesis of the right kidney, severe dysplasia in the left kidney, and a communication of the blind-ended rectal pouch and the prostatic urethra.

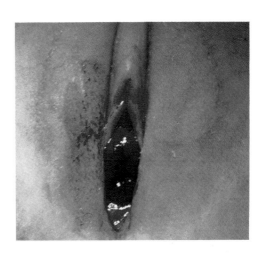

FIG. 13.16 Urethral prolapse in a 3-year-old girl.

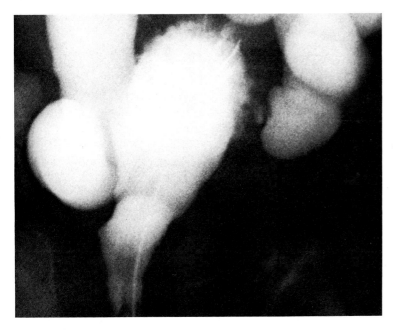

FIG. 13.17 Posterior urethral valves. Voiding cystourethrogram of a 3-week-old male infant who presented with renal failure demonstrates the valves as well as the elongation and ballooning of the posterior urethra and a trabeculated bladder. Also seen is severe bilateral dilatation and tortuosity of the ureters secondary to outflow obstruction and vesicoureteral reflux.

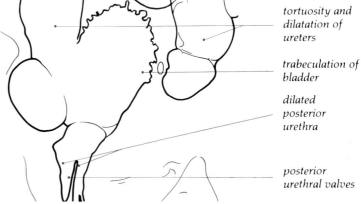

tortuosity and dilatation of ureters

trabeculation of bladder

dilated posterior urethra

posterior urethral valves

tracts, children with imperforate anus have a high incidence of genitourinary and lower spinal abnormalities. A high imperforate anus (at or above the supralevator muscle) (Fig. 13.15) is associated with a 50 percent incidence of genitourinary anomalies, mainly unilateral renal agenesis, neurogenic bladder, or vesicoureteral reflux. In males one usually finds a fistulous communication between the blind end of the rectal pouch and the prostatic urethra. In females, the rectum communicates with the vagina or posterior fourchette. All children with imperforate anus should undergo evaluation of the genitourinary tract with renal ultrasound and voiding cystourethrography, and must be monitored for urinary tract infection.

Urethral Prolapse

This is an uncommon condition seen primarily in black prepubertal girls who present with mild introital bleeding (Fig. 13.16). Therapeutic excision of the prolapsed segment is usually curative.

Posterior Urethral Valves

The most common obstructive lesions of the lower urinary tract in infants are posterior urethral valves. Such folds traverse the urethra from a point just distal to the verumontanum to the proximal limit of the membranous urethra and cause obstruction to urinary flow with consequent enlargement of the prostatic urethra, hypertrophy of the bladder neck, trabeculation of the bladder, and significant dilatation of the upper urinary tract. Children with posterior urethral valves may present as infants with renal failure and profound electrolyte imbalance. Older children may present with abdominal masses, voiding disturbances, or infection. Diagnosis is made radiologically by voiding cystourethrography (Fig. 13.17) and confirmed endoscopically. Although urinary diversion is frequently required, some patients can be treated directly with transurethral valve ablation. Surgery is usually successful in achieving urinary drainage, but in many cases associated renal dysplasia may lead to chronic renal failure during infancy or childhood.

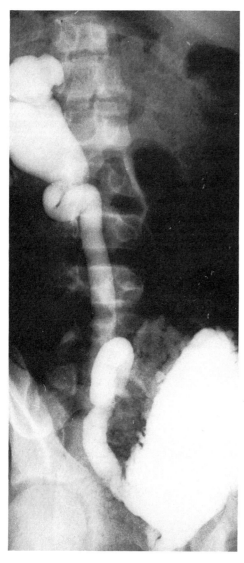

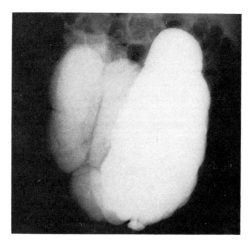

FIG. 13.19 Voiding cystourethrogram demonstrates severe hydronephrosis which was due to primary nonobstructive megaureter.

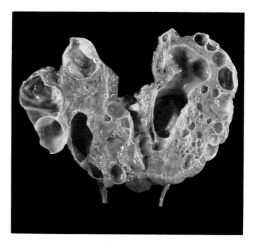

FIG. 13.20 Bilateral cystic renal dysplasia. Multiple cysts of variable size are seen throughout the cortex and medullary regions.

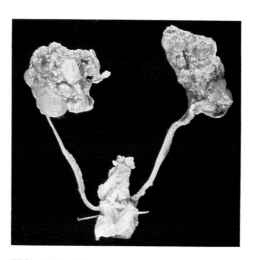

FIG. 13.21 Bilateral, severe renal dysplasia causes renal failure and death in the neonatal period.

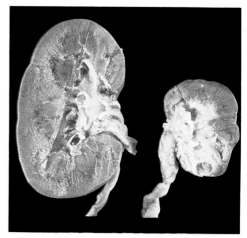

FIG. 13.22 Unilateral renal hypoplasia/dysplasia. In contrast to the normal right kidney, the left is markedly small. The parenchyma in the upper pole is normal, but microscopic examination of the lower pole showed several morphologic features of dysplasia.

FIG. 13.18 Neurogenic bladder. Intravenous pyelogram of a 14-year-old boy in whom the removal of a sacral tumor affected bladder innervation demonstrates an enlarged bladder and dilatation of the upper genitourinary tract secondary to incomplete bladder emptying.

Neurogenic Bladder

Urinary tract dysfunction may result from abnormal innervation of the bladder. Such deranged innervation may result from congenital abnormalities of the spinal cord (myelomeningocele, sacral dysgenesis), trauma to the spinal cord or sacral innervation, tumors, or systemic neuropathies (diabetes, multiple sclerosis). The consequence of incomplete bladder emptying is progressive obstruction and dilatation of the upper genitourinary tract, which in severe cases can lead to renal failure (Fig. 13.18). In addition, incomplete bladder emptying promotes stasis which may cause urinary infection.

Infants with neurogenic bladder may present with abnormal voiding patterns or abdominal distention secondary to their massively enlarged bladder. Older patients may present with incontinence or urinary tract infection. Assessment of patients with neurogenic bladder focuses upon the diagnosis of underlying neurologic deficits and the detailed assessment of urinary tract anatomy with complete radiographic evaluation. The goals of urologic management of neurogenic blad-

der are to ensure bladder emptying (and thus decrease the risk of renal impairment from obstructive uropathy) and to prevent urinary tract infections. Such goals may often be attained with intermittent manual expression of the bladder (Credé maneuver) or intermittent catheterization regimens, but may require urinary diversion procedures which permit free external drainage of the genitourinary system (cutaneous vesicostomy or supravesicular diversion).

Hydronephrosis

Hydronephrosis, or enlarged kidney, along with multicystic kidneys represent the most common abdominal masses found in newborn infants. Although hydronephrosis can occur in many of the genitourinary disorders described in this chapter, it occasionally occurs in the absence of any obstruction. As seen in Figure 13.19, the ureters and renal pelvis have become markedly enlarged as a result of inadequate peristalsis in one or more segments of the ureters. This condition is known as primary nonobstructive megaureter and requires no surgical

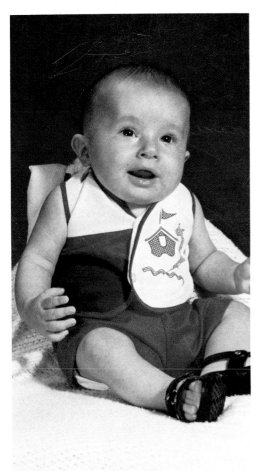

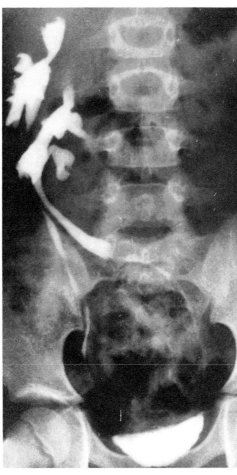

FIG. 13.23 An infant with Klippel-Feil syndrome (left) demonstrates a short neck (fused cervical vertebrae) and nonfunctioning right thumb due to lack of tendons to this digit. Intravenous pyelogram (right) reveals crossed renal ectopia of the left kidney, while the ureter from the left kidney crosses the midline and inserts into the left side of the trigone.

treatment unless there is obstruction or recurrent urinary tract infections which can damage the kidney. Obstruction can be demonstrated by a diuretic renogram, or by infusing fluid at a rate of 10 cc/minute through a needle positioned in the renal pelvis and showing a rise in intrapelvic pressure above 12 mmHg (Whitaker test).

Multicystic Kidney (Cystic Dysplasia)

This condition is more often unilateral than bilateral, and is often diagnosed during the neonatal period after palpation of a "lumpy" intra-abdominal mass of variable size which often transilluminates (Fig. 13.20). Since atresia of the ureter is usually present, urine output and renal function will depend on the presence of bilateral involvement as well as the degree of associated renal dysplasia (presence of primitive nephrons, fibrosis, and cartilage in between the cysts). Very large multicystic kidneys can interfere with respiration or produce mechanical intestinal compression. Oligohydramnios and Potter facies may be found in patients with bilateral involvement and severe renal dysfunction. Renal ultrasonography and retrograde urography are usually sufficient to establish the diagnosis. Although somewhat controversial, the prevailing opinion is that unilateral and asymptomatic multicystic kidneys do not need to be removed. However, correction of any associated obstructive abnormalities that may be present in the contralateral kidney is of vital importance.

Renal Hypoplasia/Dysplasia

Abnormal renal morphogenesis includes processes leading to both deficient parenchyma (hypoplasia) and abnormally differentiated parenchyma (dysplasia) (Fig. 13.21). These conditions often coexist and give rise to small, abnormally developed kidneys (Fig. 13.22). When bilateral, these renal disorders are frequently detected during the first few weeks of life. The infant usually demonstrates poor weight gain, pallor, emesis, and tachypnea. Many of the early symptoms are secondary to metabolic acidosis resulting from renal insufficiency. The amount of urine output bears little relationship to the degree of renal failure as reflected by the serum creatinine and blood urea nitrogen concentrations. Together, these conditions constitute the most common cause of chronic renal failure in children. Fortunately, they are rarely inherited, although familial cases have been reported.

Patients with renal hypoplasia often have gastrointestinal, central nervous system, cardiac, and pulmonary abnormalities, but other abnormalities of the genitourinary tract are rarely present. Obstruction of the excretory tract is commonly found in patients with dysplasia, while less common anomalies may include Down syndrome, as well as tracheoesophageal fistula, ventriculoseptal defect, and lumbosacral dysraphias which together make up the VATER association.

Crossed Renal Ectopia

Children with this developmental anomaly generally present with an abdominal mass or with hematuria following minor trauma. Obstruction at the ureteropelvic junction is quite common. The location of the ectopic kidney may be cryptic, and can be best demonstrated by a renal radionuclide scan. Crossed renal ectopia is often found in association with Klippel-Feil syndrome (Fig. 13.23), but has also been associated with cervicothoracic vertebral anomalies and with müllerian duct aplasia in females.

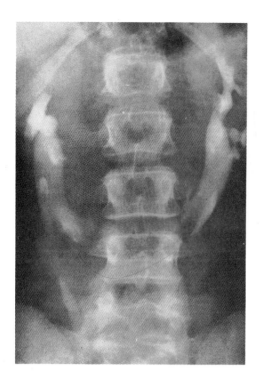

FIG. 13.24 Horseshoe kidney. This excretory urogram was performed as part of the evaluation for gross hematuria following abdominal injury in the child. Notice the unusual and oblong configuration of the collecting system resulting from fusion of the lower renal poles.

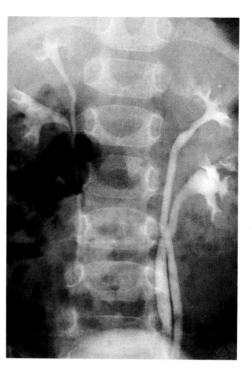

FIG. 13.25 Excretory urogram shows bilateral duplication of the urinary collecting system. This child had recurrent urinary tract infections due to vesicoureteral reflux in the ureter from the left lower pole. Ureteral duplication is incomplete on the right side (Y-type).

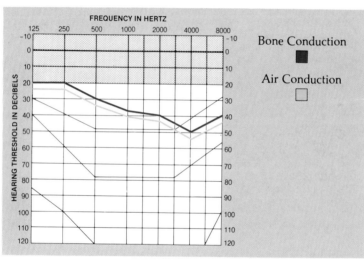

FIG. 13.26 In Alport syndrome, a loss of high-frequency auditory perception may be found in 40 percent of patients. Since the hearing deficit may be most marked at frequencies between 4000 and 8000 Hz, it may be initially detected only by audiometric testing.

Horseshoe Kidney

This condition results from fusion of the lower renal poles during development (Fig. 13.24). Although generally asymptomatic, patients with horseshoe kidney may present with (1) hematuria after trauma to the pelvic area, (2) a midline abdominal mass, or (3) a ureteropelvic junction obstruction, a common associated finding in this condition.

Duplication of the Urinary Collecting System

This is one of the most common of all genitourinary abnormalities. It is sometimes familial and more common in females than in males. About 30 percent of the duplications are bilateral (Fig. 13.25), but with much variation in the extent of duplication. This condition occurs when the kidney is penetrated by two separate ureteral buds during nephrogenesis. When present, vesicoureteral reflux usually occurs in the ureter from the lower pole, while ureteral obstruction almost exclusively occurs in the ureter from the upper renal segment. Reflux into a duplicated system is unlikely to resolve spontaneously. These associated problems may predispose patients to recurrent infection or hydronephrosis necessitating surgical correction.

HEREDITARY AND METABOLIC DISORDERS

Alport Syndrome

Alport syndrome, or hereditary progressive nephritis, is characterized by recurrent hematuria, progressive renal failure, and neurosensory deafness. It is transmitted by autosomal-dominant inheritance with variable penetrance. The most common clinical feature is persistent or recurrent hematuria which may be recognized early in childhood. Proteinuria is absent or mild in the early stages of the disease but increases as the disease progresses. The course is commonly one of slowly progressive renal failure, often accompanied by hypertension which is more severe in males than in females. The majority of patients with Alport syndrome have neither deafness nor ocular defects, but loss of high-frequency auditory perception occurs in as many as 40 percent of patients and thus may be used as a clinical marker in family studies. The acoustic loss is most often in the range of 4000 to 8000 Hz and may only be detectable by audiometric testing (Fig. 13.26).

Alport syndrome must be differentiated from the many benign forms of childhood hematuria as well as from other pro-

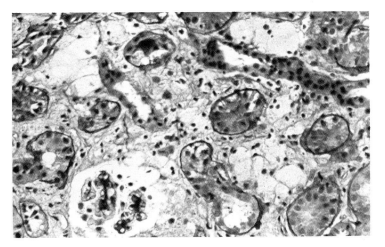

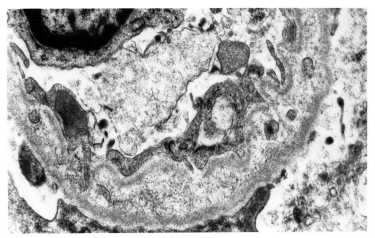

FIG. 13.27 Renal biopsy of a 6-year-old male with high-frequency hearing loss and persistent hematuria and proteinuria reveals multiple aggregations of foam cells and areas of glomerular sclerosis.

FIG. 13.28 Ultrastructural studies on renal tissue from the patient in Figure 13.27 reveal the characteristic lamellation and irregularities of the glomerular basement membrane, diagnostic of Alport syndrome.

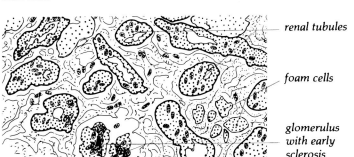

renal tubules

foam cells

glomerulus with early sclerosis

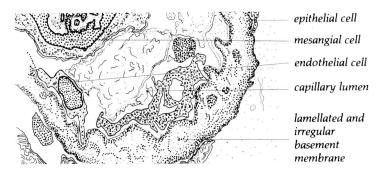

epithelial cell

mesangial cell

endothelial cell

capillary lumen

lamellated and irregular basement membrane

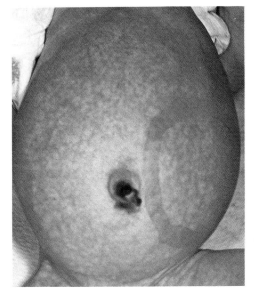

FIG. 13.29 This infant with infantile polycystic kidney disease shows marked abdominal distention and bilaterally enlarged kidneys, as indicated by the outlined areas.

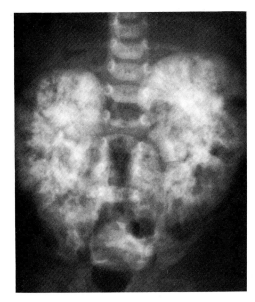

FIG. 13.30 Intravenous pyelogram of the patient in Figure 13.29 shows the characteristic mottled nephrogram, with brushlike medullary opacification secondary to retention of contrast material in dilated cortical and medullary collecting ducts.

gressive glomerular disorders. Diagnosis relies on careful family history, audiologic or ocular abnormalities, and renal histopathologic features such as the presence of foam cells and glomerular sclerosis on light microscopy (Fig. 13.27), and diagnostic ultrastructural alterations of the glomerular capillary basement membrane (Fig. 13.28). There is no specific treatment for this disorder, and progressive end-stage renal disease is supported with dialysis and/or renal transplantation.

Infantile Polycystic Kidney Disease

Infantile polycystic kidney disease is a disorder transmitted by autosomal-recessive inheritance in which there is diffuse cystic involvement of both kidneys. Though it may occasionally present in older children, the disease most commonly presents in newborns or infants with greatly enlarged kidneys and abdominal distention (Fig. 13.29). It may be differentiated from bilateral hydronephrosis of any etiology by thorough radiologic evaluation which may include sonography, cystography, and intravenous pyelography. The intravenous pyelogram in Figure 13.30 shows a characteristic mottled nephrogram, with the retention of contrast material in dilated medullary and cortical collecting ducts producing brushlike medullary opacification with streaks radiating to the outer portion of the kidney. This correlates well with the pathologic findings in such kidneys of cystic dilation localized

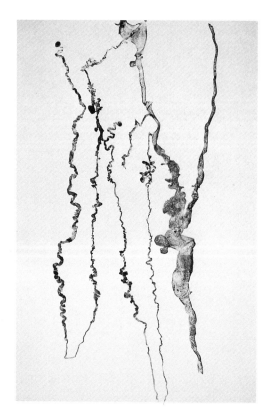

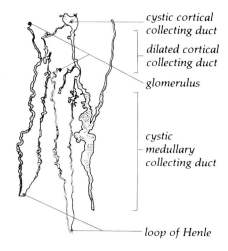

FIG. 13.31 The cystic areas are apparent in the microdissected nephron tree shown in this photograph. (Courtesy of Dr. G. Fetterman)

cystic cortical collecting duct

dilated cortical collecting duct

glomerulus

cystic medullary collecting duct

loop of Henle

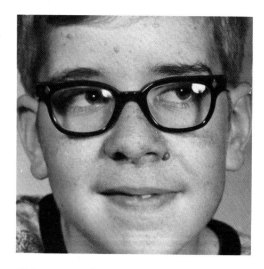

FIG. 13.32 This 6-year-old patient with tuberous sclerosis demonstrates characteristic papules distributed across the bridge of the nose and the nasolabial folds. This same patient was originally diagnosed as having polycystic kidney disease because of abdominal distention and bilateral renal enlargement prior to the onset of any skin lesions.

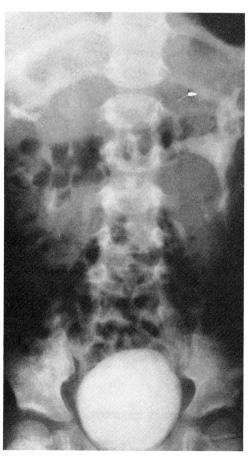

FIG. 13.33 Intravenous pyelogram of the patient in Figure 13.32 shows enlarged kidneys with the collecting system stretched and distorted by multiple soft-tissue masses, later found to be renal angiomyolipoma.

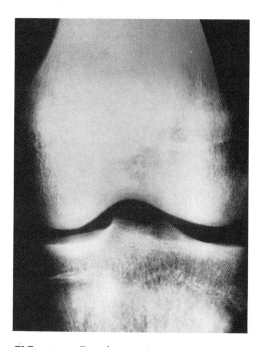

FIG. 13.34 Renal osteodystrophy in the knee of a child. Note the increased thickness and fraying in the region of the growth plate, as well as subperiosteal erosion of the femoral cortex. In addition, osteoporosis and coarsening of the trabecular pattern of the femur and tibia are evident.

to the medullary and cortical collecting ducts. This localization is best demonstrated by the technique of isolated nephron microdissection (Fig. 13.31).

Systemic hypertension develops in almost all children with infantile polycystic kidney disease, and the clinical course is one of progressive renal insufficiency. Progressive hepatic fibrosis also occurs to some degree in all children with the disease and may lead to portal hypertension in some patients.

Tuberous Sclerosis

Tuberous sclerosis is a neurocutaneous syndrome inherited as an autosomal-dominant trait with marked variability of expression. The full syndrome is characterized by seizures, mental deficiency, foci of intracranial calcification, and pathognomonic skin lesions which are fibroangiomatous nevi (adenoma sebaceum). The latter may be present during the

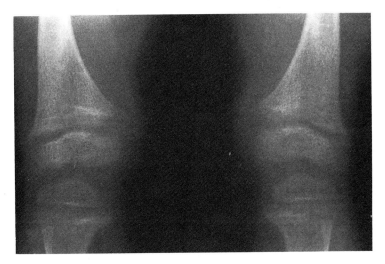
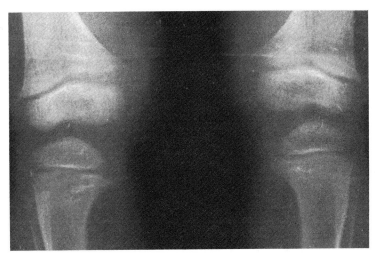

FIG. 13.35 Hypophosphatemic rickets. (Left) Radiograph of the knees of a 2-year-old female who presented with bow legs. Note the widened space between the metaphyses and epiphyseal ossification center, cupping and splaying of the metaphyses of the femur and tibia, and an overall decreased density of bone.

(Right) Radiograph taken 6 months following the initiation of treatment with oral phosphorus and vitamin D analogues reveals resolution of the rachitic conditions. In this patient, healing was accompanied by an increase in growth velocity. (Courtesy of Dr. M. Goodman, Children's Hospital of Pittsburgh)

first year of life, but may not be noted until the age of 4 to 7 years when they take the form of discrete yellowish papules distributed along the bridge of the nose and the nasolabial folds (Fig. 13.32). Patients with tuberous sclerosis may have hamartomas in many organs and tissues. Renal angiomyolipoma causing genitourinary symptomatology may suggest the diagnosis of polycystic kidney disease in patients with minimal skin or central nervous system involvement (Fig. 13.33). In such instances, the diagnosis of tuberous sclerosis is confirmed by family history and the development of other features of the syndrome.

Renal Osteodystrophy

Renal osteodystrophy is the osseous manifestation of chronic renal failure and results primarily from two major pathologic processes: (1) relative deficiency of 1,25-dihydroxyvitamin D which leads to impaired mineralization of cartilage and bone, resulting in rickets and osteomalacia; and (2) an excess of parathyroid hormone which leads to osteitis fibrosa cystica, the classic bone disease of primary hyperparathyroidism. In any given patient, each of these pathologic processes may occur with varying severity giving a wide range of clinical and radiologic presentation. In children, renal osteodystrophy is clinically characterized by growth retardation, bone pain, and deformity of long bones. The radiologic features in children include increased thickness and fraying of the radiolucent zone in the region of growth plates, subperiosteal erosion of the cortices of long bones and phalanges, and changes in bone density including osteoporosis, osteosclerosis, or coarsening of the trabecular pattern of long bones (Fig. 13.34). Studies indicate that aggressive medical control of mineral imbalance, acidosis, malnutrition, and hormone replacement with 1,25-dihydroxyvitamin D may control hyperparathyroidism and slow, if not completely ameliorate, the osseous manifestations of chronic renal failure.

Hypophosphatemic Rickets

Rickets is a disturbance of growing bone in which defective mineralization of matrix leads to an abnormal accumulation of uncalcified cartilage and osteoid. Hypophosphatemic vitamin D–resistant rickets is an X-linked inherited disorder which clinically presents during the first year of life with hypophosphatemia, short stature, and rickets. Normal muscle tone and strength, the absence of tetany or convulsions, and the predominance of rachitic changes in the lower extremities help in the clinical differentiation of this specific disorder from other forms of childhood rickets. Biochemically, this disorder is differentiated from the other forms of childhood rickets by the characteristic profile consisting of low plasma phosphorus, normal or borderline low plasma calcium, a normal parathyroid hormone level, the absence of aminoaciduria, a normal 25-hydroxyvitamin D level, and a 1,25-dihydroxyvitamin D level which is low for the level of hypophosphatemia. The pathogenesis of the disorder is believed to involve a renal tubular phosphate leak which is accompanied by an inappropriately low 1,25-dihydroxyvitamin D synthesis by renal tubular cells. The characteristic radiologic features of hypophosphatemic rickets, as in all forms of childhood rickets, include early widening of the space between the end of the metaphyses of long bones, and an overall decreased bone density. Treatment with oral phosphorus and vitamin D analogues promotes rapid healing (Fig. 13.35) as well as marked increases in growth velocity.

Cystinosis

Cystinosis is an autosomal-recessive metabolic disorder which is characterized by the intralysosomal accumulation of cystine in most body tissues. In its nephropathic form, the disease presents with global proximal tubular dysfunction (Fanconi syndrome) and progressive glomerular damage. The clinical manifestations of such renal tubular dysfunction of any etiology include failure to thrive, renal tubular acidosis, and rickets which results from persistent urinary losses of bicarbonate and phosphorus. Also associated with such disorders are low molecular weight proteinuria and glycosuria.

Cystinotic children show a number of clinical features not obviously related to the renal abnormalities. The majority have blonde hair and a fair complexion; this, in association

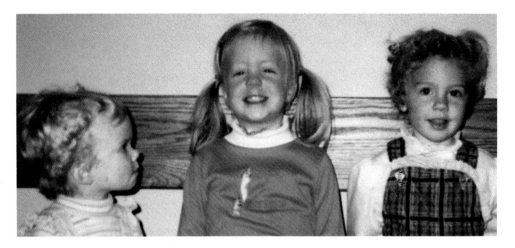

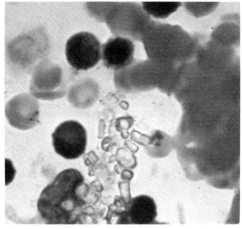

FIG. 13.36 These three children, all with blonde hair, fair complexion, and growth failure, are unrelated patients with nephropathic cystinosis.

FIG. 13.37 Diagnosis of cystinosis is often confirmed by the finding of cystine crystals in bone marrow aspirate from affected individuals, as seen here.

FIG. 13.39 The urinary calculus is quite evident in this excretory urogram, which underscores the value of this study in the evaluation of patients with suspected urolithiasis.

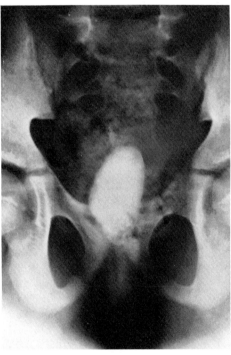

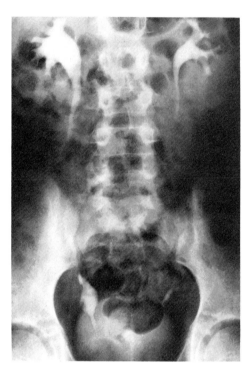

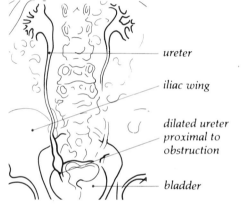

ureter

iliac wing

dilated ureter proximal to obstruction

bladder

FIG. 13.38 Radiograph shows a large, calcified, endemic bladder calculus.

with growth failure and rickets, results in striking physical similarities between unrelated patients (Fig. 13.36). Clinical diagnosis is established by ophthalmologic examination which detects a characteristic peripheral retinopathy, and by slit-lamp examination which detects the deposition of crystalline material in the conjunctiva and cornea. Diagnosis is confirmed by the finding of cystine crystals in the bone marrow of affected patients (Fig. 13.37), and by the presence of elevated levels of cystine in fibroblasts or peripheral leukocytes.

Treatment of nephropathic cystinosis consists of treatment of the metabolic abnormalities induced by the tubular dysfunction. Patients thus receive alkali, phosphorus, potassium supplements, and often vitamin D analogues. Despite such therapy, renal function progressively deteriorates, and most patients require end-stage renal disease therapy in the first decade. Although there is no specific treatment available for this metabolic disorder, treatment with cysteamine is now undergoing extensive clinical studies.

Urinary Calculi

A number of metabolic and genitourinary conditions predispose to calculus formation, including disorders of uric acid, oxalate, and cystine metabolism; hypercalciuria with or without hypercalcemia; distal (type I) renal tubular acidosis; urinary stasis in obstructive uropathy; and urinary tract infections. The most common calculi found in American children contain calcium oxalate followed by uric acid. On occasion, so-called "endemic" or bladder stones are seen primarily in young boys, and are composed of ammonium acid urate (Fig. 13.38). The cause of endemic stones is unknown.

In children, renal colic is poorly localized and described only as abdominal pain. Thus a strong index of suspicion is required on the part of the clinician so that appropriate diagnostic studies may be undertaken. In some patients with small stones, the disorder may be totally painless and may be suspected only after an episode of gross hematuria, pyuria, or urinary tract infection. The type of crystals in the urine is usually not helpful in establishing the underlying diagnosis.

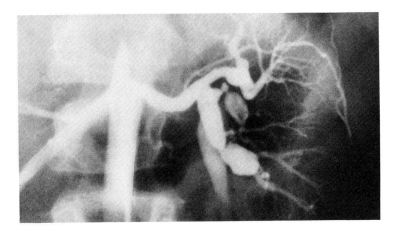

FIG. 13.40 *Arteriogram of a 12-year-old patient who presented with malignant hypertension shows multiple areas of stenosis alternating with aneurysmal dilatation in the distal segment of the renal artery, characteristic of fibromuscular dysplasia.*

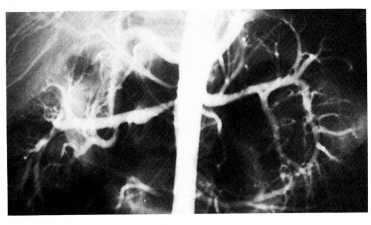

FIG. 13.41 *Arteriogram of a 13-year-old patient with neurofibromatosis who presented with mild mental retardation and a blood pressure of 140/100 shows narrowing of the renal artery close to its origin from the aorta, in contrast to the distal involvement of fibromuscular dysplasia.*

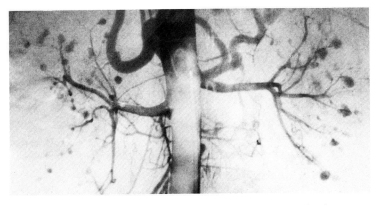

FIG. 13.42 *This arteriogram is from a 12-year-old girl who presented with weight loss, fever, abdominal pain, and malignant hypertension. Note the diagnostic features of renal involvement with polyarteritis nodosa, characterized by multiple thrombi and aneurysms.*

The finding of a calcium/creatinine ratio greater than 0.2 in a random urine specimen strongly suggests the presence of hypercalciuria and is often regarded as a precalculous condition in a patient with recurrent asymptomatic gross hematuria. An intravenous pyelogram frequently shows the area of obstruction even though the calculi may be radiolucent, as in the case of uric acid, urates, matrix, and xanthine (Fig. 13.39).

RENOVASCULAR HYPERTENSION
Renal Artery Stenosis

Although only 5 percent of pediatric hypertension is caused by renal artery stenosis, detection of this abnormality is particularly important since surgical correction is usually curative. The basic pathophysiology of all renovascular hypertension involves activation of the renin-angiotensin-aldosterone system. If a lesion in the minor or major branches of the renal artery significantly decreases renal perfusion pressure, it causes an increased renin release from the affected kidney. The high plasma renin activity leads to increases in angiotensin II levels with subsequent increases in total peripheral vascular resistance, and also leads to increased adrenal aldosterone production with resultant renal sodium and water retention and expansion of extracellular fluid volume.

Renovascular hypertension should be suspected in any hypertensive child with the physical finding of high-pitched bruits heard in the flank or abdominal areas, or when stigmata of syndromes in which arterial abnormalities are known to occur are present (e.g., homocystinuria, Marfan syndrome, and the phakomatoses). Patients with renovascular hypertension may show abnormalities on intravenous urography (delayed appearance of contrast in the affected kidney, difference in renal length, ureteric notching), abnormalities on radionuclide renal scans, or elevated plasma renin activity. Renal arteriography together with selective renal vein renin sampling is the definitive diagnostic procedure for all pediatric patients with suspected renovascular hypertension.

Intrinsic diseases of the renal artery include fibromuscular dysplasia, thrombotic and embolic lesions, aneurysms, arteritis, and arteriosclerosis. The lesions of fibromuscular dysplasia involve multiple areas of stenosis alternating with aneurysmal dilatation in the distal two-thirds of the main renal artery (Fig. 13.40). Pheochromocytoma and neurofibromatosis may also be associated with renal artery disease. Although difficult to differentiate from fibromuscular dysplasia histologically, narrowing of the renal artery associated with neurofibromatosis generally begins within 1 cm of the origin from the aorta and thus may be distinguished from distal involvement of fibromuscular dysplasia (Fig. 13.41). The majority of pediatric patients with polyarteritis nodosa have renal involvement with hypertension, which leads to arterial lesions characterized by multiple thrombi and aneurysms (Fig. 13.42). Such arteriographic findings are diagnostic in the child with hypertension accompanied by weight loss, fever, and systemic manifestations of diffuse arteritis.

Therapies for renovascular hypertension with intrinsic disease of the renal artery include surgical revascularization of the kidneys or dilatation of discrete stenoses by transluminal angioplasty. Diffuse arteritis, which may cause renovascular hypertension in children with underlying systemic diseases, is treated medically with corticosteroids, immunosuppressives, or anticoagulants depending on the nature of the primary disease process.

Hirsutism

Although there are many endocrinologic causes of hirsutism, a number of drugs used in children with renal disorders are capable of producing this condition. Marked hirsutism generally accompanies the use of minoxidil, a potent antihypertensive agent causing direct relaxation of arteriolar smooth muscle (Fig. 13.43). Cyclosporine, a newer immunosuppressive agent used to combat tissue allograft rejection after organ transplantation, has a dose-dependent effect on hair growth. Hirsutism related to drugs may be a major determinant of drug-effectiveness. Since it alters body image, it can have a marked influence on medical compliance, particularly in adolescent females.

BIBLIOGRAPHY

Belman AB, Kaplan GW: Genitourinary Problems in Pediatrics. Saunders, Philadelphia, 1981.
Edelman CM (ed): Pediatric Kidney Disease. Little Brown, Boston, 1978.
Ingelfinger JR: Pediatric Hypertension. Saunders, Philadelphia, 1982.

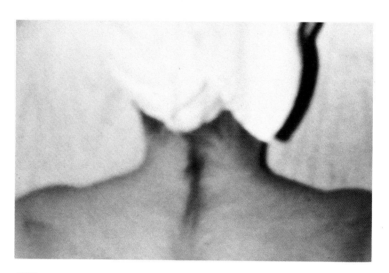

FIG. 13.43 Hirsutism in an adolescent girl who required a large dosage of minoxidil for the control of hypertension.

PEDIATRIC NEUROLOGY

Henry B. Wessel, M.D.

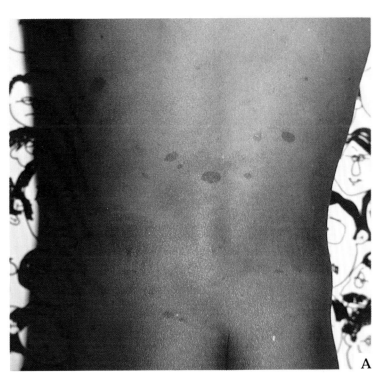

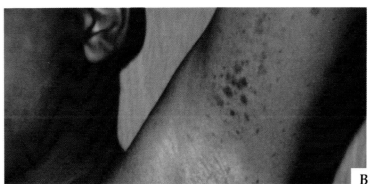

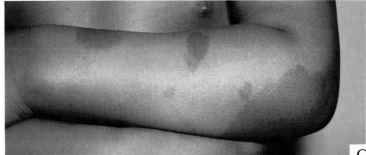

*Fig. 14.1 Neurofibromatosis: Clinical manifestations of cutaneous pigmentary abnormalities. Most common are multiple café au lait spots over the trunk (**A**). Also seen are axillary freckling (**B**) or extensive areas of hyperpigmentation (**C**). (Courtesy of Dr. M. Sherlock)*

The primary objective of the traditional systematic neurologic examination is to determine the functional integrity of the central and peripheral nervous systems. This cornerstone of neurologic physical diagnosis permits detection and localization of neurologic dysfunction, the first step in neurologic differential diagnosis. Neurologic evaluation also includes careful inspection for skin lesions, abnormalities of head shape and volume, disturbances of gait and posture, and abnormalities of muscle bulk, findings which may provide important additional diagnostic clues. This chapter will concentrate on selected neurologic disorders which are accompanied by physical signs that can be detected on visual inspection.

NEUROCUTANEOUS SYNDROMES

The neurocutaneous syndromes or phakomatoses are congenital, often inherited disorders with prominent cutaneous and neurologic manifestations. This simultaneous involvement of skin and nervous system, both derivatives of embryonic ectoderm, suggests that these disorders may be caused by an unknown abnormality of the embryonic epiblast. Although the clinical and pathologic features of the phakomatoses are diverse, these syndromes share a propensity for malformations and hamartomatous tumors of multiple organs. Among the more frequently encountered phakomatoses are neuro-

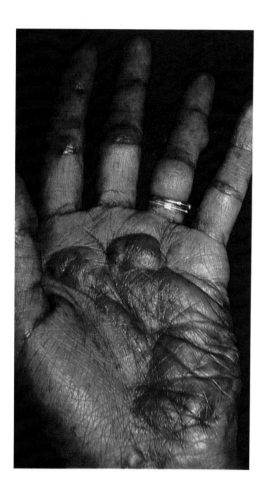

Fig. 14.2 Neuro-fibromatosis: Extensive plexiform neurofibroma of the palm. (Courtesy of Dr. M. Sherlock)

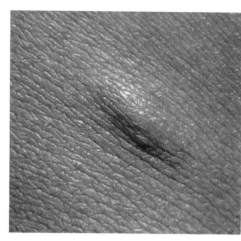

Fig. 14.3 Neuro-fibromatosis: Sub-cutaneous neuro-fibroma along the course of a nerve trunk. (Courtesy of Dr. M. Sherlock)

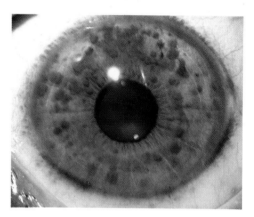

Fig. 14.4 Neurofibromatosis: Pigmented hamartomas of the iris (Lisch nodules).

fibromatosis, tuberous sclerosis, Sturge-Weber syndrome, ataxia telangiectasia, and linear sebaceous nevus.

Neurofibromatosis (von Recklinghausen Disease)

Neurofibromatosis, an autosomal-dominant disorder, is the most common of the neurocutaneous syndromes and is characterized by multiple tumors of spinal and cranial nerves, subcutaneous neurofibromas, and abnormal cutaneous pigmentation. While the fully developed clinical syndrome is rare, abortive forms are common. Overall incidence is estimated at 1 in 2000.

The most frequently encountered cutaneous abnormalities are multiple café au lait spots. These are brown hyperpigmented macules, usually most numerous over the trunk (Fig. 14.1). Although solitary café au lait spots may be seen in normal individuals, the occurrence of four or more such lesions is uncommon. Of patients with neurofibromatosis, 95 percent will have six or more café au lait spots greater than 1 cm in diameter. Other abnormalities of cutaneous pigmentation include axillary freckling or extensive areas of hyperpigmentation. These lesions almost always precede the development of neurologic symptoms. However, they are not necessarily present at birth and are often inconspicuous in early childhood, becoming more prominent at puberty.

Additional cutaneous manifestations of neurofibromatosis may include extensive plexiform neuromas at the terminal distribution of nerve fibers (Fig. 14.2) or small subcutaneous nodules, neurofibromas, scattered along the course of nerve trunks (Fig. 14.3).

Pigmented hamartomas of the iris, termed Lisch nodules, constitute an important ocular finding in neurofibromatosis (Fig. 14.4). They are found in over 90 percent of patients with neurofibromatosis who are 6 years of age or older, and occur in nearly one-third of younger patients. They do not occur in normal individuals. These hamartomas are asymptomatic and do not correlate with the extent or severity of other manifestations, but are helpful in establishing diagnosis.

Skeletal abnormalities are found in 51 percent of affected individuals. The characteristic findings include (Fig. 14.5):

1. Severe angular scoliosis with dysplasia of vertebral bodies
2. Defects of the posterior-superior wall of the orbit
3. Congenital bowing and pseudarthrosis of the tibia, fibula, femur, or clavicle
4. Disorders of bone growth associated with elephantoid hypertrophy of overlying soft tissue
5. Erosive bony defects produced by contiguous neurogenic tumors
6. Scalloping of the posterior margins of the vertebral bodies corresponding to saccular areas of dilatation of the spinal meninges

Other manifestations of neurofibromatosis may include hemihypertrophy of the tongue, face, or extremities; optic nerve glioma; endocrine disturbances; and an increased incidence of meningioma and pheochromocytoma.

Tuberous Sclerosis

Tuberous sclerosis is another autosomal-dominant neurocutaneous disorder whose more prominent features include seizures (96 percent), mental retardation (60 percent), intracranial calcifications (49 percent), tumors of various organs including the brain, and cutaneous lesions. Seizures are the most frequent presenting complaint. The reported prevalence of the disorder is 1 in 150,000, though this may be an underestimate since manifestations can be inconspicuous.

The characteristic skin lesion of tuberous sclerosis is angio-

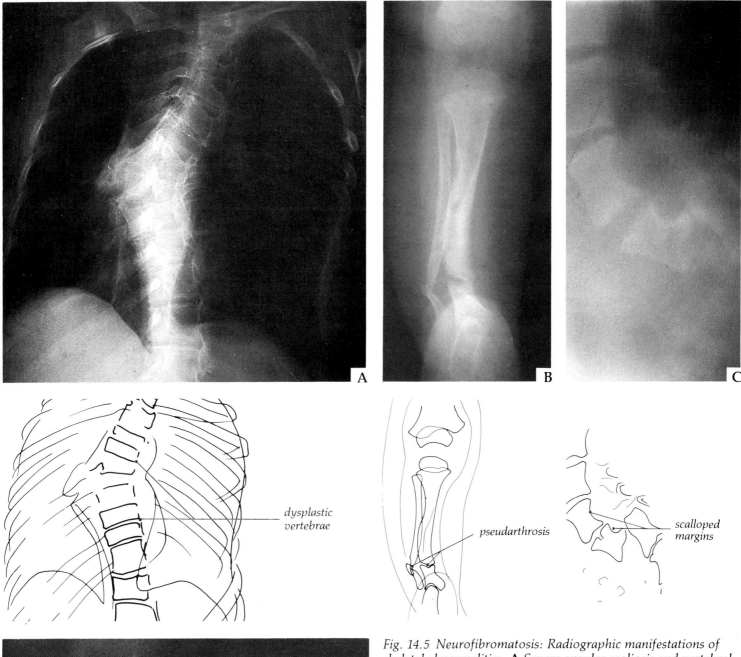

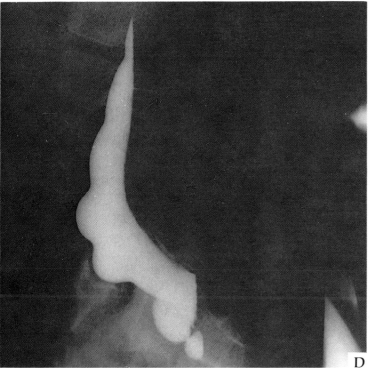

dysplastic vertebrae

pseudarthrosis

scalloped margins

Fig. 14.5 Neurofibromatosis: Radiographic manifestations of skeletal abnormalities. **A** Severe angular scoliosis and vertebral dysplasia. **B** Congenital bowing and pseudarthrosis of the tibia and fibula. **C** Scalloping of posterior margins of the vertebral bodies. A pantopaque myelogram demonstrates underlying dural ectasia (**D**). (Courtesy of Department of Radiology, Children's Hospital of Pittsburgh)

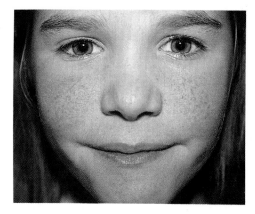

Fig. 14.6 Tuberous sclerosis: Patient, age 9, demonstrates adenoma sebaceum in characteristic malar distribution.

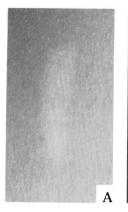

Fig. 14.7 Tuberous sclerosis: An ash-leaf spot, clinical presentation (**A**) and under Wood's light (**B**). (Courtesy of Dr. M. Sherlock)

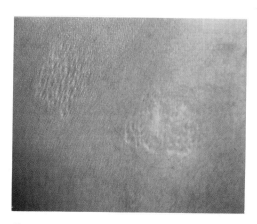

Fig. 14.8 Tuberous sclerosis: Shagreen patch. This plaque of thickened skin with a cobblestone texture is distinctive, but is one of the less common cutaneous manifestations of tuberous sclerosis. (Courtesy of Dr. M. Sherlock)

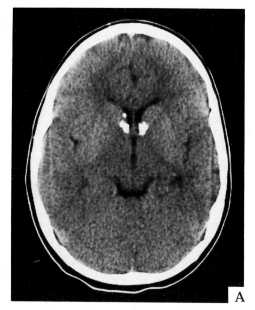

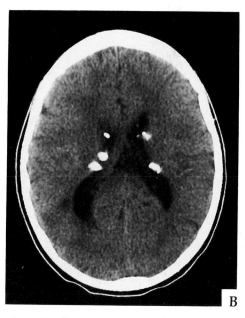

Fig. 14.9 Tuberous sclerosis: CT scans through the foramina of Monro (**A**) and bodies of the lateral ventricles (**B**) show the multiple periventricular calcific deposits characteristic of this disorder. (Courtesy of Division of Neuroradiology, University Health Center of Pittsburgh)

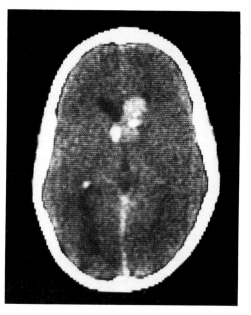

Fig. 14.10 Tuberous sclerosis: CT scan demonstrates a large subependymal astrocytoma which intermittently obstructed the ventricular system, producing episodic symptoms of increased intracranial pressure. (Courtesy of Division of Neuroradiology, University Health Center of Pittsburgh)

fibroma (adenoma sebaceum). These are seen as erythematous papules distributed over the nose and malar region (Fig. 14.6). Approximately 40 percent of children with tuberous sclerosis demonstrate these lesions by 3 years of age.

Ovoid depigmented nevi with irregular borders, termed "ash-leaf" spots, are another common cutaneous manifestation (Fig. 14.7). These generally appear earlier than adenoma sebaceum and may be present at birth. They are detectable by 2 years of age in over half of affected children. While resembling vitiligo, they differ in that they are not completely devoid of melanin. In fair-skinned infants, these nevi may be demonstrable only under Wood's light.

Another valuable cutaneous marker is the shagreen patch, a plaque of thickened skin with a cobblestone or orange peel texture (Fig. 14.8). Histologically, the shagreen patch is a connective tissue nevus.

Additional dermatologic manifestations of tuberous sclerosis include periungual and dental fibromas and macular areas of hyperpigmentation. Recognition of the cutaneous features can suggest an etiologic diagnosis in some patients presenting with mental retardation or seizures.

The majority of patients with tuberous sclerosis have intracranial calcifications demonstrable by CT scan. These appear as multiple scattered areas of increased density adjacent to the walls of the lateral and third ventricles (Fig. 14.9). The CT scan is of particular value in demonstrating intracranial calcifications in young children at a time when plain skull films are often negative. It may also demonstrate typical intracranial calcifications in asymptomatic relatives who have no external manifestations of the disorder. This has led to the identification of many subclinical cases, and can play an important role in genetic counseling.

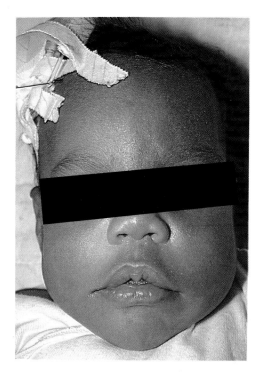

Fig. 14.11 Sturge-Weber syndrome: Nonelevated purple cutaneous hemangioma in a trigeminal distribution.

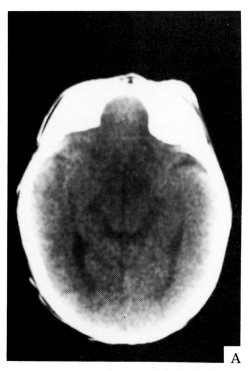

Fig. 14.12 Sturge-Weber syndrome: **A** Normal CT scan at birth. Subsequently, findings such as gyriform contrast enhancement, seen here in the left occipital, temporal, and parietal lobes (**B**), and associated hemispheric atrophy (**C**) may be observed by age 4 months. Serpiginous parenchymal calcifications may be observed in the older child (**D**). (Courtesy of Division of Neuroradiology, University Health Center of Pittsburgh)

A

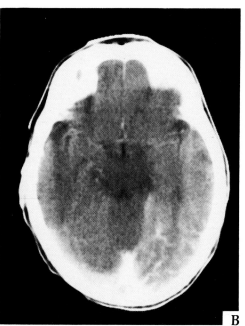

B

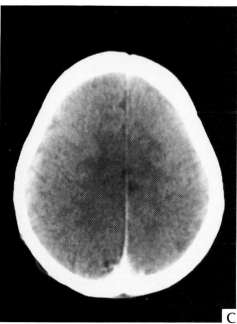

C

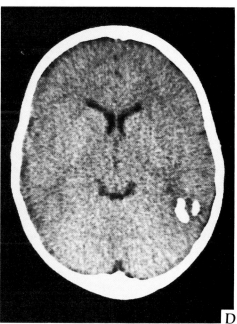

D

The characteristic gross abnormality of the brain is the presence of multiple gliotic nodules of varying size, which constitute the tubers for which this disorder is named. These are located over the convolutions of the cerebral hemispheres and beneath the ependymal lining of the lateral and third ventricles. Heterotopic nodules of identical structure may be found in the central white matter. Tumors may arise from either the cortical or subependymal tubers, complicating the course of the disease by producing increased intracranial pressure and other symptoms associated with intracranial mass lesions (Fig. 14.10).

Visceral lesions associated with tuberous sclerosis include cardiac rhabdomyomas, renal hamartomas and mixed embryonal tumors, and hepatic hamartomas. The cardiac rhabdomyomas are usually asymptomatic, but occasionally an affected newborn may present with obstructive congestive heart failure. Renal lesions are often unimportant functionally, but can produce albuminuria or hematuria. Chronic renal failure and malignant transformation of renal tumors are quite rare. Hepatic hamartomas are clinically insignificant.

Sturge-Weber Syndrome

The cardinal manifestations of Sturge-Weber syndrome are:
1. A vascular nevus or "port wine" stain involving the face, most commonly in the trigeminal distribution
2. Ipsilateral leptomeningeal angiomatosis with associated intracranial calcifications
3. A high incidence of mental retardation

The vascular nevus (Fig. 14.11) is usually present at birth and consists of a pink to purple macular cutaneous hemangioma. Seizures occur in 90 percent of cases and generally begin before 1 year of age. Contralateral hemiparesis eventually develops in 30 percent of patients.

The coincidence of seizures and facial vascular nevus should suggest the diagnosis of Sturge-Weber syndrome, which can be confirmed by CT scan (Fig. 14.12). These scans may be normal at birth, but subsequently will show areas of

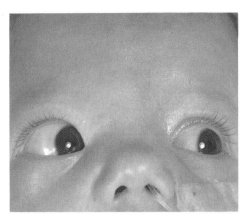

Fig. 14.13 Buphthalmos: Enlargement of the right eye, one of the associated ocular findings in Sturge-Weber syndrome. (From Booth IW, Wozniak ER: Pediatrics. Williams & Wilkins, Baltimore, 1984, p 32)

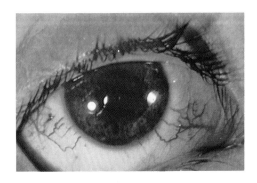

Fig. 14.14 Ataxia telangiectasia: Such telangiectases in the bulbar conjunctiva usually develop between 3 months and 6 years of age.

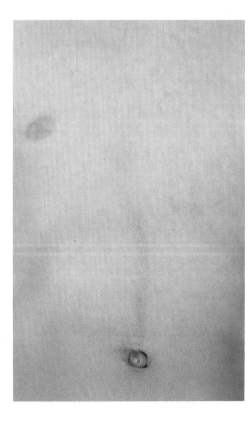

Fig. 14.15 Linear sebaceous nevus: Clinical photograph shows a linear, yellow-tan, waxy-appearing lesion, in this case associated with seizures and mental retardation.

gyriform contrast enhancement corresponding to the leptomeningeal angiomatosis. Serial examinations often demonstrate progressive ipsilateral cerebral atrophy. Additional findings may include serpiginous calcifications of brain parenchyma underlying vascular malformations of the pia. These intracranial calcifications are first seen on CT scan but become evident on plain skull films by the end of the second decade.

Associated ocular abnormalities are often encountered. Buphthalmos or coloboma may be present at birth, and glaucoma frequently develops in infancy or later childhood (Fig. 14.13). Dilated vessels in the sclera, conjunctiva, and retina are common, while angiomatous malformations of the choroid occasionally occur.

The estimated incidence of facial cutaneous angioma is 1 in 5000, and the estimated frequency of the complete syndrome is 1 in 30,000. While most cases are sporadic, genetic determination has not been ruled out. There are, however, no reported cases of direct transmission from parent to child.

Ataxia Telangiectasia

Ataxia telangiectasia is a multisystem, autosomal-recessive degenerative disorder characterized by ataxia, oculocutaneous telangiectasia, immunodeficiency, and a high incidence of neoplasia. The nature of the basic underlying defect is unknown. Ataxia is the usual presenting feature and the course of the neurologic disturbance is rather stereotypic. Tremors of the head may be seen before 1 year of age, and unsteadiness of gait is evident when the child first walks. Progressive global ataxia and slurred, scanning, dysarthric speech are typical during the early school-age years. Loss of deep-tendon reflexes and impairment of position and vibratory sensation are evident by the end of the first decade. Adolescence is marked by choreoathetosis, dystonic posturing, gaze apraxia, and progressive dementia.

The characteristic cutaneous manifestations of this disorder appear by 6 years of age. Telangiectases first appear on the bulbar conjunctiva (Fig. 14.14), and develop later over the malar regions, ears, antecubital fossae, neck, and upper chest.

Neuropathologic changes are widespread, with the cerebellum being the site of maximal degeneration. Loss of Purkinje and basket cells, thinning of the granular cell layer, and mild changes in the molecular layer are characteristic findings. Systemic manifestations include major defects in both cellular and humoral immunity. Deficiencies of IgA and IgM are characteristic, and together with impaired cellular immunity contribute to susceptibility to the recurrent respiratory infections which mark this disorder.

Linear Sebaceous Nevus

The sebaceous nevus of Jadassohn is usually present at birth, presenting as a yellow-tan, waxy-appearing linear lesion (Fig. 14.15) which contains a papillomatous excess of sebaceous glands. This nevus may be found on the scalp, face, neck, trunk, or extremities. With time, the lesion becomes unsightly. This phenomenon as well as a 15 to 20 percent risk of malignant degeneration has led practitioners to recommend early surgical excision. While this lesion usually occurs as an isolated abnormality in otherwise normal individuals, an association with seizures and mental retardation is reported. The risk of associated neurologic abnormalities is greatest when the cutaneous lesion is located in the midfacial area.

CAUSES OF MACROCEPHALY

Early Infantile (Birth to 6 Months)

Hydrocephalus (progressive or arresting)
  Induction disorders (congenital malformations)
    Spina bifida cystica, cranium bifidum, Chiari
    malformations (types I, II, and III), aqueductal
    stenosis, holoprosencephaly
  Mass lesions
    Neoplasms, A-V malformations, congenital cysts
  Intrauterine infections
    Toxoplasmosis, cytomegalic inclusion disease,
    syphilis, rubella

Peri- or postnatal infections
  Bacterial, granulomatous, parasitic
Peri- or postnatal hemorrhage
  Hypoxia, vascular malformation, trauma
Hydranencephaly
Subdural Effusion
  Hemorrhagic, infectious, cystic hygroma
Normal Variant (often familial)

Late Infantile (6 Months to 2 Years)

Hydrocephalus (progressive or arresting)
  Space-occupying lesions
    Tumors, cysts, abscesses
  Postbacterial or granulomatous meningitis
  Dysraphism
    Dandy-Walker syndrome, Chiari type I
    malformation
  Posthemorrhagic
    Trauma or vascular malformation
Subdural Effusion
Increased Intracranial Pressure Syndrome
  Pseudotumor cerebri
    Lead, tetracycline, hypoparathyroidism, steroids,
    excess or deficiency of vitamin A, cyanotic
    congenital heart disease
Primary Skeletal Cranial Dysplasias (thickened or
  enlarged skull), Osteogenesis Imperfecta, Hyperphos-
  phatemia, Osteopetrosis, Rickets

Megalencephaly (increase in brain substance)
  Metabolic CNS diseases: Leukodystrophies (e.g.,
    Canavan, Alexander), lipidoses (Tay-Sachs),
    histiocytosis, mucopolysaccharidoses
  Proliferative neurocutaneous syndromes
    von Recklinghausen, tuberous sclerosis,
    hemangiomatosis, Sturge-Weber
  Cerebral gigantism
    Soto syndrome
  Achondroplasia
  Primary megalencephaly
    May be familial, and unassociated or associated
    with abnormalities of cellular architecture

Early to Late Childhood (After 2 Years)

Hydrocephalus (arrested or progressive)
  Space-occupying lesions
  Preexisting induction disorder
    Aqueductal stenosis, Chiari type I malformation
  Postinfectious
  Hemorrhagic

Megalencephaly
  Proliferative neurocutaneous syndromes
  Familial
Pseudotumor cerebri
Normal variant

Fig. 14.16 Causes of macrocephaly. (From Gabriel RS: Malformations of the central nervous system. In Menkes JH (ed.) *Textbook of Child Neurology, 2nd ed. Lea & Febiger, Philadelphia, 1980)*

CENTRAL NERVOUS SYSTEM MALFORMATIONS

Malformations of the central nervous system are a leading cause of neurologic and developmental disability in infants and children. Although CNS malformations are not necessarily accompanied by external dysmorphic features, disturbances of cranial volume, abnormalities of head shape, and skin lesions overlying the dorsal midline should alert the physician to the possibility of associated CNS dysmorphogenesis.

Macrocephaly

Macrocephaly is defined as a head circumference greater than two standard deviations above the mean for age, sex, and gestation. It is a phenomenon which can be caused by a myriad of conditions (Fig. 14.16), including excessive accumulation of cerebrospinal fluid (hydrocephalus); intracranial mass lesions (tumors, subdural effusions); thickening or enlargement of the skull (primary skeletal dysplasias); or a true increase in brain substance (megalencephaly) such as is seen in Soto syndrome, achondroplasia, the neurocutaneous

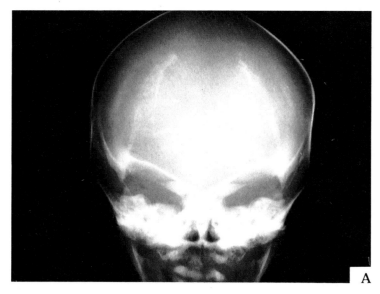
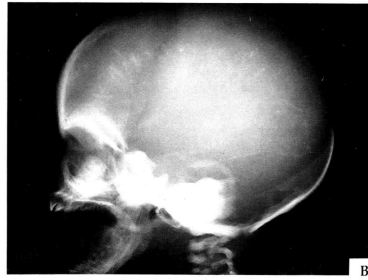

A

B

Fig. 14.17 Macrocephaly: Frontal (**A**) and lateral (**B**) radiographs reveal bilaterally symmetrical, paraventricular cerebral calcifica-

tions in association with cranial enlargement. (Courtesy of Department of Radiology, Children's Hospital of Pittsburgh)

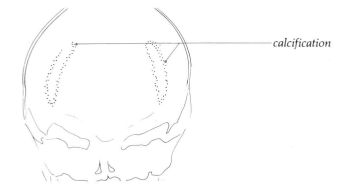

calcification

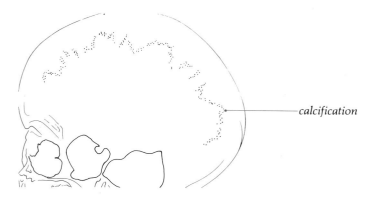

calcification

syndromes, and certain lipidoses, leukodystrophies, and mucopolysaccharidoses. Primary megalencephaly may occur as a benign familial trait.

Evaluation of the child with a head which is abnormally large or which appears to be growing at an excessive rate should include:

1. Evaluation of serial measurements of head circumference
2. Measurement of the parents' head circumferences and exploration of family history for evidence of macrocephaly or neurologic and cutaneous abnormalities
3. Developmental history
4. Careful examination for evidence of increased intracranial pressure, developmental delay, skeletal dysplasia, abnormal transillumination, cranial bruits, ocular abnormalities, or organomegaly

Plain skull X-rays may provide evidence of increased intracranial pressure, identify intracranial calcifications (Fig. 14.17), or detect primary skeletal dysplasias (Fig. 14.18). CT scan allows assessment of ventricular size, and permits detection of intracranial mass lesions and subdural effusions.

HYDROCEPHALUS

Hydrocephalus is an imbalance between cerebrospinal fluid (CSF) production and resorption of sufficient magnitude to result in a net accumulation of fluid within the ventricular system. Impaired CSF resorption may occur secondary to obstruction of CSF pathways within the ventricular system

(noncommunicating hydrocephalus) or as a result of obstruction of the subarachnoid space (communicating hydrocephalus). Hydrocephalus secondary to CSF overproduction is rare, but does occur in some cases of choroid plexus papilloma. Noncommunicating hydrocephalus is often due to aqueductal stenosis or congenital malformations of the fourth ventricle, and accompanies tumors or vascular malformations of the posterior fossa which compress the cerebral aqueduct or obstruct outflow from the fourth ventricle. Causes of communicating hydrocephalus include intracranial hemorrhage, meningitis, cerebral venous or dural sinus thrombosis, and diffuse infiltration of the meninges by malignant cells.

The clinical manifestations of hydrocephalus in infancy are stereotypic (Fig. 14.19). The head is either excessively large at birth or grows at an abnormally rapid rate, becoming macrocephalic over the first few months. The forehead is disproportionally large, and the face appears small in relation to the calvarium. The scalp is thin and glistening; its veins are distended, often becoming strikingly dilated when the infant cries. The anterior fontanelle is large, tense, and nonpulsatile, and the sutures are excessively wide. Divergent strabismus, abducens nerve paresis, and impaired upgaze are important ocular findings. With severe hydrocephalus there may be involuntary, forced conjugate downward deviation of the eyes so that the inferior half of the iris is hidden by the lower eyelid, producing the "sunsetting" sign. Neurologic abnormalities include developmental delay, persistence of early infantile automatisms, and spasticity and hyperreflexia of the lower extremities.

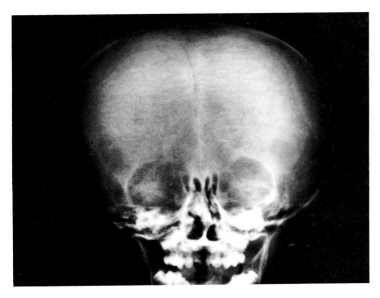

Fig. 14.18 Macrocephaly: Plain skull radiographs allow detection of primary skeletal dysplasias. In this case note the mosaic rarification of the cranial vault and multiple wormian bones characteristic of osteogenesis imperfecta. (Courtesy of Department of Radiology, Children's Hospital of Pittsburgh)

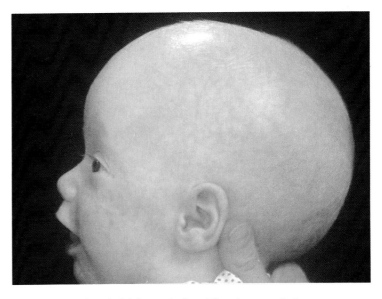

Fig. 14.19 Infantile hydrocephalus: The characteristic appearance is an enlarged head, thinning of the scalp, distended scalp veins, and a full fontanelle. (From Booth IW, Wozniak ER: Pediatrics. Williams & Wilkins, Baltimore, 1984, p 108)

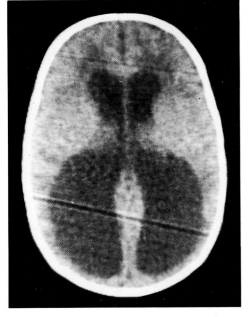

Fig. 14.20 Infantile hydrocephalus: CT scan demonstrates a dilated ventricular system and thinning of the cortical mantle. (Courtesy of Division of Neuroradiology, University Health Center of Pittsburgh)

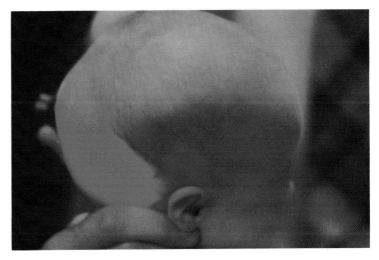

Fig. 14.21 Dandy-Walker malformation: Transillumination demonstrates a posterior fossa cyst. Note also the bulging occiput, prominent scalp veins, and enlargement of the head. (Courtesy of Dr. M.J. Painter)

The CT scan will demonstrate enlargement of the ventricular system and thinning of the cortical mantle, and may provide additional anatomic information concerning etiology (Fig. 14.20).

Infantile hydrocephalus must be distinguished from other causes of macrocephaly in infancy such as chronic subdural hematoma, expanding porencephalic cyst, and certain degenerative disorders which may produce abnormal enlargement of the head (see Fig. 14.16). In premature infants with suspected hydrocephalus, the normally rapid postnatal head growth of the premature must be taken into account.

DANDY-WALKER MALFORMATION
Dandy-Walker malformation is a primary developmental abnormality characterized by progressive cystic enlargement of the fourth ventricle beginning early in fetal life. This is accompanied by enlargement of the posterior fossa and upward displacement of the tentorium, torcula, and transverse sinuses. Associated hydrocephalus is almost universal, and may be present at birth or develop later during infancy or childhood. Of affected individuals, 60 percent show signs of hydrocephalus and increased intracranial pressure by 2 years of age.

Clinical manifestations of Dandy-Walker malformation are variable, and depend upon the severity and rate of progression of the associated hydrocephalus. Symptomatic children often have an unusually prominent bulging occiput in addition to the usual findings of hydrocephalus. In children under 1 year of age, transillumination of the skull effectively demonstrates the posterior fossa cyst (Fig. 14.21). Ataxia, nystagmus, and cranial nerve deficits may also be prominent.

Plain skull X-rays demonstrate posteroinferior enlargement of the cranial vault, thinning and ballooning of the occipital squama, and upward displacement of the torcula. A CT scan will confirm the presence of a large posterior fossa

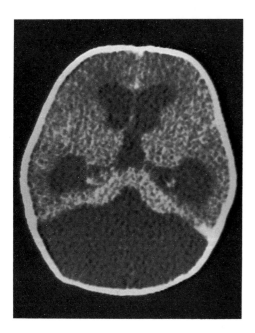

Fig. 14.22 Dandy-Walker malforma-tion: CT scan shows a posterior fossa cyst, a small cere-bellar remnant, and associated hydro-cephalus.

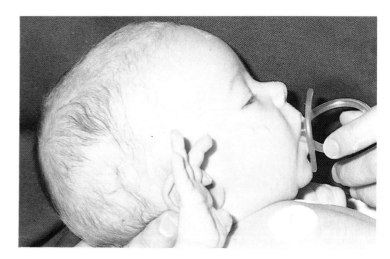

Fig. 14.23 Hydranencephaly: Patient, age 3 weeks, has a decep-tively normal appearance with little to suggest a severe brain abnormality.

cyst along with a small cerebellar remnant and associated hydrocephalus (Fig. 14.22).

Hydranencephaly

Hydranencephaly is a severe anomaly of the brain character-ized by the absence of the cerebral hemispheres despite intact meninges and a normal skull. Affected children often appear deceptively normal at birth, with little to suggest the presence of a severe brain abnormality (Fig. 14.23). Since newborn in-fants function at a subcortical reflex level, even complete absence of the cerebral hemispheres may not interfere with normal reflexes. However, within the first few weeks of life, developmental arrest, decerebration, hypertonia, and hyper-reflexia become apparent in the hydranencephalic infant. Most do not live beyond 6 to 12 months, although survival for several years is occasionally reported. Seizures are common, and progressive enlargement of the head may complicate nursing care.

Diagnosis may be suggested if, on transillumination of the skull, the entire calvarium is lit up (Fig. 14.24). It must be noted, however, that severe hydrocephalus and bilateral sub-dural hygromas may present a similar appearance.

CT scan demonstrates a large water-dense cavity replacing the cerebral hemispheres with islands of residual brain tissue at the base (Fig. 14.25). To distinguish this disorder from massive bilateral subdural hygromas, cerebral angiography is required to confirm absence of the cerebrum.

Microcephaly

Microcephaly is defined as a head circumference which is more than two standard deviations below the mean for age, sex, and gestation. Apart from cases due to premature closure of the sutures (generalized craniosynostosis), microcephaly reflects an abnormally small brain and can be a symptom of any disorder which impairs brain growth (Fig. 14.26). The neurologic manifestations range from minor (poor fine motor skills, mild intellectual impairment) to profound (decerebra-tion, chronic vegetative state). Diagnostic evaluation should include family history, prenatal history, search for associated congenital anomalies, karyotyping, amino acid screening,

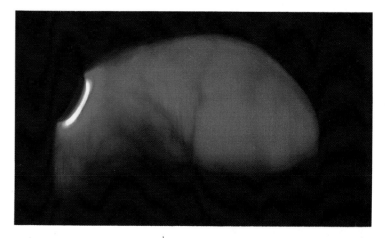

Fig. 14.24 Hydranencephaly: Transillumination of the skull lights up the calvarium, suggesting the diagnosis.

and serologic studies for intrauterine infection. Plain skull X-rays can detect craniosynostosis, while the CT scan is useful in identifying intracranial calcifications.

Occult Spinal Dysraphism

Development of the human nervous system begins early in the third week of gestation with proliferation of ectodermal cells in the dorsal midline to form the neural plate. By the end of the fourth week, the neural plate has invaginated and then fused in the midline to form the neural tube. The cerebrum, diencephalon, midbrain, and brainstem will develop from the rostral portion of the neural tube. The caudal portion separ-ates from the overlying ectoderm forming the precursor of the spinal cord and becomes surrounded by mesodermal ele-ments destined to form the vertebral bodies and supporting soft-tissue structures. Midline spinal cord/vertebral skeletal defects, termed "spinal dysraphism," result from defective closure of the caudal neural tube. Abnormal neural tube closure beginning early in the embryologic sequence produces dysraphic states which involve both neural and skeletal ele-ments (myelomeningocele), while later-occurring closure defects produce congenital anomalies restricted to the pos-terior elements of the vertebrae (spina bifida occulta).

Occult spinal dysraphism is a defect of intermediate sever-ity in which vertebral anomalies are associated with underly-

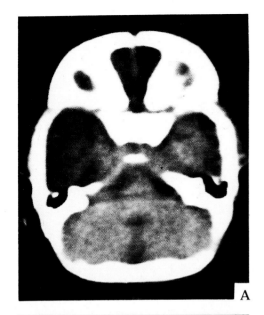

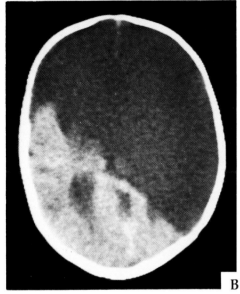

Fig. 14.25 Hydranencephaly: CT scan demonstrates a normal cerebellum and posterior fossa structures (**A**) as well as replacement of the cerebral hemispheres by a large water-dense cavity with residual islands of brain tissue in regions of the occipital poles and right inferior temporal lobe (**B**). (Courtesy of Division of Neuroradiology, University Health Center of Pittsburgh)

CAUSES OF MICROCEPHALY

Genetic Defects
    Autosomal-recessive
    Autosomal-dominant
Disorders of Karyotype
    Trisomies
    Deletions
    Translocations
Intrauterine Infections
    Rubella
    Cytomegalic inclusion disease
    Toxoplasmosis
    Congenital syphilis
    Herpes virus

Prenatal Irradiation
Exposure to Drugs and Chemicals
    during Gestation
        Ethyl alcohol (fetal alcohol
            syndrome)
        Phenytoin
        Trimethadione
        Methyl mercury
Maternal Phenylketonuria
Perinatal Insults
    Traumatic
    Anoxic
    Metabolic
    Infectious

Fig. 14.26 Causes of microcephaly.

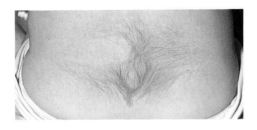

Fig. 14.27 Occult spinal dysraphism: Note hairy patch over lumbar region, here associated with diastematomyelia. (Courtesy of Dr. M.J. Painter)

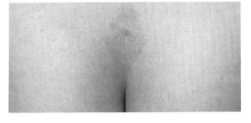

Fig. 14.28 Occult spinal dysraphism: Sacral sinus tract associated with intraspinal dermoid tumor. (Courtesy of Dr. M.J. Painter)

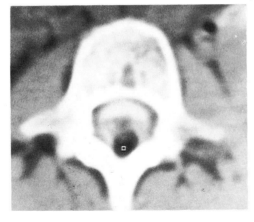

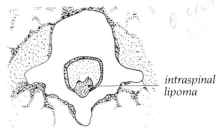

Fig. 14.29 Occult spinal dysraphism: CT scan demonstrates an intraspinal lipoma in a child who presented with a subcutaneous lipoma over the lumbar spine.

intraspinal lipoma

ing intraspinal tumors or developmental abnormalities. Its presence is often betrayed by cutaneous abnormalities such as a hairy patch (Fig. 14.27), skin tag, "port wine" stain, hemangioma, subcutaneous lipoma, or sinus tract (Fig. 14.28). Patients found to have such skin lesions overlying the lumbosacral spine should have spinal radiographs taken. If these reveal underlying vertebral abnormalities, neuroradiologic investigations (i.e., myelography, spinal CT scan) are indicated, as early surgical intervention can prevent the development of progressive neurologic deficits. Common intraspinal lesions include dermoid tumors, intraspinal lipomas (Fig. 14.29), and diastematomyelia.

While some patients with occult spinal dysraphism may show signs of neurologic dysfunction and talipes equinovarus from birth, most develop symptoms insidiously after a symptom-free interval. Dysfunction usually begins at around 3 years of age, but many do not develop problems until school age or adolescence. Presenting complaints may include back or leg stiffness, clumsiness, mild weakness or numbness of the lower extremities, or problems with bladder dysfunction. Objective findings may consist of decreased tone and deep-tendon reflexes in the lower extremities; patchy decreases in sensation; and foot deformities consisting of broadening and shortening, deepening of the arch, and contractures of the toes. Patients with associated tethering of the spinal cord tend to present during a period of rapid growth with back, leg, or buttock pain; signs of lower limb spasticity; and, on occasion, bowel and bladder dysfunction.

	Duchenne	Becker	Fascioscapulo-humeral	Limb-Girdle	Myotonic
Inheritance	X-linked recessive	X-linked recessive	Autosomal-dominant	Autosomal-recessive	Autosomal-dominant
Age of Onset	Early childhood	Late childhood, adolescence	Variable, childhood through early adult life	Childhood to early adult	Highly variable
Pattern of Weakness	Pelvic girdle, shoulder girdle	Pelvic girdle, shoulder girdle	Face, shoulder girdle	Pelvic girdle, shoulder girdle	Face, distal limbs
Rate of Progression	Rapid	Slow	Very slow	Variable	Variable
Associated Features	Pseudohyper-trophy of calves	Pseudohyper-trophy of calves	None	Pseudohyper-trophy rare	Myotonia
Systemic Features	Mental retardation, abnormal EKG, cardio-myopathy	Occasional mental retardation	None	None	Frequent mental retardation, heart block, cataracts, pre-mature balding, testicular tubu-lar atrophy, diabetes

Fig. 14.30 Clinical features of the muscular dystrophies.

NEUROMUSCULAR DISORDERS

Weakness is the most common presenting symptom of neuro-muscular disease. If time is taken to determine the ways in which the weakness interferes with normal activities and un-cover the types of tasks that the patient finds difficult, the distribution and severity of muscle weakness can be predicted from the clinical history. Determining the mode of onset and pattern of progression of the symptoms is essential in differen-tial diagnosis and selection of diagnostic studies. Since many neuromuscular disorders are genetically determined, a com-plete family history must be obtained.

Essential components of the physical examination of pa-tients with neuromuscular disease include inspection, palpa-tion, percussion, evaluation of the deep-tendon reflexes, and assessment of muscle strength. Inspection can reveal muscle wasting and atrophy, abnormal spontaneous activity, and ab-normal resting postures. Palpation permits assessment of muscle consistency, determination of muscle tone, and detec-tion of muscle tenderness. Percussion is useful in detecting myotonia. Assessment of muscle strength includes both indi-vidual muscle testing and functional evaluation. The strength

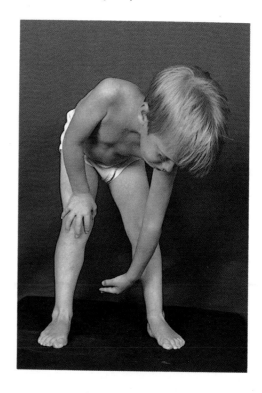

Fig. 14.31 Duchenne muscular dystrophy: This child, age 5, has difficulty rising. Unilateral hand sup-port on the knee is required to get erect.

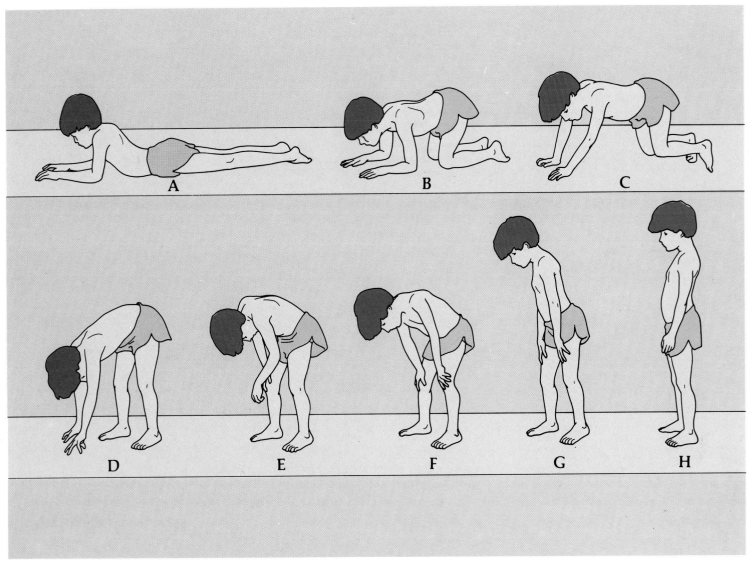

Fig. 14.32 *The Gower maneuver. This series of diagrams illustrates the sequence of postures used in attaining the upright position. First the legs are pulled up under the body, and the weight is shifted to rest on the hands and feet (A–C). The hips are then thrust in the air as the knees are straightened and the hands are brought close to the legs (D). Finally, the trunk is slowly extended by the hands walking up the thigh (E–G) until the erect position is attained (H).*

of individual muscles is recorded using a standardized system:

  0 — no contraction
  1 — flicker or trace contraction
  2 — active movement with gravity eliminated
  3 — active movement against gravity
  4 — active movement against gravity and resistance
  5 — normal power

Functional evaluation of muscle strength is accomplished by observing the patient rising from the floor, rising from a chair, stepping onto a stool, climbing stairs, walking on heels, hopping on toes, and raising the arms above the head. This permits rapid detection of proximal weakness of the hips and shoulders, and distal weakness of the legs.

Duchenne Muscular Dystrophy

The muscular dystrophies are genetically determined disorders characterized by progressive degeneration of skeletal muscle, usually following a latency period of seemingly normal development and function. The various clinical types of muscular dystrophy are distinguished on the basis of pattern of inheritance, distribution of initial weakness, age of onset of clinical manifestations, and rate of progression (Fig. 14.30).

Duchenne muscular dystrophy is the most frequently encountered disorder, with an incidence of 13 to 33 cases per 100,000 male live births. It is characterized by X-linked recessive inheritance; symmetrical and initially selective involvement of the pelvic and pectoral girdles; pseudohypertrophy of the calves; relentlessly progressive weakness leading to loss of ambulation within 10 years of onset of symptoms; and very high levels of activity of certain serum enzymes, notably creatine kinase.

Clinical manifestations of Duchenne muscular dystrophy do not usually appear until the second year of life. Early developmental milestones are normally attained, although the first attempts at walking may be delayed. Gait is often clumsy and awkward from the start, and the ability to run is never normally attained. Difficulty climbing stairs, frequent falls, and progressive difficulty rising from the floor are early features. In order to rise from the floor, the child may, at first, need only to push with one hand on a knee (Fig. 14.31). However, as weakness of the extensors of the hips becomes more pronounced, rising from the floor becomes increasingly difficult and requires the use of the hands to "climb up the legs" (the Gower maneuver) (Fig. 14.32).

Progressive gluteal weakness leads to the assumption of a

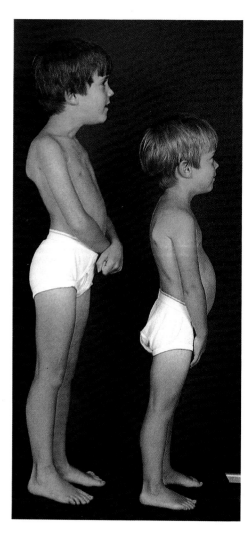

Fig. 14.33 Duchenne muscular dystrophy: These brothers, ages 5 and 8, show progressive compensatory postural adjustments, with broadening of stance, accentuated lumbar lordosis, and forward thrusting of the abdomen.

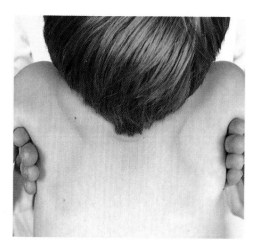

Fig. 14.34 Duchenne muscular dystrophy: This child, age 5, demonstrates weakness and hypotonia of shoulder girdle musculature. Upward displacement of shoulders and abnormal rotation of scapulae are seen when the child is lifted with the examiner's hands under his arms.

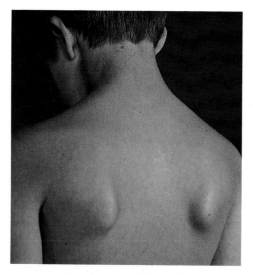

Fig. 14.35 Duchenne muscular dystrophy: Spontaneous winging of the scapulae can be noted in this 8-year-old.

compensatory posture characterized by a broadened base, accentuated lumbar lordosis, and forward thrusting of the abdomen (Fig. 14.33). Although weakness of the arms is not a common early symptom, proximal upper extremity weakness is easily detected on clinical examination when the child is lifted with the examiner's hands placed beneath the arms. There is marked laxity of the shoulder girdle musculature associated with upward displacement of the shoulders and abnormal rotation of the scapulae (Fig. 14.34). In addition, spontaneous winging of the scapulae may be prominent (Fig. 14.35).

Weakness of the neck flexors, as evidenced by marked head lag when pulled to sit from the supine position (Fig. 14.36), is an early finding. Enlargement of muscles, particularly in the calves (Fig. 14.37), is a common feature by 5 or 6 years of age. The abnormally enlarged muscles have an unusually firm rubbery consistency on palpation. Early in the clinical course this increase in muscle volume may be due to true hypertrophy, with muscle strength proportional to bulk. Later, infiltration by fat and connective tissue sometimes maintains this bulk in spite of loss of muscle fibers. This is called "pseudohypertrophy."

Charcot-Marie-Tooth Disease (Hereditary Motor-Sensory Neuropathy, Type I)

Charcot-Marie-Tooth disease is an autosomal-dominant demyelinating form of peroneal muscular atrophy. Onset of symptoms is usually in the second decade, the presenting complaints being foot deformities and gait abnormalities.

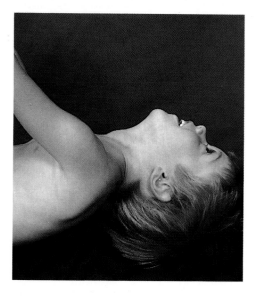

Fig. 14.36 Duchenne muscular dystrophy: This 5-year-old has neck flexor weakness. Note marked head lag when the patient is pulled to sit from the supine position.

Often, pes cavus or hammer-toe deformities develop in early childhood long before more overt symptoms appear. The clinical picture is quite variable, and as most affected persons do not consult a physician for their neurologic problems, the majority remain undiagnosed. The astute physician will consider the diagnosis when a patient who presents with unrelated symptoms is found to have pes cavus or hammer toes and symmetrical distal weakness.

Muscle weakness and atrophy begin insidiously in the foot and leg muscles. The intrinsic muscles of the foot are often affected first, followed by involvement of the peronei, anterior tibial muscles, long toe extensors, intrinsic hand muscles, and

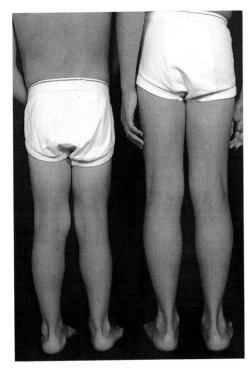

Fig. 14.37 Duchenne muscular dystrophy: Enlargement of calves in brothers ages 5 and 8.

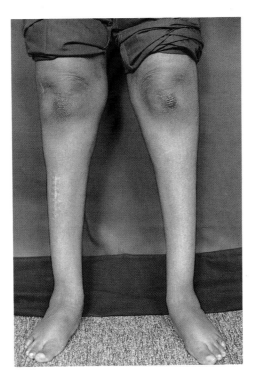

Fig. 14.38 Charcot-Marie-Tooth disease: Patient, age 15, with distal muscular atrophy of the lower extremities ("stork-leg" appearance).

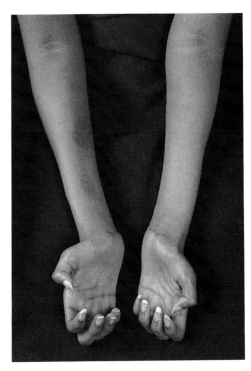

Fig. 14.39 Charcot-Marie-Tooth disease: This 15-year-old demonstrates atrophy of forearm and intrinsic hand muscles and "claw-hand" deformity.

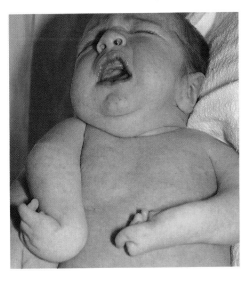

Fig. 14.40 Congenital cervical spinal atrophy: This 2-day-old infant has flaccid paresis limited to the upper extremities and associated congenital flexion contractures.

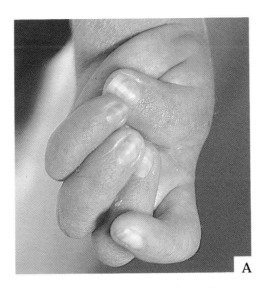

Fig. 14.41 Congenital cervical spinal atrophy: Wasting and atrophy of intrinsic hand muscles with flexion contractures of

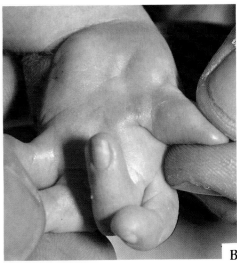

the fingers (**A**) and poorly developed transverse palmar creases (**B**) can be seen in this 2-day-old.

gastrocnemius. Weakness and atrophy may spread to the more proximal muscles of the leg and forearm. The degree of muscle wasting is often mild; however, in some cases the loss of muscle mass in the distal lower extremities is severe, giving rise to a striking "stork-leg" appearance (Fig. 14.38). With involvement of the distal upper extremities there may be obvious wasting of the intrinsic hand muscles and development of secondary "claw deformities" (Fig. 14.39). Deep-tendon reflexes are first lost in the gastrocnemius and soleus, and subsequently in the quadriceps femoris and upper limbs. Sensation may be mildly impaired in the distal lower extremities.

Congenital Cervical Spinal Atrophy

This rare disorder presents at birth with dramatic flaccid paresis of the upper extremities (Fig. 14.40). The presence of congenital flexion contractures suggests chronic denervation which must have occurred in utero, and allows this syndrome to be distinguished from injury to the cervical spine or brachial plexuses during delivery. Abnormalities in the formation of the transverse palmar creases are present in all cases (Fig. 14.41), suggesting a prenatal insult during the first trimester. The disorder is nonprogressive.

Myotonia Congenita

Myotonia congenita is an inherited disorder of skeletal muscle in which muscle stiffness is the only complaint. Both autosomal-dominant and autosomal-recessive forms occur. The clinical symptoms are rather stereotypic. After a period of inactivity, the muscles stiffen and are difficult to maneuver; however, with continued activity, the stiffness diminishes and movement becomes almost normal. Typically, the child moves clumsily with a stiff awkward gait and often falls. However, as activity continues, he begins to walk freely, and with "warm-up" is able to run without difficulty.

Generalized muscular hypertrophy is a frequent finding on examination, with affected children often presenting an unusually well-developed athletic appearance (Fig. 14.42). This belies their sedentary habits and physical ineptitude due to muscle stiffness. Clinically, the myotonia may be demonstrated following sustained contraction of a group of muscles, as produced by clenching the hand or by percussion of the thenar eminence (Fig. 14.43).

BIBLIOGRAPHY

Brooke MH: A Clinician's View of Neuromuscular Diseases. William & Wilkins, Baltimore, 1977.

Menkes JH: Textbook of Child Neurology, 2nd ed. Lea & Febiger, Philadelphia, 1980.

Warkany J, Lemire RJ, Cohen MM: Mental Retardation and Congenital Malformations of the Central Nervous System. Yearbook, Chicago, 1981.

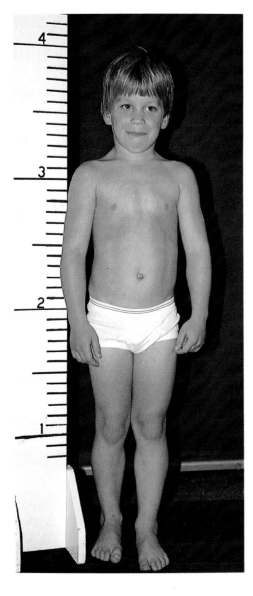

Fig. 14.42 Myotonia congenita: Patient, age 8, demonstrates generalized muscular hypertrophy, giving a well-developed athletic appearance.

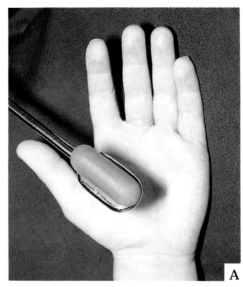

A

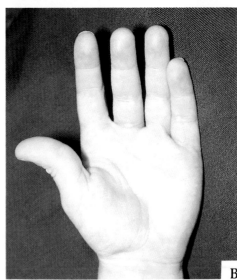

B

Fig. 14.43 Myotonia congenita: Percussion of the thenar eminence (**A**) is followed by involuntary opposition of the thumb and visible contraction of the thenar muscles (**B**) which lasts for several seconds.

PEDIATRIC SURGERY

David A. Lloyd, M.D.

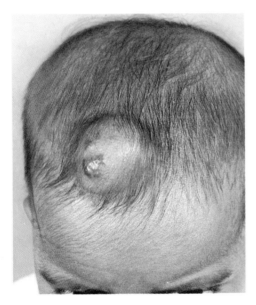

FIG. 15.1 Cavernous hemangioma of the scalp, with involvement of the overlying skin.

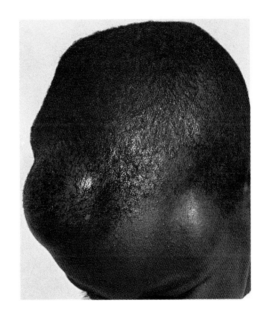

FIG. 15.2 Scalp metastases from a primary intra-abdominal neuroblastoma.

This chapter encompasses general pediatric surgical disorders not discussed elsewhere in this book, but is not intended to be an exhaustive survey. Emphasis is on surgical conditions likely to be encountered in general pediatric practice, amplified by the inclusion of some uncommon and rare disorders.

HEAD AND NECK

Swellings and abnormal openings in the skin of the head and neck in childhood usually represent congenital abnormalities; most are benign. Of practical importance is the fact that lesions which appear to be superficial may communicate with underlying deep structures; this may lead to difficulties for the unwary surgeon.

Scalp

Common swellings encountered on the scalp in infancy include hemangioma, encephalocele, and teratoma. The caver-

nous hemangioma (Fig. 15.1) is a firm, raised mass which blanches and shrinks somewhat when compressed, only to re-expand when released. The overlying skin may be involved by capillary hemangioma. The typical "mixed" hemangioma enlarges during the first year of life and then undergoes partial regression. An encephalocele communicates with the underlying meninges and brain, becoming tense when the baby cries. A skull defect is seen radiographically. A cystic swelling on the forehead may indicate a frontal encephalocele.

Scalp masses appearing in childhood include sebaceous cysts, dermoid cysts, and benign or malignant tumors such as rhabdomyosarcoma or metastatic neuroblastoma (Fig. 15.2). A sebaceous cyst is a well-circumscribed, firm lesion, somewhat movable in the subcutaneous tissue. One may note a small punctum in the overlying skin. The cyst is not tender unless there is secondary infection. A dermoid cyst resembles a sebaceous cyst but lacks the skin punctum and is often tense and hard. Dermoid cysts characteristically occur in the lateral part of the eyebrow or at the lateral angle of the orbit

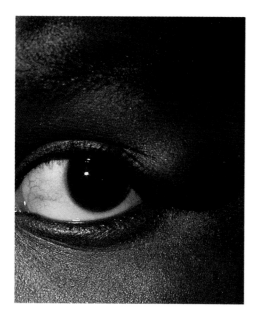

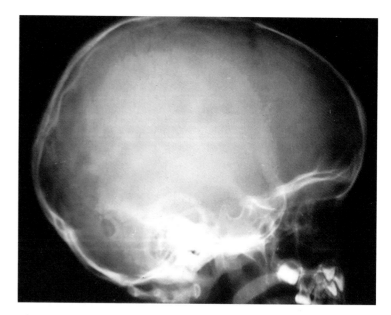

FIG. 15.3 Dermoid cyst at the lateral corner of the eye. Such cysts are also found in the eyebrow.

FIG. 15.4 Lateral skull radiograph shows a circular defect in the occipital region of a patient who presented with a superficial dermoid cyst over the occiput. The cyst extended through this bone defect into the intracranial cavity.

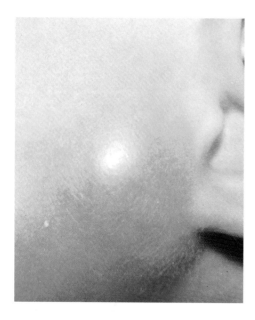

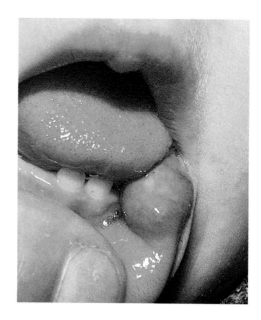

FIG. 15.5 Parotid gland cyst.

FIG. 15.6 Mixed hemangioma of the lip.

(Fig. 15.3). The rare meningocele occurring in the same position is softer and becomes tense when the child cries. If a meningocele is suspected, a skull film is indicated to detect a bony defect. Swellings on the cranium, especially those over the occiput or in the midline of the scalp or forehead, pose a special risk as they may extend through the calvarium. For example, a superficial dermoid cyst may communicate with an intracranial component (Fig. 15.4). A skull radiograph is therefore always indicated for a midline swelling or a suspicious occipital mass, and if a bony defect is identified, computerized tomography should be done.

Face

Preauricular sinuses, pits, and discrete swellings, often containing cartilage, are encountered anterior to the ear. These are ectodermal inclusions related to the formation of the external ear. The lesion is often ignored until infection occurs, causing pain and swelling and a purulent discharge from the sinus. Remnants of the first branchial arch are rare and may present as a fistula or mass lying in the preauricular area or below the angle of the mandible (see Fig. 15.10). A tender, preauricular swelling is usually due to acute inflammation of the preauricular lymph nodes; there is no overlying skin pit, and a regional source of infection may be apparent.

The parotid gland is situated in front of the lower half of the external ear. Diffuse parotid enlargement with tenderness occurs with inflammatory lesions of the gland, as in mumps or parotitis. A circumscribed nodule in this area is more likely to be an enlarged lymph node, but may represent a parotid tumor or cyst (Fig. 15.5). Parotid tumors vary in consistency from soft to hard and are painless, elevating the lobe of the ear as they expand. Associated facial nerve palsy is rare. Sialography may demonstrate a space-occupying mass in the parotid gland. Excision or biopsy of a mass in this area should be undertaken with caution because of the risk of damage to the seventh cranial nerve. Other lesions occurring in this area are hemangioma and lymphangioma, which present acutely

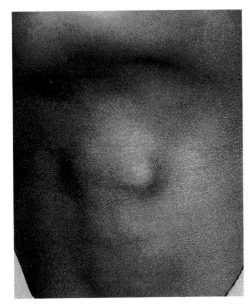

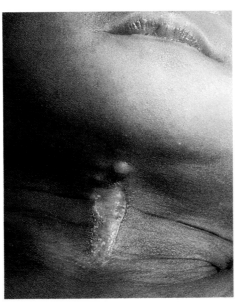

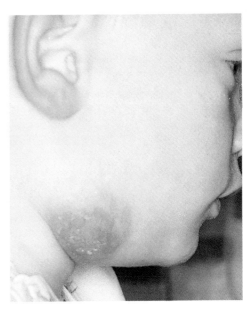

FIG. 15.7 Thyroglossal duct cyst, slightly to the left of the midline. Typically these cysts occur in the midline.

FIG. 15.8 Midline cervical cleft.

FIG. 15.9 Tuberculous lymphadenitis.

if there is secondary infection or hemorrhage, and tumors such as lymphoma and rhabdomyosarcoma. The latter occasionally presents as a tender mass and may be misdiagnosed as an abscess. Burkitt's lymphoma arises more anteriorly, in the maxilla. A well-defined swelling behind the ear is usually an enlarged, posterior auricular lymph node, but a soft-tissue sarcoma is a rare alternative. Mastoiditis causes diffuse swelling, with tenderness maximal over the mastoid bone.

A smooth, cystic swelling of the lip with normal overlying skin indicates a mucous retention cyst. Hemangiomas of the lip are also common; these are not as well-circumscribed, and the overlying skin is frequently involved by hemangioma (Fig. 15.6). A mucous retention cyst may also occur in the floor of the mouth under the tongue, where it is termed a ranula. Rarely, it extends below the mandible to present as a cystic swelling in the midline of the neck (plunging ranula), and must be distinguished from a cystic hygroma.

Midline of the Neck

Characteristic anomalies occur in the midline of the neck. An enlarged submental lymph node will be situated behind the point of the mandible. It is often confused with a thyroglossal duct cyst, which is usually found lower in the neck. With lymph node enlargement there is usually a preceding history of acute, painful swelling of the node, and a source of infection may be apparent on the chin or around the mouth. The lymph node does not move with swallowing or with protrusion of the tongue. The embryonic thyroglossal duct extends from the foramen cecum on the posterior aspect of the tongue, through or around the hyoid bone, to the thyroid isthmus. Remnants of the duct may enlarge, forming a cyst situated in or near the midline of the neck anywhere from just above the hyoid bone to the thyroid gland (Fig. 15.7). Usually a smooth, discrete, painless mass, a thyroglossal duct cyst may become infected and present as an acute abscess. Typically, the cyst moves upward when the tongue is protruded. A patent thyroglossal duct, originating at the foramen cecum, may communicate with a cyst or may present as a small opening in the midline of the neck, with a mucoid or purulent discharge. Rarely, ectopic thyroid tissue occurs along the line of the thyroglossal duct as a firm nodule. Localized enlargement of the isthmus or pyramidal lobe results in a midline mass. Characteristically, the thyroid gland moves upward with swallowing. Epidermoid cysts occur in the midline of the neck and do not move with swallowing or protrusion of the tongue. Ultrasonography will demonstrate the cystic or solid nature of the mass and its relationship to the thyroid gland. A radionuclear scan of the thyroid gland will further elucidate the nature of the lesion. A midline cervical cleft is a vertical red streak of thinly epithelialized tissue situated in the anterior midline of the neck, probably the result of defective midline fusion of the branchial arches (Fig. 15.8).

Side of the Neck

Enlarged cervical lymph nodes are the most frequent cause of a lateral neck mass. Acute lymphadenitis anterior to the sternocleidomastoid muscle is usually associated with infection of the face, mouth, or pharynx. There may be symptoms referable to the primary lesion, such as the painful throat of tonsillitis. An acutely enlarged lymph node is tender and firm; early antibiotic therapy may abort the infection. Continued infection leads to suppuration of the lymph node, which then becomes fluctuant. Aspiration at this stage will reveal pus; incision and drainage is usually required.

With chronic cervical adenopathy due to infections such as cat-scratch disease, the enlarged node is usually discrete and slightly tender. There may be fever and leukocytosis. Tuberculous lymph nodes are not clearly defined and are frequently matted together. Aspiration may be followed by suppuration, with abscess and fistula formation (Fig. 15.9). Atypical mycobacterial infection is associated with asymptomatic, painless lymph node enlargement; spontaneous softening of the nodes with sinus formation may occur. Diagnostic evaluation should include skin testing for tuberculosis and a chest radiograph. Lymphoma is an ever-present possibility

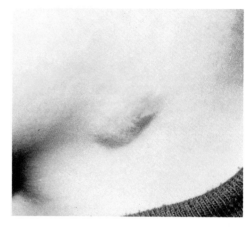

FIG. 15.10 First branchial arch fistula, previously diagnosed as an infected lymph node, after treatment by incision and drainage.

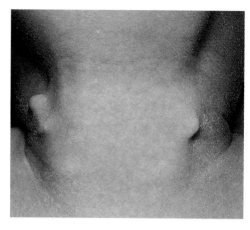

FIG. 15.11 Remnants of the second branchial arch may appear as swellings anterior to the sternocleidomastoid mus-

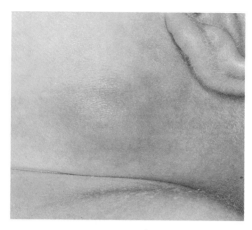

cle. (Left) Bilateral cartilaginous remnants; (right) infected second branchial arch cyst.

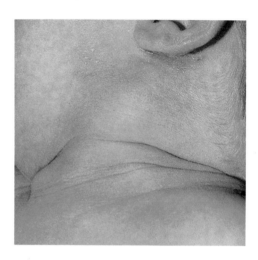

FIG. 15.12 Sterno-cleidomastoid tumor in the new-born infant.

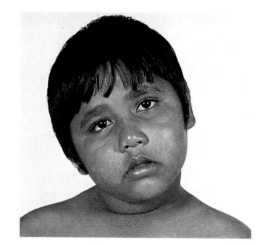

FIG. 15.13 Long-standing torticollis (wry-neck) with shortening of the affected side of the face.

when an enlarged, painless lymph node is discovered in the neck or axilla. The involved nodes are usually discrete, firm, and rubbery. Excisional biopsy is indicated when studies fail to confirm an infective etiology or when there is progressive enlargement of the nodes.

The rare first branchial arch fistula appears as a swelling below the angle of the mandible, and usually cannot be distinguished from an enlarged cervical lymph node (Fig. 15.10). The fistula runs deep to the facial nerve, to the external auditory canal, and may be associated with a discharge from the ear. The submandibular salivary gland also lies beneath the horizontal ramus of the mandible; enlargement may be accompanied by pain and tenderness, especially during meals. A calculus in the submandibular gland duct may be palpated under the tongue.

Lateral neck swellings occurring anterior to the sternocleidomastoid muscle include remnants of the second branchial arch. These present as a cyst, fistula, or cartilaginous nodule anywhere along the anterior border of the sternocleidomastoid muscle (Fig. 15.11). There may be a mucoid or purulent discharge from a fistula. Enlargement of the lateral lobe of the thyroid will also manifest as a mass anterior to the sternocleidomastoid muscle. A sternocleidomastoid tumor presents within a few weeks of birth as a mass in the middle third, and less commonly in the lower third, of the muscle (Fig. 15.12). The fusiform swelling can be moved from side to side but not upward or downward. In the early stages there is no associated deformity; later, torticollis becomes ap-

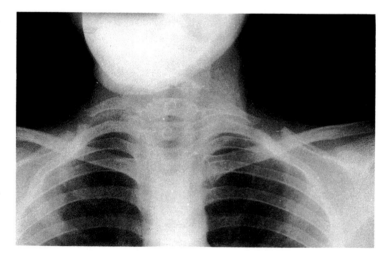

FIG. 15.14 Bilateral cervical ribs.

parent with rotation of the face toward the opposite side (Fig. 15.13). A firm mass in the posterior triangle of the neck, behind the sternocleidomastoid muscle, may represent an enlarged lymph node, a soft-tissue sarcoma, or a cervical rib (Fig. 15.14).

Cystic hygromas are common in the neck and axilla. The soft, cystic lesion may arise as a small, localized swelling, but more often is lobulated, multicystic, and irregular and typically transilluminates brilliantly. A sudden increase in size is usually the result of hemorrhage into a cyst, or infection.

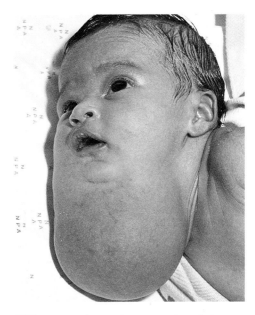

FIG. 15.15 Cystic hygroma involving the neck and floor of the mouth.

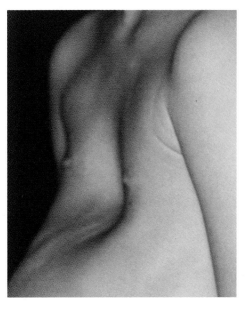

FIG. 15.16 Pectus excavatum (funnel chest).

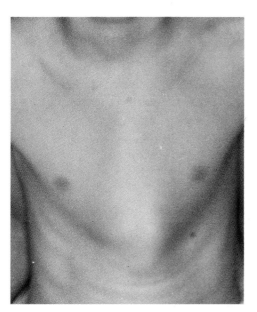

FIG. 15.17 Pectus carinatum (pigeon chest).

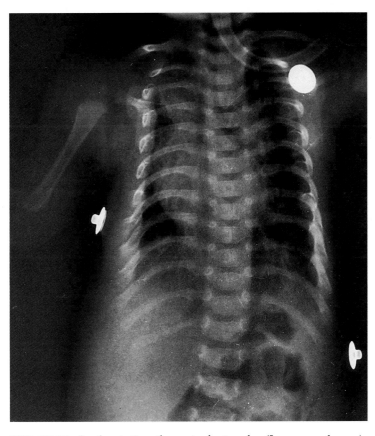

FIG. 15.18 Asphyxiating thoracic dystrophy (Jeune syndrome).

A large cervical cystic hygroma may extend into the floor of the mouth, resembling a ranula, and may obstruct the pharynx leading to difficulty with breathing and swallowing (Fig. 15.15). Aspiration is not helpful as the lesions are multicystic, and the procedure carries the risk of introducing infection. There may be a solid component to the mass if there is associated lymphangiomatous tissue. A cervical teratoma is an uncommon congenital abnormality presenting as a large mass in the neck. There are solid and cystic components, and the mass seldom transilluminates as clearly as a cystic hygroma.

CHEST WALL

Pectus excavatum (funnel chest), the most common congenital deformity of the sternum, is characterized by concavity of the sternum from above-downward as well as from side to side (Fig. 15.16). The costal cartilages are also involved in the deformity. The concavity, which varies in shape from a deep cup to a wide saucer, may be asymmetrical and is occasionally rotated toward the right. The deformity is usually present at birth, although it may not be noticed for several weeks or months, and becomes progressively more pronounced until the child is fully grown. Cardiorespiratory compromise is uncommon, but the psychological effects may be significant, leading the child to withdraw from social events that will expose the deformity (such as swimming).

Pectus carinatum (pigeon chest) manifests in two forms. Pouter pigeon chest consists of prominent forward protrusion of the manubrium, followed by a sharp depression of the sternum, which in its lowest part turns forward again. Seen in profile, the sternum is Z-shaped. Some consider this deformity a form of pectus excavatum. True pigeon chest is a prominent keel-shaped deformity of the sternum, with depression of the costal cartilages on each side (Fig. 15.17). Asymmetrical variations are common. The deformity usually becomes apparent at about the age of 3 or 4 years and increases progressively with the growth of the child. There are no functional side effects.

Sternal cleft is due to failure of midline fusion of the embryonic sternum, with vertical separation of the left and right halves of the sternum. If only the upper or lower sternum is involved, a U-shaped deformity results. The cardiac impulse is clearly seen through a lower sternal cleft. Ectopia cordis, where the naked heart is completely exposed on the chest wall, is usually associated with a sternal cleft. The pentalogy of Cantrell includes a lower sternal cleft, an omphalocele, a ventral diaphragmatic defect, free pericardial-peritoneal communication, and an intrinsic cardiac defect.

Asphyxiating thoracic dystrophy (Jeune syndrome) is a rare deformity which may present in infancy with acute respiratory distress (Fig. 15.18). The characteristics of the deformity are short, broad, horizontal ribs terminating in the

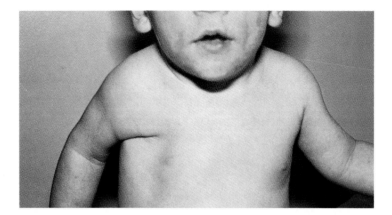

FIG. 15.19 *Poland syndrome.*

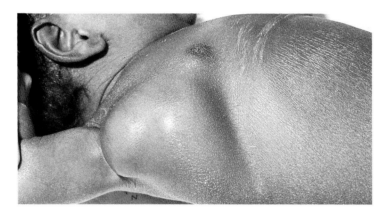

FIG. 15.20 *Cystic hygroma of the chest wall.*

axillary line; a solid sternum; and a rigid, bell-shaped chest. There may be associated anomalies of the hands and pelvis. The degree of respiratory embarrassment varies; in severe cases it is progressive and the outlook is poor.

Poland syndrome (Fig. 15.19) consists of unilateral absence of the second, third, and fourth cartilages and adjacent ribs, absence of the pectoralis minor muscle and the costosternal part of pectoralis major muscle, hypoplasia or absence of the breast and/or nipple, and hypoplasia of the subcutaneous tissue. The breast, when present, is displaced upward. In the complete syndrome, short, webbed fingers are present on the affected side (brachysyndactaly).

Swellings of the chest wall most commonly develop in or below the axilla. In infants, cystic hygroma typically occurs in this region (Fig. 15.20) and is distinguished from a hemangioma, lipoma, or other soft-tissue lesions by its cystic nature and clear transillumination. A firm, solid lesion may be a malignant soft-tissue tumor arising from the chest wall or extending from an intrathoracic tumor. A chest radiograph should be obtained.

Abnormalities of the breast are uncommon before puberty. The normally developing breast bud or disc may be mistaken for an abnormal nodule. Biopsy must be avoided except in rare circumstances, as this may result in abnormal growth of the breast. In a postpubertal girl, a discrete breast mass is usually a fibroadenoma or cyst, which may be impossible to distinguish except with ultrasonography or aspiration. A discharge from the nipple should be tested for the presence of blood, which is usually a manifestation of mammary dysplasia but may be due to an intraduct papilloma. In a teenage boy, gynecomastia may cause severe psychological problems, justifying subcutaneous mastectomy.

SURGICAL CAUSES OF RESPIRATORY DISTRESS

In the Newborn Infant	In the Older Child
Posterior choanal atresia	Foreign body aspiration
Pierre Robin syndrome	Pneumothorax
Esophageal atresia	Thoracic empyema
Laryngeal web	Mediastinal lymphoma
Congenital lung anomalies	
Posterolateral diaphragmatic hernia	
Pneumothorax	
Congenital cardiac anomalies	

FIG. 15.21 *Surgical causes of respiratory distress.*

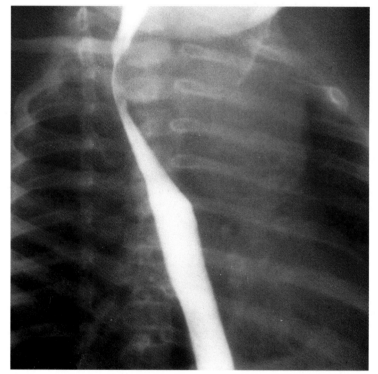

FIG. 15.22 *Barium swallow shows displacement and compression of the esophagus by an intrathoracic neuroblastoma.*

MEDIASTINUM

In general, the important abnormalities in the mediastinum manifest as cysts or solid masses, which become apparent clinically when they compress adjacent mediastinal structures. An enlarging mass in the superior mediastinum will obstruct the superior vena cava, leading to venous congestion and edema of the head, neck, and upper extremity; it may also compress the trachea, causing stridor, dyspnea, and increasing respiratory distress (Fig. 15.21). Esophageal displace-

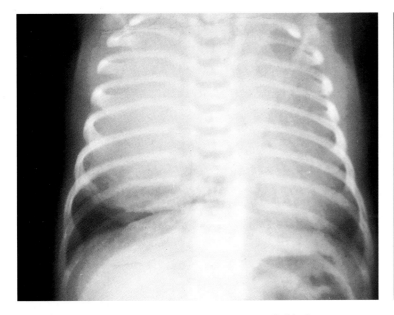 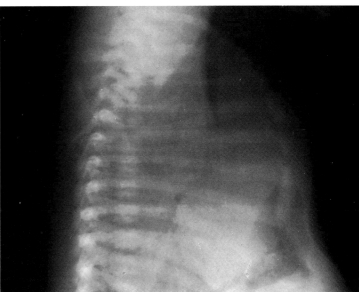

FIG. 15.23 Foregut duplication. On AP view (left) there is a large mass in the right side of the chest. A lateral view (right) demonstrates that the mass is in the posterior mediastinum, anterior to the vertebral column, displacing the trachea anteriorly.

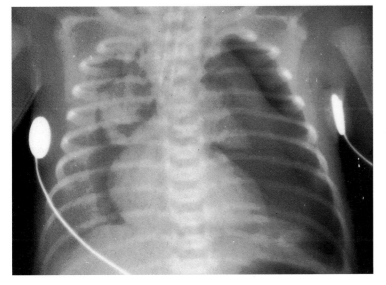 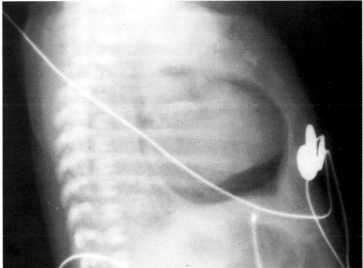

FIG. 15.24 AP chest radiograph reveals left pneumothorax and pneumomediastinum in an infant receiving positive-pressure ventilation.

FIG. 15.25 Pneumopericardium.

ment may cause difficulty with swallowing, and progressive obstruction will lead to the accumulation of saliva in the upper esophagus and pharynx. Secondary bacterial infection of a mediastinal cyst causes an abscess and a severe pyrexial illness. Chest radiographs demonstrate a widened mediastinum, and barium swallow examination may show displacement and compression of the esophagus (Fig. 15.22). Ultrasonography and computerized tomography can distinguish cystic from solid lesions, and the mass can be accurately localized (see Fig. 15.30). Abnormalities of the superior and anterior mediastinum include enlargement of the thymus (a normal finding in the newborn infant; see Fig. 15.32), cystic hygroma, lymphadenopathy (including lymphoma), teratoma, and dermoid cysts. In the middle mediastinum, lymphadenopathy, anomalies of the heart and great vessels, and pericardial cysts may occur. A mass in the posterior mediastinum may represent foregut duplication (Fig. 15.23), enteric cyst, neurogenic tumor, bronchogenic cyst, extralobar sequestration of the lung, or anterior meningocele.

Acute mediastinitis, a grave condition resulting from bacterial invasion of the mediastinum, may follow perforation of the pharynx, esophagus, trachea, or bronchus by disease or trauma (including endoscopic injury), or it may complicate retropharyngeal or cervical infections. Acute mediastinal infection evokes a severe systemic response with pain, dyspnea, high fever, and tachycardia. Air escaping from the esophagus or trachea produces mediastinal emphysema, and dissects upward into the neck resulting in crepitation in the supraclavicular fossae. A chest radiograph will demonstrate widening of the mediastinum which is outlined by extravasated air. Pneumomediastinum (Fig. 15.24) and pneumopericardium (Fig. 15.25) are also seen in association with pneumothorax in infants receiving positive-pressure ventilation.

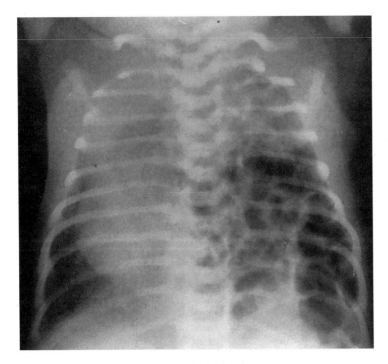

FIG. 15.26 Left congenital Bochdalek's hernia.

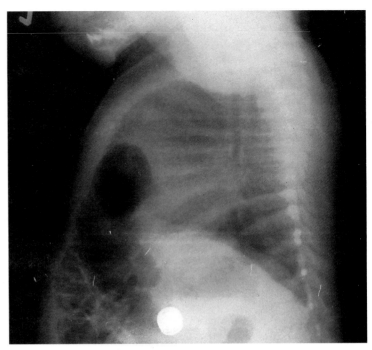

FIG. 15.27 Herniation of intestine through the foramen of Morgagni.

DIAPHRAGM

Posterolateral diaphragmatic hernia (Bochdalek's hernia), an important cause of neonatal respiratory distress syndrome, is due to persistence of the embryonic pleuroperitoneal canal. Severe, progressive respiratory distress may be present at birth or may develop hours or days later. Other clinical features include diminished breath sounds on the affected side, displacement of the cardiac impulse toward the opposite side, and a scaphoid abdomen. Anteroposterior and lateral chest radiographs are usually diagnostic (Fig. 15.26), showing gas-filled bowel loops in the chest with compression of the ipsilateral lung, and extreme mediastinal shift compressing the contralateral lung. Differential diagnosis includes cysts and dysplasias of the lung.

Eventration of the diaphragm mimics Bochdalek's hernia. The hypoplastic diaphragm is stretched upward into the pleural cavity by the abdominal viscera, compressing the lung. Respiratory distress may be present at birth or may not manifest until months later. Diagnosis is usually apparent on the chest radiograph, which shows loops of intestine in the chest but, unlike a congenital diaphragmatic hernia, the bowel is surrounded by a thin membrane representing the diaphragm.

A hernia through the foramen of Morgagni, situated immediately behind the xiphisternum, is an uncommon defect and is usually an incidental finding on a chest radiograph (Fig. 15.27). Small hernias are asymptomatic, but a rare, large Morgagnian hernia may be associated with epigastric pain or intestinal obstruction.

Paralysis of a hemidiaphragm results from phrenic nerve injury. A difficult delivery may injure the brachial plexus and phrenic nerve of the newborn, leading to the characteristic upper limb deformity (Erb's palsy) and varying degrees of respiratory distress. In older children, phrenic nerve injury

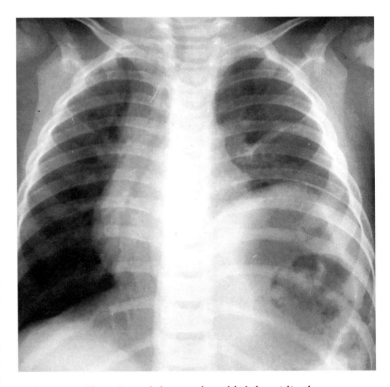

FIG. 15.28 Elevation of the paralyzed left hemidiaphragm following iatrogenic injury to the left phrenic nerve.

may follow accidental or iatrogenic trauma to the nerve as it passes through the neck or mediastinum. A chest radiograph will show elevation of the paralyzed diaphragm (Fig. 15.28), seen by fluoroscopy to move paradoxically. Often the diagnosis is not made until a radiograph is taken for persistent or recurrent respiratory infection.

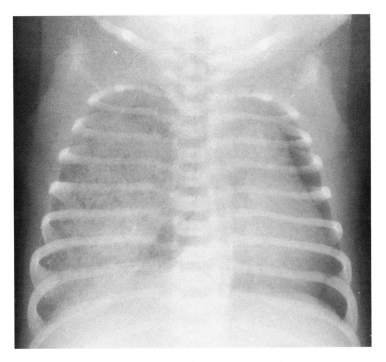

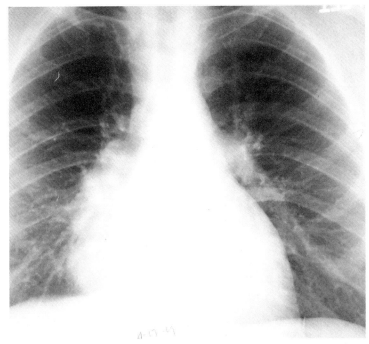

FIG. 15.29 *Congenital cystic adenomatoid malformation of the right upper lobe.*

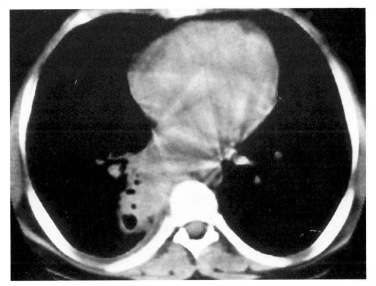

FIG. 15.30 *Extralobar sequestration. Chest radiograph (top) shows a right mediastinal mass. CT scan (bottom) localizes the mass to the right posterior mediastinum and demonstrates cystic and solid components. An aortogram confirmed the diagnosis by showing the arterial supply to the sequestration arising directly from the aorta.*

LUNGS AND PLEURA

Developmental abnormalities of the lung include congenital cystic adenomatoid malformation, congenital cystic disease of the lung, and congenital lobar emphysema. Cystic adenomatoid malformation presents in three forms: fetal anasarca, with prematurity and perinatal death; acute progressive respiratory disease in the newborn; and a less severe course characterized by recurrent respiratory infection. Expansion of cystic lesions leads to progressive respiratory distress, and with secondary infection and abscess formation there is fever and toxemia. A chest radiograph is usually diagnostic (Fig. 15.29).

Pulmonary sequestration is an uncommon congenital malformation characterized by a mass of lung tissue which usually has no communication with the normal bronchial tree. The sequestration may be within the normal lung (intralobar sequestration) or separate from the normal lung (extralobar sequestration). Rarely, it becomes infected or may lead to congestive cardiac failure if there is significant left to right shunting. Sequestration is usually identified as an incidental finding on a chest radiograph (Fig. 15.30), appearing as a homogenous density; cysts are more often seen with the intralobar variety. Of practical importance is the fact that the blood supply to the sequestration is derived from an anomalous systemic artery (often arising below the diaphragm) and not from the pulmonary arterial system. Aortography will establish the diagnosis by demonstrating the aberrant arterial supply. Differential diagnosis includes bronchogenic cyst and thoracic neuroblastoma.

A pneumothorax may cause acute respiratory distress and therefore demands urgent diagnosis and treatment. Pneumothorax may follow blunt or penetrating trauma; spontaneous pneumothorax may occur with cystic fibrosis and in patients on high pressure ventilation. Inspiration is severely limited, and there is restricted movement of the affected side of the thorax, which remains expanded and tympanitic. Breath sounds are greatly diminished on the affected side; in a newborn infant this sign is often absent, as breath sounds from the normal side may be transmitted through the thorax. The trachea is deviated toward the opposite side. A chest radiograph will confirm the diagnosis. In an emergency situation where there is no time for a chest radiograph, a needle attached to a 20-ml syringe containing 5 ml of sterile water or saline is inserted through the second intercostal space anteriorly. On aspirating the syringe, air is seen to bubble freely through the water. The plunger is completely removed from the syringe, allowing the pneumothorax to decompress until proper chest drainage can be accomplished.

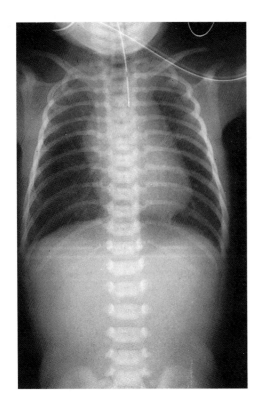

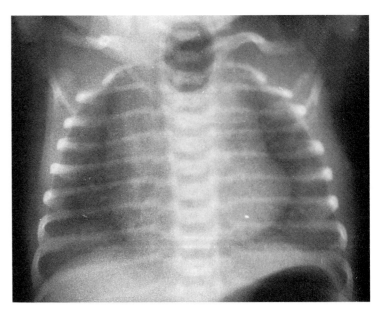

FIG. 15.31 Esophageal atresia, with a feeding tube in the air-filled proximal esophageal pouch. The absence of gas in the abdomen excludes the presence of a distal tracheoesophageal fistula.

FIG. 15.32 Esophageal atresia, with the proximal pouch clearly outlined by air. Air in the stomach indicates the presence of a distal tracheoesophageal fistula. The wide superior mediastinum represents the normal thymus of the newborn.

ESOPHAGUS

Esophageal atresia, with or without a tracheoesophageal fistula, typically presents soon after birth with mild respiratory distress. Occasionally the diagnosis is not suspected until an attempt is made to feed the child. Saliva accumulates in the oropharynx, and frequent suctioning is required. Bubbles form in the mouth as the infant breathes, leading to episodes of cyanosis and choking. Attempts to pass an orogastric tube reveal obstruction in the esophagus (a firm catheter should be used, as a soft tube may coil in the proximal pouch giving a false impression that the stomach has been entered). A plain radiograph will demonstrate the tip of the catheter in the blind proximal pouch, usually at the level of T2–T3 (Fig. 15.31). The upper pouch is usually outlined by the air within it (Fig. 15.32). Rarely, radiopaque contrast material is necessary to delineate the upper pouch; a maximum of 0.25 ml of contrast is adequate and must be withdrawn as soon as the film has been exposed. The diagnostic "test feed" is to be condemned, as this may lead to aspiration and pneumonia.

A tracheoesophageal fistula without esophageal atresia usually presents with a long history of recurring bouts of respiratory infection. Diagnosis is made by contrast radiographic studies and endoscopy, but a small fistula may be difficult to identify. A tracheobronchial cleft is a rare deformity, difficult to demonstrate radiographically but readily seen on endoscopy. It presents with choking during feeding and with aspiration, leading to recurrent respiratory tract infection.

In the older child, esophageal stenosis occurs as a complication of gastroesophageal reflux or ingestion of corrosive liquids. Gastroesophageal reflux, the repeated reflux of gastric contents into the esophagus, results in esophagitis and recurrent aspiration pneumonitis. Severe reflux with vomiting leads to undernutrition and failure to thrive; hematemesis may also occur. Chronic anemia and esophageal stricture with inability to swallow are late complications. In the new-

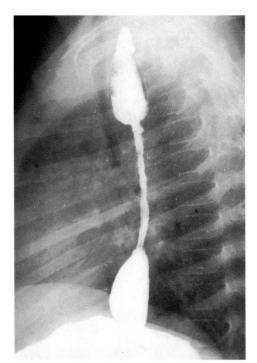

FIG. 15.33 Lateral view of the esophagus during barium contrast examination demonstrates a sliding hiatal hernia immediately above the diaphragm, and a long stricture of the midesophagus secondary to reflux esophagitis.

born, gastroesophageal reflux may be associated with apnea. Hiatal hernia is not common in childhood, and when present is usually associated with gastroesophageal reflux. An upper GI barium study will demonstrate reflux of barium into the esophagus (Fig. 15.33). Reflux can also be identified by esophageal pH monitoring, and by scanning the lungs following a radioisotope-labeled meal. Esophagitis is confirmed by endoscopic examination and esophageal biopsy. Ingestion of corrosive liquids requires urgent treatment if esophageal stricture is to be prevented. Esophagoscopy is required to identify the acute esophageal injury.

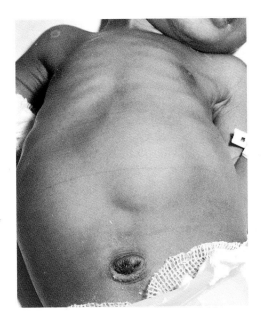

FIG. 15.34 Hypertrophic pyloric stenosis. This patient demonstrates epigastric distention due to the dilated stomach, with prominent peristaltic waves moving along the stomach from left to right.

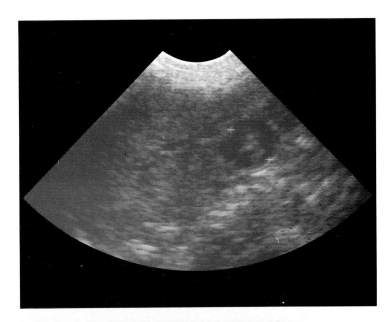

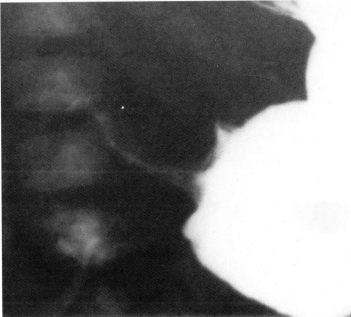

STOMACH

Hypertrophic pyloric stenosis occurs more commonly in male infants, and presents at 3 to 6 weeks of age with vomiting of feedings. The vomiting is typically projectile and does not contain bile, but in the later stages—if gastritis develops—may contain altered blood. Continuous vomiting leads to dehydration, lethargy, and oliguria. Epigastric distention is a common finding; peristaltic waves in the distended, thickened stomach may be seen moving from the left subcostal region toward the right (Fig. 15.34). The hypertrophic pyloric muscle is palpable as an olive-sized mass, commonly deep to the right rectus muscle approximately midway between the xiphisternum and the umbilicus. The mass is most easily palpated when the child is relaxed and the stomach empty, usually after a vomit or after nasogastric tube decompression. A glucose water feed during the examination will help relax the abdominal wall and often stimulates gastric peristalsis, accentuating the pyloric tumor. When a mass is not palpable, the thickened pylorus may be visualized by ultrasonography, and an upper GI barium study will demonstrate gastric retention and a narrow, elongated pyloric canal (Fig. 15.35). Pyloromyotomy is the established method of treatment. Obstruction by a duplication cyst of the gastric antrum or proximal duodenum mimics the clinical features of pyloric stenosis and can usually be identified by ultrasonography.

FIG. 15.35 Hypertrophic pyloric stenosis. Ultrasonographic scan of the upper abdomen (top) demonstrates the thickened pyloric muscle, indicated by the cursors. Barium study of the stomach (bottom) shows thin streaks of barium in the pyloric canal. The hypertrophic pyloric muscle bulges into the gastric antrum producing a "reversed 3" configuration with a central beak projecting into the pyloric canal.

OBSTRUCTION OF THE SMALL INTESTINE

The cardinal features of intestinal obstruction are vomiting, abdominal distention, failure to pass stools, and cramping abdominal pain. Blood-stained stools may indicate intestinal ischemia and should never be ignored. The clinical picture is related to the level of obstruction. With obstruction of the proximal small intestine, vomiting is an early symptom. The vomitus is bile-stained, except when the obstruction is proximal to the ampulla of Vater. The abdominal distention is confined to the epigastrium. One or two small stools may be passed before stools cease altogether. Distal small-bowel obstruction causes vomiting of the bile-stained intestinal content, which later becomes brown and offensive (feculant).

There is generalized abdominal distention and failure to pass stool. Colonic or rectal obstruction leads to failure to pass stool and early onset of generalized abdominal distention. Vomiting occurs later and is bile-stained or feculant. Plain abdominal radiographs in the erect or lateral decubitus positions show air-fluid levels and will usually indicate the level of obstruction.

Intestinal Obstruction in the Newborn Infant

ATRESIA

Atresia of the duodenum is the most common cause of duodenal obstruction in the newborn infant and is often associated with other abnormalities. Infants with complete

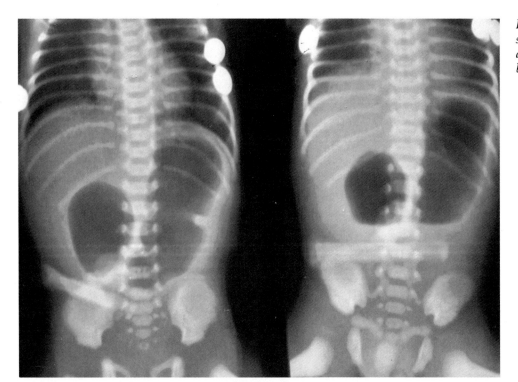

FIG. 15.36 Duodenal atresia. These supine (left) and erect (right) radiographs demonstrate the characteristic "double bubble."

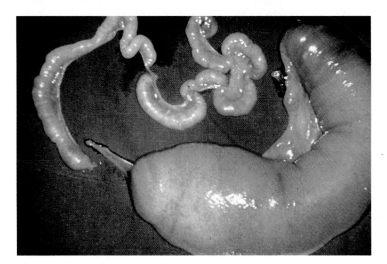

FIG. 15.37 Resected small intestine with two atretic segments. The grossly dilated proximal intestine contrasts with the narrow, empty distal bowel.

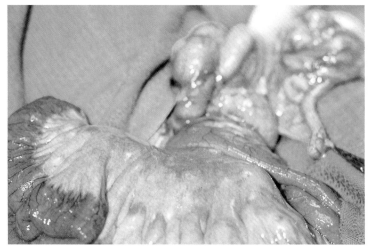

FIG. 15.38 Malrotation of the intestine with midgut volvulus. The midgut is seen twisted around the base of the mesentary. The cecum and appendix, indicated by the instrument on the right of the picture, are on the patient's left.

obstruction present shortly after birth with vomiting, usually bile-stained. The abdomen is not distended. With incomplete obstruction, as with a fenestrated diaphragm, there is intermittent vomiting; the diagnosis may not be recognized for several weeks or even months. Radiographs show the typical double-bubble representing gas and fluid in the stomach and proximal duodenum (Fig. 15.36). Annular pancreas is associated with partial or complete duodenal obstruction and clinically resembles duodenal atresia. Jejunal and ileal atresia (Fig. 15.37) present with bile-stained or feculant vomiting and generalized abdominal distention. One or two meconium stools may be passed before stooling ceases altogether. Radiographs show multiple loops of distended bowel containing air-fluid levels. Christmas tree deformity (apple peel deformity) is a form of intestinal atresia associated with a major arterial defect in the small-bowel mesentery. The small intestine distal to the atresia receives its blood supply in a retrograde direc-

tion from the ileocecal artery; the distal small bowel spirals around this marginal artery and is susceptible to volvulus.

MALROTATION

Malrotation is failure of the midgut (small intestine and right half of colon) to achieve its normal anatomic position in the abdominal cavity during embryonic development, with the result that the cecum and colon lie toward the left upper quadrant, and the duodenum and small intestine are on the right side. The mesenteric pedicle is narrow, and this predisposes to volvulus of the midgut (Fig. 15.38), with the risk of intestinal ischemia and gangrene. Volvulus is therefore a surgical emergency. Peritoneal bands overlying the duodenum (Ladd's bands) may cause duodenal obstruction in the absence of volvulus. Clinically, midgut volvulus causes high intestinal obstruction, with vomiting and minimal abdominal distention in the early stages. With the development of

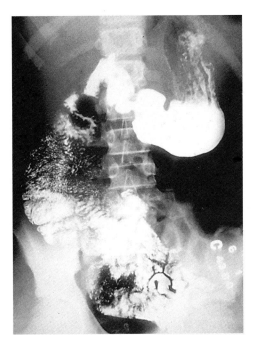

FIG. 15.39 Malrotation of the intestine. This upper GI barium study shows the duodenum and small intestine on the right side of the abdomen. Compression of the duodenum by Ladd's peritoneal bands can be observed at approximately the level of the ampulla of Vater, causing partial obstruction of the proximal duodenum.

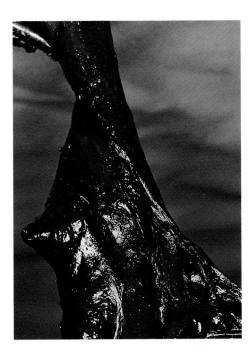

FIG. 15.40 Meconium ileus. This thick, tenacious meconium was removed during surgery.

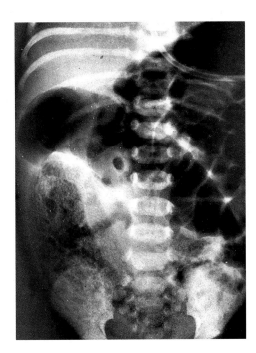

FIG. 15.41 Meconium ileus. In the right lower quadrant one can observe a large dilated loop of bowel containing meconium and gas, producing the "soap-bubble" sign typical of meconium ileus. Proximally, the bowel is distended with gas.

midgut ischemia, there is progressive abdominal distention with tenderness and involuntary guarding. The patient is lethargic, and has fever and tachycardia. Stools may be passed during the early stage of illness and may contain blood, an important sign of mucosal ischemia. Erythema and edema of the abdominal wall are late indications of underlying intestinal gangrene. Plain abdominal radiographs show features of high small intestinal obstruction; the obstructed midgut may be filled with fluid and appear relatively gasless. If there is no clinical evidence of intestinal ischemia mandating urgent surgery, contrast studies are done to establish the diagnosis of malrotation. An upper GI series shows partial duodenal obstruction and absence of the duodenal loop, with the jejunum situated on the right side of the abdomen (Fig. 15.39). Barium enema examination shows the cecum in an abnormal position in the upper or left abdomen.

MECONIUM ILEUS

Meconium ileus is due to the abnormally thick, tenacious, tarry meconium (Fig. 15.40) associated with cystic fibrosis impacting in the ileum, producing complete obstruction. The ileum distal to the obstruction is narrow, containing "rabbit pellet" concretions of meconium, and the colon is narrow and empty ("microcolon"). With simple (uncomplicated) meconium ileus there is progressive abdominal distention during the first 24 to 48 hours of life, accompanied by bilious vomiting and failure to pass meconium. Distended loops of intestine may be visible, and the putty-like, meconium-filled intestine can be palpated. The anus and rectum are unusually narrow and are often misinterpreted as anal stenosis. A family history of cystic fibrosis is an important diagnostic factor, found in up to one-third of patients. Complicated meconium ileus occurs when progressive meconium impaction causes ischemia of the bowel wall, or when the heavy, meconium-filled loop twists, forming a volvulus. The consequences of these events include intestinal stenosis, atresia, volvulus, necrosis, perforation, meconium peritonitis, and pseudocysts. In newborn infants with complicated meconium ileus, there is rapid, severe abdominal distention within 24 hours after birth, sometimes leading to respiratory distress, especially if there is perinatal perforation with pneumoperitoneum. Vomiting is bilious and no stools are passed. The veins of the abdominal wall are distended; edema and erythema indicate an underlying pseudocyst or intestinal infarction.

Abdominal radiographs often do not show the typical features of intestinal obstruction because the thick meconium filling the intestine does not form air-fluid levels. Bubbles of air mixed with the impacted meconium produce a "soap-bubble" appearance, often in the right iliac fossa (Fig. 15.41). Gas-filled intestinal loops may vary considerably in diameter. A few air-fluid levels may be seen in the proximal small intestine where the contents are more liquid. Air-fluid levels are more likely to be seen in complicated meconium ileus with atresia or volvulus, but there may be no radiologic evidence that a volvulus is present. Abdominal calcification signifies meconium peritonitis. A pseudocyst manifests as a large, radiopaque

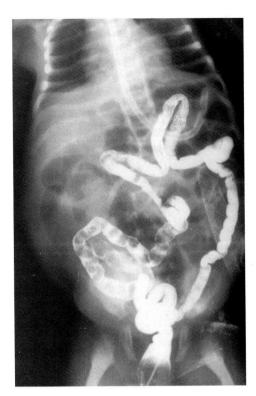

FIG. 15.42 Meconium ileus. Barium enema examination shows the empty "microcolon." The cecum is in the center of the abdomen, and barium has entered the distal ileum. The filling defects in the ileum represent "rabbit pellet" concretions of meconium.

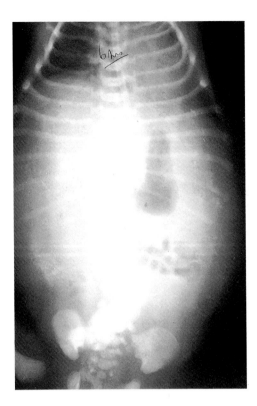

FIG. 15.43 Meconium peritonitis. Intraperitoneal calcification, seen here on the left and right sides of the abdomen, is characteristic of this condition.

mass, often with calcification. Barium enema examination demonstrates the narrow, empty "microcolon," and if there is reflux into the ileum, the "rabbit pellet" meconium concretions are outlined (Fig. 15.42). This latter examination will exclude other causes of distal obstruction, notably meconium plug, Hirschsprung's disease, small left colon syndrome, functional intestinal ileus of the newborn, and colonic stenosis. Hyperosmolar contrast agents must never be used for diagnosis because they may be misleading and, in addition, may cause acute hypovolemic shock. Having established the diagnosis by barium enema, simple meconium ileus may be successfully managed by hyperosmolar enema, but only after the infant has been fully resuscitated with intravenous fluids, complications have been excluded, and a surgical evaluation obtained. Failure to relieve the obstruction by hyperosmolar enema or evidence of complications are indications for surgery.

MECONIUM PERITONITIS

Meconium peritonitis is the result of intrauterine intestinal perforation, with leakage of meconium into the peritoneal cavity, resulting in an aseptic inflammatory reaction. There is complete intestinal obstruction, either as a result of the primary abnormality leading to the perforation or as a result of the inflammatory reaction. The clinical features are those of intestinal obstruction, with abdominal distention. Abdominal radiographs show distended loops of bowel with air-fluid levels, and linear or speckled calcification which is pathognomonic of the condition (Fig. 15.43).

DUPLICATION OF THE INTESTINE

Duplications of the intestine may be cystic or tubular (Fig. 15.44), and occur from the mouth to the anus, though the duodenum and ileum are most commonly affected. Usually the duplication is intimately attached to the normal alimentary tube by a common muscular wall and shares a common blood

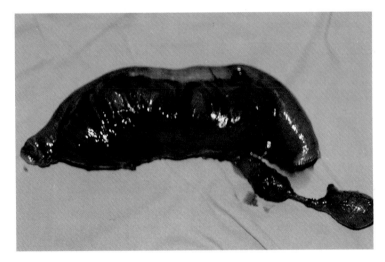

FIG. 15.44 A tubular duplication of the intestine, situated along the mesenteric margin of the normal intestine. Attached to it are two smaller duplication cysts.

supply; in addition, tubular duplications may communicate with the adjacent normal lumen. Intestinal duplications are situated on the mesenteric aspect of the adjacent intestine—between the leaves of the mesentery—and, like thoracic duplications, often contain gastric mucosa.

In the abdomen, duplications often present as an asymptomatic mass. Compression of the normal lumen causes gastric or intestinal obstruction; other possible complications are volvulus, intussusception, or perforation. Acid secretions from ectopic gastric mucosa may cause ulceration of the adjacent intestinal mucosa, with hemorrhage or perforation. Hemorrhage in tubular duplications communicating with the

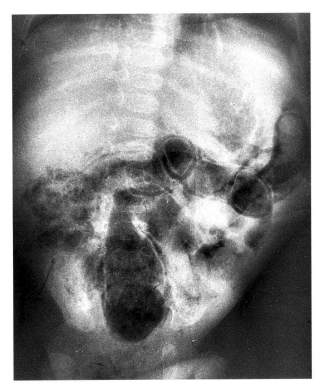

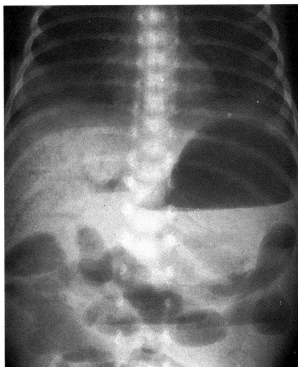

normal intestine is an uncommon cause of gastrointestinal hemorrhage, which may be severe. An intestinal duplication should therefore be suspected in a patient with an abdominal mass associated with pain or rectal bleeding. Ultrasonography or computerized tomography will demonstrate the cystic mass, and barium contrast studies will show indentation of the adjacent normal bowel and exclude intussusception.

In the thorax, duplication cysts occur in the posterior mediastinum and may compress the tracheobronchial tree, causing respiratory distress; or the esophagus, causing dysphagia. An abnormal thoracic vertebra is a common associated finding; the combined abnormality is termed a neurenteric cyst. Rarely, a fistula from the duplication passes through a bifid vertebra and spinal cord to open onto the skin of the back. Tubular duplications in the thorax may extend through the diaphragm to communicate with the stomach, duodenum, or jejunum. Asymptomatic thoracic duplications are usually first identified on a chest radiograph as a mediastinal mass. Computerized tomography may help localize the lesion, but the diagnosis is usually not confirmed until surgery.

NEONATAL NECROTIZING ENTEROCOLITIS

Neonatal necrotizing enterocolitis mimics intestinal obstruction, with bilious vomiting and abdominal distention. The stools are frequently heme-positive or frankly bloody. The disease is common in premature infants, particularly those recently starting to feed. Progressive transmural disease is associated with septicemia, leading to septic shock. Abdominal radiographs often show nonspecific air-fluid levels resembling intestinal obstruction; the diagnostic features are intestinal pneumatosis (linear streaks or bubbles of gas in the bowel wall) and gas in the portal venous system (Fig. 15.45). With intestinal perforation, localized or generalized pneumoperitoneum is seen (Fig. 15.46). Signs of septicemia include tachycardia or bradycardia, falling blood pressure, apneic epi-

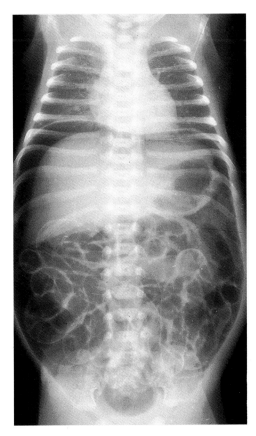

sodes, temperature instability, and hypoglycemia; the platelet count decreases and the white count may rise. Colonic stenosis, a late complication in patients recovering from acute necrotizing enterocolitis, causes progressive abdominal distention and decreasing passage of stools. The diagnosis is confirmed by barium enema examination.

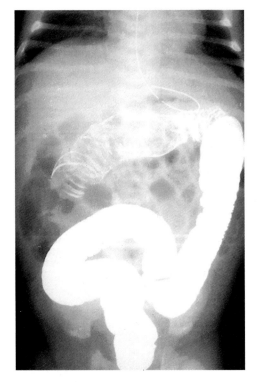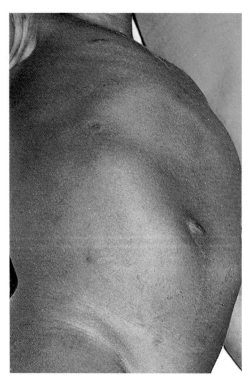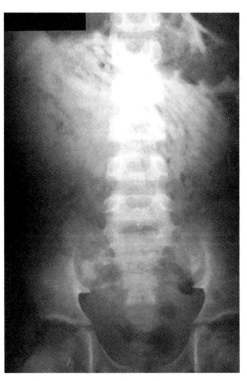

FIG. 15.47 Acute intussusception. Barium enema study outlines the head of the intussuscepted bowel (intussuscipiens) in the transverse colon. The "watch-spring" pattern is characteristic of this condition.

FIG. 15.48 Intestinal obstruction due to infestation by Ascaris lumbricoides. (Left) A visible abdominal mass representing the impacted bolus of worms.

(Right) On a plain abdominal radiograph, the worms are seen as parallel linear shadows.

Intestinal Obstruction in Infancy and Childhood

INTUSSUSCEPTION

Intussusception occurring between the ages of 3 and 18 months is usually idiopathic; in older children there is frequently an underlying abnormality such as an intestinal polyp, Meckel's diverticulum, lymphoma, small-bowel tumor, or parasitic infestation. Intussusception is characterized by intermittent colicky abdominal pain during which the infant turns pale, screams, and draws up his knees. Between attacks, which last 2 or 3 minutes, the child is symptom-free and relaxed. Abdominal examination during periods of quiet may reveal a sausage-shaped mass lying along the line of the colon, usually in the upper or left side of the abdomen. During the early stages the stools are normal or loose; later, blood and mucus resembling red current jelly are passed per rectum. Also later, there is bilious vomiting and abdominal distention. The presence of blood in the stool is confirmed on rectal examination, and the tip of the intussusception may be palpated in the rectum. Occasionally, the intussusception presents at the anus and must be distinguished from rectal prolapse.

Plain abdominal films are not diagnostic but may indicate intestinal obstruction. Barium enema examination will outline the head of the intussuscepted bowel in the colon, producing a characteristic "watch-spring" or "coil-spring" pattern (Fig. 15.47). Hydrostatic reduction of the intussusception may be possible during this examination; an intravenous infusion should be commenced prior to the procedure. A tender abdominal mass strongly suggests secondary ischemic changes in the intussuscepted bowel and is a contraindication

to hydrostatic reduction; treatment then is by surgery. Ileoileal intussusception secondary to intramural hematoma associated with Henoch-Schönlein purpura or Peutz-Jegher intestinal polyps will not be demonstrated by barium enema if the ileocecal valve is competent. The diagnosis is suspected clinically and confirmed at laparotomy.

In warm climates, where intestinal infestation by Ascaris lumbricoides is common, a bolus of worms in the small or large intestine may cause severe intestinal colic with vomiting, and this must be distinguished from intussusception. The bolus is visible or palpable as a sausage-shaped mass which alters in position; often there are several masses. Blood will not be found in the stools in the absence of complications. On plain abdominal radiographs, the mass of worms may be identified as a collection of linear or curved shadows (Fig. 15.48). Barium enema examination will exclude ileocolic intussusception.

OTHER CAUSES OF INTESTINAL OBSTRUCTION IN INFANCY AND CHILDHOOD

Intestinal obstruction may be caused by volvulus of a loop of intestine around a congenital intraperitoneal band, such as a persistent omphalomesenteric duct extending from the umbilicus to a Meckel's diverticulum. The volvulus produces complete obstruction and, if untreated, ischemia and gangrene of the intestine ensue, resulting in acute peritonitis. An internal hernia occurs when a loop of intestine becomes snared under a fold of mesentery or is trapped by an intraperitoneal adhesion following previous surgery or peritonitis. An incarcerated hernia—usually inguinal and rarely umbilical or hiatal—may become strangulated, causing complete intestinal obstruction. Obstruction of the terminal ileum may be due to Crohn's disease, tuberculosis, or lymphoma; in these conditions a mass may be palpated in the right lower quadrant.

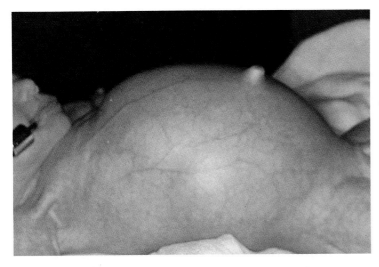

FIG. 15.49 Hirschsprung's disease. This newborn infant presented with progressive abdominal distention and failure to pass meconium.

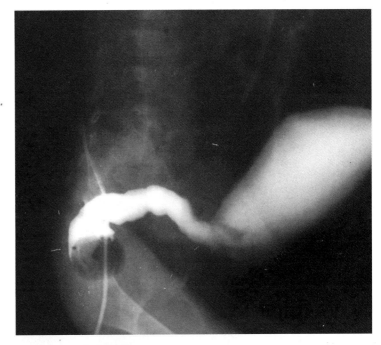

COLON AND RECTUM

Hirschsprung's Disease

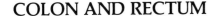

Hirschsprung's disease always affects the distal rectum and extends proximally for a variable distance. The basic abnormality is the absence of intramural ganglion cells, resulting in functional obstruction of the colon. Diagnosis is confirmed by demonstrating the absence of ganglion cells on rectal biopsy. There are three clinical manifestations of this disease:

1. The newborn infant with failure to pass meconium and progressive abdominal distention
2. Acute enterocolitis
3. The older child with chronic constipation, abdominal distention, and failure to thrive

The newborn infant may present with failure to pass meconium and progressive abdominal distention (Fig. 15.49). Later, bile-stained vomiting may develop. Plain abdominal radiographs show severe gaseous distention of the intestine; frequently it is not possible to distinguish large bowel from small bowel. Barium enema examination demonstrates a distended normal ganglionic colon tapering at the transitional zone to the narrow aganglionic distal bowel (Fig. 15.50). Rectal biopsy is performed without anesthesia by suction biopsy of the mucosa and submucosa, or by full-thickness muscle biopsy under general anesthesia. Anorectal manometry may suggest the diagnosis by demonstrating failure of the internal anal sphincter to relax with rectal distention. In the newborn, Hirschsprung's disease must be differentiated from meconium plug syndrome and small left colon syndrome. Total colonic aganglionosis, where the whole colon and occasionally the distal ileum are abnormal, must be distinguished from ileal atresia and meconium ileus.

Acute enterocolitis is a potentially lethal complication in infants with Hirschsprung's disease. The patient presents with an acute severe illness, abdominal distention, and fulminating diarrhea. Profound hypovolemia may develop rapidly. Occasionally the onset is less severe, with chronic diarrhea and failure to thrive. Hirschsprung's disease should be suspected in a child with profuse diarrhea associated with abdominal distention. Plain radiographs show intestinal distention with air-fluid levels, and a transitional zone may be identified on

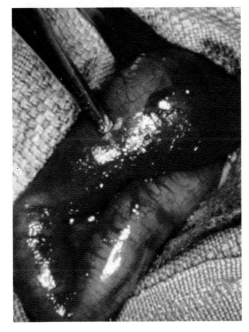

FIG. 15.50 Hirschsprung's disease. Barium enema study (top) shows the dilated proximal colon, the conical transitional zone, and the narrow, distal aganglionic colon. On the bottom we see the gross appearance at surgery. The pointer indicates the transitional zone leading into the narrow aganglionic colon.

barium enema examination. Urgent rectal biopsy is required to confirm the diagnosis.

In older children, Hirschsprung's disease may present with chronic constipation, abdominal distention, and failure to thrive. It is distinguished from habitual or acquired constipation by a history of constipation starting at or soon after birth, absence of abdominal pain or discomfort, lack of fecal soiling, and an empty rectum on digital rectal examination. Diagnosis is made by barium enema examination and rectal biopsy.

Meconium Plug Syndrome

Meconium plug syndrome refers to failure of the newborn infant to pass meconium as a result of an impacted plug of inspissated meconium in the rectum. This may occur in an otherwise normal baby or may be associated with Hirschsprung's disease or cystic fibrosis. The abdominal distention

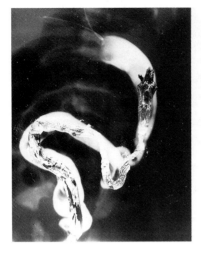
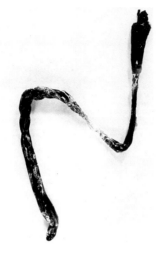

FIG. 15.51 Meconium plug syndrome. (Left) On barium enema examination, the meconium plug is outlined in the rectum and distal colon. After instilling Gastrografin into the rectum, the entire meconium plug was passed (right).

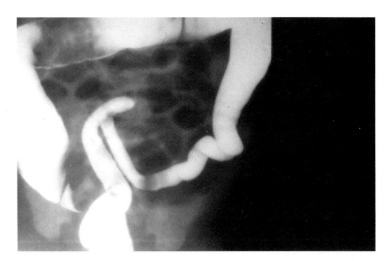

FIG. 15.52 Small left colon syndrome.

may be severe, resembling Hirschsprung's disease, with vomiting and refusal to feed. On barium enema examination, the plug is seen as a filling defect in the rectum and colon; it may be expelled after digital examination or Gastrografin enema (Fig. 15.51). Typically, the presenting tip of the plug is composed of desquamated epithelial cells and is gray-white in color; the remainder of the plug is a firm, sometimes sticky cord of thick meconium.

Other Causes of Colorectal Obstruction

Small left colon syndrome is functional obstruction of the descending colon, usually seen in infants of diabetic mothers. The clinical features are abdominal distention, failure to pass stools, and vomiting. Barium enema examination shows a narrow left colon and dilated transverse and right colon (Fig. 15.52). The clinical and radiologic features resemble Hirschsprung's disease, which is excluded by rectal biopsy. Atresia of the colon or rectum is a rare congenital cause of distal intestinal obstruction. Acquired colonic stenosis may occur as a late complication of necrotizing enterocolitis.

Rectal Prolapse

Rectal prolapse is the circumferential descent of one or more layers of the rectal wall through the anus. It is most common during the first 2 years of life, and is precipitated by conditions producing sudden increases in intra-abdominal pressure or by excessive straining while passing stools, particularly in ill or undernourished infants. Predisposing conditions include chronic respiratory infections, constipation, diarrhea, polyps, and worm infestation. Specific disorders associated with rectal prolapse are cystic fibrosis and neurologic abnormalities related to myelomeningocele or sacral agenesis. Rectal prolapse is distinguished from intussusception by the fact that with prolapse, the mucosal covering of the prolapsed rectum merges with the anal skin, whereas with intussusception there is a space between the mucosa of the intussuscepted bowel and the rectal mucosa.

ANUS

Congenital Malformations: Imperforate Anus

The different forms of imperforate anus can usually be diagnosed by simple inspection of the perineum. Since continence depends on the rectum being contained within the levator ani muscle sling, it is important to determine whether the rectum terminates above or below this muscular sphincter.

In females, the anomaly usually occurs in three forms:

1. If only one orifice is noted, the probable diagnosis is a persistent cloaca. The urethra, vagina, and rectum open into the common orifice, the rectum ending above the levator sling.

2. When two openings are present, one the urethra and the other the vagina, the rectum usually communicates with the vagina as a rectovaginal fistula (Fig. 15.53). The fistula may be situated high in the vagina, or low, just above the hymenal ring.

3. The presence of three openings signifies an ectopic anus, where the rectum has passed through the puborectalis sling but terminates in an anus which is anterior to its normal position. Usually the ectopic anus is visible at the vaginal fourchette, but it may lie in the introitus close to the hymen where it is easily overlooked, leading to the incorrect diagnosis of rectovaginal fistula.

In the male with a high lesion, the perineum is more or less flat, and the rectum usually communicates with the posterior urethra above the levator ani musculature or ends as a blind pouch. The passage of meconium or gas in the urine is diagnostic of a rectourethral fistula (Fig. 15.54).

There are two forms of low lesion in the male. The anterior ectopic anus or perineal fistula presents as an opening anterior to the normal position of the anus. The "covered anus" is situated at the normal site but is covered either partially or completely by a membrane or thick ridge of skin. When the ridge is well-defined, it is often termed a "bucket handle." A small fistulous track containing meconium may extend from the covered anus anteriorly in the midline over the scrotum to the ventral surface of the penis (Fig. 15.55).

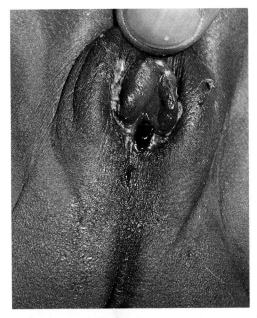
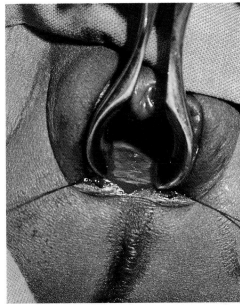

FIG. 15.53 Imperforate anus with a rectovaginal fistula. (Left) Meconium is passed through the vagina. (Right) Vaginoscopy reveals the fistula on the posterior wall of the vagina well above the hymen. This is a high or supralevator lesion.

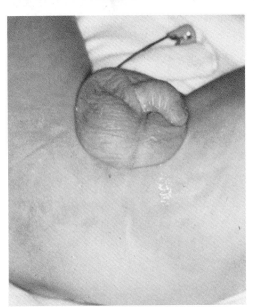
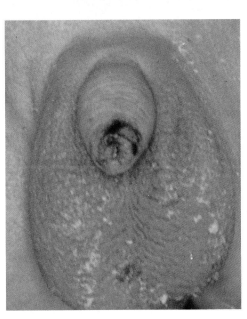
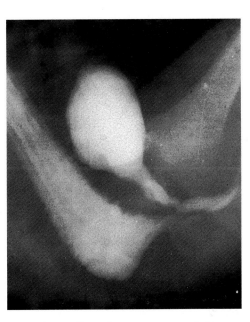

FIG. 15.54 Imperforate anus with a high (supralevator) lesion in a male infant. (Left) The perineum is flat with no external opening or fistula. (Center) Meconium is passed through the urethra.

(Right) Cystogram demonstrates reflux of contrast material into the rectum through a rectourethral fistula.

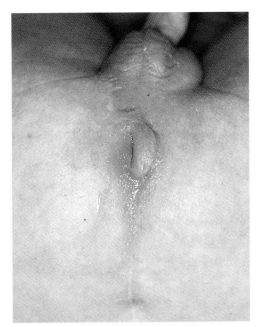
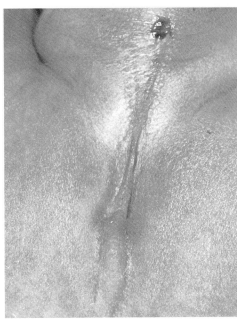

FIG. 15.55 Imperforate anus with a low (infralevator) lesion in a male infant. (Left) The "bucket-handle" type of covered anus, with a thick ridge overlying the anus. There may be an adjacent opening into the anus. (Right) Covered anus with a superficial fistula running anteriorly from the anus along the midline of the perineum and scrotum. Meconium is draining from the fistula.

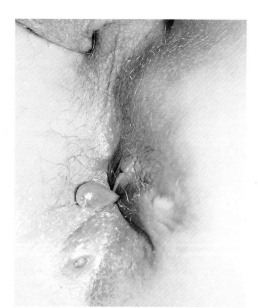

FIG. 15.56 Fissure-in-ano. Chronic fistulas at 4 and 7 o'clock. A perianal skintag can also be seen.

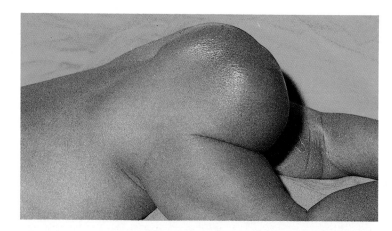

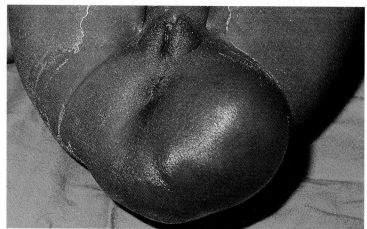

FIG. 15.57 Sacrococcygeal teratoma. (Top) Characteristic relationship to the perineum and sacrum. (Bottom) In this view we see the anus is pushed anteriorly.

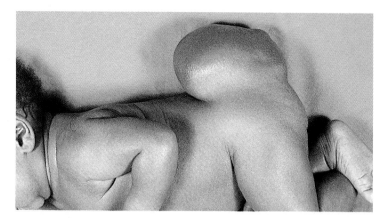

FIG. 15.58 Sacral meningocele.

Acquired Anomalies

Fissure-in-ano is a superficial longitudinal tear of the anal mucosa, usually in the anterior or posterior midline. It is caused by the passage of a large, hard fecal mass or as the result of digital examination of the anus. In infancy and early childhood, fissures are the most common cause of rectal bleeding. Pain and anal spasm lead to retention of stool, constipation, and eventual passage of another hard stool with further trauma and bleeding. The presenting features are painful defecation with bleeding, the blood typically on the surface of the stool rather than mixed with the fecal matter. The fissure can usually be seen by gently spreading the buttocks and inspecting the everted anus. With a chronic anal fissure there is an external skintag at the anal verge (Fig. 15.56).

A perianal abscess originates in the anal crypts and spreads to the perianal subcutaneous tissues where it presents as an acute painful swelling. If the abscess ruptures through the skin, a fistula results. This is a painful lesion characterized by persistent purulent drainage and recurrent infection. Usually the external perineal opening is easily seen. The internal opening can often be identified on anoscopy, best performed under general anesthesia. Perianal disorders may be associated with chronic granulomatous disease, and in the older child the possibility of Crohn's disease must be considered.

Sacrococcygeal Teratoma

A sacrococcygeal teratoma is a prominent congenital mass arising from germinal tissue associated with the coccyx. The teratoma grows between the coccyx and rectum, characteristically displacing the anus anteriorly and pushing the coccyx posteriorly (Fig. 15.57). While the bulk of the mass lies in the perineum and projects posteriorly over the sacrum, the abnormal tissue may also extend behind the rectum into the pelvis and enter the sacral canal. By contrast, a sacral meningocele is situated posteriorly on the sacrum and does not displace the anus forward (Fig. 15.58). Most sacrococcygeal teratomas are benign at birth, but the incidence of malignancy increases with the age of the infant.

GASTROINTESTINAL HEMORRHAGE

Gastrointestinal bleeding may occur at any age (Fig. 15.59). The first step should be to ascertain that it is indeed a true hemorrhage, since red dyes or foods such as beets cause red stools, and ingested iron produces melena-like stools. Bleeding is often a consequence of a generalized bleeding disorder, particularly in the newborn infant, and appropriate coagulation studies must be done. GI bleeding most commonly originates in the lower esophagus, stomach, duodenum, and colon as a result of a mucosal erosion or tear, or as a complication of portal hypertension or a congenital vascular malformation of

CAUSES OF GASTROINTESTINAL BLEEDING

In the Newborn Infant	In the Infant and Young Child	In the Older Child
Hemorrhagic disease of the newborn (Vitamin K₁ deficiency)	Intussusception	Peptic ulceration
	Meckel's diverticulum	Esophageal varices
Anal fissure	Esophagitis	Intestinal polyps
Neonatal necrotizing enterocolitis	Intestinal polyps	Inflammatory bowel disease
Milk allergy	Duplication of the alimentary tract	Henoch-Schonlein purpura
Intestinal infarction (volvulus, strangulated hernia)	Peptic ulceration	Vascular malformation
	Rectal prolapse	
Peptic ulceration		
Intestinal or liver trauma		
Thrombocytopenia		

FIG. 15.59 Causes of gastrointestinal bleeding.

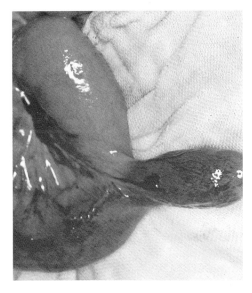

FIG. 15.60 Meckel's diverticulum. Gross appearance at surgery.

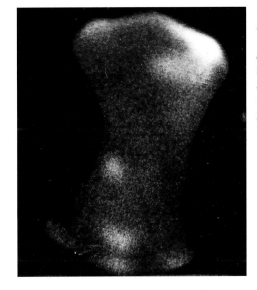

15.61 Meckel's diverticulum. Technetium scan demonstrates gastric mucosa in a Meckel's diverticulum. The patient presented with intestinal bleeding.

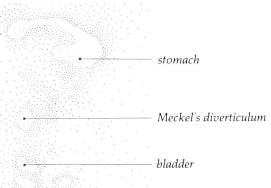

stomach

Meckel's diverticulum

bladder

the intestinal mucosa. When the bleeding site is in the esophagus, stomach, or duodenum, blood may be vomited (hematemesis); blood exposed to gastric and intestinal secretions becomes dark and manifests as black, heme-positive stools (melena). The passage of red blood in the stools (hematochezia) indicates massive upper GI bleeding with rapid transit, or a bleeding site in the distal colon, rectum, or anus.

Meckel's Diverticulum

Meckel's diverticulum is a remnant of the omphalomesenteric duct (vitelline duct) (Fig. 15.60). It exists as an isolated diverticulum, and may be complicated by inflammation (diverticulitis), which clinically resembles acute appendicitis and is diagnosed at surgery. Bleeding occurs when acid secreted by ectopic gastric mucosa in the diverticulum leads to ulceration of the adjacent intestinal mucosa. Usually there are no accompanying symptoms, and the bleeding presents with the passage of altered blood per rectum. Diagnosis is made by excluding other causes of GI hemorrhage. Radioactive technetium may be taken up by the ectopic gastric mucosa and is identified as a

"hot spot" on abdominal scanning (Fig. 15.61). Inversion of the diverticulum may lead to ileoileal intussusception. Meckel's diverticulum may communicate with the umbilicus as a granuloma, with discharge of mucous or small-bowel content. At times, the diverticulum is attached to the umbilicus by a fibrous cord representing the obliterated vitelline duct. Small-bowel volvulus around the fibrous band leads to intestinal obstruction.

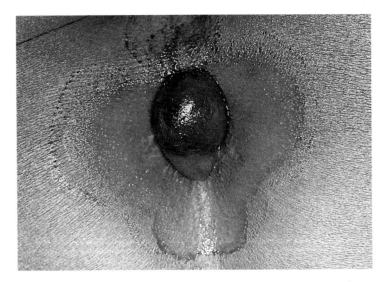

FIG. 15.62 A rectal juvenile polyp, prolapsed through the anus.

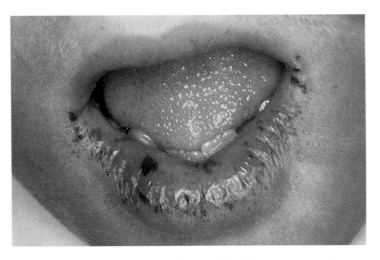

FIG. 15.63 Peutz-Jegher syndrome. The characteristic melanotic spots are seen on the lips (and are also found around the anus).

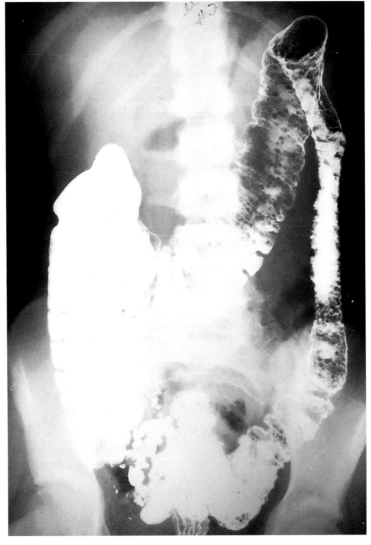

FIG. 15.64 Familial adenomatous polyposis. Barium enema study demonstrates multiple small polyps throughout the colon.

Polyps

Intestinal polyps are a common cause of rectal bleeding and, less commonly, of intussusception. Juvenile polyps comprise 80 to 90 percent of childhood polyps and usually present between the ages of 3 and 8 years with the passage of fresh blood per rectum. The rectal bleeding may not be related to passing stools, and the blood is not well mixed with the stool. Juvenile polyps occur throughout the large intestine and may be palpated in the rectum. A pedunculated polyp may prolapse through the anus and is often misdiagnosed as a hemorrhoid (Fig. 15.62). Sigmoidoscopy or colonoscopy reveals a smooth, shiny, round mass, the color of the adjacent intestinal mucosa. A rectal polyp is easily removed per rectum using a snare. Juvenile polyps are benign, and further evaluation of the patient is not necessary.

Peutz-Jegher polyps are multiple, benign hamartomatous polyps found in the small intestine. Bleeding causes the passage of altered blood in the stool. Intestinal peristaltic activity may drag the polyps distally, causing intermittent colicky abdominal pain; frank intussusception may also occur. Characteristically, melanin pigmentation of the skin and mucosa surrounding the mouth and anus will be observed (Fig. 15.63).

Barium contrast studies show multiple filling defects in the small intestine.

Adenomatous polyps are often multiple and may be associated with hereditary (familial) polyposis, which is transmitted as an autosomal-dominant disease. The polyps usually appear during the second decade of life. Initially benign, they become aggressive, invasive tumors during the fourth decade, making early diagnosis imperative. These colonic or rectal polyps usually present with bleeding, and less commonly with intermittent pain; they should be removed for histologic diagnosis. Barium enema examination or colonoscopy is essential to identify polyps in the colon (Fig. 15.64). Gardner syndrome is the association of familial polyposis with benign connective tissue neoplasms, notably desmoid tumors, fibromas, and chondromas.

Other Causes of GI Hemorrhage

Acute peptic ulceration may also result in GI bleeding. This may occur at any age, particularly in patients severely stressed by illness or injury. Portal hypertension with esophageal varices is common in children with chronic liver disease due to biliary atresia, hepatitis, or metabolic disorders. (For further discussion of liver diseases, see Chapter 10.)

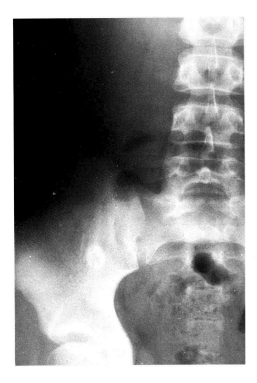

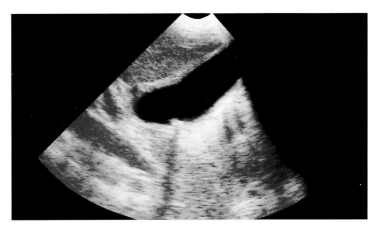

FIG. 15.65 This patient had acute appendicitis due to intraluminal obstruction of the appendix by a fecalith, seen here as a calcified density overlying the right iliac bone.

FIG. 15.66 Ultrasonogram of the right upper quadrant shows a distended gallbladder containing a gallstone. The dense gallstone has produced an acoustic shadow below it.

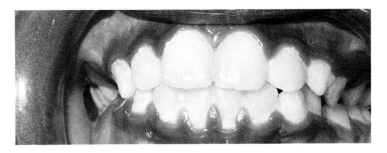

FIG. 15.67 Chronic lead poisoning, with typical discoloration of the gingival margins.

ACUTE ABDOMINAL PAIN

Acute appendicitis is the most common acute abdominal surgical problem of childhood, affecting children of all ages. Characteristically, the child will initially experience vague, periumbilical abdominal pain associated with anorexia and vomiting. Over a matter of hours the pain gradually localizes in the right iliac fossa and increases in severity. The patient begins to feel unwell, and a low-grade fever develops. With progressive inflammation there is increasing pain and the vomiting continues. On examination the patient is feverish and has a dry, furred tongue. There is tenderness in the right iliac fossa localized to McBurney's point. In the early stages there is voluntary guarding, but deep palpation may be possible if the patient is distracted, and rebound tenderness can be elicited. Later, involuntary guarding develops. Sudden movements such as coughing or walking precipitate severe right iliac fossa pain, and the patient prefers to lie on one side with the right hip flexed. Rectal examination reveals tenderness on the right side; this may be difficult to elicit in an apprehensive child. With perforation of the appendix there is sudden relief of the pain in the right iliac fossa, followed by generalized abdominal pain as peritonitis develops. This results in boardlike rigidity of the abdomen, cessation of bowel sounds, and a pyrexial, toxemic state. As the inflamed appendix becomes walled off by the omentum and adjacent loops of intestine in the later stages of appendicitis, a palpable, tender appendix mass develops. Rectal examination at this stage reveals a boggy swelling on the right. Leukocytosis is often absent in the early stages of appendicitis, but there is usually an increasing white cell count as the inflammatory process progresses. Abdominal radiographs are frequently normal. A fecalith may be seen in the right iliac fossa and will help to establish the diagnosis in a doubtful case (Fig. 15.65). Two or three fluid levels may be localized to the right iliac fossa. When perforation has occurred, there is generalized intestinal distention, with scattered air-fluid levels typical of paralytic ileus. In childhood, the differential diagnosis includes Meckel's diverticulitis,

Crohn's disease, salpingitis, and primary peritonitis. With the latter two conditions, the pain and tenderness is often present on the left as well as the right side of the abdomen, and there may be a purulent vaginal discharge. Crohn's disease may be associated with a mass in the right iliac fossa and perianal fistulas.

Intussusception, a common cause of colicky abdominal pain in infants and young children, was discussed earlier. An ovarian tumor or cyst may cause the ovary to twist (torsion of the ovary), resulting in acute, lower abdominal pain. If the torsion leads to ovarian ischemia and infarction, there is increasing pain with progressive signs of peritoneal irritation. If the ovary is large, a tender mass is palpable.

Acute right upper quadrant pain occurs with biliary tract disorders, including biliary colic due to gallstones or parasitic infestation of the bile ducts, acute cholecystitis, or cholangitis associated with choledochal cyst or following operation for biliary atresia. The pain is intermittent and, in the case of cholecystitis, is localized to a point below the costal margin in the midclavicular line. A tender, distended gallbladder or choledochal cyst may be palpated, and there is often mild jaundice and fever. Ultrasonographic examination will demonstrate dilatation of the gallbladder and bile ducts, and biliary calculi or roundworms may be seen (Fig. 15.66). The differential diagnosis includes acute hepatitis, pyelitis, or renal colic, the latter associated with pyuria or hematuria. Acute pain in the epigastrium or left upper quadrant may signify acute pancreatitis (identified by a raised serum amylase level), peptic ulcer disease, or renal disorders.

Other causes of acute abdominal pain include acute tonsillitis, pneumonia, diabetes mellitus, acute porphyria, and lead poisoning (Fig. 15.67).

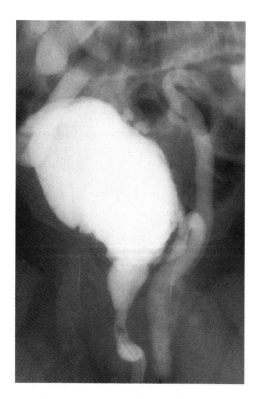

FIG. 15.68 The posterior urethral valves seen in this film resulted in a large trabeculated bladder, bilateral ureteric reflux with tortuosity of the ureters, and hydronephrosis. The infant presented with a suprapubic mass (the distended bladder) and palpable kidneys.

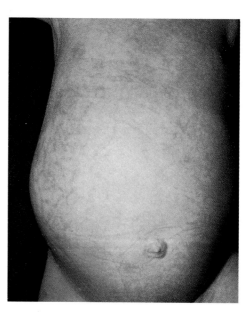

FIG. 15.70 The mass seen in the right upper abdomen of this infant, initially thought to be a liver tumor, proved on ultrasonography to be cystic and was found to be a large hepatic abscess.

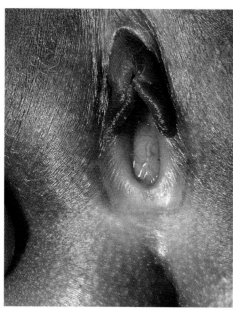

FIG. 15.69 Imperforate hymen. Accumulated secretions in the vagina and uterus caused bulging of the hymen and a pelvic mass.

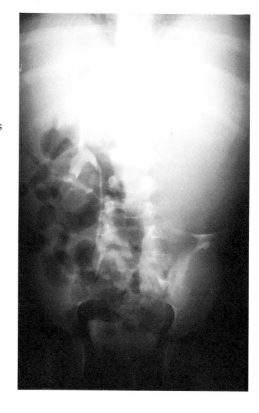

FIG. 15.71 Wilms tumor. This intravenous pyelogram shows distortion of the upper pole of the left kidney by a large nephroblastoma

ABDOMINAL MASSES

The discovery of a mass in the abdomen is a cause for anxiety because of the possibility of malignancy. It is imperative that urgent steps be taken to establish the diagnosis so that, if malignancy is confirmed, treatment can be commenced without delay. Most benign and malignant tumors are not recognizable at birth, even though they may be present at that time, and may not become sufficiently large to be appreciated until the child is 3 or 4 years of age or until metastases develop.

Ultrasonography is the most useful method for initial evaluation of an abdominal mass. Cystic and solid lesions can be distinguished, and the origin of the mass and its relationship to adjacent structures can often be demonstrated. This is less true of large lesions which compress and distort neighboring organs. Abdominal radiographs are seldom diagnostic, although the presence of calcification is of value if neuroblast-

oma is suspected. Computerized tomography usually follows ultrasonography when more precise information is required, and will visualize para-aortic lymph nodes and liver metastases. The inferior vena cava is best seen by ultrasonography. Intravenous injection of contrast during computerized tomography will provide a simultaneous pyelogram. Arteriography is seldom required for diagnosis, but may provide information of value to the surgeon.

In the newborn infant, a mass in the right upper abdomen usually represents an enlarged liver; if associated with a low hematocrit, a subcapsular hematoma due to birth trauma should be suspected. A mass in the left upper abdomen may indicate an enlarged spleen or left lobe of liver. A localized, smooth mass in the renal area is most likely to be a congenital renal abnormality such as cystic disease, renal dysplasia, or hydronephrosis. Mesoblastic nephroma is an uncommon, relatively benign variant of nephroblastoma, often present at

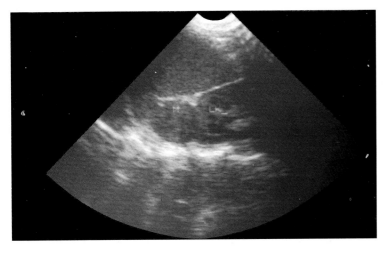
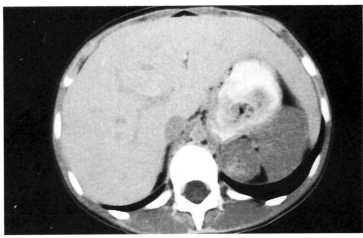

FIG. 15.72 Adrenal adenoma in a 6-year-old girl who presented with virilization. A sagittal ultrasonogram (left) reveals a well-circumscribed mass (M) superior to the left kidney. CT scan (right) demonstrates the suprarenal mass lying between the vertebral column and the left kidney.

birth. If hematuria is present, and especially if the child has congenital cardiac disease and has undergone cardiac catheterization, renal venous thrombosis should be suspected. Adrenal hematoma in the newborn resembles a renal mass, and calcification may be seen on the abdominal radiograph. A tense, hard suprapubic mass in a male child is usually a distended urinary bladder, obstructed as the result of posterior urethral valves (Fig. 15.68). In severe cases there is accompanying bilateral, tense hydronephrosis which manifests as a hard mass in each loin. In the female newborn infant, a smooth, round pelvic mass may represent distention of the vagina or uterus by secretions which have accumulated because of congenital vaginal obstruction (Fig. 15.69). Cystic abdominal lesions in the newborn infant include retroperitoneal lymphangioma or hemangioma, cysts of the ovary or mesentery, or, in the upper abdomen, a choledochal cyst.

Most masses become apparent during infancy and early childhood. The most common mass in the right upper quadrant is an enlarged liver due to cardiac, infective, or metabolic disorders. A tumor, cyst, or abscess in the liver may expand upward, displacing the diaphragm into the thoracic cavity, or downward toward the right iliac fossa (Fig. 15.70). The lower edge of the mass and its continuity with the liver can usually be appreciated, and the mass moves with the liver during respiration. A hydatid cyst of the liver may present with jaundice and fever due to compression of adjacent biliary ducts or release of daughter cysts into the bile ducts. Hepatic neoplasms are usually asymptomatic. With hepatoblastoma or hepatic carcinoma, the usual malignant liver tumors in children, the serum alpha-fetoprotein level is elevated.

On the left side, splenic enlargement is commonly encountered secondary to portal hypertension, hematologic disorders, or as a manifestation of an acute or chronic infective process. As in the newborn, renal enlargement is common and may be due to multicystic or polycystic renal disease, urinary obstruction with hydronephrosis, and neoplasms. The polycystic kidney is enlarged, irregular, usually bilateral, and associated with renal failure. Hydronephrosis presents as a smooth, cystic lesion; as with unilateral multicystic disease, renal function is not affected provided the opposite kidney is normal. A nephroblastoma (Wilms tumor) presents as a mass arising from the renal area and may reach large proportions,

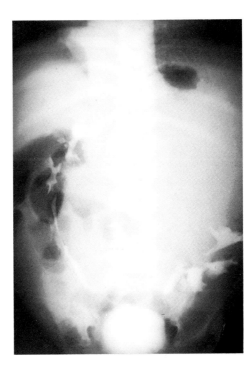

FIG. 15.73 Neuroblastoma. This intravenous pyelogram shows the left kidney displaced downward and laterally and the right ureter stretched laterally by a large neuroblastoma.

extending across the midline (Fig. 15.71). Hematuria, hypertension, and polycythemia are uncommon associated findings. Varicocele may be present in the left scrotum if the left renal vein is obstructed by tumor. Bilateral nephroblastoma occurs in 5 percent of patients. The lungs are the first organ to be involved with metastases, and a chest radiograph showing spherical lung metastases in association with a loin mass should make one highly suspicious of nephroblastoma.

Functioning tumors of the adrenal cortex are usually small, and patients present with the clinical manifestations of the hormonal abnormality. Tumors arising from the adrenal medulla range from benign ganglioneuroma to highly malignant neuroblastoma. In the early stages, these tumors are confined to the capsule of the adrenal gland (Fig. 15.72). Large neuroblastomas are irregular and nontender, varying in consistency from firm to soft, and displacing the kidney downward and laterally (Fig. 15.73). Acute enlargement with tenderness may be the result of hemorrhage into the tumor. Calcification

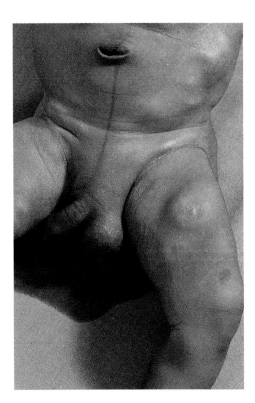

FIG. 15.74 Neuro-blastoma. Multiple skin metastases in a patient with stage IV-S disease.

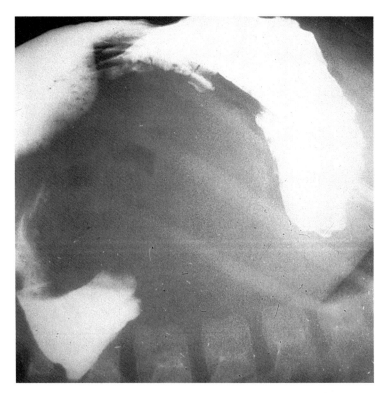

FIG. 15.75 Pancreatic pseudocyst. An upper GI series shows anterior displacement of the stomach and duodenum by the pseudocyst.

in the tumor may be seen on the abdominal radiograph, and the urinary levels of catecholamine metabolites are elevated. Neuroblastomas characteristically metastasize early, and patients frequently present with overt metastases before the primary abdominal lesion becomes apparent. Common sites for metastases are the liver, bone marrow, bone, and skin. A unique variety of neuroblastoma occurring in infants under 1 year of age is the stage IV-S lesion, which consists of a small, primary suprarenal tumor with metastases to soft tissues and bone marrow but not the skeleton. Despite the metastases, these infants generally have a good prognosis. Typical presentations include a grossly enlarged liver and impaired ventilation, or multiple, prominent skin nodules (Fig. 15.74) which may be misdiagnosed as lymphangioma or hemangioma.

In the epigastrium, a smooth, nontender mass may be a choledochal cyst, a gastric or duodenal duplication cyst, a pancreatic pseudocyst (Fig. 15.75), or a liver cyst or tumor. A choledochal cyst is situated toward the right of the midline, and is often associated with recurrent attacks of cholangitis, which manifests with fever, pain, and jaundice. Duplication cysts frequently cause partial or complete obstruction of the gastric outlet or proximal duodenum. With a pancreatic pseudocyst, there may be a preceding history of pancreatitis or blunt abdominal trauma.

A lower abdominal mass in a female child is most likely ovarian in origin (Fig. 15.76). An ovarian cyst may become very large before being detected and is typically mobile in all directions. An advanced ovarian tumor may be adherent to the surrounding viscera and presents as an irregular, fixed intra-abdominal mass. Frequently, there is associated ascites.

As in the newborn, enlargement of the uterus occurs in association with vaginal atresia or stenosis or an imperforate hymen. In the latter case, examination of the introitus will reveal the bulging, intact hymen. The bladder may be distended due to outlet obstruction by an intrinsic bladder tumor such as a rhabdomyosarcoma, which is usually associated with hematuria, or by extrinsic compression from a pelvic tumor or a loaded rectum due to chronic constipation. Neurologic disorders such as myelomeningocele may lead to a distended neurogenic bladder. In the male child, bladder outlet obstruction occurs as a result of posterior urethral valves or congenital and acquired urethral strictures; in the female, a uterocele may obstruct the bladder neck and opposite ureter. An ectopic (pelvic) kidney presents as an asymptomatic mass in the right or left iliac fossa, usually toward the midline, and is demonstrated by ultrasonography or intravenous pyelography.

An irregular mass arising in the center of the abdomen is likely to be a malignant tumor, a lymphoma involving the mesenteric lymph nodes, or a neuroblastoma arising from the para-aortic sympathetic chain. Both result in large, lobulated masses which vary in consistency from firm to soft and are associated with weight loss. Chronic constipation resulting in a grossly distended, impacted colon may present as an abdominal mass. The fecal matter can usually be indented, and rectal examination reveals a loaded, impacted rectum. A mesenteric cyst is a large, smooth mass in the abdomen which is usually mobile along an oblique line drawn from the right iliac fossa to the left upper quadrant. With large cysts there may be symptoms of partial intestinal obstruction if the adjacent intestine is compressed.

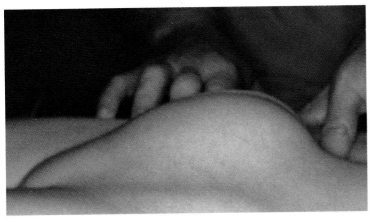

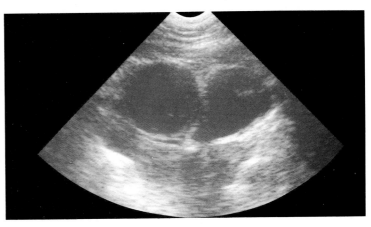

FIG. 15.76 Ovarian mass. (Left) A large ovarian mass arising out of the pelvis. (Right) A transverse ultrasonogram shows an ovarian cyst to the right of the bladder.

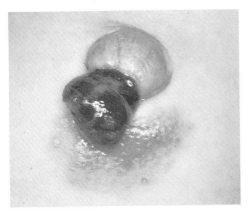

FIG. 15.77 Umbilical remnant of the omphalomesenteric duct. Secretions from the ectopic mucosa have excoriated the adjacent skin.

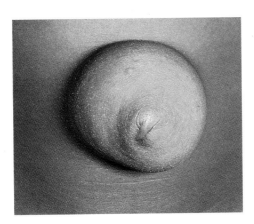

FIG. 15.78 Umbilical hernia.

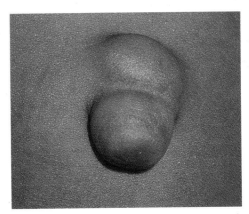

FIG. 15.79 Umbilical hernia with an adjacent supraumbilical hernia.

ABDOMINAL WALL

Umbilical Abnormalities

Abnormalities of the umbilicus are usually seen in the newborn infant as a result of infection of the cord stump or persistent remnants of the omphalomesenteric duct or urachus. An umbilical granuloma is a friable pink mass of tissue which develops at the umbilicus following separation of the cord. As a result of continued low-grade infection, the granulation tissue grows to form a polypoid lesion, with a purulent or blood-stained discharge. There are no associated abnormalities, and the granuloma responds to local treatment. An umbilical polyp, a remnant of the omphalomesenteric duct (see Meckel's diverticulum earlier in this chapter), consists of ectopic intestinal mucosa. It is red, smooth, and produces a mucoid discharge (Fig. 15.77). Subsequent inflammation results in a granulomatous appearance with a yellow or blood-stained discharge. Rarely, small intestinal content will discharge through the umbilical lesion, signifying a patent omphalomesenteric fistula. Unlike an umbilical granuloma, it does not respond to local treatment. The diagnosis is confirmed by histologic examination of the excised polyp. A patent urachus (urachal fistula), a remnant of the embryonic communication between the fetal bladder and the allantois, communicates with the dome of the bladder and opens at the umbilicus as a small fistula, often surrounded by urinary epithelium or granulation tissue. If urine drains through the fistula, there may be underlying bladder neck obstruction (such as posterior urethral valves) and a cystourethrogram should be done.

An umbilical hernia is a skin-covered bulge at the umbilicus which enlarges when intra-abdominal pressure is increased by crying or straining (Fig. 15.78). More common among black children, the hernia develops weeks or months after separation of the umbilical cord. Usually the hernia is easily reducible, allowing the abdominal wall defect to be palpated. There may be a history of intermittent colicky pain, but incarceration is surprisingly uncommon in childhood. Most umbilical hernias will resolve spontaneously by the age of 5 years. An incarcerated umbilical hernia presents as a painful, hard, tender, nonreducible mass at the umbilicus, with signs of intestinal obstruction in some patients. A supraumbilical hernia resembles an umbilical hernia but is situated in the midline above and separate from the umbilicus (Fig. 15.79). It represents a congenital abdominal wall defect, and spontaneous resolution does not occur.

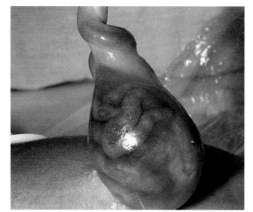
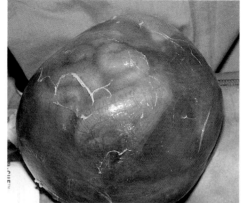

FIG. 15.80 Omphalocele. (Left) A small omphalocele with the umbilical cord attached to the apex of the sac. (Right) Giant omphalocele containing the stomach, small and large intestine, and liver.

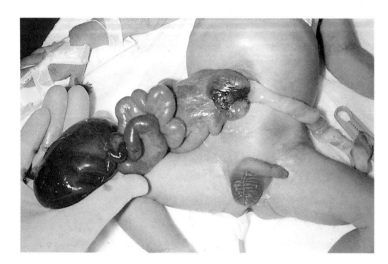

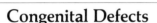

FIG. 15.81 Gastroschisis. The umbilical cord emerges from the abdominal wall to the left of the defect. Only the intestine has prolapsed, and intrauterine volvulus of the cecum has resulted in gangrene of that organ.

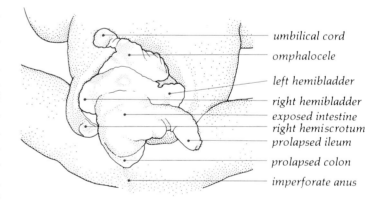

FIG. 15.82 Cloacal exstrophy consists of an omphalocele superiorly, below which the bladder is separated into halves by the exposed intestine. Proximally and distally, the bowel has prolapsed outward.

Congenital Defects

An omphalocele (exomphalos major) is an abdominal wall defect situated at the umbilicus and covered by a thin, transparent sac containing the intestine and, less commonly, the liver (Fig. 15.80). The umbilical vessels run along the side of the sac to the umbilical cord, which is usually attached to the sac near its apex. The fragile sac may rupture during the perinatal period, resulting in evisceration of its contents. Approximately 50 percent of patients with omphalocele have associated anomalies, notably cardiac and renal. An umbilical cord hernia (exomphalos minor) represents herniation of small intestine into the base of the umbilical cord. Although the hernia is not large, complete reduction is often prevented by adhesions of remnants of the omphalomesenteric duct. If unrecognized, the herniated bowel may be damaged when the umbilical cord is clamped after birth.

Gastroschisis resembles an omphalocele but does not have a sac (Fig. 15.81). The defect is typically situated to the right of the umbilical cord from which it may be separated by a narrow bridge of skin. The length of the defect varies; rarely, it extends from the sternum to the symphysis pubis. Because there is no hernia sac, the prolapsed small intestine, which has been lying free in the amniotic cavity, is usually covered by a thick fibrinous membrane. Associated intestinal stenosis, atresia, or volvulus may be found but there are usually no extra-abdominal abnormalities.

Cloacal exstrophy (vesicointestinal fissure) is due to defec-

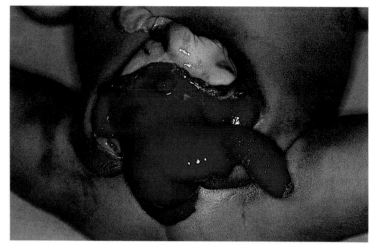

umbilical cord
omphalocele
left hemibladder
right hemibladder
exposed intestine
right hemiscrotum
prolapsed ileum
prolapsed colon
imperforate anus

tive fusion of the lower abdominal wall at the cloacal stage of embryonic development (Fig. 15.82). The defect consists of an omphalocele, below which the left and right halves of the open, everted bladder are separated in the midline by the open cecum. The latter communicates proximally with the ileum and distally with the colon. The rectum terminates in a blind pouch, and the symphysis pubis is widely separated.

Hypoplasia of the abdominal wall musculature (prune belly syndrome) is associated with malformations of the genitourinary system. A lateral abdominal wall hernia is rare (Fig. 15.83), and is easily confused with a neoplasm or hamartoma of the abdominal wall. The hernia is distinguished from these by being reducible. An abdominal wall hemangioma may enlarge when the patient strains, mimicking a hernia, but there is no muscular defect.

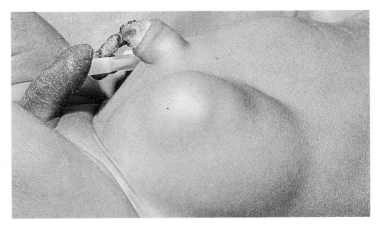

FIG. 15.83 Lateral abdominal wall hernia. A defect was palpated in the abdominal wall when the hernia was reduced.

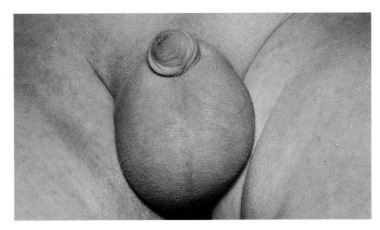

FIG. 15.84 Bilateral congenital hydroceles.

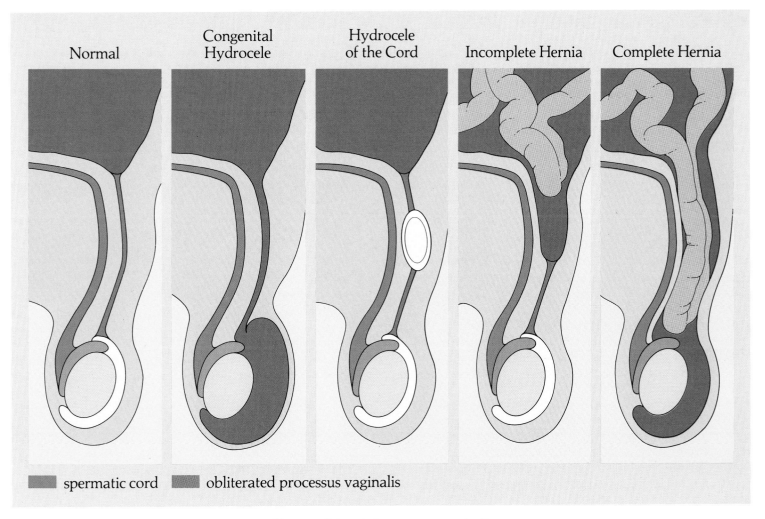

| Normal | Congenital Hydrocele | Hydrocele of the Cord | Incomplete Hernia | Complete Hernia |

■ spermatic cord   ■ obliterated processus vaginalis

FIG. 15.85 Abnormalities of the processus vaginalis.

INGUINOSCROTAL ABNORMALITIES

Congenital Hydrocele and Inguinal Hernia

The patent processus vaginalis is the basis for congenital hydrocele and congenital inguinal hernia. A narrow patent processus vaginalis allows peritoneal fluid to enter the tunica vaginalis, forming a communicating hydrocele. This manifests clinically as a swelling of the scrotum (Fig. 15.84). The fluid surrounds the testicle, making it difficult to palpate. The scrotum transilluminates brilliantly. Usually it is possible to palpate the proximal (upper) limit of the hydrocele which, unlike an inguinal hernia, does not extend into the external inguinal ring (Fig. 15.85). An encysted hydrocele of the cord is a tense, round cyst outside the external ring or in the upper scrotum, resulting from the obliteration of the processus vaginalis proximal and distal to the cyst. The equivalent abnormality in the female is a cyst of the canal of Nuck.

An inguinal hernia exists when the patent processus vaginalis is sufficiently wide to admit an intra-abdominal viscus, usually the omentum or a loop of intestine. In the female, the

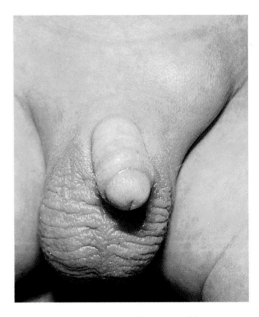 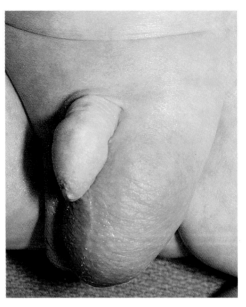 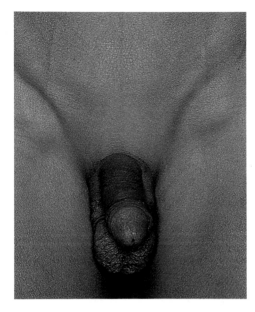

FIG. 15.86 Congenital inguinal hernia. (Left) Incomplete inguinal hernia, presenting as a mass in the groin. Both testicles are fully descended in the scrotum.

(Right) Complete inguinal hernia which has descended to the base of the scrotum, obscuring the testis.

FIG. 15.87 Bilateral femoral hernia. The swelling is below the inguinal ligament, medial to the femoral artery.

fallopian tube and occasionally the ovary enter the hernia sac. Clinically, the hernia presents as a bulge in the groin (Fig. 15.86) which increases in size when intra-abdominal pressure increases and can be reduced into the abdominal cavity by gentle pressure when the child relaxes. In an infant, the hernia can be demonstrated by making the infant cry, and in the older child by asking him to blow up a balloon or perform the Valsalva maneuver. A high retractile or undescended testis may be confused with an inguinal hernia in an infant; it is therefore important to ascertain that the testis is in the scrotum when examining for a hernia. A large inguinal lymph node is a distinct swelling, lacking continuity with the inguinal canal. Extension of the herniated viscera into the scrotum produces a complete indirect inguinal (scrotal) hernia. This is distinguished from a hydrocele by its failure to transilluminate brightly, although exceptions occur when the hernia contains gas-filled loops of intestine. Furthermore, with a hernia, the thickened spermatic cord continues proximally into the external ring. In the female with a gonad in the hernia sac, the possibility of testicular feminization syndrome must be considered. At surgery, the gonad is carefully examined and biopsied if at all abnormal.

An incarcerated hernia is one which cannot be reduced into the abdominal cavity. In infancy there may be no associated symptoms, or there may be partial or complete intestinal obstruction with associated colicky abdominal pain, distention, and vomiting. The risk of incarceration is highest in newborn infants less than 1 month of age. The chief complication of incarceration is strangulation, which occurs as the result of the trapped bowel being constricted at the internal and external inguinal rings, causing impairment of its blood supply. Left untreated, this leads to gangrene and perforation. The local signs of strangulation are a tender groin swelling with edema and redness of the overlying skin. The patient is febrile and has signs of intestinal obstruction. Abdominal films will show signs of intestinal obstruction, and air may be seen within loops of bowel in the scrotum. The testicle on the affected side may be enlarged and tender due to compression of the testicular vessels by the hernia. In the female, the herniated ovary may strangulate. A femoral hernia is rare in childhood and presents as a bulge below the medial end of the inguinal ligament (Fig. 15.87).

Undescended Testis (Cryptorchidism)

Cryptorchidism may be unilateral or bilateral. On examination, one or both sides of the scrotum are empty, and typically flat and "unused" (Fig. 15.88). There are several reasons for an empty scrotum, the most common being the retractile testis. This is a normal testis which is pulled out of the scrotum by an active cremaster muscle. The testis and epididymis can be manipulated completely into the scrotum, although they usually retract back into the groin when released. Permanent descent occurs before or at puberty. Failure of the testis to develop (anorchia) is a rare cause of cryptorchidism. Testicular atrophy may follow orchitis, testicular torsion, or trauma.

True undescended testis results from failure of normal testicular descent. The testis may be found anywhere along its normal route of descent from the abdominal cavity to the scrotum and cannot be brought completely into the scrotum. Frequently the testis can be moved around inside a sac and is mistaken for a nonreducible inguinal hernia. There may be an associated inguinal hernia. In some patients with incompletely descended testis, the testis is situated within the abdominal cavity and cannot be detected clinically. There is no reliable method of identifying an intra-abdominal testis before surgery.

An ectopic testis is one which has deviated from its normal route during descent and lies in an abnormal position. The most common ectopic position is the superficial inguinal pouch, lateral to the external ring and superficial to the external oblique aponeurosis. The perineum (Fig. 15.89), femoral triangle, and base of the penis are other sites where an ectopic testis may be found.

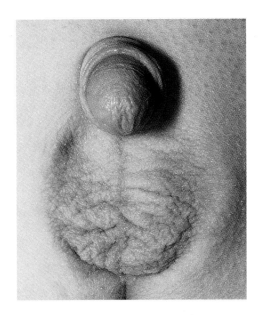

FIG. 15.88 Cryptorchidism. A flat, "unused" scrotum in a patient with bilateral undescended testes.

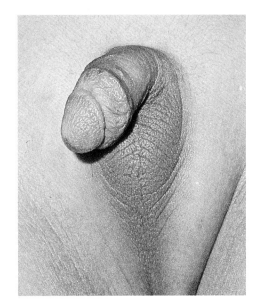

FIG. 15.89 Perineal ectopic testis. This patient presented with an undescended left testis. An ectopic testis is located in the left side of the perineum between the scrotum and the inguinal skinfold.

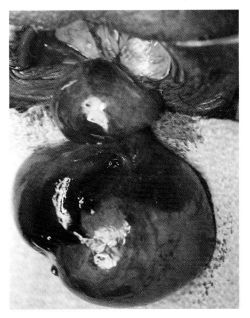

FIG. 15.90 Torsion of the testicle. Twisting of the spermatic cord has resulted in ischemia of the testis, to the left of which the dark, congested epididymis is seen.

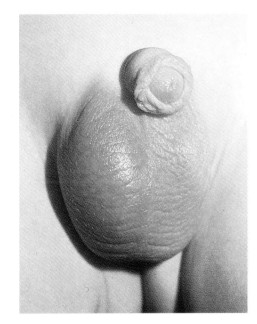

FIG. 15.91 Inflammation of the scrotum may be due to primary cellulitis, but may also be secondary to torsion of the testicle with gangrene. When the latter cannot be excluded, this is a surgical emergency.

Acutely Painful Testis

Torsion of the testicle occurs when the testis and spermatic cord twist, resulting in testicular ischemia (Fig. 15.90). If left untreated, this leads to gangrene of the testis. Typically there is acute onset of severe, unremitting testicular pain associated with nausea and vomiting. Careful palpation reveals a slightly enlarged, extremely tender testis and epididymis, which may have retracted to the upper scrotum. In infancy, pain is not prominent, but the infant is restless and may refuse feeding. The overlying skin may be inflamed, depending on the degree of testicular ischemia (Fig. 15.91). Radionuclear scanning of the testis or Doppler examination of the cord may indicate decreased or absent blood flow through the affected testis. Whenever torsion is diagnosed or cannot be excluded with certainty, emergency surgery is required to establish the diagnosis and relieve the torsion. Clinically, torsion of the testicular appendage mimics torsion of the testis. On examination, the testis is moderately tender; at its superior pole a small, hard, very tender nodule approximately 3 mm in diameter can be palpated—this is the infarcted appendage. The

scrotum may be enlarged on the affected side due to an associated inflammatory hydrocele.

Acute epididymo-orchitis is uncommon in a child with a normal urinary tract, and is usually associated with instrumentation of the urethra or infection in a patient with urinary tract abnormalities. The patient presents with acute pain and enlargement of the testis; on examination, the epididymis is usually considerably more tender than the testis, although both may be enlarged. The spermatic cord is also tender, and on rectal examination the tender seminal vesicles can be palpated. There is pyrexia and leukocytosis; the urine may contain leukocytes and, rarely, bacteria are identified on Gram stain. Diagnosis is made on the history and clinical findings. If torsion of the testicle cannot be conclusively excluded, emergency surgery is necessary to establish the diagnosis. Blunt trauma may cause acute, severe pain, tenderness, and swelling of the testis due to edema and hemorrhage. A hydrocele or hematocele may develop. An underlying tumor must be suspected if progressive resolution does not take place, in which case exploration and biopsy are indicated.

Painless Testicular Enlargement

Neoplasms of the testis and paratesticular tissues generally occur as a painless solid mass in the scrotum (Fig. 15.92). They are asymptomatic in children, often discovered on routine examination. A patient with a functional tumor may present with precocious puberty. Older children may be aware of a vague discomfort or dragging sensation in the scrotum. The absence of symptoms of acute inflammation distinguishes testicular tumors from testicular trauma, torsion, and epididymo-orchitis. The lack of continuity of the mass with the inguinal canal and negative transillumination exclude inguinal hernia and hydrocele. Metastases may be palpable in the para-aortic nodes and the left supraclavicular fossa.

Diagnosis is made by direct examination and biopsy of the testis through an inguinal incision, with the spermatic cord occluded.

BIBLIOGRAPHY

Holder TM, Ashcraft KW: Pediatric Surgery. Saunders, Philadelphia,1980.

Knight PJ, Reiner CB: Superficial lumps in children: What, when and why? Pediatrics 72:147–153, 1983.

Rickman PP, Soper RT, Stauffer UG: Synopsis of Pediatric Surgery. Georg Thieme Verlag, Stuttgart, 1975.

Welch KJ, Randolph JG, Ravitch MM, O'Neill, Jr. JA, Rowe MI: Pediatric Surgery, 4th ed. Year Book, Chicago, 1986.

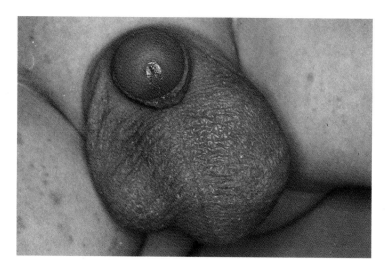

FIG. 15.92 Testicular tumor. Painless enlargement of the left testicle produced a hard mass which proved to be a teratoma of the testis.

PEDIATRIC AND ADOLESCENT GYNECOLOGY

16

Holly W. Davis, M.D.
Melissa Hamp, M.D.

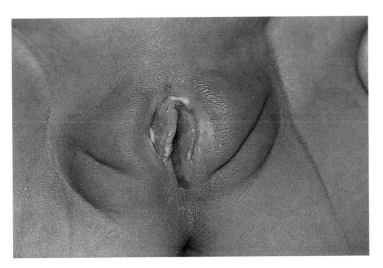

FIG. 16.1 *Normal appearance of the genitalia in a newborn female. The labia majora are full and the thickened labia minora protrude between them. The mucosa is pink and a milky white discharge is seen, reflecting stimulation by maternal hormones. (Courtesy of Dr. Ian Holzman)*

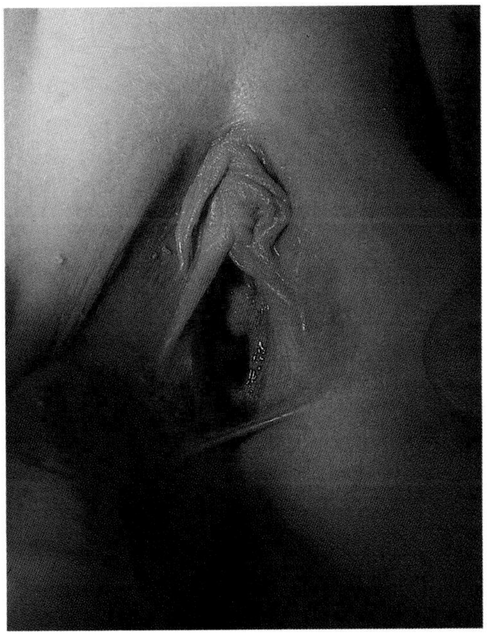

FIG. 16.2 *Normal appearance of the genitalia of a prepubertal female. The labia majora are flattened and the labia minora and hymen are thin and flat. The vaginal orifice is easily seen and the mucosa is thin, relatively atrophic, and reddish.*

Pediatricians and other primary care physicians who treat children and adolescents are finding themselves faced with gynecologic complaints with ever increasing frequency. This increase stems in part from the trends to earlier age of menarche, earlier onset of sexual activity, and to the high frequency of teenage pregnancy and venereal disease. Advances in the understanding of vulvovaginitis and in the recognition of sexual abuse have added to the need for practitioners to develop expertise in pediatric gynecology. Toward that end, this chapter will emphasize normal anatomy, techniques of examination, and the conditions most commonly encountered: obstruction, trauma, inflammation, and infections. The reader is referred to Chapter 9 for a discussion of precocious puberty and to Chapter 6 for a more detailed description of the approach to sexual abuse.

NORMAL FEMALE GENITALIA
Newborn and Prepubertal Periods

In the newborn female the physical appearance of the genitalia reflects stimulation by maternal hormones. The labia majora appear puffy and the thickened labia minora protrude between them (Fig. 16.1). Separation of the labia minora reveals thick hymenal folds that often hide the small central vaginal opening and urethral meatus. The mucosa is pink and moist, vaginal pH is acidic, and a milky discharge (physiologic leukorrhea) is seen. The phenomenon of withdrawal bleeding during the first week of life is not uncommon.

Within 6 to 8 weeks the effect of maternal hormones abates; the labia majora lose their fullness and the labia minora and hymen become thin and flat. Separation of the labia minora usually will expose the vaginal opening (Fig. 16.2). In fact the labia do not fully cover the vaginal vestibule

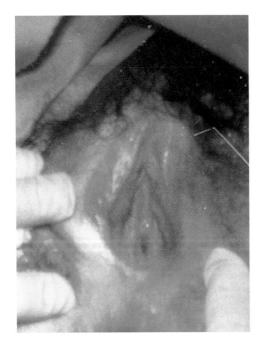

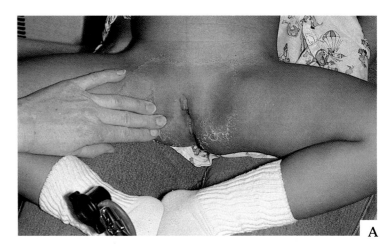

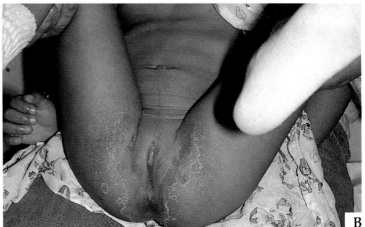

FIG. 16.3 *Normal appearance of the genitalia of a pubertal girl. The labia majora and mons pubis have filled out, the labia minora have become thickened and more rounded, and the hymenal orifice has enlarged. (Courtesy of Dr. K. Sukarochana)*

FIG. 16.4 *Optimal position for perineal inspection of the young prepubertal girl. **A**, Frog leg position on the mother's lap. **B**, Lithotomy position on the mother's lap.*

(particularly when the infant or child is sitting) and thus offer incomplete protection from external sources of irritation. The mucosa is thin, relatively atrophic, and has a reddish hue. Vaginal pH is now neutral or alkaline and secretions are minimal. From this point until puberty, the perineum, perivaginal tissues, and pelvic supporting structures will be relatively rigid and inelastic. This factor increases the likelihood of tearing as a result of trauma. The ovaries actually are intra-abdominal organs, being positioned above the pelvic brim until the onset of early puberty. Hence, ovarian disorders in the prepubertal years present with abdominal rather than pelvic symptoms and signs.

Peripubertal Period

With the onset of puberty the mons pubis begins to thicken and midline hair begins to form. Fat deposition fills out the labia majora. The labia minora thicken, become softer, and are more rounded. The clitoris enlarges slightly, and the urethra becomes more prominent. The hymen also becomes thicker as its central orifice enlarges (Fig. 16.3). The vaginal mucosa thickens and softens, becomes moist and pink, secretions increase, and pH drops. Perineal and pelvic tissues become more elastic and the ovaries gradually descend into the pelvis. In the months preceding menarche, physiologic leukorrhea recurs, consisting of a white discharge containing mature epithelial cells and vaginal secretions stimulated by estrogen (see Fig. 16.28).

GYNECOLOGIC EVALUATION
Examination of the Prepubertal Patient

INDICATIONS FOR EXAMINATION

Inspection of the external genitalia should be a part of every general physical examination. Careful attention to perineal inspection of female infants at newborn and 8-week visits facilitates early identification of major congenital anomalies. This is important because of a strong association between external congenital anomalies and other genitourinary malformations that may require early intervention. Thereafter, routine inspection during well child care visits can enable early diagnosis of new problems. The reluctance of some parents to mention concerns about possible genital disorders adds to the importance of such screening examinations. Routine pelvic examination in the patient without a complaint or abnormality on inspection is unnecessary until the onset of coital activity or until the late teens or early twenties. An exception to this rule would be the child exposed to diethylstilbestrol (DES) in utero, who having an increased risk of developing vaginal adenocarcinoma in adolescence should begin routine gynecologic evaluations at the time of menarche.

Patients presenting with certain chief complaints at acute care visits warrant inspection of the genitalia, and, on occasion, internal examination. These complaints include abdominal pain; dysuria, urinary frequency and urgency, incontinence, or enuresis; constipation and encopresis;

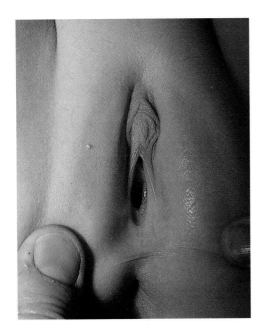

FIG. 16.5 Perineal inspection of the prepubertal child. To facilitate visualization of the introitus and lower third of the vagina, the examiner can either press down and laterally on the labia majora with the index and middle fingers of both hands (see Fig. 16.2) or can gently grasp the labia majora between thumbs and index fingers and pull down and laterally, as shown here. Use of a light facilitates inspection.

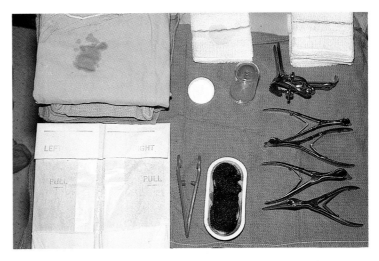

FIG. 16.6 Equipment used for examination under anesthesia. Nasal specula of varying sizes, a small pediatric vaginal speculum, Betadine-soaked and dry sponges are shown along with a specimen jar, drapes, and gloves.

perineal pruritus and/or perineal pain; vaginal discharge, or bleeding prior to menarche; and possible sexual abuse.

TECHNIQUE OF EXAMINATION

Whether the patient is being seen for a routine checkup or for a specific problem, the gynecologic portion of the assessment should occur toward the end of the examination to avoid frightening the child at the outset. Careful evaluation of physical growth and secondary sex characteristics is important for patients with precocious puberty (see Chapter 9) and for patients in the peripubertal and pubertal periods. All children with potential gynecologic problems deserve a thorough abdominal and inguinal examination. Adequate preparation is important prior to the gynecologic assessment itself. In the case of patients being seen for routine checkups the task is one of simple external inspection. In such instances, following abdominal and inguinal examination the physician generally can say to patients old enough to understand, "Now, I need to take a look at your bottom and you can help me." The patient then can be shown how to help by getting into position. Drapes generally are unnecessary and often are perceived by the patient as threatening. Young infants can be assessed easily on an exam table after being positioned by the examiner. Older infants and toddlers tend to be more relaxed when examined on their mother's lap, with the mother assisting by gently holding the child in either the frog leg or lithotomy position (Fig. 16.4). Older preschool and young school-age children usually are able to be examined on the table. Once the patient is in position, excellent visualization of the perineum and the lower portion of the vagina can be attained either by pressing down and laterally with the index and middle fingers of both hands on the lower portion of the labia majora (see Fig. 16.2) or by grasping the labia majora between thumbs and index fingers and gently pulling them down and laterally (Fig. 16.5). The maneuver should be explained first and the child reassured that the examiner is just going to look. If the child so desires or if she is mildly anxious, she may place her hands beneath the examiner's, or the mother may be en-

listed to perform the maneuver. Inspection is facilitated by use of a light held by an assistant or by a prepositioned flexible neck lamp. In addition, examination with the child in a knee-chest position can aid vaginal and cervical visualization without instruments. On deep breathing the orifice will often open widely. However, this position is not good for specimen collection and frequently is unacceptable to many patients who feel threatened by examination from behind. Nevertheless, it can be very useful for selected school-age patients.

If the patient is highly anxious about the procedure and unable to be reassured, the exam should be deferred to a later date. At no time should an anxious struggling child be physically restrained and forced to undergo examination, as yield will be minimal and the experience traumatic.

On inspection the physician can readily ascertain the presence or absence of pubic hair; note the appearance and configuration of the labia majora, labia minora, clitoris, urethra, hymen and vaginal orifice; observe the color of the mucosa and the presence or absence of rash or discharge; and visualize the distal vagina. Vaginoscopy is required only occasionally in the prepubertal child, and then only in those with specific problems. These include vaginal bleeding with or without evidence of trauma, suspected vaginal foreign body, and suspected vaginal tumors. Because of the high potential for inflicting pain, especially if the patient moves suddenly, vaginoscopy generally is best performed under anesthesia by a pediatric gynecologist or a pediatric surgeon. Figure 16.6 displays the tray used at our institution for examination under anesthesia. Heavy sedation may suffice in the child under 3 or 4 years of age but often is insufficient. Older school-age children may tolerate internal examination by a skilled examiner without sedation if preparation is careful. Again, a traumatic experience is to be avoided at all costs.

When specimens of vaginal secretions are required for cultures, wet mounts or cytology, these can be collected easily and with little or no discomfort by use of a small soft catheter or angiocath, if the patient is prepared for the pro-

LABORATORY EVALUATION OF VULVOVAGINITIS WITH VAGINAL DISCHARGE

Saline Wet Mount	For yeast, trichomonas, clue cells, inflammatory cells, pinworms, sperm
Gram Stain	For inflammatory cells, bacteria, clue cells
KOH	For yeast; "Whiff test" for gardnerella
Giemsa Stain	For herpes
Cultures	Routine for normal flora, nonvenereal pathogens, and gardnerella*
	For gonorrhea, herpes, chlamydia, ??mycoplasma†, and ureaplasma†

Primarily of use in prepubertal patients.

†*These cultures may be deferred at the initial visit and considered if no pathogens are found on initial smears and cultures and discharge persists, or if treatment for an identified pathogen fails to eradicate the discharge.*

FIG. 16.7 Laboratory evaluation of vulvovaginitis with vaginal discharge.

cedure with simple explanations. After cleansing the perineum, the sterile catheter is inserted gently through the vaginal opening with care taken to avoid contact with the perineum. When a discharge is present it can be gently aspirated. In the absence of discharge, sterile nonbacteriostatic saline is instilled slowly and then aspirated back. Cotton-tipped swabs are best avoided as they tend to abrade the thin vaginal mucosa of the prepubertal child. Further, by using a soft catheter, enough material can be obtained via aspiration for multiple culture swabs and smears. This obviates the need for repeated insertion of multiple swabs and thus minimizes discomfort. However if catheters are unavailable and cotton swabs are the only means of obtaining the specimens, they should be premoistened with nonbacteriostatic saline. Figure 16.7 enumerates the specimens that should be considered in evaluating patients with vaginal discharge. Figure 16.8 shows the equipment needed for internal examination in prepubescent patients and for collection of specimens.

Patients with precocious puberty, suspected abdominal masses, suspected vaginal foreign body, and/or abdominal pain should undergo rectal bimanual examination (vaginal bimanual is virtually never necessary). In most cases this can be accomplished readily in the office with good preparation. If the patient is unable to cooperate, the procedure should be deferred and an examination under anesthesia considered, if the results of ancillary studies such as sonography or CT scan warrant it.

Examination of the Adolescent or Pubertal Patient

INDICATIONS FOR EXAMINATION

A pelvic examination is indicated for any postmenarchial adolescent as part of the evaluation of complaints of vaginal discharge, pelvic pain, abnormal bleeding or menstrual disorders, and for all sexually active adolescents as a part of routine care. The nature of the initial experience of this procedure may greatly affect a young woman's comfort with her body and the ease with which she experiences routine gynecologic care throughout her adult life. Thus the examiner's approach should be sympathetic, unhurried, and sensitive to the modesty of the patient.

TECHNIQUE OF EXAMINATION

Successful examination depends on adequate patient preparation and use of appropriate instruments. For virginal adolescents, the narrow-bladed Huffman speculum (½ in. by 4¼ in.) is ideal. While long enough to expose the cervix, its narrow blades are inserted easily through the virginal introitus. Most sexually active adolescents can be examined with the Pedersen (1 in. by 4½ in.) or Graves (1⅜ in. by 3¾ in.) speculum. These instruments are shown in Figure 16.9. The examiner should carefully explain the various parts of the procedure—inspection of the external genitalia, speculum examination of the vagina and cervix, and bimanual palpation—before beginning. Use of anatomic drawings or models can be very helpful. The patient should be shown the speculum and be allowed to touch it if she so desires. Before and during examination, the examiner should talk to the patient, explaining what he or she is seeing. The patient should be told that she will feel "a sense of pressure," not pain, and should be reminded to breathe at a steady and regular rate to avoid breath-holding and the resulting tensing of abdominal and pelvic muscles, which can produce discomfort.

The teenager will generally prefer to have her mother out of the room during the pelvic examination. However, if she wishes her mother present, this should be respected. In general, particularly with a male examiner, the presence of a chaperone (such as a nurse or an aide) is optimal, both for propriety as well as to facilitate the handling of specimens.

With the patient in the lithotomy position, the external genitalia are inspected first. Pubic hair pattern and clitoral size are assessed. The presence of vulvar lesions or of vaginal discharge on the perineum should be noted. The introital opening is inspected and its edges palpated for any swellings in the regions of Bartholin's glands. The urethral opening is then inspected, and if erythema or discharge are noted the urethra is gently stripped with a gloved finger along the vaginal roof. Any purulent material obtained should be cultured.

The examiner then should gently insert the index finger into the vagina to assess the size of the introital opening and to locate the cervix. Vaginal muscle tone can be assessed by asking the patient to "tighten her muscles" around the examiner's finger. Then, with the index finger partially withdrawn but gently pressing on the vaginal floor, the specu-

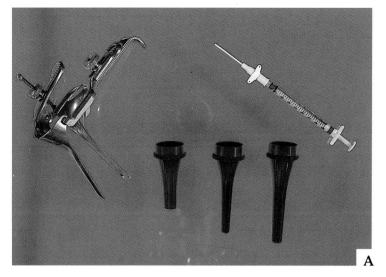
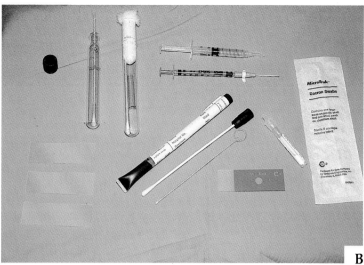

FIG. 16.8 Equipment needed for internal examination of prepubertal patients and for collection of specimens. **A**, A narrow pediatric speculum and three veterinary otoscope specula are shown. Specimen collection is easier and less traumatic if a soft angiocath (as shown) is used to aspirate vaginal secretions. **B**, Materials needed for collecting and processing a vaginal discharge may include (clockwise from upper left): test tube with a small aliquot of saline for wet mounts, a standard culture tube, a syringe with saline for lavage, a syringe with attached angiocath, chlamydia culture and slide kit, Neisseria gonorrhoeae culture and transport pack, and glass slides for wet mount, KOH prep, and Gram stain. Swabs can be used to collect all specimens in postmenarchial patients.

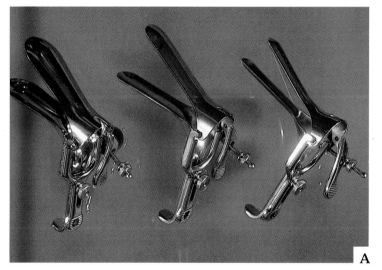
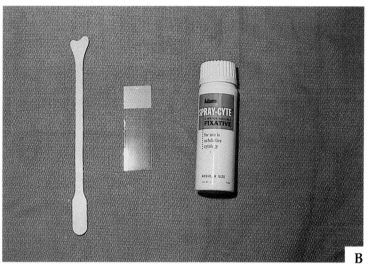

FIG. 16.9 Equipment needed for pelvic examination of adolescent patients. **A**, From left to right, a Graves (1⅛-in. by 3¾-in.) speculum, a Pedersen (1-in. by 4½-in.) speculum and a narrow-bladed Huffman (½-in. by 4¼-in.) speculum are shown. The Graves and Pedersen specula are useful for examining sexually active patients while the Huffman is ideal for virginal adolescents. **B**, The spatula used for obtaining a Pap smear is shown along with a glass slide and spray fixative.

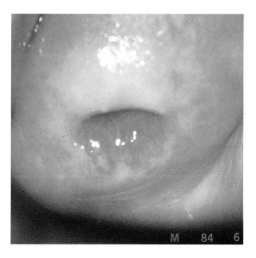

FIG. 16.10 Normal nulliparous cervix. The surface is covered with pink squamous epithelium that is uniform in consistency. The os is small and round. (Courtesy of C. Stevens)

lum (premoistened with warm water, not lubricant) is inserted over the finger into the vagina. Excess pressure on the anterior vaginal wall, and hence on the urethra, is to be avoided.

With the speculum in place the vaginal walls are inspected for erythema, lesions, or the presence of discharge. Visible vaginal secretions from the posterior vaginal pool should be sampled with a cotton swab and placed in a small amount of normal saline for wet mount and KOH examination. The cervix is then inspected. Any vaginal pool secretions should be removed from the cervical surface, using cotton swabs, prior to inspection of the cervix or sampling of cervical secretions. The normal nulliparous cervix has a small round os and is covered with squamous epithelium that is pink and uniform in consistency (Fig. 16.10). Cervical lesions (cysts,

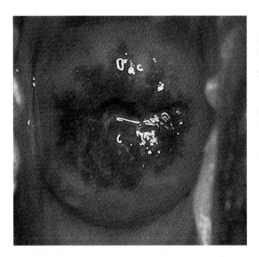

FIG. 16.11 Ectropion. Columnar mucosal cells usually found in the endocervical canal have extended out onto the surface of the cervix creating a circular raised erythematous appearance. Note the normal nonpurulent cervical mucus. This normal variant is not to be confused with cervicitis. (Courtesy of Dr. E. Jerome)

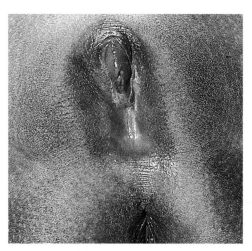

FIG. 16.12 Labial adhesions. Agglutination and adhesion of the labia minora, as a result of healing following erosion or inflammation, produce the appearance of a smooth flat surface overlying the introitus, divided centrally by a thin lucent line. (Courtesy of Dr. D. Lloyd)

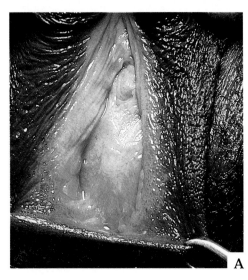

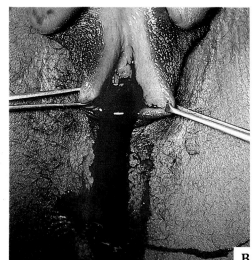

A   B

FIG. 16.13 Imperforate hymen/hematocolpos. This child presented with a 2-month history of intermittent crampy lower abdominal pain, which had acutely worsened. She had well-developed secondary sex characteristics but was premenarchial by history. **A**, Examination revealed midline fullness and tenderness of the lower abdomen and a smooth bulging mass at the introitus. **B**, Incision of the imperforate membrane just inside the hymenal ring allowed the accumulated menstrual blood and vaginal secretions to drain. (Courtesy of Dr. D. Lloyd)

polyps, vesicles) should be noted. An ectropion (or eversion) of the endocervical columnar epithelium onto the cervical surface is not uncommon in adolescents, and by itself is not abnormal (Fig. 16.11). Ectropion should be distinguished from cervicitis, the latter being suggested by the presence of erythema, friability, and mucopurulent cervical discharge (see Fig. 16.39B). If the endocervical epithelium extends onto the vaginal walls or if the cervical shape is abnormal or hypoplastic, this raises the possibility of in utero DES exposure, and gynecologic referral is warranted.

A Pap smear should then be obtained by rotating a wooden Ayre spatula around the cervical os. Ideally the squamocolumnar junction is sampled. If this junction is not visible or if a spatula is not available, a saline-moistened cotton swab may be inserted and rotated in the os. Upon collection, samples are applied to glass slides and are sprayed with Pap fixative (see Fig. 16.9B).

The speculum is then removed and the bimanual (vaginal-abdominal) examination is performed. The examiner should note the size, consistency, position and mobility of the uterus, and should check for tenderness on cervical or fundal motion. The adnexa should be palpated for enlargement or tenderness. Rectal bimanual examination should be reserved for patients in whom the vaginal bimanual is not sufficient for palpation of pelvic structures (e.g., when the uterus is retroflexed). Once the assessment is completed, the patient should be assisted to the sitting position. The results are then explained to her and positive feedback regarding her cooperation is given.

GENITAL TRACT OBSTRUCTION
Labial Adhesions

The most common form of vaginal obstruction in prepubertal patients is that produced by fusion of the labia minora as a result of labial adhesions. It is postulated that inflammation and erosion of the inner surfaces—whether due to mechanical trauma, infection, or noninfectious dermatitis—result in agglutination of the apposed labia minora by fibrous tissue upon healing. The process typically begins posteriorly and extends forward, ultimately covering the vaginal vestibule and occasionally the urethra. On inspection there is a smooth flat surface overlying the introitus, divided centrally by a thin lucent line (Fig. 16.12). While most patients with labial fusion are asymptomatic, some present with symptoms of lower urinary tract inflammation. The problem responds readily to application of estrogen cream once or twice daily, for 2 to 3 weeks. The patient's mother should be informed that topical estrogen may cause transient hyperpigmentation that will regress once therapy is completed. Treatment of the primary process and instructions on good perineal hygiene tend to prevent recurrence. Manual separation is painful and therefore traumatic. Furthermore, it is frequently followed by a recurrence of fusion. Thus, the practice should be abandoned.

Imperforate Hymen

In actuality the anomaly referred to as imperforate hymen consists of an imperforate membrane located just inside the

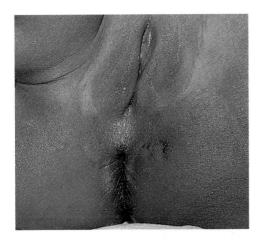

FIG. 16.14 Superficial blunt trauma. Healing abrasions are seen in this patient who was a victim of sexual abuse.

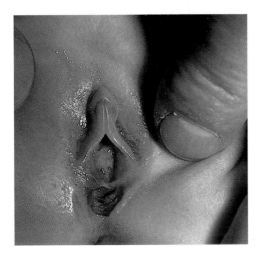

FIG. 16.15 Superficial penetrating injury. This infant presented with a chief complaint of blood spotting on the diaper. Inspection revealed a perineal tear just posterior to the hymenal ring, with no evidence of internal extension on vaginoscopy under anesthesia. Sexual abuse was suspected.

hymenal ring. This is likely to be missed on newborn examination because of the redundancy of the hymenal folds. It should become evident however by 8 to 12 weeks of age on perineal inspection. Occasionally young infants with this anomaly have unusually copious vaginal secretions stimulated by maternal hormones, and will develop *hydrocolpos*. They present with a cystic swelling of the lower abdomen (especially noticeable when the bladder is full) and upon perineal inspection are found to have a whitish bulging membrane at the introitus. Treatment consists of incision of the membrane and removal of redundant portions.

If undetected in infancy, the patient with imperforate hymen frequently presents in early puberty with *hematocolpos*. The major complaint is one of intermittent lower abdominal pain. If not diagnosed promptly, difficulty in urination ensues and a lower abdominal swelling may become noticeable. On occasion acute urinary retention may prompt the visit. The patient has well-developed secondary sex characteristics but is premenarchial by history. Perineal inspection reveals a tense bulging bluish membrane at the introitus (Fig. 16.13A). A low cystic swelling is palpable anteriorly on rectal examination. Operative incision allows drainage of the accumulated blood and vaginal secretions (Fig. 16.13B). Patients found to have an imperforate hymen, regardless of age at diagnosis, should have follow-up radiologic studies of the genitourinary tract because of a significant frequency of associated anomalies.

Other forms of genital tract obstruction are rare and beyond the scope of this chapter. It is important to note, however, that early routine genital inspection will usually reveal absence of a vaginal orifice and enable appropriate early evaluation to delineate the nature of the anomaly and thus facilitate planning for corrective surgery.

GENITAL TRAUMA

As mentioned earlier the genital structures and pelvic supporting tissues of the prepubescent girl not only are smaller but also are considerably more rigid than those of the adolescent or adult female. This inelasticity significantly increases the risk of tearing with either blunt or penetrating trauma, and of internal extension of injury especially in cases of penetrating injury. Appropriate assessment and management necessitate appreciation of this factor along with recognition that serious internal injuries of the vagina, rectum, urethra, bladder, and peritoneal structures may underlie deceptively mild external abnormalities. Careful attention must be given to vital signs, abdominal examination and evaluation of the urethra, hymen, lower vagina, perineal body, and rectum. Clues to internal extension of injury include hymenal tears, vaginal bleeding and/or vaginal hematoma, tears of the perineal body, inability to urinate or gross hematuria, and abnormal sphincter tone or rectal bleeding. When injuries have extended to involve peritoneal structures, lower abdominal tenderness is seen, and at times is associated with signs of hypovolemia. Direct tenderness may range from mild to marked and may or may not be accompanied by rebound tenderness. Adolescents, in contrast, are more likely to have contusions than tears and are much less likely to have internal extension of injury unless the applied force is very great.

The role of the primary care or emergency physician is one of assessing the patient's general status and determining the likely extent of injury. This can be accomplished largely with a good general examination, careful perineal inspection, and urinalysis. The physician must at all times be patient and sensitive to the patient's physical discomfort and emotional distress, providing emotional support and reassurance whenever possible. Patients should also be protected from having to undergo multiple examinations, a particular risk in teaching hospitals. When external inspection suggests that the prepubertal patient's injury is more than superficial, internal examination under anesthesia (by a pediatric surgeon or gynecologist) should be arranged. This enables meticulous inspection and wound exploration under optimal conditions without traumatizing the child further. Most adolescents are able to tolerate inspection and internal examination as outpatients. However if injuries are severe or if the postmenarchial patient is too anxious to undergo pelvic examination when indicated, examination under anesthesia is the better course.

Superficial Perineal Injuries

The majority of cases of superficial perineal trauma are the result of mild blunt force incurred via straddle injury, minor falls, and sexual abuse. Typical lesions include superficial abrasions, mild contusions, and occasionally superficial lacerations (Fig. 16.14). The latter are found most frequently at the junction of the labia majora and minora and usually are only 1 to 3 mm deep. Minor falls onto or scrapes against sharp objects tend to produce simple perineal and vulvar lacerations. As in cases of mild blunt trauma the junction of the labia minora and majora is the site most frequently involved; however, tears of the labia majora or perineal body are not uncommon (Fig. 16.15).

Whether blunt or penetrating, when injuries are truly superficial, bleeding if present at all tends to be scant. The ex-

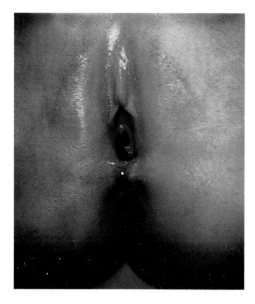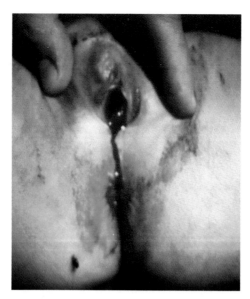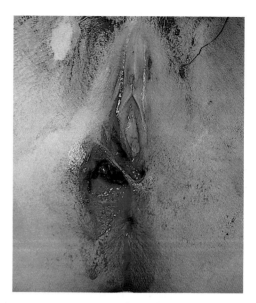

FIG. 16.16 Moderate blunt trauma. Following a straddle injury on a diving board, this 9-year-old girl presented with vaginal bleeding. External inspection revealed a superficial tear of the anterior portion of the perineal body, a small hematoma to the right of the introitus, and blood trickling through the vaginal orifice. Examination under anesthesia disclosed a tear of the lateral vaginal wall. (Courtesy of Dr. K. Sukarochana)

FIG. 16.17 Moderate genital trauma. This 6-year-old girl presented with painless vaginal bleeding, which had soaked three sanitary pads in 2 hours. Inspection disclosed a hematoma of the right labia majora and contusions of the introitus with clotted blood protruding through the vaginal opening. A small superficial laceration is present on the left, between the labia majora and minora, and another on the right between the superior portion of the introitus and the labium minora. At vaginoscopy under anesthesia a vaginal tear involving the right lateral wall was found. Sexual abuse was strongly suspected. (Courtesy of Dr. K. Sukarochana)

FIG. 16.18 Moderately severe penetrating genital trauma. This youngster fell while roller skating and slid on her bottom for several feet, tearing her perineum on an object projecting up from the ground. A laceration involving the right labia majora and minora and extending through the perineal body to the anus is evident on inspection. The patient complained of only minor discomfort. Examination under anesthesia revealed vaginal and rectal extension of the tear with complete transection of the external anal sphincter. The peritoneum was intact.

ception to this is a penetrating injury involving the corpus cavernosum of the labia majora, in which case hemorrhage may be profuse. Patients may experience mild perineal discomfort and pain on urination but otherwise are asymptomatic. Most of these injuries can be managed supportively with topical bacteriostatic ointment, sitz baths, and careful perineal cleansing. Application of the ointment prior to urinating relieves dysuria as does urinating in a tub of water. Deeper tears of the labia majora necessitate control of bleeding vessels and suturing under anesthesia.

Moderate Genital Trauma

Moderately forceful blunt trauma often results in perineal tears and in venous disruption and hematoma formation. Hematomas of the perineum appear as tense round swellings with purplish discoloration, which are tender on palpation (Fig.16.16). When large, these may cause intense perineal pain. Those located in the periurethral area may interfere with urination. Moderate blunt force also can produce submucosal tears and vaginal mucosal separation with resultant vaginal bleeding or vaginal hematoma formation (Fig. 16.17). In some cases, the associated external injuries can be deceptively mild (see Fig. 16.16). Vaginal hematomas are the source of significant pain that usually is perceived as perineal and/or vaginal but at times is referred to the rectum or buttocks. Inspection through the vaginal orifice reveals a bluish swelling involving one of the lateral walls.

This also may be evident as a tender swelling anterolaterally on rectal examination.

Moderate penetrating injuries result primarily from falls onto sharp objects ("picket fence injury"), rape, sexual molestation with phallic-shaped objects, and occasionally auto accidents. Lesions include perineal tears that extend into the vagina, rectum or bladder but do not breach the peritoneum. While many patients present with external lacerations that obviously are extensive on inspection (Fig. 16.18; see also Chapter 6, Fig. 6.21), a significant proportion have deceptively minor external injuries. It is important to bear in mind that in the absence of associated hematomas extensive tears may produce little pain. Furthermore, while most such injuries result in moderate bleeding some patients have remarkably little blood loss.

Whether the mechanism of injury involves blunt force or penetration, when physical findings include bleeding through the vaginal orifice, a vaginal hematoma, rectal bleeding, rectal tenderness or abnormal sphincter tone, gross hematuria or inability to urinate, internal extension of injury is probable. All such patients warrant exploration and repair in the operating room. This obviates the need for extensive examination in the office or emergency department.

Severe Genital Trauma

Severe falls from heights onto flat surfaces can produce major perineal lacerations simulating penetrating injury. In ad-

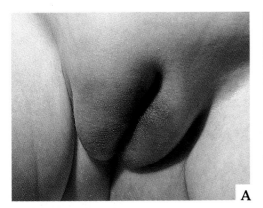
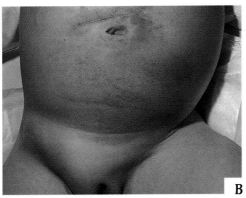

FIG. 16.19 Severe blunt perineal trauma. Following a fall from a height in which she had landed on her bottom, this young child presented with **(A)** labial contusions and hematomas, lower abdominal tenderness, and signs of hypovolemia. The force of the fall ruptured pelvic vessels, resulting in retroperitoneal bleeding that **(B)** ultimately extended along the anterior abdominal wall. These photographs were taken a few days after the injury. (Courtesy of Dr. Marc Rowe)

A

B

CATEGORIES OF PREPUBERTAL VULVOVAGINITIS

Noninfectious	Infectious	
	Nonvenereal Pathogens	Venereal Pathogens
Poor hygiene	Bacterial respiratory and/or skin pathogens	Bacterial pathogens
Poor perineal aeration and maceration	Group A beta-hemolytic streptococcus*	*Chlamydia trachomatis**
Chemical irritant	*Streptococcus pneumoniae**	*Gardnerella vaginalis**
Contact dermatitis (allergic vulvitis)	*Haemophilus influenzae**	*Neisseria gonorrhoeae**
Frictional trauma	Viral pathogens	?Genital mycoplasmas
Sympathetic inflammation and fistulas*	Varicella-Zoster virus	Protozoans
Vaginal foreign body*	Adenovirus*	*Trichomonas vaginalis**
Physiologic leukorrhea*	Echovirus*	Viral pathogens
	Urinary tract pathogens	Herpes simplex
	Gastrointestinal pathogens	Papilloma virus
	Candida species	
	Shigella species*	
	Enterobius vermicularis	

*Conditions in which vaginal discharge is prominent.

FIG. 16.20 Categories of prepubertal vulvovaginitis.

dition, occasionally they can cause disruption of pelvic vessels, mesentery and intestine, with or without pelvic fracture (Fig. 16.19). Similarly, severe penetrating injury may produce tears that extend through the cul-de-sac, rupturing pelvic vessels and tearing intra-abdominal structures. While external injuries in these cases usually are extensive and are associated with significant bleeding, they can be incredibly minor in appearance, particularly when penetration is the source. These children will complain of lower abdominal and perineal pain, which may radiate down one leg. Abdominal examination should reveal at least mild direct tenderness with some guarding and possibly mild rebound tenderness early on. Patients with pelvic bleeding will ultimately have signs of hypovolemia (at a minimum, they will exhibit tachycardia with widened pulse pressure) although these signs may not be evident immediately following the injury. Any patient with clinical signs of peritoneal extension of genital trauma warrants prompt hemodynamic stabilization followed by surgical exploration and repair.

NONTRAUMATIC VULVOVAGINAL DISORDERS

Prepubertal "Vulvovaginitis"

Strictly defined, vulvovaginitis denotes an inflammatory process involving both the vulva and the vagina. In practice however, the term is applied more loosely to prepubertal patients who have symptoms consistent with vulvovaginitis (dysuria, vulvar pain or itching, vaginal discharge) regardless of the presence or absence of signs of inflammation, or to patients with vulvar irritation not involving the vagina. This process traditionally has been subdivided into specific and nonspecific types, the former having an identifiable infectious source and the latter having no identifiable pathogen and usually attributed to poor hygiene. Recent research has begun to shed more light on etiologic factors and has resulted in significant improvements in diagnostic techniques. As a result, the spectrum of known infectious agents has expanded, and specific sources of "nonspecific" vulvovaginitis are being identified with increasing frequency. Therefore, it seems more logical to reclassify the problem into noninfectious and infectious subgroups. Figure 16.20 presents the currently recognized sources of

CLINICAL AND LABORATORY FEATURES OF VAGINAL DISCHARGE IN ADOLESCENTS

	Physiologic	Candida	Trichomonas	*Gardnerella vaginalis*
Appearance	White, gray or clear; flocculent	White; curdlike, with adherent plaques	Gray, yellow or creamy; ± frothy or homogeneous	Gray, white; homogeneous
Amount	Variable	Scant	Large	Large
Vulvar and Vaginal Irritation	None	Common	Occasional	Rare
pH of Discharge	≤4.5	≤4.5	>5.0	>4.5
Amine Odor with 10% KOH (Whiff Test)	Absent	Absent	Present	Present
Microscopy	Epithelial cells, few WBCs, lactobacilli	↑WBCs, +KOH: pseudohyphae and budding yeast	↑WBCs, motile trichomonads (in saline prep) in 80 to 90% of symptomatic patients	Few WBCs, +clue cells on saline prep

FIG. 16.21 *Clinical and laboratory features of vaginal discharge in adolescents.*

ORGANISMS THOUGHT TO CONSTITUTE NORMAL OR NONPATHOGENIC VAGINAL FLORA*

Aerobes and Facultative Anaerobes

Diphtheroids
Staphylococcus epidermidis
Beta-hemolytic streptococcus group B
Lactobacilli (newborn and postmenarchial)
Escherichia coli
Klebsiella species
Group D streptococcus
Staphylococcus aureus
Pseudomonas species
Proteus species

Anaerobes

Bacteroides species
Peptococcus species
Peptostreptococcus species

It is currently unclear as to whether or not Mycoplasma hominis, Ureaplasma urealyticum, *and* Gardnerella vaginalis *can constitute normal flora or if they should be regarded as primarily pathogenic.*

FIG. 16.22 *Organisms thought to constitute normal or nonpathogenic vaginal flora.*

vulvovaginitis in prepubertal patients.

Vulvovaginitis is relatively common in prepubertal girls and accounts for nearly 90 percent of genital complaints prior to menarche. Its frequency is explained in part by the fact that the labia do not fully cover and thus do not completely protect the vestibule from friction and external irritants, especially when the child is sitting or squatting. Additionally, the unestrogenized epithelium is thin, relatively friable, and more easily traumatized. Finally, young children tend not to appreciate the importance of good perineal hygiene and are less careful than older children and adults about cleansing and avoiding contamination. Also in contrast to adolescents and adults, prepubertal girls are not at risk for internal extension of vulvovaginal infections (cervicitis and pelvic inflammatory disease) as the unestrogenized genital tract does not support the ascent of infection through the uterus and fallopian tubes.

The multiplicity of potential etiologies necessitates meticulous history taking. Questions related to symptoms and duration of problems must be supplemented by those addressing recent respiratory, gastrointestinal and urinary tract infections, and concurrent abdominal pain. Intake of medications, application of topical agents, use of bubble bath or strong soaps, quality of hygiene, presence of enuresis and day wetting, and the nature of recent activities also must be addressed. Finally, the possibility of sexual abuse has to be considered (see Chapter 6). Physical assessment must include determination of degree of pubertal development as well as inguinal, abdominal and often rectal examination, along with careful perineal and vaginal inspection. Underwear should be checked for fit, cleanliness and signs of discharge, stool, and urine. Presence of discharge necessitates specimen collection for multiple smears (wet mount,

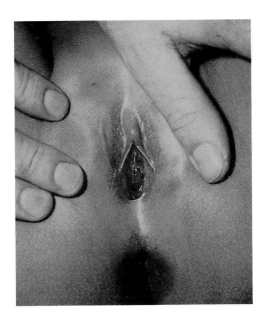

FIG. 16.23 Nonspecific vulvar irritation. On perineal inspection mild nonspecific inflammatory changes are seen. There is no associated vaginal discharge. Meticulous history taking is generally required to make the diagnosis, as smears and cultures are seldom revealing. Chemical irritants (such as bubble bath), poor perineal hygiene, and sexual abuse are the most common causes.

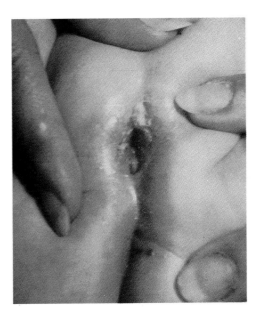

FIG. 16.24 Poor perineal hygiene. Despite prior cleansing by a nurse for a "clean-catch" urine, the initial specimen contained numerous white cells and debris. When the perineum was rechecked, the infant was found to have copious amounts of smegma adhering to the clitoris and labia minora. Urine obtained after thorough recleansing was normal.

KOH prep, Gram stain) and cultures (routine, gonorrhea, and possibly chlamydia, and mycoplasma) (see Figure 16.7). Material should be collected from the vaginal canal unless the vagina appears spared. When a vaginal foreign body is suspected, rectal examination and vaginoscopy are indicated. Urinalysis should be done on all patients.

Vulvovaginal Complaints in Adolescents

Vulvovaginal complaints are also common among adolescent females, particularly among those who are sexually active. However, in this age group infectious processes are the major source of vulvovaginal inflammation, and sexually transmitted pathogens are the predominant offending organisms. The clinical manifestations of some of these disorders in adolescent girls can be very similar to those seen in prepubertal children although estrogenization and maturation of the genital tract alter its pathophysiologic response, favoring upward spread of some infectious processes, particularly those of gonorrhea and chlamydia. As a result, subclinical infection, cervicitis and pelvic inflammatory disease, in addition to vulvovaginitis, are significant concerns following menarche. Clinically, vulvar lesions, vaginal discharge, odor, pruritus and dysuria are common presenting problems in adolescents, but dyspareunia, pelvic pain, fever, and irregular bleeding may be prominent complaints as well. These symptoms are relatively nonspecific and may represent the final common pathway of different etiologic agents of irritation, infection, or infestation. In addition to identification of specific etiologic agents, a major goal of evaluation is to differentiate vulvovaginal or cervical processes from upper tract disease (e.g., pelvic inflammatory disease, or normal or abnormal pregnancy). The presence of systemic signs and symptoms and of abnormalities on bimanual pelvic examination suggests processes involving the uterus and adnexal and peritoneal structures. In contrast, isolated vulvovaginal disorders rarely are accompanied by such findings. In the majority of cases, careful history, inspection, "bench" lab tests (such as wet mount, KOH prep, and Gram stain), and selected cultures will provide a specific diagnosis on which to base treatment decisions. Some of the clinical and laboratory features of various etiologic agents of vaginal discharge are presented in Figure 16.21.

In the ensuing sections we will address noninfectious disorders first, followed by infections that are not sexually transmitted and then sexually transmitted diseases (STDs). The readers should bear in mind that the first two categories are seen primarily in prepubertal patients while the latter category applies to patients of any age. Emphasis will be given to how manifestations differ depending on age. The introductory section on infections due to sexually transmitted pathogens details the major differences in approach and procedure that are essential to appropriate evaluation of the prepubertal and pubertal patient, respectively.

Noninfectious Vulvovaginitis

Clinical findings of noninfectious vulvovaginitis vary considerably depending on cause. In some cases the vulva and vagina appear normal while in other cases varying degrees of inflammation or irritation are noted, at times accompanied by signs of excoriation. Vaginal discharge is unusual however, and vaginal cultures grow normal or nonspecific flora (Fig. 16.22). These disorders are quite common in prepubertal children but are relatively infrequent following menarche.

IRRITATION SECONDARY TO POOR HYGIENE
Poor perineal hygiene is one of the most common sources of local irritation. Symptoms consist primarily of perineal itching and dysuria. History often is suggestive in young patients, as the mother may report infrequent bathing and the finding of fecal material on the child's underwear. Examination typically reveals mild nonspecific vulvar irritation (Fig. 16.23). Bits of stool and toilet paper may be seen adhering to the perineum and perianal areas, and smegma may be found around the clitoris and labia (Fig. 16.24). Underwear is often grossly dirty. Coliforms tend to predominate on vaginal culture when lower vaginal inflammation is associated. The search for other sources is negative, and symptoms resolve with a regimen of sitz baths, and careful

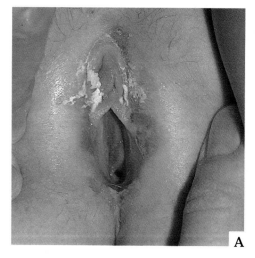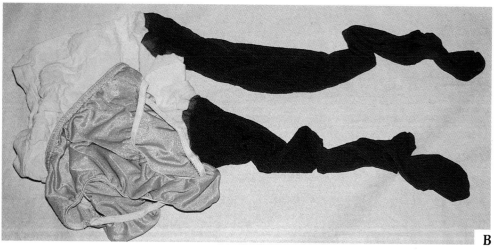

FIG. 16.25 *Maceration secondary to poor perineal aeration. This child's chief complaint was one of dysuria.* **A,** *On examination the inner surfaces of the labia were found to be macerated and mildly inflamed. Adherent smegma suggested poor perineal hygiene.* **B,** *When* her clothing was checked she was found to have been wearing nylon underpants with tights, which impeded aeration of her perineum. This condition has a significant risk of secondary infection.

cleansing after urination and defecation. Failure to improve should lead to suspicion of treatment noncompliance or of the possibility of sexual abuse.

MACERATION SECONDARY TO POOR PERINEAL AERATION

Obesity, with fat buttocks and thighs impeding aeration of the perineum, is a common predisposing factor to this form of vulvar irritation. Additional sources include wearing tights or panty hose over underwear, wearing panty hose under slacks, tight jeans, and sitting for prolonged periods in a wet bathing suit. In all these instances, moisture, whether from normal secretions, perspiration or swimming, is unable to evaporate, promoting maceration and inflammation of perineal tissues. Symptoms include perineal itching, discomfort, and dysuria. Nonspecific inflammation often with frank maceration will be the predominant finding (Fig. 16.25). Peripubertal and postmenarchial patients may have an associated increase in the volume of their physiologic leukorrhea. When maceration occurs, secondary infection is common. Some patients also have evidence of poor hygiene or of associated intertrigo. Attention to perineal hygiene, drying, alteration of predisposing habits, and treatment of secondary infection are the mainstays of management.

CONTACT DERMATITIS, ALLERGIC VULVITIS

Pruritus is the most prominent symptom of allergic vulvitis although scratching and excoriation may result in secondary burning and dysuria. When patients are seen in the acute phase, inspection of the labia and vestibule reveals a microvesicular papular eruption that tends to be intensely erythematous and somewhat edematous. Excoriated scratch marks are common, and place the patient at risk for secondary infection. When the process has become chronic, the vulvar skin has an eczematoid appearance being cracked, fissured, and lichenified. Topical ointments, creams and lotions, medicated or deodorant soaps and powders, bubble bath, laundry detergents and additives, and perfumed toilet paper are the most common sensitizing agents. In postpubertal patients vaginal deodorant sprays and douches also are possible causes. On occasion the vulvar eruption may be part of a generalized atopic dermatitis. The pattern of the rash, a history of pruritus as the initial symptom, and the presence of exposure to a likely sensitizer are the most helpful aids in diagnosis. However, excoriation and secondary infection can confuse the picture.

CHEMICAL IRRITANT VULVOVAGINITIS

Bubble bath, medicated and deodorant soaps, detergents, and additives also can provoke vulvitis by acting as chemical irritants. Affected patients tend to complain of mild perineal itching and dysuria. Examination usually discloses mild nonspecific inflammation (see Figure 16.23), at times associated with signs of scratching. On occasion findings are normal. Diagnosis is dependent on history and elimination of other causes.

FRICTIONAL TRAUMA

The wearing of pants that are too tight in the crotch, and intense rubbing or scratching—whether self-inflicted, incurred in the course of episodes of sexual abuse or as a result of consensual sexual activity in adolescents—may be the source of superficial abrasive changes. When chronic, the vulvar skin may become lichenified or even atrophic (Fig. 16.26). Although itching or mild discomfort are the major symptoms, dysuria may be prominent in acute cases.

SYMPATHETIC INFLAMMATION AND FISTULAS

Preschool and young school-age children with appendicitis commonly present for care following appendiceal rupture. Females having a pelvic appendix, who wall off the rupture in a periappendiceal abscess, may present with abdominal pain, anorexia, vomiting, fever, and a purulent vaginal discharge. In these cases the discharge usually is the result of sympathetic inflammation and is nonspecific microscopically, containing large numbers of leukocytes, epithelial cells, and mixed flora (Fig. 16.27). The antecedent clinical

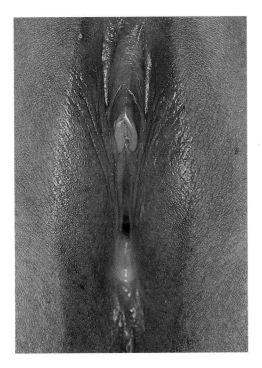

FIG. 16.26 Frictional trauma (nonspecific thickening of the vulvar skin). This patient's labial skin is thickened and mildly irritated. She had a history of recurrent vaginal foreign bodies and was strongly suspected to be a victim of chronic sexual abuse. (Courtesy of Dr. K. Sukarochana)

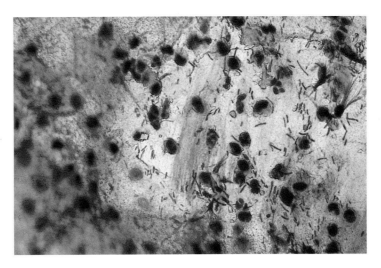

FIG. 16.27 Sympathetic purulent vaginal discharge. This photomicrograph shows numerous leukocytes and epithelial cells, with mixed flora. The patient presented with vomiting, anorexia, lower abdominal pain and a purulent vaginal discharge, and was found to have a pelvic appendiceal abscess. The vaginal discharge was the result of sympathetic inflammation.

course, consisting of anorexia and vomiting with mid-abdominal pain prior to developing lower abdominal discomfort, suggests the diagnosis. Tenderness on abdominal and rectal examination, while often bilateral, is usually more marked on the right. Finally, the fact that the unestrogenized genital tract of the prepubertal girl does not promote the ascent of venereal pathogens eliminates pelvic inflammatory disease from the differential diagnosis.

While adolescents with appendicitis usually present prior to perforation, those with pelvic appendiceal abscesses may be clinically indistinguishable from those with pelvic inflammatory disease. A history of vomiting, anorexia, and initial periumbilical pain which later localizes to the lower abdomen suggests appendicitis. In contrast, fever and pain beginning in the lower abdomen without gastrointestinal symptoms are more typical of pelvic inflammatory disease (see section on Pelvic Inflammatory Disease). However, in an occasional patient the history is not typical, and findings on examination may be consistent with either disorder. Furthermore, a nonspecific inflammatory vaginal discharge can be seen with either process. In such patients, careful observation, serial reexaminations, sonography, or even exploratory surgery may be necessary to make the diagnosis.

Vesicovaginal fistulas and *ectopic ureters* on occasion can present with symptoms of vulvovaginitis. These patients should have a history of a chronically wet perineum, however. Nonspecific inflammation and maceration are the predominant physical findings (see Figure 16.25A), and the child's underclothes should smell of urine. *Rectovaginal fistulas* also can result in vulvovaginal inflammation, but the presence of a feculent vaginal discharge usually makes diagnosis relatively easy. When rectovaginal fistulas are neither congenital nor post-traumatic in origin, patients should be investigated for inflammatory bowel disease.

VAGINAL FOREIGN BODY

The hallmark of a vaginal foreign body is the presence of a profuse brownish or blood-streaked foul-smelling vaginal discharge. The majority of patients are in the 3 to 8 year age group. While wads of toilet tissue, paper or cotton are the materials found most often, all types of small objects have been retrieved. The most common objects found in adolescents are forgotten tampons or retained condoms. The vulvar and vaginal mucosae are erythematous and may be macerated. Objects made of hard materials often are palpable on rectal examination. Since radiopaque objects generally are palpable, radiographs are unnecessary. Results of Gram stain, wet prep, and culture are nonspecific. Vaginoscopy is diagnostic and provides access for extraction, which is curative. Vaginal lavage with lukewarm saline also can help in removal of paper from young children. Shigella vaginitis in prepubertal patients, and necrotic tumors produce a discharge that is clinically indistinguishable from that of a vaginal foreign body.

When a prepubertal patient is found to have a vaginal foreign body it is important to obtain a detailed behavioral history of the child in addition to a family psychosocial history, as the problem often is recurrent and may be the result of disturbed behavior by the patient or of chronic sexual abuse.

PHYSIOLOGIC LEUKORRHEA

Physiologic leukorrhea, though manifest as a vaginal discharge, is in actuality a normal phenomenon and not a form of vulvovaginitis. It is produced in response to estrogen stimulation, and thus it is seen in the newborn period and recurs in the months preceding the onset of menses. The discharge is clear or milky, relatively thin, odorless, and nonirritating (Fig. 16.28A). When dried on diaper or underwear it may appear yellow or brown. The discharge consists of normal cervical and vaginal secretions along with desquamated vaginal epithelial cells. Perimenarchial patients often present with complaints of discharge because they and their mothers are not aware that the secretions are normal. These children are otherwise asymptomatic. Examination reveals good pubertal development and a normal perineum and distal vagina with the typical discharge. Diagnosis is confirmed by findings on wet prep and/or Gram

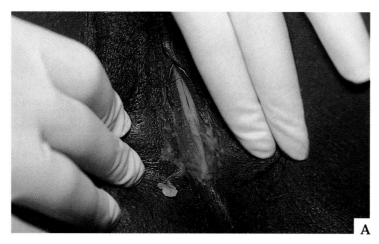

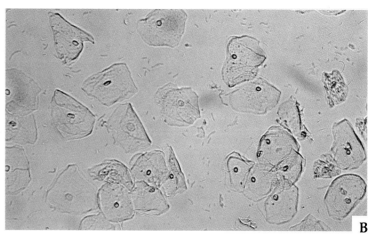

FIG. 16.28 Physiologic leukorrhea. **A**, The clinical appearance of this milky discharge is seen on the perineum of this normal adolescent. The discharge is produced in response to estrogen stimulation and is most evident in the newborn and peripubertal periods. **B**, On microscopy the discharge is found to contain sheets of estrogenized vaginal epithelial cells. There is no predominant flora and leukocytes are not increased.

CLINICAL SYNDROMES PRODUCED BY GENITAL INFECTIONS IN ADOLESCENTS

Pelvic Inflammatory Disease (Salpingitis) Present	Pelvic Inflammatory Disease Absent				
	No Symptoms	Vulvar Skin Lesions	Vulvitis	Vaginitis	Cervicitis
C. trachomatis	Chlamydia	Condyloma	Candida	(With or without	(Endocervical
N. gonorrhoeae	Gonorrhea	Herpes	Herpes	superficial	infection)
Mixed anaerobes	?Genital	Lice		cervicitis)	Chlamydia
and aerobes	mycoplasmas	Molluscum		Candida	Gonorrhea
?Genital		Scabies		Gardnerella	Herpes
mycoplasmas		Primary syphilis		Herpes	?Genital
				Trichomonas	mycoplasmas
				?Genital	
				mycoplasmas	

FIG. 16.29 Clinical syndromes produced by genital infections in adolescents.

stain, which disclose estrogenized epithelial cells with no increase in leukocytes (Fig. 16.28B). As a general rule, normally there should be approximately one polymorphonuclear leukocyte for every vaginal epithelial cell. Treatment consists of reassurance and education.

Infectious Vulvovaginitis

In contrast to most of the primarily noninfectious forms of vulvovaginitis, vaginal discharge is usually a prominent part of the clinical picture of infectious vulvovaginitis in all age groups. While some pathogens produce a fairly characteristic-looking discharge, not all patients present with this classic picture, and the discharge seen with many pathogens often is nonspecific in appearance. Furthermore, in the case of sexually transmitted infections, more than one pathogen

may be present. For these reasons, careful attention to smear and culture techniques is important.

There are two major subgroups of vulvovaginal infection. In the first subgroup genital involvement is secondary, being either a part of a systemic infection or the result of transfer of the pathogen from another primary site such as the skin, or respiratory, gastrointestinal, or urinary tracts via contaminated fingers or proximity. Infection at the primary site may precede or coexist with genital infection, and in some cases colonization of another site, without overt infection, appears to predispose. This nonvenereal infectious vulvovaginitis is not uncommon in prepubertal patients·although it is rare in adolescents because the mature female genital tract does not support these types of pathogens.

The second subgroup of infectious vulvovaginitis consists of those infections due to venereal pathogens. Both prepu-

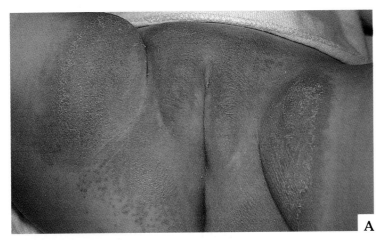

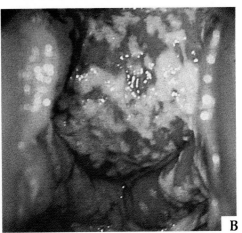

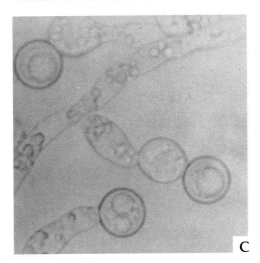

FIG. 16.30 Candida vulvovaginitis. **A,** An intensely hyperemic eruption is seen bordered by satellite lesions. In this picture the inflamed vulva is not exposed. **B,** Whitish plaques may be seen on the perineum and vaginal mucosa, and occasionally on the cervix in adolescents. A whitish cheesy or creamy vaginal discharge may be noted, as well. **C,** This wet mount specimen obtained from the perineal skin of a child without discharge contains mature yeast and pseudohyphae. (**A** courtesy of Dr. B. Cohen, **B** and **C** courtesy of Dr. E. Wald)

bertal and postmenarchial patients can present with vulvovaginitis when infected with these organisms. After puberty, however, patients can present with other clinical pictures as well, including cervicitis (with or without vulvovaginal inflammation) and salpingitis. Figure 16.29 enumerates the clinical syndromes produced by genital infections in adolescents. Regardless of age, the most frequent mode of transmission of venereal infection is sexual contact. The majority of these infections in prepubertal patients are the result of sexual abuse, although in some cases involving perimenarchial girls consensual activity is responsible. Also, in a minority of cases, transmission from a mother to her young child may be responsible. Such cases require overt infection in the mother in addition to poor hygienic practices. Hence, when venereal disease is found in the prepubertal child, the possibility of sexual abuse must

be investigated (see Chapter 6). In adolescence, consensual sexual activity is the major mode of acquisition of infection by sexually transmitted pathogens although sexual abuse remains a significant possibility. These factors necessitate obtaining a confidential history of sexual activity and case findings of sexual partners. *It also should be borne in mind that the presence of one venereal pathogen in any child or adolescent should prompt investigation for others, as multiple infections are common* (see section on Genital Infections Due to Sexually Transmitted Pathogens).

NONVENEREAL VULVOVAGINAL INFECTIONS
Candida Vulvovaginitis

Candida species are one of the more common sources of nonvenereal infectious vulvovaginitis both before and after menarche. Predisposing factors include recent antibiotic intake, seborrhea, diabetes mellitus, immunodeficiency and, in adolescents, pregnancy or use of oral contraceptives. Sites of primary involvement in young children are the mouth and gastrointestinal tract. Pruritus and dysuria are the most prominent symptoms. Examination usually discloses diffuse intense hyperemia of the vulva (Fig 16.30A). Excoriations from scratching also may be noted. Satellite lesions on the perineum are common, and on occasion whitish plaques may be seen on external genital structures. In many cases, signs of perianal dermatitis and intertrigo are found in association with vulvovaginal involvement. Inspection of the lower third of the vagina in young patients and speculum examination in adolescents may reveal a scant but thick white discharge of creamy or cheesy consistency; whitish plaques may adhere to the vaginal mucosa or to the cervix in adolescents (Figure 16.30B). KOH or wet prep will confirm the presence of budding yeast and pseudohyphae, and possibly an increase in inflammatory cells (Fig. 16.30C).

Regardless of age, topical application of antifungal cream with instillation into the lower vagina is the treatment of choice, combined with oral nystatin in prepubertal patients. In patients with recurrences, predisposing factors such as medications may have to be discontinued. An infected male partner with subacute or chronic monilial balanitis also may be the source of recurrence in sexually active patients, although this infection is not generally transmitted sexually.

Vulvovaginitis Due to Respiratory and/or Skin Pathogens

Bacterial respiratory pathogens on occasion have been found to be responsible for vulvovaginitis in prepubertal patients, presumably as a result of orodigital transmission. Both *Streptococcus pneumoniae* and *Haemophilus influenzae* have proven to be the source of purulent vaginal discharge, with associated vulvitis and vaginitis, either following or concurrent with upper respiratory tract infection. Vulvar burning and dysuria have been prominent symptoms. The most dramatic form of bacterial vulvovaginitis due to a primary respiratory (or skin) pathogen is that due to group A beta-hemolytic streptococcus. This infection may be associated with streptococcal nasopharyngitis or scarlet fever, or it may occur in apparent isolation. Nevertheless, throat cultures are positive for group A beta-hemolytic streptococcus in the majority of patients with streptococcal genital infection, even in the absence of respiratory or pharyngeal symptoms. The onset of vulvovaginal symptoms is abrupt with severe perineal burning and dysuria. Inspection reveals in-

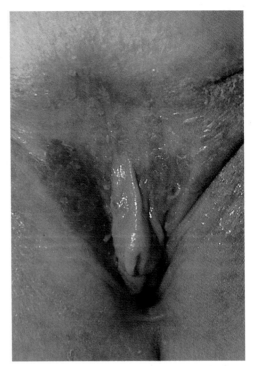

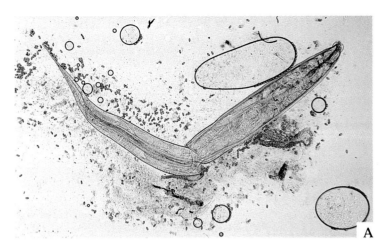

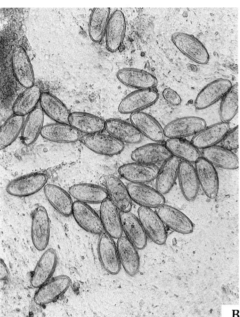

FIG. 16.31 Strepto-coccal vulvovaginitis. Severe acute perineal inflammation often with weeping charac-terizes this form of vulvovaginal infec-tion. Onset is abrupt, with intense burning vulvar pain and se-vere dysuria. Vaginal discharge when present tends to be se-rosanguineous. Gram stain may be unre-vealing,but cultures of involved skin, vag-inal discharge, and throat are positive for group A beta-hemo-lytic streptococci. (Courtesy of Dr. M. Sherlock)

FIG. 16.32 Pin-worms (Enterobius vermicularis). On this wet mount **(A)**, a mature worm is shown surrounded by eggs, which are shown more clearly at higher power **(B)**. Pa-tients with intestinal infestation may have vulvovaginal symp-toms, either as a result of scratching and excoriation or of migration of the worms into the va-gina.

tense erythema of the vulva and distal vagina (Figure 16.31). The involved skin weeps serous fluid. Most patients have a serosanguineous vaginal discharge, and about one-third will have vaginal petechiae. Gram stain may be unreveal-ing, but culture of perineal skin and/or discharge is positive. Desquamation ensues with recovery.

Impetigo and folliculitis may occur in the vulvar area of patients of any age and generally is secondary to poor hy-giene and/or mechanical irritation. Simultaneous involve-ment of the buttocks or other skin sites is common (see Chapter 12).

Viral pathogens also have been linked to vulvovaginitis in young children. Varicella is perhaps the most common, with pruritus and dysuria as its most prominent symptoms. In-spection reveals typical lesions involving the perineum and/or vagina (see Chapter 12). One report has described a patient with adenovirus and symptoms of fever, conjuncti-vitis, pharyngitis, exanthem, and vulvar erythema with a serous vaginal discharge. The virus grew on vaginal and stool cultures. Another patient with gastroenteritis, dehy-dration, and a "thick tenacious clear" vaginal discharge grew echovirus from vaginal and stool specimens.

Vulvovaginitis Due to Gastrointestinal Pathogens

In recent years a distinct form of vulvovaginitis due to shi-gella species has been identified in premenarchial patients. In the majority of cases no overt gastrointestinal symptoms precede, coincide with, or follow the onset of genital symp-toms although approximately one-third of cases have had associated diarrhea. It is thought that the neutral or alkaline pH of the vaginal mucosa in young children may predispose to infection with this organism. Adolescents and adult women prior to menopause do not appear to be susceptible. The predominant complaint is one of vaginal discharge that often is chronic. Most reported patients have been other-wise asymptomatic, although some have had complaints of dysuria. A greenish-brown, often blood-streaked, purulent and foul-smelling vaginal discharge is seen on inspection, along with vulvar and vaginal erythema. The clinical ap-

pearance of the discharge is indistinguishable from that seen with a vaginal foreign body or necrotic vaginal tumors. Gram stain reveals polymorphonuclear leukocytes and a predominance of gram-negative rods. Culture is diagnostic. Without treatment it may persist for months.

Intestinal infestation with pinworms (Enterobius vermicu-laris) is primarily associated with perianal pruritus. How-ever, the worms may crawl forward into the vagina bringing enteric flora with them and depositing eggs. Vaginal infec-tion and discharge may result. Even without this, scratch-ing may produce excoriation and secondary dysuria. In such patients (usually young children) a history of preced-ing perianal pruritus can generally be elicited. Inflammatory changes are nonspecific. Pinworm ova and/or adult worms may be found on wet mount of vaginal secretions (Fig. 16.32). In the occasional patient with associated vaginal dis-charge, culture is positive for enteric pathogens. When pin-worm infestation is suspected despite negative vaginal smears, the perianal scotch tape test should be performed by the mother during the night for the highest yield.

Vulvovaginitis Secondary to Urinary Tract Infection

On occasion a primary urinary tract infection may produce secondary vulvovaginal inflammation and masquerade as vulvovaginitis. The postulated mechanism is repeated vul-var and vaginal contamination with infected urine. Passage of part of the urinary stream into the vagina has been dem-

SEXUALLY TRANSMITTED PATHOGENS

Bacteria

*Calymmatobacterium
 granulomatis
 (granuloma
 inguinale)*
Campylobacter*
C. trachomatis
G. vaginalis
Group B streptococcus
Haemophilus ducreyi
 (chancroid)
M. hominis
N. gonorrhoeae
Neisseria meningitidis
Salmonella*
Shigella*
U. urealyticum

Fungi

Candida albicans

Viruses

AIDS virus
Cytomegalovirus
Epstein-Barr virus
Hepatitis A virus
Hepatitis B virus
Herpes simplex virus
Human papilloma
 virus (condylomata
 acuminata)
Pox virus (molluscum
 contagiosum)

Protozoa

*Entamoeba histolytica**
*Giardia lamblia**
T. vaginalis

Parasitic Insects

Pthirus pubis (lice)
Sarcoptes scabiei

Predominantly associated with enteritis in homosexual males.

FIG. 16.33 Sexually transmitted pathogens.

onstrated by voiding cystourethrography. Vulvar itching and burning along with dysuria are major complaints. When cystitis is the primary infection, frequency, urgency, and hesitancy typically are associated. Primary pyelonephritis is distinguished in part by the presence of fever, gastrointestinal symptoms, and costovertebral angle tenderness. Urine obtained by catheterization or suprapubic aspiration (obtaining a true clean catch urine generally is impossible when vulvar inflammation is present) will reveal white cells and bacteria. Perineal examination in these cases discloses nonspecific inflammation, and at times maceration, usually without discharge (see Figures 16.23 and 16.25A). Urine and vaginal cultures are positive for the same pathogen.

GENITAL INFECTIONS DUE TO SEXUALLY TRANSMITTED PATHOGENS

The number of pathogens known to be transmitted by intimate sexual contact has mushroomed in the past two decades (Fig. 16.33). The "sexual revolution" and the consequent rise in prevalence of venereal disease and neonatal infections have stimulated extensive research, leading to the recognition of an increasing array of pathogens and to a better understanding of their pathophysiology and the clinical pictures they produce. It also has made the evaluation of patients with STD considerably more complex. The majority of infections are manifested by external lesions and/or vulvovaginal inflammation with vaginal discharge. However, while some infections produce relatively specific clinical findings, many are characterized by nonspecific signs and symptoms that appear to represent a final common pathway of several different etiologic agents of irritation, infection, or infestation. A few pathogens can induce two or three different clinical pictures (or a mixed picture) in adolescents. Furthermore, the high frequency of multiple simultaneous infections adds to the complexity, and thereby necessitates more extensive laboratory evaluation. The clinical approach to these patients must not only be sensitive and individualized, but also must differ considerably depending on whether or not the patient is premenarchial or postmenarchial.

Approach to Sexually Transmitted Infections in Prepubertal Patients

Prior to menarche, lack of estrogenization inhibits ascent of infection and subclinical infection is probably unusual if not rare. Hence, manifestations of venereal infection are confined to the vulva and lower vagina. As a result, external inspection of the perineum and lower vagina and laboratory evaluation of a sample of vaginal discharge are sufficient for identification of pathogens and for institution of therapy. This does not complete the assessment, however, for whenever venereal disease is identified in a prepubertal patient, *sexual abuse must be considered as the probable source*. This necessitates obtaining an extensive psychosocial history and initiating a thorough investigation to find the person responsible for transmitting the infection to the child (see Chapter 6).

Approach to STD in Pubertal Patients

Vulvovaginitis continues to be a common mode of presentation of STD in adolescence. As is true of younger children, presenting complaints in pubertal patients include vulvar lesions, vaginal discharge, odor, pruritus or perineal discomfort, and dysuria; but these symptoms also may be associated with pelvic pain, dyspareunia, fever, and irregular bleeding. This is not the only clinical picture seen, however. A number of pathogens involve only the lower genital tract (e.g., they do not produce salpingitis), but, in contrast to the picture seen in younger patients, they may produce more extensive vaginal inflammation and may involve the cervix, as well. Herpes simplex, *Trichomonas vaginalis*, and the papilloma virus are prime examples. Infection with either *Neisseria gonorrhoeae* or *Chlamydia trachomatis* may be both asymptomatic and inapparent on examination, or may result in cervicitis, which usually is characterized by cervical inflammation and friability, with a mucopurulent discharge (see Figure 16.39B). Cervicitis, too, may be largely silent clinically, or it may be accompanied by vulvovaginitis with vaginal discharge, or, with ascent to the upper tract, may result in salpingitis.

Because of these differences in presentation, a complete pelvic examination is necessary when evaluating adolescents for vulvovaginal complaints and for the possibility of STD. Following inspection of the perineum, the vaginal mucosa and the cervix must be visualized and their appearance assessed for signs of erythema, friability, specific lesions, and mucopurulent discharge. To differentiate a true cervical discharge from normal pooled vaginal secretions adhering to the cervix, visible discharge should be removed gently with cotton swabs before inspection. If cervical secretions are then seen at the os, they should be sampled (for Gram stain and cultures) by insertion of a swab into the os.

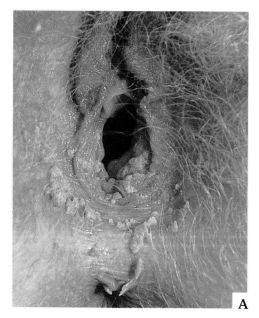

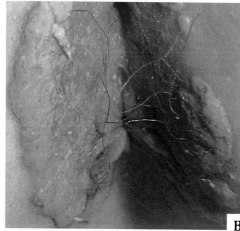

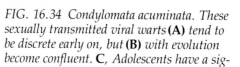

FIG. 16.34 Condylomata acuminata. These sexually transmitted viral warts **(A)** tend to be discrete early on, but **(B)** with evolution become confluent. **C**, Adolescents have a significant risk of developing vaginal and cervical lesions. (**A** and **C** courtesy of Dr. E. Jerome, **B** courtesy of Dr. M. Sherlock)

The finding of cervicitis with a mucopurulent cervical discharge suggests gonorrhea or chlamydial infection or both, and necessitates an attempt either to identify or to rule out upper tract involvement via bimanual examination. Tenderness or a palpable adnexal mass, when associated with systemic signs and symptoms, suggests this possibility (see section on Pelvic Inflammatory Disease).

A number of additional considerations are important in evaluating postpubertal patients suspected of having STD. A sexual history, obtained in confidence, is essential, and while consensual activity is common in adolescence, it must be remembered that these patients may be victims of sexual abuse. Sexual partners should be evaluated and treated whenever an STD is identified; otherwise reinfection is probable.

It also is highly important to recognize that adolescent girls with asymptomatic cervical infections may serve as silent reservoirs of venereal pathogens. This phenomenon is quite significant in the epidemiology of STD. Hence, female partners of men known to have gonorrhea or nongonococcal urethritis should be cultured and treated appropriately. The patient and partner must be counseled on abstaining from sexual activity until the course of treatment is completed. They also should be seen in follow-up for test of cure, and once cured should be seen at least every 6 months for STD surveillance because of the significant incidence of recurrent (and often subclinical) infection.

The importance of aggressive case finding, diagnosis, and treatment cannot be overemphasized because of the potential, not only for spread to others, but also for major sequelae that include ectopic pregnancy and infertility as a result of smouldering or recurrent acute upper tract disease. Finally, it is the physician's responsibility to provide education regarding STD. Patients should understand how the disease was contracted and how to prevent recurrence. Good hygiene and use of condoms should be encouraged. Education also may include discussion of responsible sexuality, including use of contraceptives, as appropriate to the patient.

Surface Infestations and Perineal Lesions
Parasitic infestations. Two parasitic infestations, *scabies* and *pubic lice*, may be transmitted via sexual contact and may present with symptoms of vulvar and inguinal pruritus and irritation. Sexual transmission is more likely in adolescents than in young children, who may acquire the parasites by close nonsexual contact. Development of pubic hair is necessary for acquisition of pubic lice. The clinical findings of both are presented in Chapter 8.

Condylomata acuminata. Venereal warts are caused by the human papilloma virus. Transmission is usually via sexual contact, especially in adolescents, although it is thought that close family contact may be responsible for some cases in young children. Passage to neonates during delivery also has been documented. The warts appear as fleshy rounded or ragged papules, often located at the posterior edge of the introitus and/or in the perianal region. Lesions may be discrete early on (Fig. 16.34A), but with evolution they tend to become confluent (Fig. 16.34B). In most cases, the lesions are asymptomatic although pruritus is reported by some patients. However, when the warts are traumatized or become secondarily infected, pain may be a complaint. Vaginal involvement is uncommon in the prepubertal child but, when present, it is accompanied by vaginal discharge. In rare cases, rapid growth is followed by necrosis, and the patient presents with a weeping mass of warts and foul-smelling discharge, which necessitates histologic examination to rule out malignancy. In adolescents, while most lesions involve the perineum, vaginal and cervical involvement are considerably more likely. Thus, when vulvar condylomata are found, inspection of the vagina and cervix should be undertaken (Fig. 16.34C) and a cervical Pap smear obtained. Patients with cervical lesions merit gynecologic referral for treatment and ongoing cytologic surveillance, because of the potential of these lesions to undergo malignant transformation.

Molluscum contagiosum. These sharply circumscribed, waxy papular umbilicated viral warts also may be spread as a result of sexual contact, in which case lesions will be found predominantly on the labia, mons pubis, buttocks, and lower abdomen. However, this mode of spread is much more likely in the adolescent than in the young child. The clinical characteristics of molluscum lesions are presented in Chapter 8.

Syphilitic chancre. Primary syphilis should be considered in any patient presenting with a genital ulcer. The typical

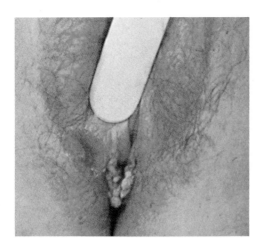

FIG. 16.35 Primary syphilis. This luetic chancre was painless and indurated on palpation. The base is smooth and the margins are rolled. This patient also has condylomata acuminata. (Courtesy of Dr. E. Wald)

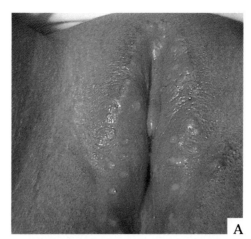

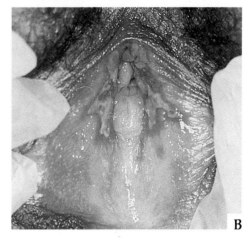

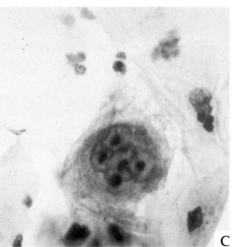

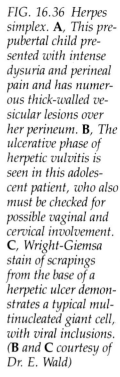

FIG. 16.36 Herpes simplex. **A**, This prepubertal child presented with intense dysuria and perineal pain and has numerous thick-walled vesicular lesions over her perineum. **B**, The ulcerative phase of herpetic vulvitis is seen in this adolescent patient, who also must be checked for possible vaginal and cervical involvement. **C**, Wright-Giemsa stain of scrapings from the base of a herpetic ulcer demonstrates a typical multinucleated giant cell, with viral inclusions. (**B** and **C** courtesy of Dr. E. Wald)

syphilitic chancre is painless and indurated, with rolled margins and a smooth base (Fig. 16.35). However, atypical lesions are common and thus all suspicious ulcers should prompt investigation either by darkfield examination of scrapings and/or by reagin serologic tests (VDRL or RPR). The latter test may be negative early in the disease course and therefore should be repeated at 1- and 3-month intervals if syphilis is strongly suspected. Positive reagin tests should always be confirmed by a fluorescent treponemal antibody (FTA) test.

Bartholin's gland abscess. This problem presents as a unilateral red hot tender mass at the posterior margin of the introitus (see Figure 16.39A). Classically it is seen in adolescents with gonorrhea but it also can occur in younger patients infected with the gonococcus. When such a mass is encountered, material should be expressed from the abscess, because, while it is usually due to gonococcal infection, other agents such as streptococci, chlamydia, and vaginal anaerobes also have been documented as pathogens. Treatment is based on Gram stain and culture results. Occasionally, incision and drainage are required.

Lower Tract Disease

A number of sexually transmitted infections that are manifest as vulvovaginitis in the prepubertal patient produce findings limited to the lower genital tract (e.g., vaginitis and superficial cervicitis) in the adolescent. A discussion of these types of infections follows. Three other venereal pathogens—*N. gonorrhoeae*, chlamydia, and mycoplasma—in addition to producing vulvovaginal findings in both prepubertal and adolescent patients, also can produce upper tract disease in the postpubertal patient. Their upper tract manifestations will be discussed later in the section on Pelvic Inflammatory Disease.

Genital herpes. Herpes simplex type 2 and, more rarely, type 1 have been confirmed as venereal pathogens in both pubertal and prepubertal girls. Genital infection is acquired almost exclusively by sexual or intimate contact with infected mucosal surfaces. Patients with primary infection frequently have systemic symptoms of fever, malaise and myalgia, in addition to severe perineal pain and dysuria. On examination tender inguinal adenopathy is prominent, and perineal inspection reveals single or clustered vesicular lesions and/or ulcers on an erythematous and edematous base (Fig. 16.36A and B). Acute ulcerations are typically covered by yellow exudate. Associated sterile pyuria may be a feature. Dysuria may be so severe as to cause acute urinary retention. The ulcerative phase gradually resolves as

the lesions scab over and heal within a period of 14 to 28 days. Recurrences are common and generally are milder, of shorter duration, and only locally symptomatic. Possible triggers include fever, menstruation, emotional stress, and friction. Occasionally prodromal tingling or burning is noticed in the area where vesicles ultimately recur. The interval between episodes varies widely. Diagnosis can usually be made on the basis of clinical appearance but it is confirmed by finding multinucleated giant cells on cytologic smears (Fig. 16.36C). The specimen is obtained by scraping the base of a lesion, smearing the specimen on a glass slide, and staining it with Wright-Giemsa stain. Viral culture of a fresh—ideally, vesicular—lesion also is confirmatory.

Postmenarchial patients with vulvar herpetic lesions require speculum examination to look for the presence of herpes cervicitis, which is characterized by ulceration, friability,

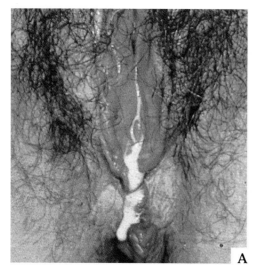 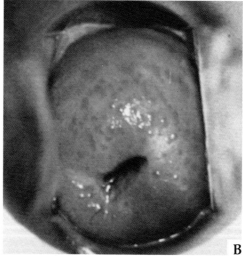 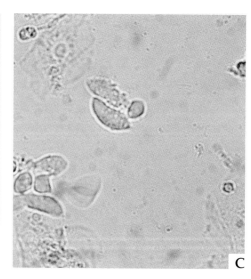

FIG. 16.37 *Trichomonas.* **A**, *T.* vaginalis *produces a profuse acrid-smelling watery discharge that usually is visible on perineal inspection. In some cases it is homogeneous, while in others it is bubbly. Vulvar pruritus often is intense.* **B**, *The vaginal mucosa is inflamed and often speckled with petechial lesions. In adolescents petechial hemor-* *rhages may also be found on the cervix, resulting in the so-called "strawberry cervix."* **C**, *Microscopic examination of a wet mount reveals multiple motile trichomonads. A sperm is seen in the upper portion of the picture.* (**A** and **B** *courtesy of Dr. E. Wald*)

and a serosanguineous discharge. Occasionally, herpetic ulcers are found on the vaginal mucosa as well. Patients with cervical involvement should be referred for gynecologic follow-up and periodic Pap smears because of the possible association between herpetic infection and the ultimate development of cervical carcinoma. Additionally, because of the risk of transmitting the virus to the newborn during vaginal delivery, pregnant girls with a history of genital herpes should have serial cultures during the last trimester. If evidence of active infection is present, elective cesarean section is recommended.

Trichomonas. *T. vaginalis* has been found in the vaginal discharge of newborns delivered of mothers infected at the time of delivery, but thereafter it tends to be an unusual finding until the peripubertal period. This is thought to be due to the unfavorable alkaline environment of the unestrogenized vaginal mucosa. Beyond the neonatal period it is acquired almost exclusively by sexual contact, often in concert with other STD pathogens. Although infection is occasionally asymptomatic in adolescents, the majority of patients, whether premenarchial or postmenarchial, have vulvar pruritus, burning and dysuria, in association with a profuse vaginal discharge. The latter may be watery, yellow-gray, or green. In some cases it is bubbly; in others it is homogeneous. Frequently the discharge has a foul acrid odor. Affected adolescents may complain of pelvic pain or heaviness.

On inspection the vulva may be hyperemic and occasionally edematous, but the degree of inflammation is highly variable. Because the discharge is profuse, it tends to be present on the perineum (Fig. 16.37A). It pools in dependent portions of the vagina and coats the vaginal walls. The vaginal mucosa is erythematous, and punctate petechial lesions may be noted. In the adolescent these hemorrhagic areas may involve the cervical mucosa, producing the so-called "strawberry cervix" (Fig. 16.37B). Ascent beyond the cervix does not occur. Diagnosis is made by finding mobile trichomonads on microscopic examination of a saline wet mount (Fig. 16.37C). On close observation, whiplike flagel-

lar movements are noted. Leukocytes are usually seen in increased numbers and may surround the organisms, making detection more difficult. The slide must be examined soon after preparation, as drying makes it uninterpretable.

Metronidazole has been shown to be effective for treatment but should be avoided in pregnant patients because of its potential for teratogenicity. Sexual partners usually are asymptomatic but occasionally have symptoms of urethritis. Treatment of the male is essential to prevent reinfection in the female.

Gardnerella vaginalis. While also found in asymptomatic children and adolescents, recent studies have confirmed *Gardnerella vaginalis* as a pathogen and as a significant source of vulvovaginitis both before and after menarche. It is now thought that the organism acts in concert with vaginal anaerobes to produce the clinical syndrome, and that many cases of vaginitis with discharge previously thought to be nonspecific were in reality caused by gardnerella. The major presenting symptom in all groups is one of vaginal discharge with a noticeable odor. Some prepubertal patients have vulvar inflammation and discomfort, but most adolescents have little in the way of vulvovaginal irritation and the cervix and upper tract are spared. On inspection, discharge is frequently present on the perineum (Fig. 16.38A) and may be seen adhering to the vaginal walls, which do not appear to be inflamed. Generally it is thin and homogeneous in consistency, grayish-white, and malodorous. In adolescents, vaginal pH is elevated to 4.5 or above. Addition of 10-percent KOH to a sample of the discharge produces a noticeable amine odor (positive "whiff test"). Saline wet prep usually reveals characteristic "clue cells," vaginal epithelial cells covered with adherent refractile bacteria (Fig. 16.38B). On Gram stain the cells appear studded with gram-negative or gram-variable rods. When clue cells are present, culture is unnecessary. If clue cells are absent but clinical suspicion of gardnerella is high, a culture is recommended. Because *G. vaginalis* is a surface pathogen and thus is rarely associated with evidence of tissue invasion, leukocytes should not be seen in increased numbers. If they are, additional pathogens should be sought.

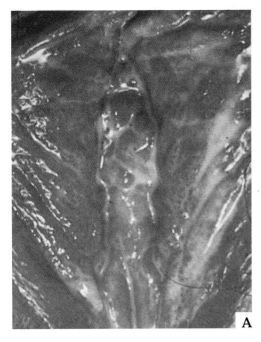

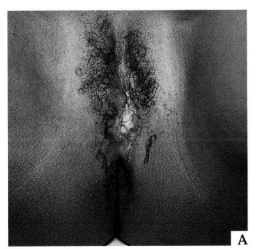

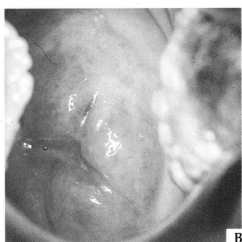

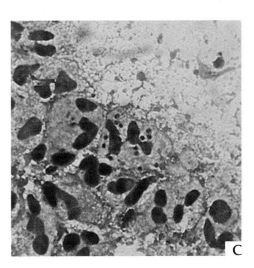

FIG. 16.39 Gonorrhea. **A**, Vulvar inflammation, edema, and a purulent vaginal discharge are seen in this peripubertal child who was a victim of sexual abuse. She also has a unilateral Bartholin's gland abscess. **B**, Adolescents are vulnerable to ascent of infection and usually have findings of cervical inflammation with mucopurulent discharge.

C, On Gram stain the vaginal discharge from the patient in **A** is found to contain sheets of leukocytes, many of which contain gram-negative intracellular diplococci. This test is highly reliable for prepubertal patients but adolescents have a significant incidence of false negatives. (**B** courtesy of Dr. L. Vontver)

In cases of recurrent infection, patients as well as their sexual partners should receive treatment.

Gonorrhea. The gonococcus is currently the most frequently identified venereal pathogen in both prepubertal and postmenarchial patients. The major complaint is one of vaginal discharge. Prior to menarche the child may be otherwise asymptomatic, but most experience some degree of vulvar discomfort, pruritus, or dysuria. Symptomatic adolescents without upper tract extension can have a similar picture, but are more likely to have lower abdominal pain—a phenomenon seen only occasionally in younger patients. Inspection reveals inflammation and sometimes edema of the vulva and a profuse purulent discharge that usually is greenish yellow but also can be creamy, yellow, green, or white (Fig. 16.39A). In about 10 percent of cases, it is malodorous. On inspection of the vaginal mucosa in younger children, the lower portion is found to be inflamed. In adolescents, the vaginal mucosa can appear normal but the cervix usually is found to be erythematous and friable, with purulent material seen draining through the os (Fig. 16.39B). Older patients also may have

evidence of urethritis manifested by erythema, edema, and tenderness of the urethra. When the latter findings are present, purulent material can be expressed by pressing along the length of the urethra through the anterior vaginal wall. A sample of this material should be sent for culture.

Laboratory studies are essential for accurate diagnosis. In prepubertal patients a Gram-stained smear of aspirated vaginal discharge will be reliably positive for large numbers of leukocytes and gram-negative intracellular diplococci and is adequate for initiation of treatment (Fig. 16.39C). Culture is important to detect the few cases with false negative Gram stain, to determine antimicrobial sensitivity, and for medicolegal confirmation. Since simultaneous throat and anal cultures commonly are positive (despite the absence of anorectal or pharyngeal symptoms), these sites should also be cultured when gonorrhea is suspected. They may, in fact, be positive when vaginal culture is negative. Both tonsils and the posterior pharyngeal wall should be swabbed in obtaining the throat specimen, and the rectal swab should be inserted no more than 1 to 2 cm past the anal orifice to avoid fecal con-

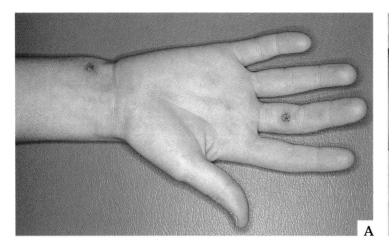
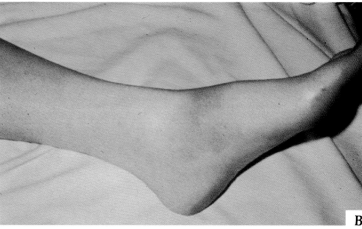

A

B

FIG. 16.40 Disseminated gonococcal infection. **A**, These pustular skin lesions with erythematous halos are characteristic of disseminated gonorrhea, which may occur at any age. **B**, Tenosynovitis and mono-articular arthritis are commonly seen in association with skin lesions in disseminated disease. (**A** courtesy of Dr. E. Wald)

tamination. Culture swabs should be placed immediately on Aime's transport medium and plated promptly on Thayer-Martin culture plates to maximize the chance for positive results.

In adolescents with symptomatic gonorrhea, Gram stain of the mucopurulent cervical discharge will reveal a predominance of leukocytes that may contain gram-negative intracellular diplococci. When results are positive, this is quite specific and treatment may be instituted. However, the incidence of false negative Gram stains is significant. Cultures are thus even more important in this age group and are processed in the same manner as described above. It also must be borne in mind that purulent cervicitis may be due to chlamydia or even to both organisms. Recent studies of women with culture-proven gonococcal cervicitis have shown concurrent chlamydial infection in up to two-thirds of these patients. Thus, when purulent cervicitis is found clinically (whether the Gram stain is positive or negative), consideration should be given either to obtaining specific cultures for chlamydia or to covering for this organism when instituting treatment, even when gonorrhea is diagnosed.

On occasion, patients with gonorrhea may develop *disseminated gonococcal infection* via hematogenous spread. Although this phenomenon may occur at any age, it appears more commonly in patients with asymptomatic (and therefore, untreated) endocervical, urethral (males), anal or pharyngeal infections, but also can be seen in patients with symptomatic vulvovaginitis or cervicitis. Following menarche females are more likely to develop symptoms during a menstrual period or during pregnancy. The clinical picture often is biphasic. Initially fever and chills are prominent, and the patient is intermittently bacteremic. During this stage, which lasts 2 to 5 days, polyarthralgias are experienced (involving knees, wrists, ankles, elbows, and hands) and characteristic skin lesions often appear. These begin as small erythematous papules or petechiae that usually evolve to form pustules surrounded by red halos (Fig. 16.40A). Later, these may necrose centrally. Lesions are often Gram stain positive, but usually are culture negative. If not diagnosed and treated promptly, patients progress to a second phase, characterized by monoarticular arthritis with effusion, or tenosynovitis (Fig.

16.40B). In up to 50 percent of these cases, culture of joint aspirate will be positive. Specialized techniques to isolate cell-wall-deficient organisms further increase culture yield. Myocarditis, pericarditis, endocarditis, and meningitis also may yield from hematogenous seeding.

Chlamydia trachomatis. Chlamydia is fast replacing the gonococcus as the most commonly identified sexually transmitted pathogen and is likely to surpass it as techniques of identification become more readily available and less expensive. Vaginal discharge specimens of prepubertal females with purulent vulvovaginitis have been found to be culture positive for chlamydia, both concurrently with and subsequent to documented gonococcal infection. In some of these cases, vaginal discharge has persisted following successful treatment for gonorrhea. In other cases, symptoms resolved but patients remained culture positive for chlamydia. Simultaneous rectal cultures also have been positive. The persistent discharge may be intermittent and has been described as thin or serous, and white or yellowish-brown. Pruritus appears to be the predominant symptom. The organism also has been linked to sexual abuse. Because of the expense, it probably is not justifiable to obtain chlamydial cultures from all prepubertal patients with vaginal discharge, but they should be considered when other venereal pathogens have been identified and discharge persists after eradication of the initially identified pathogen.

In adolescence, infection with chlamydia, while usually asymptomatic, can produce a picture that is indistinguishable from that of symptomatic gonorrhea, with purulent vaginal discharge, perineal irritation, and findings of cervicitis with mucopurulent discharge (see Fig. 16.39B). When seen as an isolated infection, the cervical discharge is found on Gram stain to contain increased numbers of leukocytes without intracellular organisms. However, patients commonly are simultaneously infected with the gonococcus and chlamydia—hence the rationale for either culturing for both organisms or covering for both with treatment, when purulent cervicitis is found on examination. Chlamydia also can produce the acute urethral syndrome in postpubertal patients. This is characterized by dysuria, urgency, frequency, and sterile pyuria.

A sample of aspirated vaginal discharge is sufficient for culture in prepubertal patients but in adolescents an endocervical swab specimen is necessary. Calginite or Dacron swabs are used for specimen collection and should be placed immediately in 2-SP transport medium and promptly inoculated. Giemsa-stained smears have not been helpful, and the sensitivity and specificity of the immunofluorescent test have not been determined as yet for premenarchial girls. Treatment is necessary to eradicate infection and the asymptomatic carrier state.

Mycoplasma hominis and *Ureaplasma urealyticum*. Although reported as growing on vaginal culture from asymptomatic prepubertal children, these two organisms have been isolated from a patient with chronic symptoms of dysuria, frequency, enuresis and intermittent incontinence, in association with signs of severe vulvar and vaginal inflammation and vaginal discharge. Symptoms had persisted for approximately 1 year despite treatment with multiple antibiotics. Cultures for other pathogens were negative, and treatment with tetracycline was curative. The child was found to have been sexually molested shortly before the onset of symptoms, implicating venereal transmission. While routine cultures for these organisms probably are not justified, they should be considered in evaluating prepubertal patients with venereal vulvovaginitis unresponsive to prior treatment, and in patients with persistent discharge that is found negative for pathogens on standard cultures.

M. hominis has been isolated from postpubertal patients with vaginitis and/or cervicitis in the absence of other organisms. Treatment with tetracycline has resulted in clinical improvement, suggesting but not as yet confirming its role as a pathogen. It also has been associated with the acute urethral syndrome.

Pelvic Inflammatory Disease

An important complication of lower genital tract infection in the postmenarchial female is pelvic inflammatory disease (PID). PID, or salpingitis, usually results from ascending spread of a cervical infection that may or may not have been symptomatic. Though classically attributed to gonorrhea, PID is being increasingly recognized as a polymicrobial infection. Pathogens implicated include *N. gonorrhoeae*, *C. trachomatis*, *M. hominis* and a host of other organisms, which are considered normal vaginal flora but are potentially pathogenic given the right circumstances. Among these are bacteroides species, other anaerobic gram-positive bacilli and cocci, and aerobes including streptococcal species, *E. coli*, klebsiella, and proteus species. In fact, the majority of cases of salpingitis may be due to mixed anaerobic and aerobic infection, rather than to the classically recognized venereal pathogens. Risk factors for developing upper tract infection include being an adolescent, having multiple sexual partners, use of an IUD, and previous PID. Long-term morbidity is significant and includes ectopic pregnancy, infertility and chronic pelvic pain, sequelae that are secondary to tubal occlusion and scarring of pelvic structures. It is estimated that for every episode of PID there is a 15-percent chance of subsequent infertility.

Diagnosis is complicated by the fact that there is a wide range in severity of the clinical picture, that acute salpingitis may mimic a number of other disorders (ectopic or intrauterine pregnancy, appendiceal abscess, torsion or hemorrhage of an ovarian cyst, septic abortion, endometriosis, pyelonephritis, cholecystitis, and pelvic tumors), and that in many instances upper tract infection is totally subclinical.

The classic picture of acute PID is that of a sexually active female who abruptly develops a high fever, often with a shaking chill, in association with intense lower abdominal pain. Nausea and vomiting may be reported, occasionally. Walking is often painful, resulting in a stooped shuffling gait. Because menstruation facilitates ascent of pathogenic organisms from the cervix, the time of onset usually is during the course of or shortly after a menstrual period. The patient appears acutely ill and uncomfortable. On abdominal examination there is prominent lower abdominal tenderness and guarding, often with rebound. Cervical visualization may disclose signs of cervicitis with mucopurulent discharge. Bimanual palpation elicits extreme pain on cervical motion and reveals marked tenderness of the fundus and adnexa. Adnexal enlargement, if present, suggests abscess formation. The sedimentation rate usually is markedly elevated, and there is generally a marked leukocytosis with a left shift on CBC and differential. This picture is seen most often as the first episode of PID and has the highest likelihood of being associated with positive cultures for *N. gonorrhoeae*. Even with this "textbook" picture (which constitutes a relatively small percentage of cases), errors in diagnosis are not uncommon and gynecologic consultation should be strongly considered when PID is suspected. Additional procedures such as culdocentesis or laparoscopy may be helpful, along with serial reexamination in questionable cases. Sonography also is of use in evaluating masses.

More commonly, the onset of symptoms is insidious and the clinical picture is more subtle. This is particularly likely with nongonococcal PID. Fever may be absent or low grade, the abdomen and pelvis may be only mildly tender, and peripheral blood work may be normal. In such cases diagnosis can be particularly difficult and requires a high index of suspicion and a low threshold for obtaining cultures on the part of the clinician.

Because of the potentially devastating sequelae, aggressive and largely empiric antibiotic treatment is warranted. Treatment should include antibiotics to cover the common organisms per current CDC recommendations. Increasingly, polymicrobial coverage is being considered from the outset, and is advisable when dramatic improvement is not seen following 2 days of first-line therapy. Patients who are suspected of having an abscess, patients in whom the diagnosis isn't clear (e.g., PID vs. ectopic vs. appendicitis), and patients who are toxic-appearing, pregnant, or unable to comply with outpatient treatment should be admitted for intravenous treatment, appropriate consultation, and observation. If treated as an outpatient, it is mandatory that the patient with PID be reexamined within 48 hours to document improvement. If no such improvement occurs, the patient should be admitted and treated parenterally. In addition to antibiotic resistance, failure to improve promptly on therapy raises the possibility of complications such as abscess formation and pelvic thrombophlebitis, or of a missed diagnosis.

Perihepatitis (Fitz-Hugh-Curtis syndrome). One of the complications of salpingitis or PID presents as a clinically distinct entity, that of perihepatitis. The infection appears to ascend from the fallopian tubes along the paracolic gutters to the right upper quadrant, resulting in inflammation of Glisson's capsule and of the adjacent peritoneum. The clinical picture is one of sudden onset of intensely sharp right upper quadrant pain in association with chills and fever. The pain often has a pleuritic component and may be referred to the right shoulder. Vomiting and headache may be additional complaints. Right upper quadrant tenderness and guarding are the major physical findings, although in some cases a friction rub is heard over the liver. Gynecologic examination in most instances will disclose findings of purulent endocervicitis and salpingitis. Laparoscopy of the right upper quadrant reveals a gray fibrinous exudate overlying the capsular surface. *N. gonorrhoeae* and *C. trachomatis* are the major pathogens associated with this syndrome. When nongonococcal in origin, the predisposing salpingitis may be silent.

BIBLIOGRAPHY

Altchek A: Vulvovaginitis, vulvar skin disease and pelvic inflammatory disease. Pediatr Clin North Am 28:397–432, 1981.

Amsel R et al: Nonspecific vaginitis. Am J Med 74:14–22, 1983.

Anonymous: Treatment of sexually transmitted disease. The Medical Letter 26(653):5–8, 1984.

Corey L: Diagnosis and treatment of genital herpes. JAMA 248:1041–1049, 1982.

Cowell CA: The gynecologic examination of infants, children, and young adolescents. Pediatr Clin North Am 28:247–266, 1981.

Dewhurst J: Genital tract obstruction. Pediatr Clin North Am 28:331–344, 1981.

Emans SJ, Goldstein DP: Pediatric and Adolescent Gynecology. Little, Brown, Boston, 1982.

Eschenback DA: Vaginal infection. Clin Obstet Gynecol 26:186–202, 1983.

Heller RH, Joseph JM, Davis HJ: Vulvovaginitis in the premenarcheal child. J Pediatr 74:370–377, 1969.

Holmes KK, Stamm WE: Chlamydial genital infections: A growing problem. Hosp Pract 105–117, October 1979.

Huffman JW: The Gynecology of Childhood and Adolescence, 2nd ed. Saunders, Philadelphia, 1981.

Paradise JE, Campos JM, Friedman HM, Frishmuth G: Vulvovaginitis in premenarchial girls: Clinical features and diagnostic evaluation. Pediatrics 70:193–198, 1982.

Pheifer TA, Forsyth PS, Durfee MA et al: Nonspecific vaginitis role of H. vaginalis and treatment with Metronidazole. N Engl J Med 298:1429–1434, 1978.

Shafer MA, Irwin CE, Sweet RL: Acute salpingitis in the adolescent female. J Pediatr 100:339–350, 1982.

Stamm WE, Guinan ME, Johnson C et al: Effect of treatment regimens for *Neisseria gonorrheae* on simultaneous infection with *Chlamydia trachomatis*. N Engl J Med 310:545–549, 1984.

US Dept. Health and Human Services: STD-treatment guidelines. MMWR Supplement 34(4S):75S–108S, 1985.

Woodlong BA, Kossosis PD: Sexual misuse: Rape, molestation and incest. Pediatr Clin North Am 28:481–499, 1981.

PEDIATRIC OPHTHALMOLOGY

David A. Hiles, M.D.

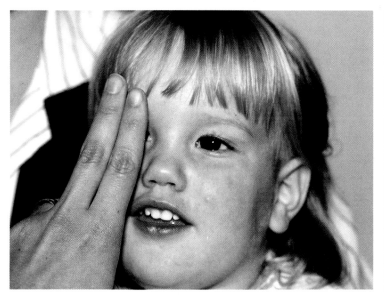 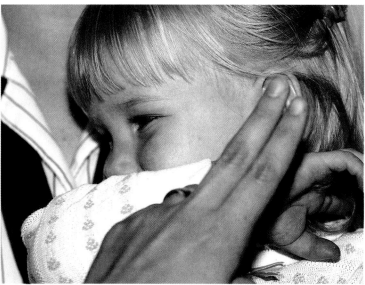

FIG. 17.1 Test for central fixation. (Left) Alert infant seated on mother's lap with one eye covered. Infant is content to fix and follow with normal eye. (Right) Cover (in this case, fingers) is then transferred to normal eye, occluding that eye. The infant now becomes disturbed, pushes hand away, and moves head to see.

Pediatric ophthalmology has evolved in recent years as a distinct subspecialty of ophthalmology, due for the most part to advances in diagnostic and surgical techniques. Consequently, there are today numerous ophthalmic physicians who are solely dedicated to child care.

Pediatric ophthalmology encompasses the evaluation of vision and therapy for refractive errors; the oculomotor system and strabismus; ocular and systemic diseases; developmental, genetic, and chromosomal disorders of the eyes; and diseases of the orbits and soft-tissue adnexa of infants and children.

EVALUATION OF VISION

The primary ocular function—vision—must be evaluated before other examinations or therapy can be instituted.

The fixation or visual reflex focuses the object onto the fovea centralis. If the fovea can steadily fixate a small target, and the eye can follow that target into all fields of gaze, a high level of vision (central fixation) is presumed. A test for central fixation is conducted by alternately covering each eye and allowing the free eye to fixate on a small object (Fig. 17.1). Normal infants fix and follow small objects by 5 to 6 months of age. More sophisticated vision tests for infants include preferential viewing, optokinetic nystagmus, and visual evoked responses (VERs). Neurologically normal infants achieve VER wave forms by 6 months of age, this being equivalent to 20/20 vision in adults. Preschool children respond to symbol matching, e.g., the Sheridan-Gardiner test, while school-aged children are able to identify illiterate "E"s, numbers, or Snellen letters. Normal visual acuity is 20/40 for a 3 year old, 20/30 for a 4 to 6 year old, and children over 8 years of age should achieve 20/20 corrected vision.

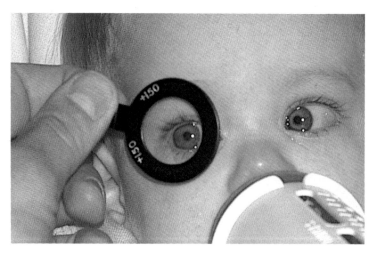

FIG. 17.2 *The examiner is viewing light emanating from the retina through the retinoscope. A lens is held in front of the patient's eye to neutralize refractive errors.*

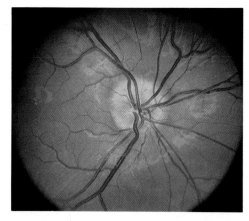

FIG. 17.3 *Funduscopic view of a pseudopapilledema in a hypermetropic child. Vessels are normal-sized; hemorrhages, exudates, and edema are absent.*

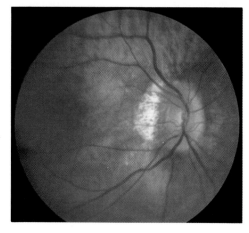

FIG. 17.4 *Funduscopic view of a myopic eye. Thinning of retinal pigment epithelium, a tessellated fundus appearance, macular cracks in Bruch's membrane (Fuch's spot), temporal crescents, and posterior staphyloma are evident.*

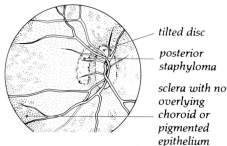

tilted disc

posterior staphyloma

sclera with no overlying choroid or pigmented epithelium

REFRACTIVE ERRORS

Abnormal vision may result from refractive errors by the cornea, lens, or from variations in the axial length of the globe. Having children view a vision chart through a pinhole is a useful test for diagnosing refractive errors. The pinhole reduces the rays of light presented to the retina, thus enhancing vision during the test. Those patients who do not indicate improved vision may have vision-reducing disorders.

Refractive errors are also determined by instilling cycloplegic-mydriatic drugs into the eyes to dilate the pupils and paralyze accommodation. The retinoscope projects a beam of light into the eye, illuminating the retina. The retina now serves as a light source and reflects light back through the pupil. The reflected light is observed through the retinoscope, and its quality is modified by the patient's refractive error. Appropriate lenses are placed before the eye to objectively neutralize these errors (Fig. 17.2).

Most children have slight hypermetropia (farsightedness), up to 1.5 diopters, which is corrected by the focusing mechanism (accommodation) of the crystalline lens. As the eye grows, hypermetropia decreases and emmetropia (no refractive error) results. If excessive growth occurs, myopia (nearsightedness) results. Hypermetropia need not be treated if the child is asymptomatic and has otherwise normal vision.

The symptoms of hypermetropia include fatigue, headaches, tired eyes, dislike of close work, and stumbling or falling in the younger child. Hypermetropia greater than 2 diopters may induce bilateral amblyopia or ametropia. Prescription glasses reduce the child's focusing need, reduce symptoms, and return vision to normal. However, if patients with very high degrees of bilateral hypermetropia are not treated by ages 6 to 8, amblyopia becomes irreversible and vision may never be returned to normal.

Hypermetropia occurs in eyes which are smaller than normal. Pseudopapilledema can also occur when nerve fibers are compressed as they pass through the small scleral canal (Fig. 17.3)

Myopia may be present in congenital or acquired forms. Congenital myopia may be unilateral or bilateral, and ranges from 8 to 25 diopters. The condition is accompanied by an increase in the axial length of the eye, producing significant retinal changes including peripapillary crescents and staphyl-

omas, decreased macular reflexes or degeneration, excavation of the optic nerve, and diminished vision (Fig. 17.4). The optic disc may appear to enter the eye at an angle.

Acquired myopia is frequently hereditary and becomes apparent following the normal reduction of hypermetropia in the preschool to teenage years. This myopic condition increases until the child is fully grown. The symptom is decreased vision at distance.

Astigmatism is an inability of the eye to focus incoming rays of light in all meridians. Symptoms are red eyes, recurring infections, headaches, dizziness, and nausea; vision may be adversely affected. Astigmatism changes during the growth of the child: it may increase or decrease, as may its meridional axis.

Anisometropia exists when each eye has different refractive errors. Usually the eye with the lesser refractive error becomes the dominant eye while the eye with the greater refractive error develops amblyopia. Anisometropia may be due to differences in farsightedness, nearsightedness, astigmatism, aphakia (absence of the lens), or combinations of these defects.

Aphakia, the unilateral or bilateral absence of the crystalline lens, is most often iatrogenic. Aphakia in children may induce amblyopia if proper postoperative optical correction does not provide clear form vision to each eye.

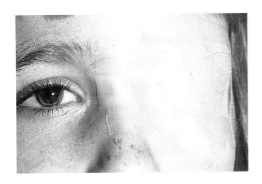 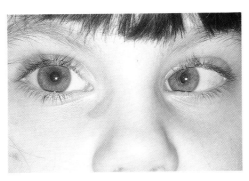 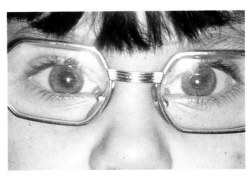

FIG. 17.5 Occlusion of the dominant eye helps to improve vision in the amblyopic eye.

FIG. 17.6 The child at left has esotropia with a high degree of hypermetropia. At right we see that corrective glasses have reduced the hypermetropia, and her esotropic eye has returned to orthophoria.

STRABISMUS

Strabismus, a malalignment of the visual axes of the two eyes, occurs in 1 to 4 percent of the population. Each of its forms has both a sensory (or visual) and a motor component.

Visual acuity, or the visual fixation reflex, is poor at birth but develops rapidly with macular differentiation into a conditioned reflex during the first 6 months of life.

Versions, or conjugate gaze movements, are the simultaneous movements of the two parallel eyes into the same fields of gaze, thus enhancing binocular vision. Normal version movements are present by approximately 4 months of age.

Vergence movements direct the visual axes of the eyes in opposite directions, creating convergence, divergence, vertical vergence, and cyclovergence. Vergences are well established by 6 months of age.

The crystalline lens within the eye produces clear vision over all viewing distances by changing its thickness during focusing or accommodation, a process well established by 6 months of age. The combination of clear vision produced by accommodation, and version and vergence movements, allows the images transmitted from the two eyes to be fused into a single image within the visual cortex. The interpretation of these images takes place in higher cerebral centers.

Because the eyes are separated horizontally within the head, the images perceived by each eye arrive from slightly different angles. These differences produce depth perception, or stereopsis, one of our most highly developed forms of binocular vision.

During normal binocular vision, the object of visual interest is projected onto the macula of each eye. When strabismus occurs, the macula of each eye observes different subjects; to avoid diplopia, a suppression scotoma (or blind spot) is physiologically created which blocks the macular area of the deviating eye. A second scotoma then blocks the image falling on the peripheral retina of the deviated eye that is simultaneously observed by the fixing eye. In the visually immature patient, suppression occurs within the first 6 weeks following the onset of strabismus. In the visually mature patient (those over 6 to 8 years of age), diplopia remains as a constant symptom.

Patients who have variable or alternating strabismus demonstrate alternating suppression scotomas. If strabismus becomes constant, the suppression scotoma becomes permanent and further visual development is prohibited. This visual loss is termed amblyopia. Amblyopia may also be produced by anisometropia (unequal refractive errors in the two eyes) or blocks to the projection of clear images onto the retina by corneal opacities, cataracts, and retinal and optic nerve abnormalities.

Amblyopia may be detected in young infants or preverbal children by observing their behavior when a cover is placed over each eye separately to test the visual fixation reflex. In older children, amblyopia exists when there is a visual acuity difference between the two eyes of at least two horizontal lines of Snellen letters (Fig. 17.5).

Phorias and Tropias

Phorias occur during periods of suspended sensory fusion of the eyes, and a motor deviation due to a disruption of motor fusion. When the obstacle to sensory fusion is removed, motor fusion returns the eyes to a straight, aligned position. With high degrees of sensory fusion, the ocular malalignment is "latent."

Phorias produce symptoms of double vision, eye fatigue, headaches, and blurring of print or moving objects. These symptoms tend to be more acute during periods of stress, emotional excitement, fatigue, or illness. Light sensitivity, dizziness, and difficulties in focusing from one distance to another may also occur.

Tropias are constant or intermittent ocular deviations during which fusion is unable to maintain the eyes in a straight position. Deviations may exist in all visual ranges, or they may increase or decrease when tested with near and distant visual targets. Double vision may persist early in the tropic phase or in patients with intermittent tropias. Abnormal head postures compensate for double vision produced by horizontal or cyclovertical muscle palsies.

Both phorias and tropias are classified according to pattern of eye deviation: esodeviations, exodeviations, hyperdeviations, and cyclodeviations.

ESODEVIATIONS

In patients with extreme farsightedness, excessive accommodation is necessary to obtain clear vision. Excessive convergence is associated with this accommodative effort in a midbrain reflex, and esotropia occurs. The onset of this deviation occurs most commonly in children between the ages of 18 months and 3 years. A family history of strabismus has been found in approximately 50 percent of these patients.

Corrective glasses or contact lenses, determined by cycloplegic refraction, can compensate for any preexisting farsightedness, and with their wear, the eyes return to an orthophoric position (Fig. 17.6). Some patients with accommodative esotropia have a greater tropia in the near range than at a

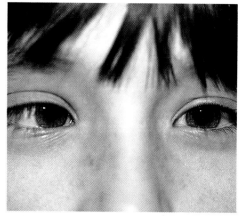
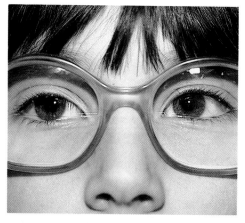
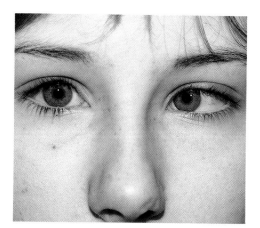

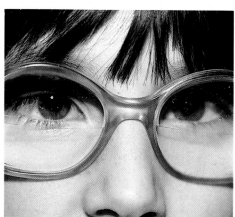
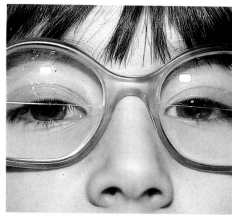
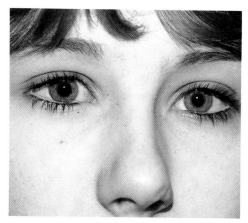

FIG. 17.7 *This child displays hypermetropia and esotropia when fixing at distance, and even greater esotropia in near range. When glasses were prescribed (bottom left), correction of hypermetropia*

occurred, and her eyes straightened at distance. However, her near esotropia remained (top right). Bifocals were then prescribed, and the near esotropia was corrected (bottom right).

FIG. 17.8 *The girl at top shows nonaccommodative esotropia, an esotropia which could not be corrected with glasses or miotics. Surgery was performed, and the 1-week postoperative photograph at bottom shows reduced esotropia with normal alignment.*

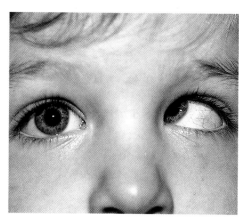
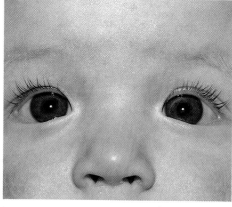
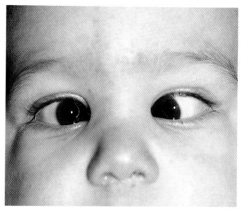

FIG. 17.9 *This deviation is due to an overacting left inferior oblique muscle or elevation in adduction associated with esotropia.*

FIG. 17.10 *This infant has pseudostrabismus, caused by a flat nasal bridge, wide epicanthal folds, and closely placed eyes.*

FIG. 17.11 *Infantile esotropia with decentered corneal light reflexes.*

distance, and an additional optical correction or bifocal can be added to their glasses to reduce this discrepancy (Fig. 17.7).

The accommodative component must be determined in all esotropic patients by the prescription of glasses or miotics before surgery can be considered. Only the nonaccommodative (nonoptical-medical) component of the esodeviation receives surgical correction. Surgery may be performed at

any time after 6 months of age (Fig. 17.8).

It is not uncommon for vertical deviations to coexist with esotropia; they consist of over- or underactions of the inferior or superior oblique muscles, the vertical recti, or dissociated vertical deviations (Fig. 17.9).

Pseudostrabismus is a phenomenon seen in infants who have wide epicanthal folds, closely placed eyes, and flat nasal

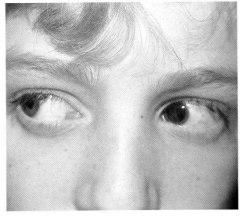 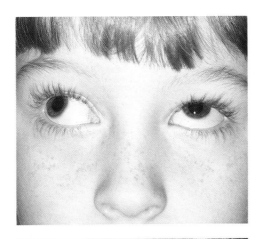

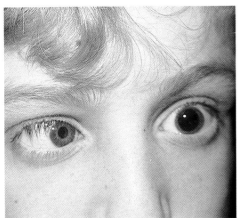 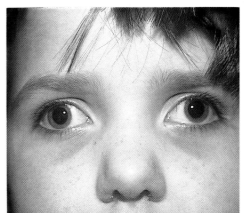

FIG. 17.12 The photograph at top shows a patient with normal ocular alignment in right gaze. However, at bottom we see the result of a total abduction defect caused by left sixth nerve palsy.

FIG. 17.13 This patient shows two manifestations of Duane syndrome. (Top) Narrowing of the palpebral fissure in adduction, with upshoot of the left inferior oblique muscle. (Bottom) Widening of the left palpebral fissure in attempting abduction of the eye. No abduction past the midline is possible in Duane syndrome.

FIG. 17.14 Exotropia, a divergent deviation of the eyes.

bridges simulating the presence of esotropia (Fig. 17.10). The cover-uncover test (described later in this chapter) confirms the absence of an ocular deviation.

Infantile esotropia, an esodeviation present at birth or arising in the neonatal period, requires surgical intervention when the infant is 6 months of age or older (Fig. 17.11). Efforts are made to achieve a normal ocular alignment early in life so that maximum benefits may be derived from binocular visual development. While none of these patients will achieve the same high degree of fusion or stereopsis that a nonstrabismic child attains, satisfactory results are frequently achieved. Infantile esotropia is often associated with cross-fixation or apparent palsies of the lateral recti, rotatory nystagmus, and large-angle strabismus.

Paretic esotropias occur following sixth nerve palsies, and are induced by diplopia, abnormal head postures, and an inability to abduct the involved eye(s) (Fig. 17.12). The abnormal muscle function may return to normal over a 6- to 12-month observation period.

Duane syndrome, a congenital neurologic defect, is characterized by the inability to abduct one or both eyes past the midline. There is often an associated up or down "shoot" upon attempting adduction of the affected eye. The palpebral

fissure narrows on adduction and widens on abduction due to contraction of both the medial and lateral rectus muscles in adduction and no contraction of these muscles in abduction (Fig. 17.13).

EXODEVIATIONS

Fleeting exodeviations arise in very young children, and are associated with fatigue, daydreaming, illness, or exaggerated emotional states. The progression of this disorder varies: Some patients continue to have nonsymptomatic exophorias while others develop an intermittent exotropia which may become constant when fixating at a distance (Fig. 17.14). Exodeviations in the near range arise as these latter children grow, and may increase to equal or surpass the distance deviation. Another group of patients may develop a constant exotropia at both distance and near range which may be associated with amblyopia in the deviated eye. Other exodeviations include congenital exotropia, third nerve palsies with exotropia, and exodeviations associated with visual deprivation, ocular organic disease, or anisometropia. Exotropic patients frequently close or cover one eye in bright light, notice blurred or double vision with prolonged close work, or complain of difficulty with night driving.

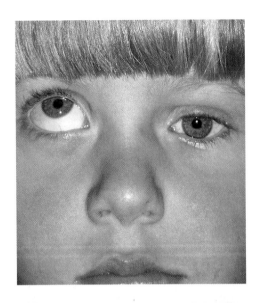

FIG. 17.15 Left third nerve palsy with ptosis and an inability to elevate and adduct the eye.

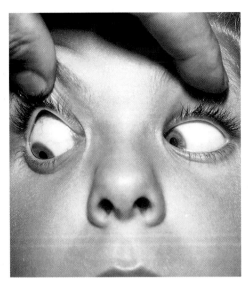

FIG. 17.16 Left fourth nerve palsy with an inability to depress the involved eye in adduction. Abnormal head posture is common, as is overaction of the direct antagonistic inferior oblique muscle.

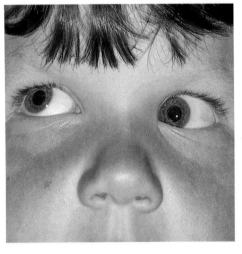

FIG. 17.17 Brown syndrome, an inability to elevate an eye in adduction due to a tight superior oblique tendon.

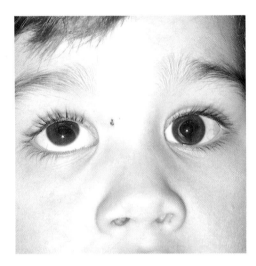

FIG. 17.18 Dissociative vertical deviation, an upward drifting of an eye without symptoms or the presence of a hypodeviation of the other eye.

HYPERDEVIATIONS

Vertical deviations where one eye is intermittently or constantly higher than the other, frequently exist in only one field of gaze. Associated torsional defects are common, and compensatory head postures are utilized to eliminate diplopia. This is a common cause of head tilt or torticollis.

Vertical deviations include congenital or acquired third (Fig. 17.15) and fourth (Fig. 17.16) nerve palsies, Brown syndrome (Fig. 17.17), elevator or depressor palsies, dissociative vertical deviations (Fig. 17.18), Duane syndrome, defects associated with craniofacial anomalies and trauma, A and V patterns associated with horizontal strabismus, external ophthalmoplegias, and defects associated with systemic disease such as myasthenia gravis, diabetes mellitus, hypertension, and thyroid ophthalmopathy.

Tests for Strabismus

The presence and amount of the motor deviation is determined by the cover-uncover test and the corneal light reflex test. The cover-uncover test requires useful vision in each eye, and the targets observed require a constant amount of accommodation. Snellen test types, illiterate "E"s, figures, or pictures, rather than lights, are used as targets. The tests are performed at 20 feet, where no accommodation is required, and in the near or reading range of 13 to 14 inches.

The cover-uncover test is performed by placing a cover over one eye, thus disrupting fusion or binocularity (Fig. 17.19). The cover is then removed, and the eye is observed. If that eye does not move, this indicates that both eyes are in an orthophoric, or straight, position. If the eye moves to regain fusion with a normal ocular alignment as the cover is removed, this indicates that a phoria exists. The test is then repeated on the other eye.

A second aspect of the cover-uncover test is performed by covering one eye and observing the movement of the other eye (Fig. 17.20). If the uncovered eye does not move to take up fixation when the other eye is covered, this indicates that the uncovered eye is orthophoric and no tropia exists. The cover is then moved to the other eye, and if a tropia is present, the now uncovered deviating eye will perform a fixation movement to come to the straight position. When the cover is again removed, either no movement will occur, indicating good vision in each eye, or the previously deviating eye will again deviate. This deviation is due to a marked dominance of the fixing eye, or to amblyopia in the deviating eye.

The corneal light reflex test is performed by having the patient fixate on a penlight held 16 inches from the eyes. Normally, the corneal light reflexes are slightly nasally displaced. However, in the presence of an ocular deviation, the light reflexes are decentered in the deviating eye (Fig. 17.21). This test is useful diagnostically for patients with poor visual acuity or poor fixation in their malaligned eye.

HETEROPHORIAS

Normally, both eyes appear to be aligned and centrally fixed

Exophoria

Cover one eye—that eye deviates away from the other eye

The cover is then removed—the now uncovered eye returns to a central position

The same procedure is then performed on the other eye

Esophoria

Cover one eye—that eye deviates toward the other eye

The cover is then removed—the now uncovered eye returns to a central position

The same procedure is then performed on the other eye

Hyperphoria

Cover one eye—that eye deviates superiorly

The cover is then removed—the now uncovered eye returns to a central position

The same procedure is then performed on the other eye

FIG. 17.19 The cover-uncover test for heterophorias.

HETEROTROPIAS

In esotropia, one eye is deviated toward the other. Note that the corneal light reflex is not centrally placed

Cover the esotropic eye—there is no movement of either eye

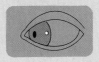

The cover is then removed—again, there is no movement of either eye— no proof of tropia

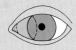

The other eye is now covered—as a result, that eye becomes esotropic and the formerly esotropic eye moves to a central position to take up fixation (Hering's law)

If the cover is removed and no eye movement occurs, this indicates that the eyes have equal visual acuity or fixation. This also indicates a relative absence of amblyopia

If the cover is removed, and both eyes move so that the original fixing eye is again centrally fixed and the originally esotropic eye is again esotropic, this indicates that there is amblyopia present

The same maneuvers can be used to determine the presence of exotropia (outward deviation), hyper- and hypotropia (upward and downward deviation), and cyclotropia (rotary displacement)

FIG. 17.20 The cover-uncover test for heterotropias.

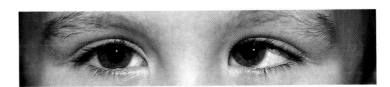

FIG. 17.21 The corneal light reflex test. The fixing right eye has a centered light reflex, while the strabismic left eye has a temporally displaced light reflex.

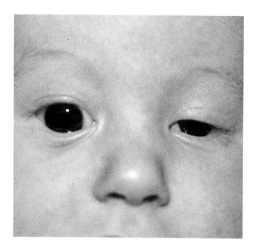

FIG. 17.22 *Unilateral congenital ptosis with lid covering pupil.*

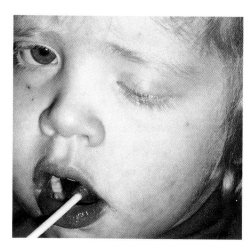

FIG. 17.23 *At left, the toddler exhibits the Marcus Gunn jaw-winking syndrome with ptosis, while at right he shows a*

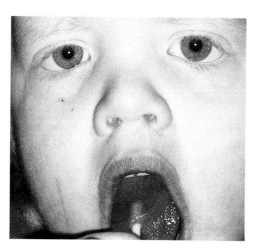

wide open ptotic lid with movements of the jaw.

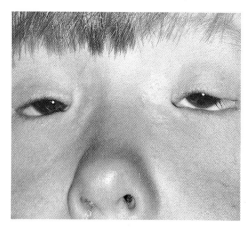

FIG. 17.24 *Komoto syndrome, a combination of blepharophimosis, ptosis, epicanthus inversus, and telecanthus.*

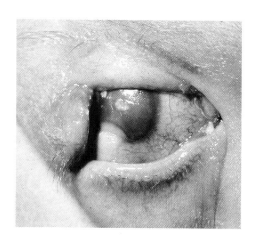

FIG. 17.25 *Goldenhar syndrome with eyelid coloboma and corneal limbal dermoid.*

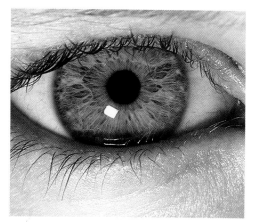

FIG. 17.26 *Districhiasis, a double row of lashes. One row, directed toward the cornea, arises from the meibomian gland orifices. The second row is directed outward in the normal position.*

DISEASES OF THE EYES AND THEIR SURROUNDING STRUCTURES

Eyelids

The eyelids and their associated cilia, glands, and muscular structures may be affected by a variety of congenital and acquired defects.

Blepharoptosis or ptosis, a drooping of one or both upper eyelids, is most frequently congenital, is often hereditary, and may be associated with other extraocular muscle or central nervous system abnormalities (Fig. 17.22). Acquired ptosis results from inflammatory and scarring diseases or injury to the levator muscle or its nerve supply.

Infants with congenital ptosis whose eyelids cover their pupils, or those patients who developed an abnormal backward head posture in order to be able to use their eyes require early surgical correction. Amblyopia rarely occurs with partial ptosis; it is usually associated with covered pupils or other extraocular muscle defects.

Patients with ptosis as well as a Marcus Gunn jaw-winking syndrome exhibit both components: jaw-winking and ptosis (Fig. 17.23). With sucking or chewing movements of the jaw, the ptotic lid elevates and descends, or winks. Even if the

ptosis is severe and covers the pupil, it will be corrected (elevated) by the jaw movements. The defect may be apparent in the newborn, but tends to decrease with age.

Ptosis is also associated with Komoto syndrome, which consists of blepharophimosis, telecanthus, epicanthus inversus, and blepharoptosis (Fig. 17.24).

Ptosis in children is also associated with microphthalmia and eyelid colobomas. Eyelid coloboma, a defect in the lid margin, tarsus, and levator muscle, may be an isolated defect or occur as part of Goldenhar syndrome, which consists of vertebral anomalies, corneal limbal dermoids, and preauricular skin tags (Fig. 17.25).

Trichiasis, or misdirected eyelashes, produces corneal irritation or abrasions, and usually follows chronic inflammations of the lids, entropion, trauma, or other scarring conditions.

Districhiasis manifests as an accessory row of lashes along the posterior border of the eyelid which rub against the eye (Fig. 17.26). Lid eversion or ectropion coexists because of defects in the tarsal plate. Districhiasis is an autosomal-dominant condition, but may occasionally follow severe ocular inflammation.

Ectropion, an outward turning of the eyelid margin, is rarely congenital. Spastic ectropion, which may be seen in children

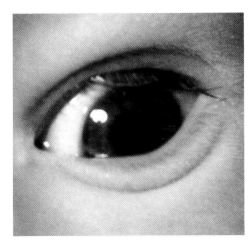

FIG. 17.27 Entropion of the upper lid.

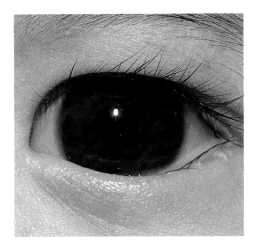

FIG. 17.28 In epiblepharon, the eyelashes are rotated upward against the globe in the medial third of the eyelid.

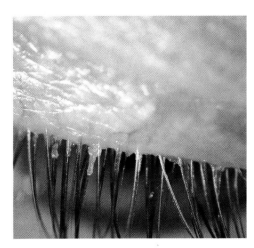

FIG. 17.29 Thickened lids with crusts around lashes in a patient with blepharitis.

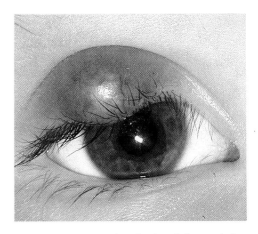

FIG. 17.30 Acute hordeola of the eyelid with swelling, induration, and purulent matter pointing externally.

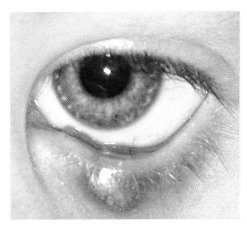

FIG. 17.31 Chalazion, a painless lid mass pointing externally or internally.

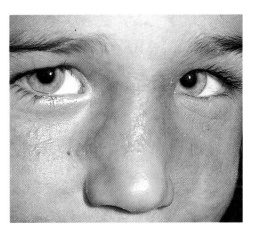

FIG. 17.32 Contact dermatitis with red, dry inflamed skin of the eyelids and face secondary to poison ivy.

following lid trauma with scarring, and burns are the most frequent cause, followed by scars from lacerations or other eyelid trauma. Ectropion may also follow seventh nerve palsies.

Entropion, rarely congenital, exists when the eyelid margin is turned inward against the globe (Fig. 17.27). Spastic entropion occurs in children and is associated with severe blepharospasm. More commonly, it follows inflammation, trauma, or eyelid surgery.

Epiblepharon is not a true entropion (Fig. 17.28); in this condition, the infant's facial fat pushes the medial third of the eyelid upward and rotates the soft lashes against the globe. The defect corrects itself spontaneously by 1 year of age, and therapy is usually not indicated. Corneal abrasion does not occur because the lashes are soft and nonirritating.

Children frequently have acute or chronic blepharitis due to staphylococcus infection; patients with seborrhea are even more prone to this entity. Allergies may precipitate episodes of itching and rubbing which leads to staphylococcal contamination. Ulcerations and thickening of the lids occur (Fig. 17.29). Hard, brittle scales are present on the lid margins and surround the bases of the cilia. Complications include lid ulceration, abscess formation, chronic conjunctivitis, and keratitis.

Acute and chronic inflammatory masses of the eyelids are hordeola or styes and chalazia, respectively. A hordeolum is a staphylococcal infection of a hair follicle or gland of Zeis which produces painful swelling and edema of the lid followed by a localization of the exudate (Fig. 17.30). Spontaneous drainage frequently occurs with conservative therapy. Orbital cellulitis is the major complication.

A chalazion is a chronic granuloma of a sebaceous gland of the tarsal plate (Fig. 17.31). There is swelling of the lid due to retention of the glandular secretion, with formation of a painless tumor of a granulation tissue or a lipogranuloma. Refractive errors are induced by the pressure of the chalazion against the cornea. The chalazion may subside spontaneously or, more frequently, may require surgical drainage.

Eyelid inflammations secondary to contact or allergic dermatitis produce redness, induration, and vesicles which rupture (Fig. 17.32); itching may be intense.

Viral diseases of the eyelids are also common in children. Primary herpes simplex of the lid is characterized by small vesicles, often unilateral, associated with mild conjunctivitis and keratitis. Varicella produces lid swelling without serious scarring. Herpes zoster is uncommon in children, but keratouveitis with glaucoma, cataracts, and macular and optic nerve inflammations may be devastating to vision. Verrucae

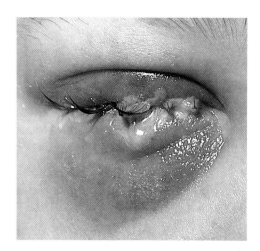

FIG. 17.33 *Vaccinia of the upper and lower eyelids with edema and secondary infection.*

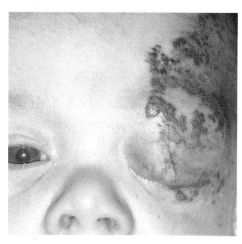

FIG. 17.34 *Hemangioma of the eyelids with occlusion of the visual axis.*

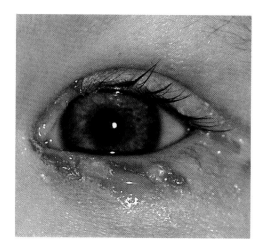

FIG. 17.35 *Unilateral stenosis of the left nasolacrimal duct with mucopurulent discharge and tearing.*

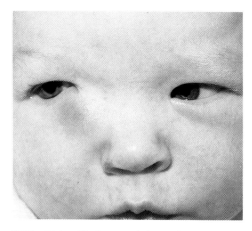

FIG. 17.36 *Hydrops of the right naso-lacrimal sac in a newborn manifests as a tense blue swelling overlying the medial canthal area. Pressure on the sac expresses a mucopurulent discharge.*

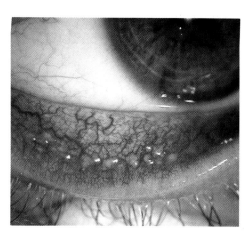

FIG. 17.37 *Follicular conjunctivitis of viral origin.*

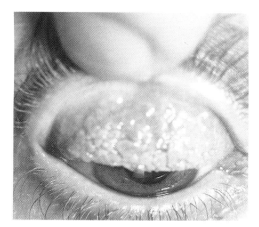

FIG. 17.38 *Papillary conjunctivitis of bacterial or allergic origin.*

on the lids are due to autoinoculation, and secondary keratitis due to the deposition of keratin flakes occurs when lid margin lesions are present. Secondary vaccinia autoinoculation leads to lid scarring or cellulitis (Fig. 17.33).

The most common eyelid tumor in children is hemangioma. Hemangiomas grow very rapidly during the first 6 months of life and diminish their growth toward spontaneous resolution over the next 5 to 6 years. They may cause marked swelling of the eyelids, with obstruction of the visual axis leading to severe amblyopia and refractive errors with high astigmatism (Fig. 17.34).

Lacrimal Gland and Nasolacrimal Drainage System

Disorders of the lacrimal gland are rare in children. Acute dacryoadenitis occurs with mumps. Chronic diseases such as sarcoid, Hodgkin's disease, leukemia, and mononucleosis produce ptosis and palpable masses. Diagnosis of the systemic disease aids in management. Conjunctival biopsy is useful for the diagnosis of sarcoid.

Stenosis of the nasolacrimal duct occurs during the first 7 days of life in 30 percent of newborns. Signs include tearing and a mucopurulent discharge present 1 to 3 weeks following

birth (Fig. 17.35). Regurgitation of the mucopurulent matter occurs with pressure over the sac. Congenital lacrimal amniotocele or hydrops of the lacrimal sac appears shortly after birth as a blue cystic mass overlying the medial canthal area (Fig. 17.36). Spontaneous resolution of the obstructed unilateral or bilateral nasolacrimal system is common before 6 months of age; between 6 months and 1 year, surgery is recommended.

Other congenital defects of the nasolacrimal duct system consist of an absence or atresia of the puncta, or the presence of epithelial membranes which cover the puctal lumen. A fistula from the nasolacrimal sac to the skin of the face may be congenital, or may occur secondary to acute dacryocystostitis. A tear or mucopurulent discharge may appear at the fistula orifice below the medial canthal ligament.

Acquired stenosis of the nasolacrimal system occurs in children secondary to infections such as trachoma, tuberculosis, or mycosis.

Conjunctiva

Conjunctivitis is common in children, but is rarely serious except in newborns. Morphologically, the conjunctiva responds with follicles or papillae. A follicle is an aggregate of lympho-

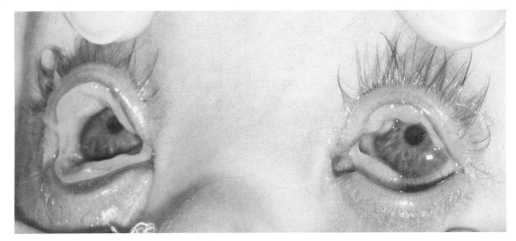

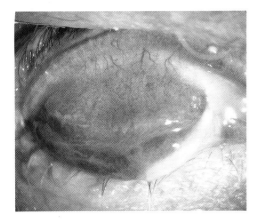

FIG. 17.40 Acute bacterial conjunctivitis with mucopurulent discharge, hyperemia, and tearing.

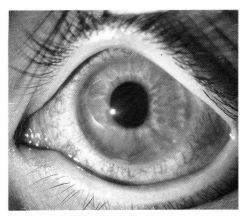

FIG. 17.41 Viral conjunctivitis with hyperemia and a thin watery discharge.

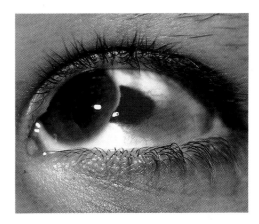

FIG. 17.42 Subconjunctival hemorrhage secondary to blunt ocular trauma.

cytes with an avascular center and a peripheral vascular network. Follicles predominate in viral diseases, except in the newborn where lymphoid tissue is not yet developed (Fig. 17.37). A papilla is a small, raised nodule with a central vascular core. Some papillae are giant-sized, measuring 1 to 2 mm in diameter. Papillary inflammation is the conjunctival response to bacterial or allergic conjunctivitis (Fig. 17.38).

Bacterial conjunctivitis may be hyperacute, acute, or chronic. Hyperacute bacterial conjunctivitis, an acute, purulent infection by *Neisseria gonorrhoeae* or *N. meningitidis*, involves both the lid and cornea. A rapid onset of a copious, purulent discharge combined with marked edema of the eyelids, pain, tenderness, conjunctival chemosis, keratitis, and regional lymphadenopathy are characteristic features (Fig. 17.39). Corneal luster is diminished, and corneal ulceration or perforation may occur.

Acute bacterial conjunctivitis is usually due to staphylococcus, pneumococcus, or hemophilus infection (Fig. 17.40). A mucopurulent discharge is associated with tearing, ocular irritation, and the lids sticking together upon awakening. Usually, one eye is involved 1 to 2 days before the other is. Conjunctival hyperemia, petechiae, punctate keratitis, and marginal corneal ulcers are frequent complications.

Chronic conjunctivitis results from the bacterial toxins of *Staphylococcus aureus*, Proteus, or Moraxella. Symptoms vary depending upon the etiologic agent. Foreign body sensations, red eyes, and mucopurulent discharge on the lids upon awakening are characteristic features. Conjunctival hyperemia, papillary hyperplasia, and thickening of the conjunctiva also occur. Mucoid or mucopurulent threads may be present in the fornices; the discharge is usually minimal.

Conjunctivitis in the newborn (ophthalmia neonatorum) is induced by silver nitrate drops which produce a purulent conjunctivitis 12 to 24 hours after instillation and last for 1 or 2 days. The latent period of gonococcal conjunctivitis is 1 to 3 days; pneumococcus, 5 to 8 days; and inclusion blennorrhea in the newborn, 10 to 15 days. Cultures and smears establish the correct diagnosis.

Viral conjunctivitis is caused by a wide variety of agents; has an acute onset; is usually bilateral; and is accompanied by minimal pain, tearing, a thin mucopurulent or watery discharge, and redness of the conjunctiva (Fig. 17.41). Photophobia may be marked. The disease is self-limited to 7 to 10 days, depending upon the virus.

Allergic conjunctivitis, an immediate hypersensitivity response to pollen, vegetable or animal protein, dust, fungus, or other airborne irritants or allergens, results in symptoms of itching eyes with photophobia, tearing, and a mucopurulent discharge. The lids and palpebral conjunctivae are hyperemic and edematous. Acute conjunctivitis may become chronic with repeated or constant exposure to an allergen. The conjunctiva is pale and boggy with a papillary reaction. Follicles occur on the palpebral conjunctiva of the lower eyelids. Complications include punctate keratitis, iritis, and neuroretinitis.

Subconjunctival hemorrhages are common in children, are secondary to trauma or infection (Fig. 17.42), and are characterized by an intense bright red color under a slightly swollen conjunctiva. The size, configuration, and color of the hemorrhage changes with the migration of blood. Spontaneous resolution occurs.

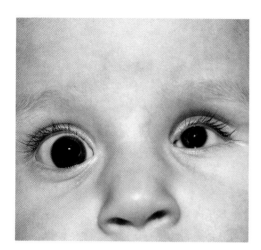

FIG. 17.43 Unilateral microcornea and microphthalmos.

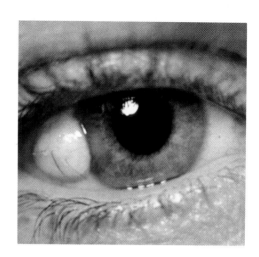

FIG. 17.44 Corneal-limbal dermoid, often associated with Goldenhar syndrome.

Cornea

The developmental anomalies of the cornea include sclerocornea, Rieger syndrome, microcornea, and corneal dermoid.

Sclerocornea, present at birth, results in a cornea whose appearance resembles sclera; the lesion is vascularized and uninflamed. Rieger syndrome, a variant of anterior segment dysgenesis, is a dominant hereditary disorder of the anterior segment of the eye, resulting in hyperplasia of the iris stroma, pupillary anomalies, anomalies of the trabecular meshwork, and early-onset glaucoma. Microcornea, whether an isolated anomaly or associated with glaucoma, cataracts, iris abnormalities, or anterior segment dysgenesis, has a corneal diameter of 9 mm or less (Fig. 17.43). Corneal dermoids occur at the limbus, grow slowly, and encroach upon the visual axis (Fig. 17.44). They are composed of fibrolipoid tissue containing hair follicles and sebaceous glands.

The cornea is also the site of many systemic diseases. Hurler syndrome, a mucopolysaccharide storage disease, produces clouding of the cornea. The cornea, clear at birth, develops an opacification by 2 to 3 years of age. Pigmentary retinopathy and optic atrophy coexist.

Cystinosis, seen in the early months of life, involves the deposition of L-cystine in the cornea (Fig. 17.45).

Corneal inflammations are associated with bacterial, viral, mycotic, and allergic diseases. Corneal ulcers are caused by the invasion of bacterial organisms into the corneal stroma, consequently leading to abscess formation (Fig. 17.46). The infection may involve the entire cornea and result in visual impairment, corneal perforation, and loss of the globe. The bacteria involved are staphylococcus, streptococcus, pneumococcus, Moraxella, *Pseudomonas aeruginosa*, *Escherichia coli*, and *Klebsiella pneumoniae*, the latter two being gram-negative agents. Appropriate smears and cultures are obtained as soon as the diagnosis is suspected.

Corneal trauma or abrasion of the epithelium produces pain, blepharospasm, and marked tearing. Diagnosis is confirmed by the application of fluorescein dye which imparts a greenish color to the abraded corneal surface (Fig. 17.47).

Herpes simplex, a severe viral infection of the cornea, is transmitted from active herpes in the maternal birth canal, or results from direct contact with infected individuals. Primary herpes is a unilateral lesion associated with regional lymphadenopathy; a few weeks after infection, half of the patients develop a punctate of typical dendritic keratitis (Fig. 17.48).

Recurrent herpes keratitis occurs in 25 percent of individuals presenting with primary herpes. The lesion appears as a typical branching dendrite. Recurrences may be complicated by stromal keratitis, keratouveitis, and anesthesia of the cornea. Stromal disease is a serious complication reducing visual recovery, and may lead to vascularization of the cornea or chronic keratitic inflammation (Fig. 17.49).

Phlyctenular or nodular keratoconjunctivitis occurs in response to an allergy. The phlyctenular lesion is a small, pinkish-white nodule in the center of a hyperemic area of conjunctiva at the limbus which evolves into a microabscess and heals in 10 to 14 days without scarring. The symptoms consist of itching, tearing, and irritation. A mucopurulent discharge may occur if secondary infection is present. Patients with corneal phlyctenulosis have more severe symptoms of pain, light sensitivity, and tearing.

Glaucoma

Infantile or congenital glaucoma occurs as an autosomal-recessive trait with incomplete penetrance. The disease, present at birth or arising several weeks or months later, is caused by an embryonic defect in the development of the trabecular meshwork or filtration area of the eye. The signs and symptoms consist of epiphora, blepharospasm, photophobia, corneal enlargement with clouding and edema, ruptures in Descemet's membrane with Haab striae, and cupping of the optic disc. Amblyopia, refractive errors, and strabismus complicate the disease (Fig. 17.50).

Juvenile glaucoma is a primary glaucoma which arises in patients between 3 and 23 years of age. Secondary glaucoma occurs in patients with aniridia, iridocorneal dysgenesis, Sturge-Weber syndrome, neurofibromatosis, Lowe syndrome, chronic uveitis, traumatic angle recession, and aphakic glaucoma.

Anterior Chamber

Hyphema, an accumulation of blood within the anterior chamber, most commonly occurs in children following ocular trauma, but may also result from juvenile xanthogranuloma and systemic hematologic disorders. Bleeding arises from the iris or from tears into the anterior face of the ciliary body, with rupture of the greater arterial circle of the iris. Blood is layered in the lower aspect of the anterior chamber when the

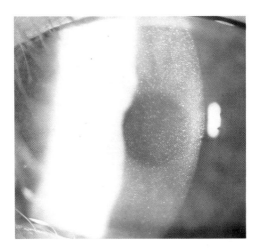

FIG. 17.45 Cystinosis of the cornea with deposition of L-cystine crystals in the stroma.

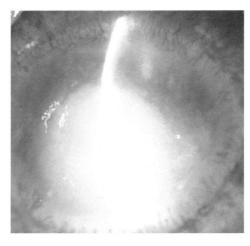

FIG. 17.46 Central corneal ulcer associated with conjunctival infection, corneal haze, and mucopurulent discharge.

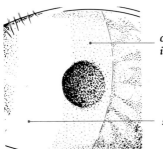

cystine crystals in cornea

slit-lamp beam

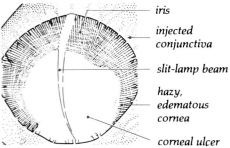

iris

injected conjunctiva

slit-lamp beam

hazy, edematous cornea

corneal ulcer

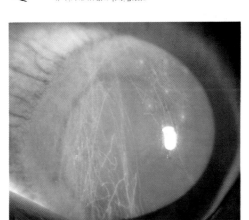

FIG. 17.47 Corneal abrasions stained with fluorescein dye and viewed under blue light. The abrasions appear green in the area of corneal epithelial loss.

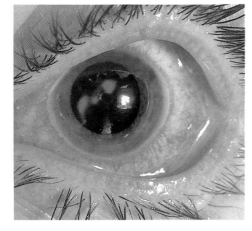

FIG. 17.48 Herpes simplex dendritic corneal ulcer stained with fluorescein.

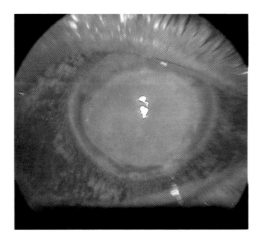

FIG. 17.49 Chronic herpes simplex corneal ulcer stained with fluorescein.

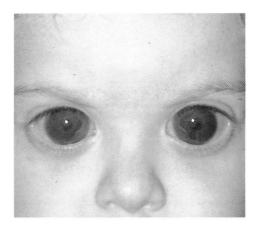

FIG. 17.50 Manifestations of infantile glaucoma. (Left) Bilateral infantile glaucoma with an enlarged but clear cornea. Note the dislocated lens that bisects the pupil. (Center) Clouded, enlarged cornea

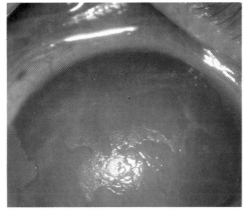

and irregular epithelial surface caused by elevated pressure in a patient with infantile glaucoma. (Right) Glaucomatous optic atrophy. In glaucoma, excavation extends

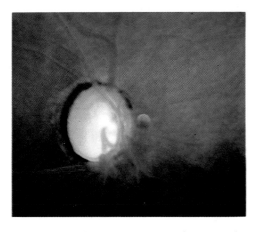

to the disc edge in contrast to the cupped disc seen in myopia where a normal rim of tissue exists. Retinal vessels emerge from under the disc edge.

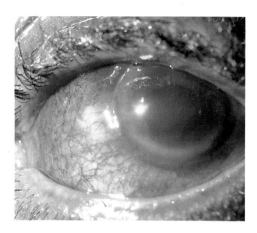

FIG. 17.51 *Layered hyphema in the anterior chamber following blunt ocular trauma.*

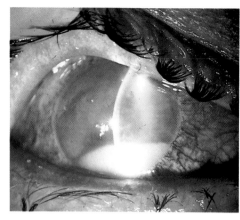

FIG. 17.52 *Hypopyon, pus layered in the inferior anterior chamber.*

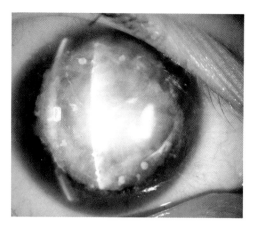

FIG. 17.53 *Aniridia with cataract.*

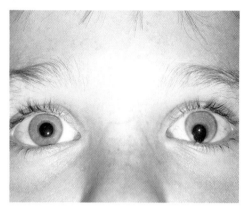

FIG. 17.54 *Typical unilateral coloboma in an otherwise normal left eye.*

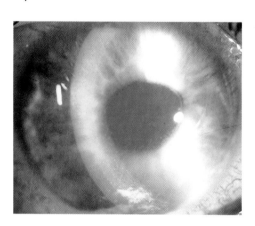

FIG. 17.55 *Iritis with circumcorneal ciliary flush.*

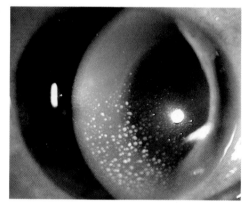

FIG. 17.56 *Keratic precipitates on the posterior corneal synechiae in a patient with chronic iritis.*

patient is sitting upright (Fig. 17.51). One to five days are required for reabsorption of blood to occur.

Complications of hyphema are increased intraocular pressure, optic atrophy, blood staining of the cornea, and blockage of the trabecular meshwork with cellular breakdown products. Rebleeding most commonly occurs on the fourth or fifth posttrauma day, may be massive, and produces a marked increase in intraocular pressure. Patients suffering hyphema must be followed periodically throughout life, for chronic open-angle glaucoma may develop in the traumatized eye for as many as 40 years posttraumatically.

Hypopyon, pus in the anterior chamber, arises from contamination following ocular trauma or surgery, corneoscleral ulcerations, or systemic metastatic inflammatory diseases (Fig. 17.52). Occasionally, the pus may be sterile.

Iris

The iris is most frequently affected by congenital defects and inflammation.

Aniridia, which presents itself as the apparent absence of the iris, has many variations and is due to a failure of the mesoderm to grow outward from the iris root during the fourth month of gestation (Fig. 17.53). The pupils appear as large as the cornea, while the ever-present iris root remains as a small residual structure. A membrane between the rudimentary iris and the trabecular meshwork pulls the iris anteriorly, and, with time, the iris may become adherent to the meshwork, inducing secondary glaucoma. This glaucoma, unlike

congenital glaucoma, rarely develops an enlarged cornea.

The visual acuity in aniridic patients is markedly decreased due to macular hypoplasia; nystagmus and photophobia are frequent. An autosomal-dominant inheritance occurs in two-thirds of patients; the remainder are sporadic. Approximately 20 percent of all infants with sporadic aniridia develop Wilms' tumor (with 90 percent of those tumors occurring by age 3), other genitourinary defects, or mental retardation. Ocular defects associated with aniridia include displaced lenses due to breakage of the inferior zonules, cataracts, corneal epithelial dystrophy commencing at the limbus and progressing centrally, and calcified band keratopathy which produces recurrent episodes of pain.

A persistent pupillary membrane is due to hyperplasia of the mesoderm of the anterior layer of the iris. Instead of terminating at the pupillary margin, iris strands cross the pupillary space from collarette to collarette or terminate to become adherent to the anterior lens capsule.

Colobomas of the iris, frequently a dominant trait, are typically found at the inferior and nasal positions and indicate an anomaly in the closure of the fetal fissure (Fig. 17.54).

Rubeosis iridis, a fibrovascular growth of tissue over the anterior surface of the iris and trabecular meshwork, impairs aqueous outflow and increases intraocular pressure. Neovascularization of the iris occurs secondary to retinal hypoxia from ocular and systemic causes, which include diabetes, central retinal vein occlusion, intraocular tumors, retinal detachment, and sickle cell anemia. Iris angiography is helpful in early diagnosis. Spontaneous hemorrhages occur in the anter-

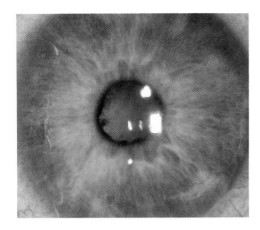

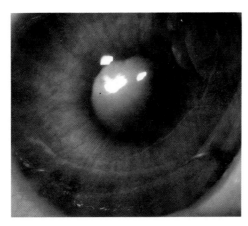

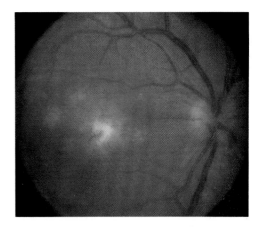

FIG. 17.57 Chronic iritis in a patient with Still disease. Posterior synechiae and complicated cataracts are also present.

FIG. 17.58 Yellow cyclitic membrane behind a clear lens in a soft phthisical eye.

FIG. 17.59 Acute toxoplasmic chorioretinitis in the macular region of a 3-year-old child. The lesion is surrounded by vitreous haze and retinal edema.

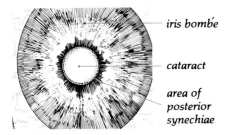

iris bombé

cataract

area of posterior synechiae

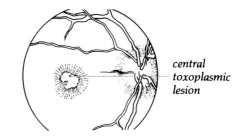

central toxoplasmic lesion

ior chamber. Associated peripheral anterior synechiae induce increased intraocular pressure with pain, corneal edema, and visual loss.

Uveitis, an inflammation of the uveal tract, is categorized by the areas which are predominantly affected: the iris, ciliary body, or choroid. Many inflammations which arise in the uveal tract of children result in diffuse and severe ocular inflammations. The inflammation may be purulent or nonpurulent, and may affect the retina, sclera, cornea, and lens. Nonpurulent or endogenous uveitis is the most common, yet is relatively rare in children. Bilateral involvement is the rule.

Children do not complain of visual impairment, and strabismus is often a presenting sign. Band keratopathy is characteristic of childhood involvement, and also occurs with juvenile rheumatoid arthritis. Posterior synechiae are frequently well formed early in the disease process, and complicated cataracts develop and mature rapidly.

Dilatation of the iris vessels with exudation of protein and inflammatory cells into the aqueous humor is characteristic of iritis (Fig. 17.55). Keratic precipitates occur on the posterior corneal surface (Fig. 17.56). Adhesions form as peripheral anterior synechiae between iris and trabecular meshwork, or as posterior synechiae between the iris and lens (Fig. 17.57). Posterior synechiae induce secondary glaucoma and iris bombe. Iris nodules are caused by tuberculosis or sarcoidosis.

Inflammations of the ciliary body produce cells and flare in the anterior chamber, a cyclitic or retrolenticular membrane, and complicated cataracts (Fig. 17.58). When the cyclitic membrane contracts, the pars plana and anterior choroid detach. The final result is ciliary body atrophy and fibrosis, which leads to phthisis bulbi.

Choroiditis produces an inflammatory exudate and cells. If the disease involves the retina, it too may be destroyed. Healing produces choroidal fibrosis, adhesions, and pigment proliferation, with white scleral patches surrounded by pigment clumps.

Toxoplasmosis is a major cause of posterior retinochoroiditis (Fig. 17.59), while Still disease, herpes simplex, and sarcoid are more prevalent in anterior uveitis. Half of childhood uveitis is of undetermined etiology. Other diseases include tuberculosis; other viral, fungal, and bacterial entities; lens-induced uveitis; and sympathetic ophthalmia following ocular trauma to the ciliary body.

Pars planitis, or peripheral uveitis, is a common type of juvenile uveitis. It starts between 6 and 10 years of age as a mild chronic cyclitis and smolders for many years. Some patients develop choroidal and retinal detachment or proceed to occlusion of the central retinal vein. A massive gray-yellow exudate which gradually becomes vascularized covers the inferior ora serrata.

Cataract

Cataract, an opacification of the crystalline lens, is derived from genetic, chromosomal, inflammatory, toxic, or syndrome-related affectations of one or both lenses from birth through childhood. In addition to opacification, subluxation or dislocation of the lens also occurs. Cataracts arising in early childhood are frequently associated with nystagmus, lending a poor visual prognosis. Early recognition and treatment is therefore mandatory. The onset of unilateral cataracts is associated with strabismus and severe deprivation amblyopia, microphthalmia, and anomalies of the trabecular meshwork producing glaucoma.

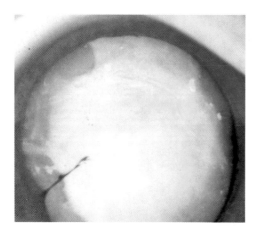

FIG. 17.60 Total cataract with no visible fundus details.

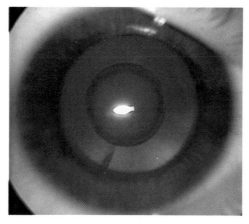

FIG. 17.61 Lamellar cataract with riders, surrounded by a clear cortex.

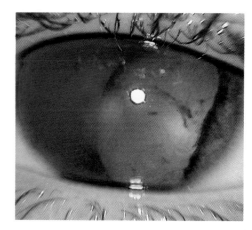

FIG. 17.62 A traumatic, dislocated cataractous lens.

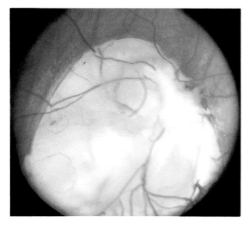

FIG. 17.63 Coloboma of optic nerve, retina, and choroid. Yellow-white sclera is visible, and retinal vessels can be seen coursing through the coloboma.

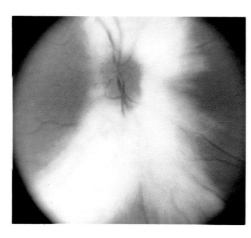

FIG. 17.64 Myelinated nerve fibers adjacent to the optic nerve.

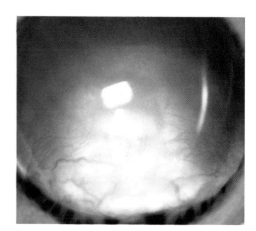

FIG. 17.65 Persistent hyperplastic primary vitreous presenting as a dense fibrovascular retrolental mass with microspherophakia, microphthalmia, and elongated inferior ciliary processes.

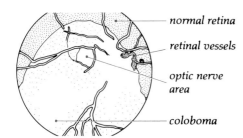

normal retina
retinal vessels
optic nerve area
coloboma

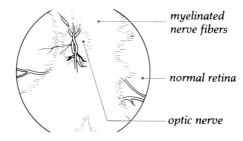

myelinated nerve fibers
normal retina
optic nerve

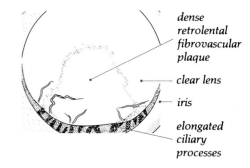

dense retrolental fibrovascular plaque
clear lens
iris
elongated ciliary processes

Total or complete cataracts (Fig. 17.60) are those in which no fundus details are present; partial or incomplete cataracts are smaller or less dense opacities. Central cataracts distort visual acuity and reduce visual development. Polar cataracts are usually small, are either anterior or posterior, and rarely affect vision. Cortical cataracts are induced by other diseases.

Lamellar or zonular cataracts occur frequently as a fetal insult at a specific time during gestation (Fig. 17.61). They have a normal, transparent, central nucleus, an affected lamellar zone, and a clear outer layer of cortex. Riders or radial extensions are frequently present. These cataracts may be autosomal-dominant, associated with vitamin A or D deficiency, or follow hypocalcemic episodes.

Rubella cataracts, characteristic opacifications of the nucleus with cortical liquefaction, are due to viral invasion of the lens. Infantile cataracts are frequently autosomal-dominant, are occasionally X-linked, and are rarely autosomal-recessive. Many cataracts are associated with a wide variety of systemic diseases which must be investigated.

Traumatic cataracts are associated with contusion or perforating injuries to the globe (Fig. 17.62). The lens capsule may be ruptured and protrude through the wound. Delayed cataracts follow contusion as well as perforating injuries.

Retina

COLOBOMAS

Colobomas of the retina and choroid are due to faulty closure of the fetal fissure within the first month of gestation. They may extend from the optic nerve forward through the ciliary

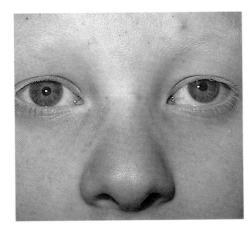

FIG. 17.66 Albinism, characterized by white hair, pale skin, and translucent irides.

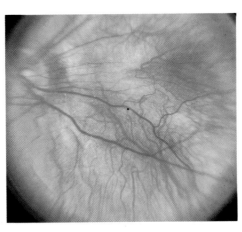

FIG. 17.67 Funduscopic view of a patient with albinism demonstrates a pale fundus, poor macular development, and prominent choroidal vasculature.

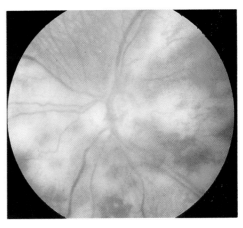

FIG. 17.68 Retinitis, with obvious hemorrhages and perivascular yellow-white exudates secondary to cytomegalic inclusion disease.

body and iris (Fig. 17.63). The coloboma is yellow-white reflecting the scleral base, and its edges are sharply demarcated from the normal retina. There is pigment along the edges, and retinal vessels course over the surface. When the coloboma involves the optic nerve and macula, visual deficits are marked. Colobomas are frequently bilateral, and are associated wtih microphthalmia, nystagmus, and marked visual loss.

MYELINATED NERVE FIBERS
Myelinated nerve fibers are a unilateral developmental defect which appear during the first year of life and remain stationary thereafter. Myelination of the optic nerve starts centrally and continues peripherally until the process reaches the lamina cribrosa at birth, at which time it ceases. Extension beyond the optic nerve produces the retinal phenomenon.

The myelinated fibers are located adjacent to the optic nerve, but some may be found in the temporal retinal periphery (Fig. 17.64). The yellow-white patches completely or partially cover the retinal blood vessels. The peripheral, feathery edges lie within the course of the retinal nerve fibers. Normal vision is usually preserved, and the macula is rarely affected. However, patients with unilateral high myopia as well as myelinated nerve fibers have very reduced vision and depressed electroretinograms.

PERSISTENT HYPERPLASTIC PRIMARY VITREOUS
Persistent hyperplastic primary vitreous is a developmental defect in which the primary vitreous does not involute during the seventh month of gestation (Fig. 17.65). The primary vitreous becomes a fibrovascular mass which extends from the optic disc to the retrolental space. A fibrovascular plaque attaches to the posterior aspect of the lens which then erodes, ruptures the posterior lens capsule, and produces a cataract and intralenticular hemorrhages. Behind the lens, traction may be exerted by the mass upon the peripheral retinal and ciliary processes, which are drawn toward the pupillary space and become elongated. The lens itself is microspherophakic. Retinal complications consist of traction upon the retina with subsequent destruction and distortion of the macular area,

retinal detachment, and optic nerve gliosis with irretrievable visual loss. The disease is progressive, and cataract surgery should be performed early to prevent glaucoma secondary to peripheral anterior synechiae or anterior displacement of the iris-lens diaphragm.

ALBINISM
Albinism, an X-linked trait, is characterized by a congenital deficiency in the pigment of the hair, skin, and eyes which may be partial or total (Fig. 17.66). Absence or deficiency of pigment in the uvea, retina, and retinal pigment epithelium produces photophobia, defective vision, nystagmus, pink pupils, translucent irides, and high refractive errors. The fundus appears orange-red, with the large choroidal blood vessels providing a characteristic background pattern and color. In the periphery, the white scleral background becomes more prominent as the choroidal vessels enlarge. The macula is incompletely developed (Fig. 17.67).

RETINITIS
Inflammations of the retina may be primary, occurring during the course of a systemic disease, or may be secondary as an extension of inflammation in other parts of the eye, particularly the uveal tract.

Primary Retinitis
Primary retinitis originates in the retina, is often bilateral, and may be secondary to bloodborne organisms, the most common being meningococcal meningitis. The disease produces gray, hazy areas with an overlying vitreous haze and retinal hemorrhage (Fig. 17.68). If the disease process continues, endophthalmitis or panaphthalmitis results. The end result is fibrosis, retinal detachment, and phthisis bulbi.

Toxocariasis
Toxocariasis is a roundworm infection, transmitted by dogs, which involves many organs. The eye frequently becomes infected via the retinal arterial circulation. A localized chorioretinal granuloma located in the posterior pole without active visible inflammation is a characteristic feature. Other forms may have severe inflammation with intense vitreous reaction. The process resolves into a white elevated mass, surrounded

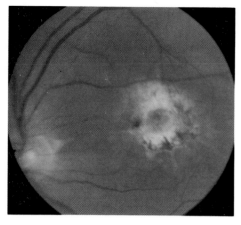

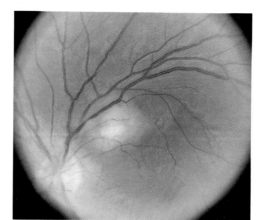

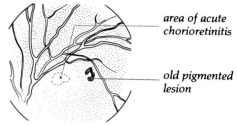

FIG. 17.70 Acute, recurrent, toxoplasmic chorioretinal inflammation adjacent to a healed pigmented lesion.

area of acute chorioretinitis

old pigmented lesion

FIG. 17.69 A retinal toxocariasis lesion appears as a white elevated mass with surrounding pigmentation.

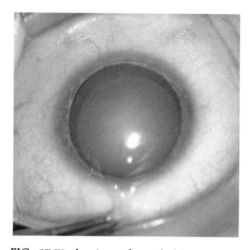

FIG. 17.72 Pigmentary retinopathy in rubella syndrome.

FIG. 17.71 A microspherophakic cataractous lens in rubella syndrome.

with areas of retinal pigmentation and depigmentation (Fig. 17.69). The diagnosis is confirmed by the ELISA titer.

Toxoplasmosis

Toxoplasmosis, a protozoal infestation of the cytoplasm of retinal cells, is, regardless of onset time, most often considered to be congenital in origin. Transplacental infection is the mode of transmission.

A necrotizing neuroretinopathy consisting of focal, circumscribed, yellow lesions associated with a vitreous haze resolves into white or pigmented scar formation (Fig. 17.70). A secondary chronic recurrent diffuse inflammatory process with progressive visual loss also occurs. When severe, congenital involvement induces microphthalmia, posterior uveitis, optic atrophy, nystagmus, strabismus, and visual loss. Bilateral macular enlargment is also characteristic of the congenital form.

Rubella

Rubella, a mild communicable disease of childhood, induces few significant ocular signs other than occasional conjunctivitis. An exposure to rubella virus during pregnancy may result in a chronic intrauterine infection manifested as the congenital rubella syndrome. The ocular findings of congenital rubella syndrome include conjunctival infection, corneal clouding, microcornea, microphthalmia, anterior uveitis, iris atrophy or hypoplasia, nuclear cataract with microsphero-

phakia (Fig. 17.71), pigmentary retinopathy (Fig. 17.72), strabismus, nystagmus, and poor pupillary dilation. Children must be observed throughout life for the development of chronic glaucoma and recurrent uveitis. Rubella retinopathy does not preclude a good visual result.

RETROLENTAL FIBROPLASIA

Retrolental fibroplasia is a bilateral disease of immature retinal vessels seen in premature infants (under 5 pounds birth weight) who were temporarily exposed to high oxygen concentrations during their first days of life. The disease is divided into an active and cicatricial phase. The active phase begins during the third to fifth weeks of life and lasts from 3 to 6 months. It is characterized by retinal neovascularization, vascular changes in the retinal periphery, vitreous hemorrhage, and retinal detachment. Spontaneous regression may occur at any point in the active phase. The cicatricial phase begins at 1 to 2 months of age, and is characterized by retinal pigmentary changes, vitroretinal membranes, high myopia, distortion of the optic disc with pallor, traction of the retinal vessels to the temporal retinal periphery, retinal folds, and incomplete or complete retinal detachment resulting in diminished visual acuity or complete blindness (Fig. 17.73). It may evolve over a prolonged period of time, although it is usually complete during the first year of life.

A funduscopic examination for retrolental fibroplasia is not productive during the course of oxygen therapy, but the

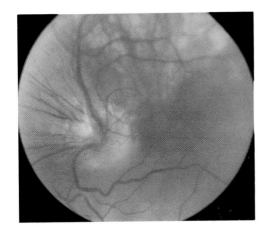

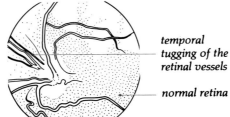

FIG. 17.73 Retrolental fibroplasia with temporal tugging of the disc.

temporal tugging of the retinal vessels

normal retina

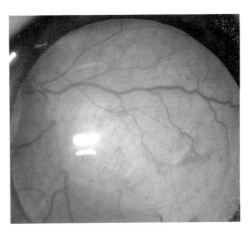

FIG. 17.74 The yellow-white mass characteristic of leukokoria observed in the pupil of a child with retinoblastoma.

FIG. 17.75 Funduscopic manifestations of Coat disease. (Left) A yellow-white slightly elevated exudate covering the macular area. (Right) Peripheral telangiectasis along the course of the retinal veins.

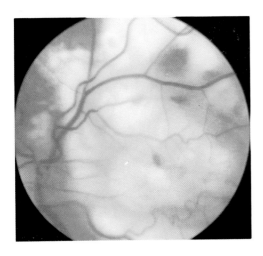

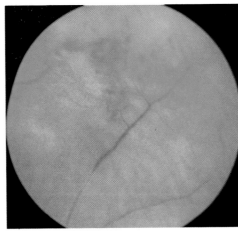

child should be examined at the conclusion of oxygen therapy and prior to discharge from the neonatal intensive care unit. Continued vascular proliferation, retinal hemorrhage, and neovascularization may require one or more of the following treatments: vitamin E therapy, photocoagulation of abnormal retinal vessels that may or do bleed, cryosurgery to coagulate these vessels, retinal detachment surgery and vitrectomy to remove traction membranes in the vitreous body, to prevent retinal detachment, and to clear the visual axis.

RETINOBLASTOMA

Retinoblastoma is a highly malignant tumor arising in one or both retinas of young children, usually under age 2. Somatic mutations or autosomal-dominant genes of high but incomplete penetrance produce this tumor. Retinoblastoma occurs in approximately 1 in 20,000 new births, and is bilateral in 30 percent of patients. Of the unilateral cases, 20 percent are new mutations, a fact proved by transmission of the disease. The remaining 80 percent are somatic mutations. Patients with bilateral disease transmit to their progeny at a 50 percent rate, while patients with unilateral involvement transmit the disease to only 10 percent of their children.

The most common presenting sign of retinoblastoma is leukokoria, a condition characterized by a white reflex in the pupil (Fig. 17.74). The second most common sign is strabismus, due to macular involvement by the tumor. Inflammatory signs of a red, painful eye without glaucoma are rare. Following a quiescent period, the disease metastasizes by various routes, including the optic nerve via the subarachnoid space to the brain, choroidal hematologic dissemination from within the globe, and by direct extension from the globe. Tumor extends outside the globe to the orbit and through the lymphatics to the regional nodes. Untreated tumor is 99 percent fatal, with spontaneous regression occurring in only 1 to 2 percent of patients.

The tumor may present as one or more elevated, round, white or yellow masses. A large lesion may be surrounded by small satellites in the retina or within the vitreous. Normal vessels may enter the mass or pass over it. The retina may be elevated, producing a retinal detachment, or the tumor may grow within the anterior or inner layers of the retina. Vitreous seeds occur, and these may deposit on the iris or cornea. The pupil may become enlarged. The inflammatory reaction may become acute, with both iritis and ciliary and conjunctival injection. Glaucoma may occur secondarily. Hemorrhages are rare.

COAT DISEASE

Coat disease is a congenital retinal vascular abnormality, characterized by peripheral telangiectasia with transudation of fluid from the anomalous vessels producing a unilateral, insidious, painless loss of vision in children. Funduscopy reveals an elevated yellow-white mass over the macula, and peripheral telangiectatic dilations of the retinal veins can be observed (Fig. 17.75). A serous retinal detachment may develop, and visual loss may be profound if left untreated.

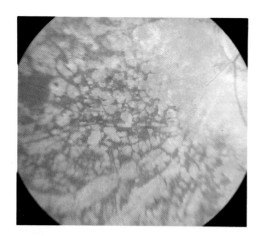

FIG. 17.76 Retinitis pigmentosa, characterized by retinal pigment deposition, narrow arterioles, and a pale disc.

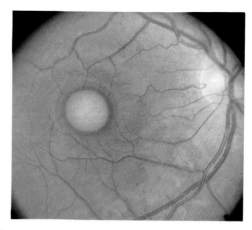

FIG. 17.77 Vitelliform macular degeneration manifests in its early phase as a sharply demarcated, homogeneous, yellow macular lesion.

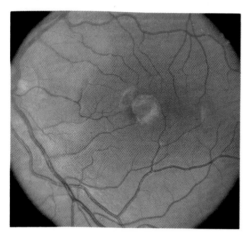

FIG. 17.78 This late vitelliform lesion shows pigmentation of the macula. Visual loss occurs in this stage.

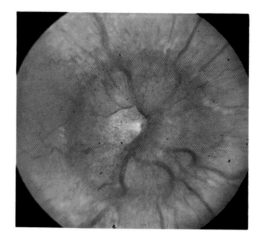

FIG. 17.79 Acute papilledema, characterized by blurred disc edges, an absent physiologic cup, and enlarged, tortuous vessels.

RETINITIS PIGMENTOSA

Retinitis pigmentosa is an inherited progressive disease of the retina, characterized by night blindness, depressed or extinct electroretinograms, and early involvement with the retinal pigment epithelium which leads to severe visual loss or blindness. The symptoms become apparent during the second decade of life, but may be present in childhood. Night blindness is the earliest symptom, followed by a progressive loss of the peripheral visual fields. Color vision and, occasionally, central vision deteriorate early.

Morphologic changes observed in the fundus depend upon genetic predisposition. The optic nerve is characteristically pale, the arteries are attenuated, depigmentation of the pigment epithelium occurs, and fine pigment stippling characterized by bone corpuscular figures is deposited in the periphery (Fig. 17.76). The choriocapillaris disappears, and there is a later loss of larger choroidal vessels. Cataracts are also a late complication.

VITELLIFORM MACULAR DEGENERATION

Vitelliform macular degeneration, or Best disease, is characterized by a sharply defined, discoid, yellow mass lesion in the macula, 1.5 to 4.0 disc diameters in size (Fig. 17.77). There are no blood vessels over the lesion. The abnormality is subretinal, and has its onset between ages 5 and 15. It is autosomal-dominant with decreased penetrance, bilateral, and slowly progressive. Later in the disease, the homogeneous vitelliform lesion becomes fragmented, leaving an area of pigmentation or chorioretinal atrophy (Fig. 17.78). Visual loss occurs at this point.

Stargardt disease is a slowly progressive, autosomal-recessive condition which manifests between ages 8 and 14 and is associated with macular degeneration. The foveal reflex is absent, pigment spots develop and accumulate irregularly, and vision is decreased centrally.

Optic Nerve

PAPILLEDEMA

Papilledema is due to congestion of the optic nerve head secondary to increased intracranial pressure. Initially, visual acuity is normal or there may be a history of intermittent blurring of vision. Visual fields show only an enlarged blind spot, with papulomacular bundle involvement and central or cecocentral scotomas. Late nasal field defects combined with an enlargement of the blind spot occur, or other field defects based upon intracranial pathology become evident.

The characteristic ophthalmoscopic signs vary from slight blurring of the disc margin to measurable disc edema. The physiologic cup is filled early, and hyperemia of the disc occurs with lack of venous pulsations. Late splinter hemorrhages and exudates surround the disc and extend toward the macula to form a star figure. Concentric folds in the retina surround the optic disc (Fig. 17.79).

Acquired papilledema may be secondary to trauma, vascular and infectious disease, tumor expansion, or of toxic origin. Trauma includes subdural and subarachnoid hematomas. Vascular etiologies include hypertension, leukemia, and hydrocephalus. Infections may be due to cerebral abscess or meningitis. Tumors create expanding intracranial lesions. Papilledema of toxic origin may be induced by dexamethasone, tetracycline, chloramphenicol, or vitamin A.

Pseudopapilledema is marked by anomalous optic disc elevations unaccompanied by vision changes, hemorrhages,

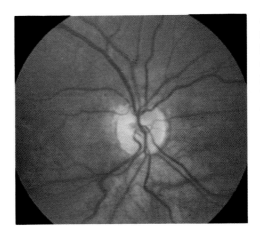

FIG. 17.80 Optic atrophy, characterized by a sharply demarcated, pale yellow-white disc, with an absence of small vessels and disc substance.

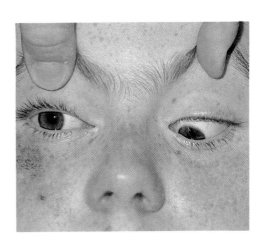

FIG. 17.81 Blowout fracture of the right orbit leading to the inability to depress the right eye.

edema, venous congestion, or exudates (see Fig. 17.3). Blind spot size appears normal on field examination, and appearance does not change from year to year, in contrast to the clinical findings in papilledema.

OPTIC ATROPHY

Optic atrophy is the partial or complete loss of small vessels over the surface of the optic nerve, creating a white or yellow-white color in these areas and indicating a permanent loss of part or all of the functions of the nerve (Fig. 17.80). The clinical signs are loss of visual acuity and a visual field defect. Optic atrophy is a difficult diagnosis to substantiate in the first 6 months of life due to the continued presence of excessive glial tissue on the optic nerve surface. With growth, resolution of this tissue takes place, and the optic nerve assumes a more normal-appearing color and configuration. At this point, the onset of atrophy becomes visually apparent, allowing for more easy diagnosis.

Optic atrophy is associated with diseases of the retina, demyelinating diseases, inflammations of the nerve, congenital and traumatic lesions, hereditary defects, blood dyscrasia, and metabolic disorders.

Cavernous optic atrophy, a marked loss of the nerve substance, occurs with advanced glaucoma and postintraorbital and intracranial lesions. Children have the ability to regenerate the structure of the optic nerve if the intraocular pressure is normalized before a permanent loss of tissue occurs.

Orbit

The primary manifestation of orbital disease is exophthalmos. Diseases of the orbit may be unilateral or bilateral, slowly or rapidly progressive, inflammatory or noninflammatory, and related to malignant or benign masses. Ocular motility may be restricted, and visual fields may be affected. The fundus may show optic nerve venous congestion, refractive changes, papilledema, or retinal striae. Bony invasion may be demonstrated radiographically.

If the eye is absent or markedly microphthalmic, its orbit may be smaller than that of the other eye since ocular development induces orbital development. Therefore, insertion of an orbital implant results in less contraction of an anophthalmic orbit. Radiologic therapy to the orbit may induce bony orbital changes and late sarcomas. Enucleation in infants is seldom recommended, except in patients with retinoblastoma.

Tumors of the orbit consist mainly of cavernous or capillary hemangiomas, though aneurysms and arteriovenous malformations sometimes occur. Malignant tumors of the orbit are uncommon, with rhabdomyosarcoma the most frequent. The most common metastatic lesion is neuroblastoma, which occurs bilaterally with proptosis and chemosis of the skin of the lids.

Trauma

Ocular or adnexal trauma results from contusions, concussion, perforations, or lacerations.

Blowout fractures of the orbit are caused by round objects striking the orbital rim, increasing the hydrostatic pressure of the orbital contents, and rupturing of the weakest wall of the orbit, usually the inferior or medial wall (Fig. 17.81). Entrapment of the inferior rectus muscle within the bony floor resulting in an inability of the patient to elevate the eye is a common complication.

BIBLIOGRAPHY

Harley RD (ed): Pediatric Ophthalmology, 2nd ed. Saunders, Philadelphia, 1983.

Helveston EM, Ellis FD: Pediatric Ophthalmology Practice. Mosby, St. Louis, 1980.

Metz HS, Rosenbaum AL: Pediatric Ophthalmology. Medical Outline Series. Medical Examination Publishing Co., Garden City, New York, 1982.

Von Noorden GK: Binocular Vision and Ocular Motility. Mosby, St. Louis, 1980.

Von Noorden GK: Von Noorden's-Maumanee's Atlas of Strabismus. Mosby, St. Louis, 1977.

ORAL DISORDERS

M. M. Nazif, D.D.S.
Mary Ann Ready, D.M.D.

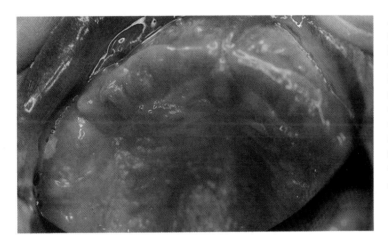

FIG. 18.1 Normal oral cavity in the newborn. Extension of the maxillary labial frenulum across the midline of the alveolar ridge and the flat-appearing posterior alveolar ridge with an anteroposterior groove are evident.

NORMAL ORAL STRUCTURES

The oral cavity, including the teeth, gingivae, and periodontal ligament, is in a constant state of evolution during infancy and childhood. From the early teething stage, through the eruption and exfoliation of the primary dentition, and finally to the eruption of all permanent teeth, the oral cavity provides one of the most visible signs of development.

Normal Oral Cavity in the Newborn

The lips of an infant reveal a prominent line of demarcation at the vermilion border. The mucosa may look wrinkled and slightly purple at birth, but within a few days exhibits a dryer appearance, with the outer layer forming crusty "sucking calluses." This callus formation affects the central portion of the mucosa and persists for only a few weeks.

The maxillary alveolar ridge is separated from the lip by a shallow sulcus. In the midline, the labial frenulum extends posteriorly across the alveolar ridge to the palatine incisive papilla. Two lateral miniature frenula are also evident. The alveolar ridge peaks anteriorly and gradually flattens as the ridge extends posteriorly, forming a pseudoalveolar groove medial to the ridge along its palatal side (Fig. 18.1). This flattened appearance is seen in young infants, and gradually

disappears with the growth of the alveolar process and the formation and calcification of posterior tooth buds. The mandibular alveolar ridges also peak anteriorly and flatten posteriorly. The mandibular labial frenulum connects the lower lip to the labial aspect of the alveolar ridge. Careful visual inspection and palpation of the ridges should confirm the presence and location of tooth buds. Anterior tooth buds are located on the labial side of the alveolar ridges, while posterior tooth buds are often located closer to the crests of the alveolar ridges. Palatal morphology and color are variable. The tongue and the floor of the mouth differ only slightly from those of older children.

Normal Primary Dentition

Development of the alveolar bone is directly related to the formation and eruption of teeth, and normal patterns of dental development occur symmetrically. At approximately 6 months of age, the mandibular central incisors erupt. This stage is often preceded by a period of increased salivation, local gingival irritation, and irritability. These symptoms may vary in intensity and usually subside when the last primary tooth erupts into the oral cavity. Other symptoms such as fever or diarrhea have never been proven to be directly related to teething. The lower incisors are soon followed by the max-

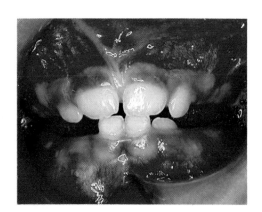

FIG. 18.2 Early primary dentition. The mandibular and maxillary central and lateral incisors are the first to erupt.

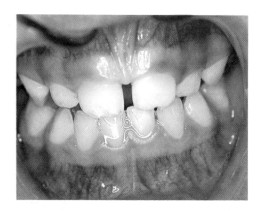

FIG. 18.3 Full primary dentition. By age 2½, all 20 primary teeth have erupted.

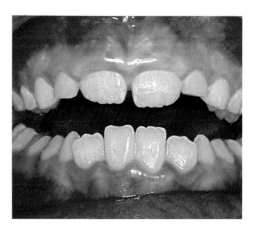

FIG. 18.4 Mixed dentition. This transitional stage from primary to permanent dentition begins at age 6 and lasts for about 6 years.

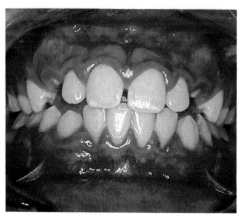

FIG. 18.5 The earliest stage of permanent dentition begins with the eruption of the 6-year molars and central incisors. The cuspids and second molars are the last to erupt.

illary central incisors and the maxillary and mandibular lateral incisors (Fig. 18.2). By the end of the first year, all eight anterior teeth are usually visible. At 2 years, all primary teeth have erupted with the exception of the second primary molars which erupt shortly thereafter. By the age of 3 years, the primary dentition is fully present and functional (Fig. 18.3).

Any variation in the time and sequence of eruption in an otherwise normal infant may call for early dental referral. In most instances, careful observation is the best course of action. For instance, delayed eruption of primary teeth for up to 8 months is occasionally observed and is considered a normal variation. Rarely, retarded eruption is associated with Down syndrome, hypothyroidism, hypopituitarism, achondroplastic dwarfism, osteopetrosis, rickets, or chondroectodermal dysplasia. A significant variation affecting a single tooth or only a few teeth should also be carefully investigated.

Spacing during this stage is normal and desirable, and often indicates that more space is available for the larger permanent teeth. The completed primary dentition establishes a baseline which dictates to a great extent the future alignment of permanent teeth and the future relationship between the maxillary and mandibular arches.

During most of the primary dentition stage, the gingiva appears pink, firm, and not readily retractable. A well-defined zone of firmly attached keratinized gingiva is present, extending from the bottom of the gingival sulcus to the junction of the alveolar mucosa. Rarely, local irritation may develop into acute or subacute pericoronitis, with elevated temperature and associated lymphadenopathy. Treatment may require topical and/or systemic therapy; however, lancing the gingiva to relieve such symptoms is not usually indicated.

Normal Mixed Dentition

This stage of development begins with the eruption of the first permanent molars at about 6 years of age and continues for approximately 6 years. During this period, the following teeth erupt from the gums in this sequence: the mandibular central incisors, the maxillary central incisors, the mandibular lateral incisors, the maxillary lateral incisors, the mandibular cuspids, the maxillary and mandibular first premolars, the maxillary and mandibular second premolars, the maxillary cuspids, and the mandibular and maxillary second molars (Fig. 18.4).

The dentition during this stage undergoes certain physiologic changes including resorption and exfoliation of primary teeth, eruption of their successors, and eruption of the posterior permanent teeth. Minor complications may occur during resorption and exfoliation of primary teeth and eruption of permanent teeth. Gingival irritation is often associated with increased mobility of primary teeth, but usually disappears spontaneously when the tooth is lost or extracted. Two transient deviations of eruption pattern may occur: the mandibular incisors may erupt in a lingual position behind the primary incisors ("double teeth"), and the maxillary incisors may assume a widely spaced and labially inclined position ("ugly duckling" stage).

Normal Early Permanent Dentition

This stage marks the beginning of a relatively quiescent period in dental development. Activities are limited to root formation of a few permanent teeth and the calcification of the third molars. By this time the length and width of the dental arches are well-established (Fig. 18.5); however, the jaws will undergo a major growth spurt during puberty which will alter their sizes and relative position. The gingiva begins to assume adult characteristics, becoming firm, pink in color, with an uneven, stippled surface texture and a thin gingival margin. Puberty is occasionally associated with gingivitis secondary to hormonal changes, necessitating good oral hygiene for control.

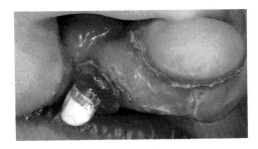

FIG. 18.6 A natal tooth associated with cleft palate. Extraction is only necessary if it is of abnormal morphology or causes feeding difficulties.

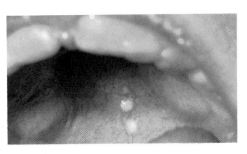

FIG. 18.7 Gingival cysts. The small, whitish cystic lesions along the midpalatine raphe are called Epstein pearls.

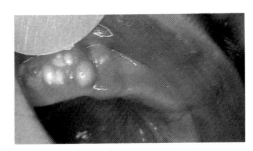

FIG. 18.8 Gingival cysts. The firm, grayish white mucous gland cysts on the buccal aspect of the alveolar ridges are called Bohn nodules.

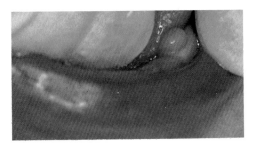

FIG. 18.9 Dental lamina cyst. The cysts are found on the alveolar ridge and usually occur singly.

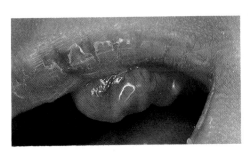

FIG. 18.10 Congenital epulis. This 4-day-old patient presented with a benign tumor of the anterior maxilla which affected both jaws.

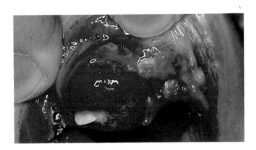

FIG. 18.11 Melanotic neuroectodermal tumor. This benign but locally aggressive tumor of the anterior maxilla has produced elevation of the lip and displaced a primary tooth.

NATAL AND NEONATAL ABNORMALITIES

Natal and Neonatal Teeth

Teeth which are present in the oral cavity at birth are called natal teeth, while those erupting during the neonatal period are called neonatal teeth. The incidence of natal teeth has been reported to be approximately 1 in 2000 births. Though seen in normal infants, this anomaly is more frequent in patients with cleft palate (Fig. 18.6) and is often associated with the following syndromes: Ellis-van Creveld, Hallermann-Streiff, and pachyonychia congenita. The vast majority of such teeth are true primary teeth, but occasionally they are supernumerary. Some are abnormal, with either hypoplastic defects or poor crown or root development. Natal teeth may cause feeding problems for both the infant and mother. Ulceration of the ventral surface of the tongue by sharp tooth edges (Riga-Fede disease) may develop if natal teeth remain in the oral cavity. This condition is usually transient, but in persistent cases appropriate reduction of incisal edges or other symptomatic treatment may be indicated. Most normal-appearing natal teeth can be retained, but those that are supernumerary, abnormal, or loose should be removed.

Gingival Cysts in the Newborn

Gingival cysts of the oral cavity are small, single or multiple superficial lesions which are formed by trapped tissues during embryologic growth and occur in about 80 percent of newborn infants. They are asymptomatic, do not enlarge, seldom interfere with feeding, and exfoliate within a few weeks.

Three types of cysts exist:
1. Epstein pearls are keratin-filled cystic lesions lined with stratified squamous epithelium. They appear as small, whitish lesions along the midpalatine raphe and contain no mucous glands (Fig. 18.7).
2. Bohn nodules are mucous gland cysts, often found on the buccal or lingual aspects of the alveolar ridges and, occasionally, on the palate. They are multiple, firm, and grayish white in appearance. Histologically, they show mucous glands and ducts (Fig. 18.8).
3. Dental lamina cysts are found only on the crest of the alveolar mucosa. Histologically, these lesions are different since they are formed by remnants of dental lamina epithelium. They may be larger, more lucent, and fluctuant than Epstein pearls or Bohn nodules, and are more likely to occur singly (Fig. 18.9).

Congenital Epulis in the Newborn

This benign, soft-tissue tumor is seen on the alveolar mucosa at birth or shortly after. It is usually found on the anterior maxilla as a pedunculated swelling (Fig. 18.10), but may appear on the mandible or occasionally on both jaws. The mass is firm on palpation, and the overlying mucosa appears normal. Histologically, sheets of large granular cells are seen. Differential diagnosis should include rhabdomyoma and melanotic neuroectodermal tumor of infancy. The lesion is amenable to conservative surgical excision, and recurrence is infrequent.

Melanotic Neuroectodermal Tumor of Infancy

This benign yet aggressive tumor occurs during the first year of life, and is often found on the anterior maxilla in association with unerupted or erupted teeth. It often bulges and destroys the alveolar bone, thus displacing the associated primary tooth (Fig. 18.11). The tumor mass is grayish blue, firm on palpation, and spherical in shape. Careful surgical removal is effective, and recurrence is unusual.

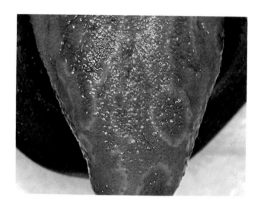

FIG. 18.12 Geographic tongue. This condition is marked by inflamed, irregularly shaped lesions on the dorsum of the tongue which give a migrating appearance.

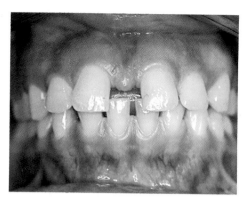

FIG. 18.13 Diastema. Rarely, the maxillary frenulum persists and contributes to excessive spacing between the maxillary central incisors in the permanent dentition.

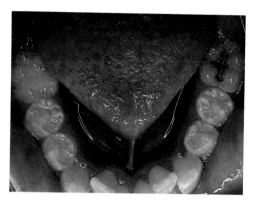

FIG. 18.14 Ankyloglossia. A shortened lingual frenulum is seen attached to the tongue near the tip. This condition rarely interferes with function and therefore does not require treatment.

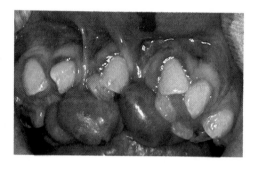

FIG. 18.15 Multiple hyperplastic frenula are seen in this patient with orofaciodigital syndrome. These frenula interfered with the eruption of teeth, causing rotations and crowding.

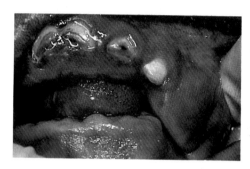

FIG. 18.16 Phenytoin-induced gingival overgrowth. The firm hyperplastic gingival tissues have completely covered the posterior teeth and are interfering with mastication.

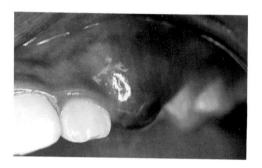

FIG. 18.17 Eruption hematoma. A bluish, fluid-filled fluctuant swelling can be seen over the crown of an erupting maxillary cuspid. The lesion resolved without treatment when the tooth erupted.

DEVELOPMENTAL ABNORMALITIES
Soft-Tissue Abnormalities

GEOGRAPHIC TONGUE
(BENIGN MIGRATORY GLOSSITIS)

This painless condition is characterized by inflamed, irregularly shaped areas on the dorsum of the tongue which are void of filiform papillae. Lesions are red, slightly depressed, and bordered by a whitish band (Fig. 18.12). Spontaneous healing followed by the formation of similar lesions elsewhere on the tongue results in a migrating appearance. Etiology is unknown; however, strong association with stress and allergies is suspected. Although benign, the course of this disorder may be prolonged for months, and it may recur.

ABNORMALITIES OF THE FRENULUM

During embryonic life, the maxillary labial frenulum extends as a band of tissue from the upper lip over and across the alveolar ridge and into the incisive (palatine) papilla. Postnatally, as the alveolar process increases in size, the labial frenulum separates from the incisive papilla and becomes relatively smaller. With the eruption of primary and later permanent teeth, the frenulum attachment moves apically and further atrophies as a result of vertical growth of the alveolar process. The developmental gap (diastema) between the maxillary central incisors tends to close with the full eruption of the maxillary permanent canines. The mandibular midline frenulum only rarely maintains a lingual extension and therefore only rarely causes a diastema between the mandibular central incisors (Fig. 18.13).

The lingual frenulum extends almost to the tip of the tongue in early infancy and then gradually recedes. Occasionally, ankyloglossia (tongue tie) is seen, but is rarely associated with feeding or speech difficulties (Fig. 18.14). Various surgical procedures have been advocated to correct this condition. In general, frenectomy is seldom indicated and should be recommended only after appropriate justification. Congenital anomalies may include an enlarged frenulum, labiolingual frenulum extensions, or supernumerary frenula as seen in orofaciodigital syndrome (Fig. 18.15).

PHENYTOIN-INDUCED GINGIVAL OVERGROWTH
(DILANTIN HYPERPLASIA)

Dilantin administration may result in the formation of a firm, hyperplastic gingival overgrowth in certain patients (Fig. 18.16). The gingiva may become inflamed, edematous, and boggy especially if proper oral hygiene is not practiced; therefore, dental referral at the onset of dilantin therapy is appropriate. As hyperplasia tends to recur following surgical excision, gingivectomy is reserved for those patients whose overgrowth interferes with function and for those whose therapy has been discontinued.

ERUPTION CYSTS (ERUPTION HEMATOMA)

An eruption cyst is a fluid-filled swelling over the crown of an erupting tooth. When the follicle is dilated with blood, the lesion takes on a bluish color and is termed an eruption hema-

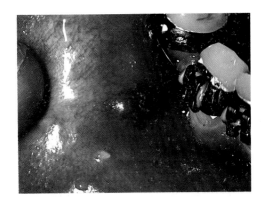

FIG. 18.18 Mucocele. These translucent, fluid-filled lesions resulted from trauma to minor salivary glands of the lower lip.

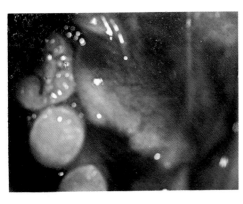

FIG. 18.19 Ranula. This bluish, fluctuant swelling in the floor of the mouth is a retention cyst associated with trauma to a salivary duct.

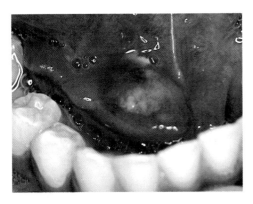

FIG. 18.20 Salivary calculus. This sialolith obstructing a salivary duct is observed in the floor of the mouth.

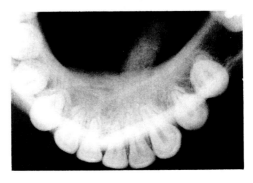

FIG. 18.21 A dental radiograph of the sublingual space reveals the size and location of the salivary calculus.

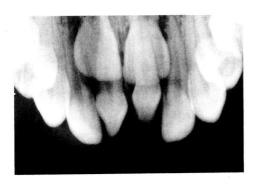

FIG. 18.22 Hyperdontia. Radiograph reveals supernumerary teeth in the anterior midline of the palate. These teeth blocked the permanent central incisors and required surgical treatment.

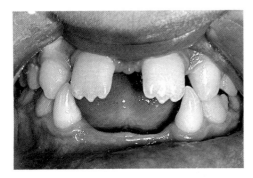

FIG. 18.23 Hypodontia. The congenital absence of teeth is seen in this patient with hereditary ectodermal dysplasia. This phenomenon may be an isolated anomaly or a manifestation of several syndromes.

toma (Fig. 18.17). Although the eruption cyst is a superficial form of dentigerous cyst, it rarely impedes eruption, and surgical exposure of the crown is seldom necessary.

MUCOCELE AND RANULA

A mucocele is a painless translucent or bluish lesion of traumatic origin, most often involving minor salivary glands of the lower lip (Fig. 18.18). The lesion may alternately enlarge and shrink. The treatment of choice is surgical excision of the lesion and the associated minor salivary gland.

A simple ranula is a retention cyst in the floor of the mouth which is confined to sublingual tissues superior to the mylohyoid muscle. It appears clinically as a bluish, transparent, thin-walled fluctuant swelling (Fig. 18.19). Herniation of the ranula through the mylohyoid muscle results in a cervical or plunging ranula which becomes more apparent in the oral cavity with the muscle contraction associated with jaw opening. Simple excision and drainage of the ranula is not an acceptable treatment since healing is followed by recurrence. Marsupialization by suturing the edges of the opened cystic wall to the mucous membrane is the recommended treatment. The plunging ranula must be removed in its entirety along with the associated salivary gland to avoid recurrence.

SALIVARY CALCULUS (SIALOLITHIASIS)

Formation of a salivary calculus is rare in the pediatric population, but when it does occur it may affect either Wharton's or Stenson's duct (Fig. 18.20). Partial obstruction of the duct results in pain and enlargement of the gland, especially at mealtime. While palpation of the stone may be possible, dental radiographs confirm the diagnosis and give appropriate information about its size and location (Fig. 18.21). Larger salivary stones wedged within the ducts may cause localized irritation and secondary infection. If the calculus cannot be milked from the duct, surgical intervention may be necessary.

Hard-Tissue Abnormalities

HYPER- AND HYPODONTIA

Variations in tooth number include both hyper- and hypodontia. Supernumerary teeth occur in about 3 percent of the normal population, but patients with cleft lip and/or cleft palate and cleidocranial dysostosis have a significantly higher incidence. The most common site is the anterior palate (Fig. 18.22). Supernumerary teeth may have the size and morphology of adjacent teeth or may be small and atypical in shape. They may erupt spontaneously or remain impacted. Early consideration of removal is justified due to complications such as impeded eruption, crowding, or resorption of permanent teeth; cystic changes; or ectopic eruption into the nasal cavity, the maxillary sinus, or other sites.

Congenital absence of teeth is more often seen in the permanent dentition than in the primary. Most frequently missing are third molars, second premolars, and lateral incisors. Hypodontia is frequently associated with several ectodermal syndromes such as anhidrotic ectodermal dysplasia and chondroectodermal dysplasia (Fig. 18.23).

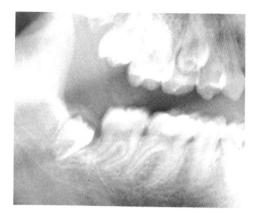

FIG. 18.24 A microdont can be seen on this panoramic radiograph near the second molar. Microdonts are often seen in the maxillary lateral incisor region.

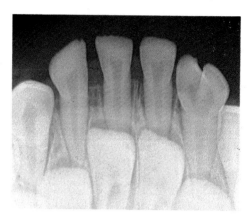

FIG. 18.25 Radiograph demonstrates gemination (twinning), the incomplete division of a tooth bud resulting in a tooth with a large notched crown and a single root.

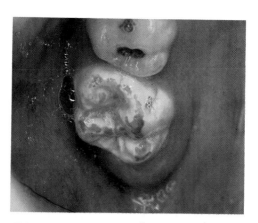

FIG. 18.26 Hypocalcification. This 6-year-old patient exhibits early signs of hypocalcification of his permanent molars. Chalky white spots indicate poor calcification of the enamel.

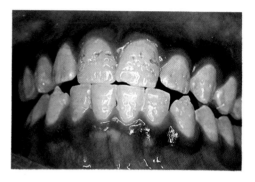

FIG. 18.27 Amelogenesis imperfecta, hypoplastic type. This process results in generalized pitting of the enamel.

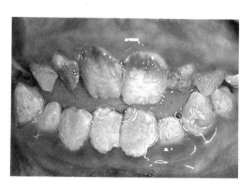

FIG. 18.28 Amelogenesis imperfecta, hypocalcified type. The enamel defects result in discoloration and erosion due to errors in the mineralization stage of tooth development and secondary staining.

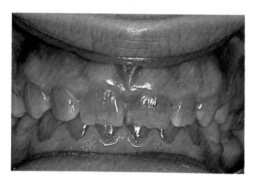

FIG. 18.29 Dentinogenesis imperfecta. The bluish opalescent sheen on several of these teeth results from genetically defective dentin. This condition may be associated with osteogenesis imperfecta.

ALTERATION IN SIZE AND SHAPE

Teeth which are smaller or larger than normal are termed microdonts and macrodonts, respectively. These teeth are genetic anomalies. It is remarkable when a discrepancy in tooth size and dental arch length results in severe crowding or spacing of the teeth. Size abnormalities are often localized to one tooth or to a very small group of teeth (Fig. 18.24).

Variations in shape also result from the joining of teeth or tooth buds. Fusion is the joining of two tooth buds by the dentin. Concrescence is the joining of the roots of two or more teeth by cementum. Gemination (twinning) results from the incomplete division of one tooth bud, resulting in a large crown with a notched incisal edge and a single root (Fig. 18.25).

HYPOPLASIA AND HYPOCALCIFICATION

Numerous local and systemic insults are capable of causing the enamel defects of hypoplasia and hypocalcification. The most common etiologic factors are local infections such as an abscessed primary tooth, systemic infections with associated high fever, trauma such as intrusion of the primary tooth, and chemical injury such as that due to excessive ingestion of fluoride. Other etiologic factors are nutritional deficiencies, allergies, rubella, cerebral palsy, embryopathy, prematurity, and irradiation. Hypoplasia results from an insult during active matrix formation of the enamel, and clinically manifests as pitting, furrowing, or thinning of the enamel (see Fig. 18.27). Hypocalcification results from an insult during mineralization of the tooth, and is seen as opaque, chalky, or white lesions (Fig. 18.26).

HERITABLE DEFECTS OF ENAMEL AND DENTIN

Amelogenesis imperfecta is the term used to describe a group of genetically determined defects which involve the enamel of primary and permanent teeth without affecting dentin, pulp, or cementum. While the types of amelogenesis imperfecta are numerous, the major defect in each is hypoplasia, hypomaturation, or hypocalcification. The hypoplastic type results in thin, pitted, or fissured enamel (Fig. 18.27). Hypomaturation manifests as discolored enamel of full thickness but decreased hardness which tends to chip away slowly, exposing underlying dentin. Radiographic evaluation will demonstrate the decreased density of enamel. Hypocalcified enamel is chalky, variable in color, and quickly erodes away (Fig. 18.28). For all types of amelogenesis imperfecta, inheritance may be autosomal-dominant, autosomal-recessive, or X-linked.

Dentinogenesis imperfecta results in dentin defects, and is usually inherited as an autosomal-dominant trait. The most common manifestation is opalescent dentin, which may be associated with osteogenesis imperfecta. The teeth are blue to pinkish brown in color and have an opalescent sheen (Fig. 18.29). Despite normal enamel morphology, there is rapid attrition of the crowns. The roots are shortened and the pulp cavities are calcified. Primary teeth are more severely affected than the permanent.

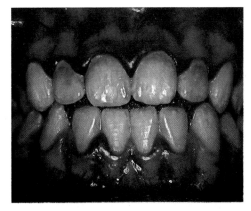

FIG. 18.30 Extrinsic discoloration. The green stain seen on the gingival third of the incisors is associated with poor oral hygiene.

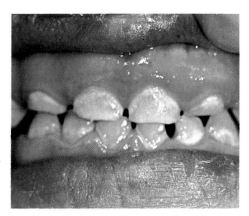

FIG. 18.31 Hepatic discoloration. Generalized intrinsic discoloration of the primary teeth is seen in this patient with biliary atresia.

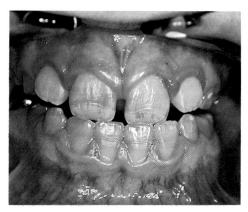

FIG. 18.32 Tetracycline discoloration. The severe discoloration seen in this patient is due to tetracycline administration during calcification of the permanent teeth.

DISCOLORATION

Two major types of tooth discoloration are frequently observed: (1) discoloration from stains that adhere externally to the surfaces of the teeth (extrinsic), and (2) discoloration from various pigments that are incorporated into the tooth structure during development (intrinsic).

Extrinsic Discoloration

Extrinsic discoloration is primarily limited to patients with poor oral hygiene, those on certain medications, those who heavily consume stain-containing foods or drinks, or those who smoke or chew tobacco or other substances. It occurs more often at certain locations, especially on the gingival third of the exposed crown and on a limited number of teeth. Diagnosis requires appropriate medical, dental, and dietary histories with emphasis on oral hygiene, food and drug intake, and smoking habits. Treatment includes scaling, dental prophylaxis and polishing, avoidance of abrasive toothpastes, and the practice of regular oral hygiene.

Brown/black stain on the lingual surfaces of anterior as well as posterior teeth is most common among smokers and tea drinkers. Green stain on the labial surfaces of the anterior maxillary teeth is common among children with poor oral hygiene. The source is usually chromogenic bacteria and fungi (Fig. 18.30). Orange/red stain is unusual, but when it does occur it can be found around the gingival third of the exposed crown. This stain often results from antibiotic intake which causes a temporary shift in the oral flora.

Intrinsic Discoloration

Intrinsic discoloration is usually induced during the calcification of dentin and enamel by the body's natural pigments such as hemoglobin and bile or by pigments introduced by the intake of chemicals such as fluorides or tetracyclines. Occasionally, *isolated* intrinsic discoloration takes place as a result of pulpal necrosis, pulpal calcification, or internal resorption.

HEPATIC DISCOLORATION

Generalized intrinsic discoloration of primary teeth is seen in patients with advanced hepatic diseases associated with persistent or recurrent jaundice and hyperbilirubinemia (Fig. 18.31). The intensity of the discoloration varies and may be somewhat related to the intensity of the hepatic disorder. The color ranges from brown to grayish brown and usually has no clinical significance unless it is associated with significant hypoplasia of the dentition.

TETRACYCLINE DISCOLORATION

Teeth stained as a result of tetracycline therapy may vary in color from yellow to brown to dark gray. Staining occurs when the tetracycline is incorporated into calcifying teeth and bone. Both the enamel and, to a greater degree, the dentin which are calcifying at the time of intake incorporate tetracycline into their chemical structures. The severity of discoloration depends upon the dose, duration, and type of tetracycline administered. The initial yellow or light brown pigmentation tends to darken with age (Fig. 18.32). Tetracyclines readily cross the placenta, so staining of primary teeth is possible if tetracycline is taken during pregnancy. Therefore, tetracycline should not be prescribed to pregnant women and to children under 10 years of age.

ERYTHROBLASTOSIS FETALIS

Children born with congenital hemolytic anemia due to Rh incompatibility may exhibit distinct discoloration of their primary teeth due to the deposition of bilirubin in the dentin and enamel during primary tooth development. The color ranges from green to blue to orange. No treatment is usually indicated unless discoloration is associated with significant hypoplasia or hypocalcification. The permanent dentition is usually not affected.

PORPHYRIA

This hereditary disturbance of porphyrin metabolism may produce a reddish or brownish discoloration of the primary and permanent teeth secondary to deposition of porphyrin in developing teeth.

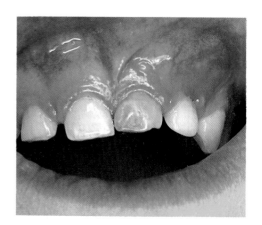

FIG. 18.33 Isolated intrinsic discoloration. The central incisor is discolored secondary to trauma. Often such a change is a manifestation of pulpal necrosis.

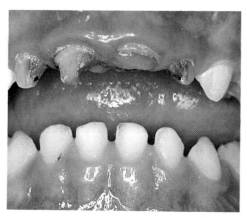

FIG. 18.34 Nursing bottle caries. Prolonged nocturnal bottle-feedings are responsible for the caries seen on the maxillary incisors and molars. The mandibular incisors were spared by the protective position of the tongue.

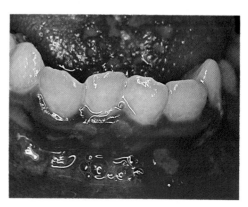

FIG. 18.35 Herpetic gingivostomatitis. The ulcerations seen on the oral mucosa were preceded by fever, headache, and lymphadenopathy. Note the erythematous halos around the ulcerations.

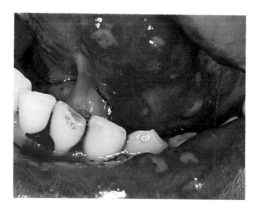

FIG. 18.36 Recurrent herpetic stomatitis. This generalized form is seen in the immunocompromised host.

ISOLATED INTRINSIC DISCOLORATION

Teeth with necrotic pulps develop an opaque appearance with discoloration ranging from light yellow to gray (Fig. 18.33). Such teeth may develop abscesses, periapical cystic lesions, or chronic fistulas. Pulpal calcification is often associated with a localized yellow discoloration. Internal resorption manifests clinically as a pink discoloration secondary to loss of dentin thickness.

CARIES

The interaction of microorganisms, especially *Streptococcus mutans*, and fermentable carbohydrates results in acid demineralization of susceptible enamel. Untreated carious destruction progresses through the enamel and dentin, and with bacterial contamination of the pulp ultimately renders the pulp necrotic. The deep pits, fissures, and grooves of newly erupted teeth are at high risk for developing carious lesions. Prevention of dental caries includes brushing and flossing on a daily basis to remove bacteria-containing plaque, implementation of systemic fluoride via the water supply or prescribed supplements, and control of the frequency of intake of fermentable carbohydrates, especially those high in sugar content and adhesiveness.

Nursing bottle caries involves the primary dentition of the child who is habitually put to bed with a bottle containing milk or another cariogenic liquid. This form of caries was originally associated with bottle-feeding only; however, an association with frequent and prolonged nocturnal breast-feeding has become apparent. Carious lesions initially develop on the maxillary incisors, and later on the molars and cuspids (Fig. 18.34). The mandibular incisors are spared by the protective position of the tongue during nursing. The deleterious effect of nocturnal nursing is due not only to the frequency of carbohydrate intake but also to the decreased rate of swallowing and salivation during sleep.

INFECTIONS

Viral Infections

HERPETIC GINGIVOSTOMATITIS

Primary herpetic gingivostomatitis, caused by herpes simplex, type I, is an extremely painful disease which affects children, especially those between the ages of 6 months and 3 years. The vesicular lesions of the lips, tongue, gingiva, and oral mucosa are preceded by fever, headache, regional lymphadenopathy, and gingival hyperemia and edema. These lesions tend to rupture quickly, leaving shallow ulcerations covered by a gray membrane and surrounded by an erythematous halo (Fig. 18.35). The inflamed gingiva is friable and bleeds easily. Lesions heal spontaneously in 1 to 2 weeks without scarring. Treatment is palliative. Since inflammation makes brushing too painful, oral hygiene should be maintained using a preparation such as Gly-oxide to decrease the incidence of secondary infection. A bland diet and rinsing with viscous lidocaine or a solution of equal parts of Benadryl and Maalox may be indicated for a patient with severe pain.

Recurrent infections due to reactivation of latent herpes simplex virus are fairly common. Lesions are few in number and more localized; systemic symptoms are absent unless the host is immunocompromised. Lesions are usually located on the lips, with prodromal symptoms of itching and burning preceding the development of thin-walled vesicles which rupture and become crusty in appearance. When intraoral lesions occur, they manifest as small vesicles in a localized group on mucosa that is tightly bound to periosteum (Fig. 18.36).

HERPES ZOSTER (SHINGLES)

Herpes zoster results from activation of the varicella zoster virus and inflammation of the dorsal root or extramedullary cranial nerve ganglion. While the disease is occasionally seen in otherwise healthy children, it is more likely to occur in the

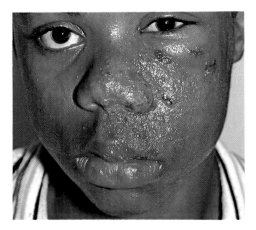

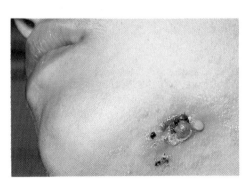

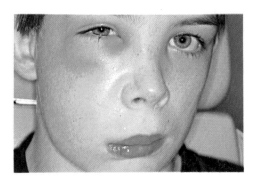

FIG. 18.37 Herpes zoster. This patient's infection involved the trigeminal nerve, including the nasociliary branch. Both the

extraoral (left) and the intraoral (right) lesions stop at the midline.

FIG. 18.38 Recurrent aphthous ulcers. The ulceration seen on the labial mucosa is surrounded by a characteristic erythematous halo.

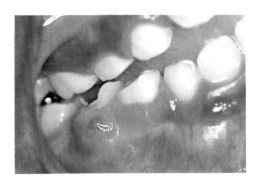

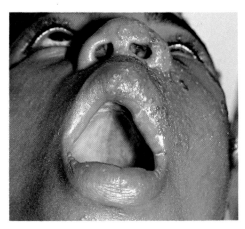

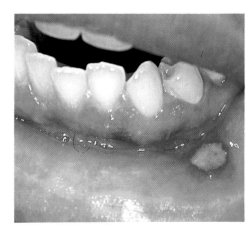

FIG. 18.39 An untreated, abscessed, mandibular posterior tooth (left) can be responsible for the type of extraoral lesion seen at right. Infection spreads by way of

a cutaneous fistulous tract. Extraction of the offending tooth is necessary for resolution of the extraoral lesion.

FIG. 18.40 Facial cellulitis. This patient's facial cellulitis is associated with an abscessed maxillary tooth. Hospital admission for intravenous antibiotics, incision and drainage, and extraction of the abscessed tooth was necessary.

severely debilitated or immunosuppressed child. The patient presents with a prodrome of malaise, fever, headache, and tenderness along the affected dermatome followed by the extraoral formation of painful grouped vesicular lesions which rupture to form ulcerations. The oral cavity may also be affected with erosions following a unilateral distribution of maxillary and mandibular divisions of the trigeminal nerve (Fig. 18.37).

RECURRENT APHTHOUS ULCERS (CANKER SORES)
Aphthous ulcers are similar to herpetic ulcers but are not of viral origin. Precipitating factors include trauma, stress, sunlight, endocrine disturbances, hematologic disorders, and allergies, alluding to a multifactorial etiology. Onset is during adolescence or young adulthood. Unlike herpetic lesions, these ulcerations are not preceded by vesicle formation. They are extremely painful, and have a pseudomembrane and erythematous halo (Fig. 18.38). They can vary in size, number, and distribution. Small aphthae may coalesce into larger lesions. While any oral mucosal surface may be involved, freely movable mucosa is more frequently involved than tightly bound. Lesions heal in 1 to 2 weeks without scarring.

Bacterial Infections

Odontogenic infections are caused by both aerobic and anaerobic microorganisms. Streptococcus and Staphylococ-

cus are most frequently isolated; however, any oral flora or opportunistic microorganism may be involved. Periapical infections resulting from pulpal necrosis of a carious or traumatized tooth are most commonly seen in the pediatric population and usually require endodontic therapy or extraction of the offending tooth. Left untreated, the chronic infection may result in abscess formation, apical granuloma, or a radicular cyst. In addition, the infection may escape the alveolar bone through oral or cutaneous fistulous tracts, causing extraoral lesions (Fig. 18.39). The acute periapical infection may localize as an abscess or spread through the soft tissues causing facial cellulitis (Fig. 18.40). Involvement of lateral pharyngeal, retropharyngeal, or sublingual spaces may necessitate airway maintenance, vigorous antibiotic therapy, and incision and drainage. Septic thrombosis of the cavernous sinus may result from infections originating in the maxillary teeth or sinuses.

A pericoronal infection is a bacteria-induced inflammation of the gingival soft tissue surrounding the crown of an erupting tooth. The third molars are most commonly involved. Symptoms include fever, malaise, localized redness, tenderness, swelling, and trismus.

ACUTE NECROTIZING ULCERATIVE GINGIVITIS
(VINCENT'S INFECTION, TRENCH MOUTH)
This is a fusospirochetal disease seldom seen before the age of 10. The gingiva is reddened, edematous, and painful with

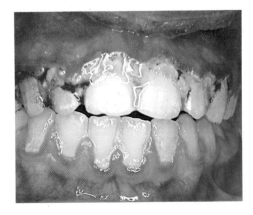

FIG. 18.41 Acute necrotizing ulcerative gingivitis. The infected gingiva exhibits localized necrosis, hemorrhage, and is covered with pseudomembranes.

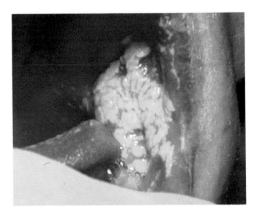

FIG. 18.42 Candidiasis. (Left) Involvement of buccal mucosa with white plaque.

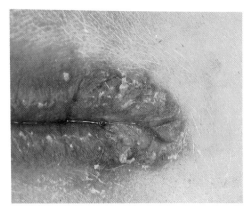

(Right) Mucocutaneous infection of the commissures of the lips.

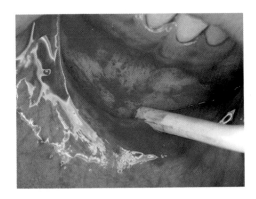

FIG. 18.43 Degloving injury, before (left) and after (right) repair. Such an injury to the oral mucosa requires immediate

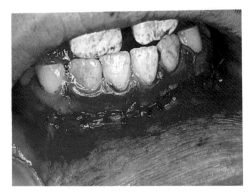

inspection, irrigation, approximation, and suturing.

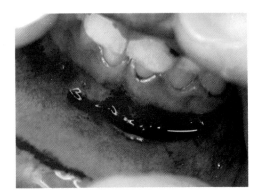

FIG. 18.44 This laceration of the oral mucosa—deep and not well-approximated —requires immediate treatment.

necrotic punched-out craters in the interdental papillae. Involved areas hemorrhage readily and become covered with a pseudomembrane (Fig. 18.41). In addition to oral symptoms, the patient presents with fetid breath, malaise, fever, and regional lymphadenopathy. Treatment generally consists of gentle dental prophylaxis followed by improved oral hygiene measures and topical peroxide applications. In most cases resolution occurs within several days without the use of antibiotics. Occasionally, secondary infection or severe involvement may necessitate the use of antibiotics; penicillin is then the antibiotic of choice.

Fungal Infections

CANDIDIASIS (MONILIASIS, THRUSH)
Candidiasis results from the opportunistic pathogen *Candida albicans*. This infection is seen in infants, in patients with underlying systemic diseases, in the immunosuppressed, or in those on antibiotic treatment. Common sites of involvement are the buccal mucosa, the tongue, the palate, and the commissures of the lips (Fig. 18.42). Intraoral lesions are soft, elevated, creamy white plaques which do not scrape off easily. While culturing is difficult and not reliable, diagnosis may be made on the basis of clinical findings or examination of a KOH preparation. Treatment consists of local application of nystatin (miconazole or ketoconazole for severe or chronic cases), and control of the underlying causes.

TRAUMA

Trauma to Soft Tissues

A variety of soft-tissue injuries including lacerations, contusions, abrasions, perforations, avulsions, and burns may occur. The injured area is initially cleansed of blood clots, debris, and foreign material, then carefully examined to determine the extent of tissue involvement. Mechanical debridement of any ragged, necrotic, or beveled margins may be necessary. Appropriate tetanus prevention should also be considered.

ABRASIONS
Superficial abrasions usually heal without complications. Extensive abrasions should be covered with a water-soluble medicated gauze following irrigation. Some may require skin grafting.

CONTUSIONS
A contusion, or bruise, usually requires no treatment, and healing proceeds favorably in most instances. Contusions are often associated with underlying injuries; therefore, a careful examination of adjacent structures is indicated.

PERFORATIONS
These small deep wounds caused by sharp objects are fairly common in children. Careful examination of the wound as well as the object is essential. Following careful inspection and

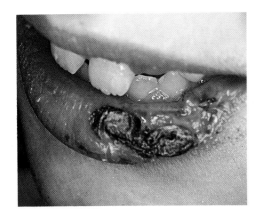

FIG. 18.45 This electrical burn healed with scarring and contractures.

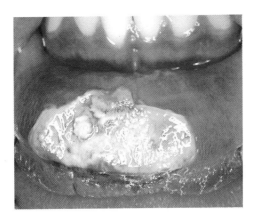

FIG. 18.46 This traumatic lip ulceration was caused by lip-biting following the administration of anesthesia.

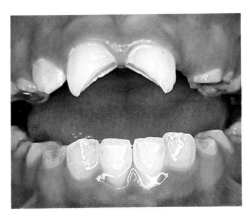

FIG. 18.47 These crown fractures demonstrate involvement of enamel and dentin, without exposure of the pulp. Immediate dental referral is necessary to prevent contamination of the pulp through the dentinal tubules.

irrigation, larger wounds should be closed in layers; smaller wounds may not require closure. If doubt exists concerning foreign bodies and/or contamination, a drain should be left in situ and proper antibiotics prescribed. The possibility of damage to large vessels should be recognized.

AVULSIONS (DEGLOVING INJURIES)
Avulsions of soft tissues are uncommon injuries, yet when they do occur they may involve deep as well as superficial tissues (Fig. 18.43). Small avulsions can be treated by undermining and suturing surrounding tissues. Larger avulsions can be treated either by reattaching the avulsed tissues or by use of a graft. The former procedure is preferable whenever possible.

LACERATIONS
Lacerations to facial and oral tissues are common in children. Small intraoral lacerations with well-approximated margins do not require suturing. Bleeding usually subsides spontaneously, and healing proceeds satisfactorily. Large lacerations, through-and-through lacerations, and those associated with extensive, recurrent, or uncontrolled bleeding require careful assessment (Fig. 18.44). Soft-palate lacerations require a thorough pharyngeal inspection. The possibility of foreign body entrapment, immediate or delayed vascular injury, or formation of pharyngeal abscesses should be seriously considered. Lacerations involving the labial frenulum of infants are common and usually require only restriction of lip manipulation and a soft diet.

BURNS
Burns involving the oral cavity usually heal, but with contracture and scarring (Fig. 18.45). Splints fabricated from dental materials can prevent or minimize contracture by maintaining proper anatomic relationships during healing.

TRAUMATIC ULCERS
This painful ulceration results from mechanical, chemical, or thermal trauma. Injury may be secondary to irritation by objects, trauma during mastication, toothbrush trauma, or abnormal habits. Large ulcerations involving the buccal mucosa or lower lip may be associated with cheek or lip biting following inferior alveolar nerve block (Fig. 18.46). Topical Glyoxide application is useful in cleansing the area. Lesions usually heal without scarring, but secondarily infected lesions may require antibiotic therapy. Identification and elimination of the habit is necessary for resolution of habit-related lesions.

Trauma to the Dentition

Traumatic injuries to the face often involve the teeth and supporting structures. The risk of such injuries is relatively high in (1) children involved in contact sports; (2) children with protruding maxillary anterior teeth, and (3) children with a deviant anatomic relationship such as an anterior open bite or a hypoplastic upper lip. Such injuries may also result from car, bicycle, skateboard, or other similar accidents. Preventive measures such as the use of helmets, mouthguards, and seatbelts should significantly reduce the incidence as well as the severity of such injuries.

Several extensive classifications of tooth injuries have been suggested, but for the purpose of this text a more simplified descriptive classification will now be presented.

CROWN CRAZE OR CRACK
A significant number of children are discovered during routine physical examination to have "cracks" within their teeth. Such cracks are presumably caused by relatively minor trauma or temperature change. The overwhelming majority of such teeth are asymptomatic and require no treatment.

CROWN FRACTURES WITHOUT PULPAL EXPOSURE
Minor fractures may not require treatment if they remain asymptomatic; however, any significant fracture of the crown which results in exposure of the dentin must receive treatment (Fig. 18.47). The treatment of choice is to seal the exposed dentin with calcium hydroxide and to protect it with an acid-etched resin bandage for a minimum of 2 to 3 months to enhance pulpal healing. This procedure should be performed as soon as possible following the injury. Dental fragments are occasionally embedded in the soft tissues of the lip or tongue; therefore, appropriate examination and palpation of these areas is indicated. The presence of such fragments may be confirmed by radiographic examination.

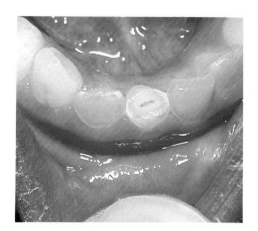

FIG. 18.48 This crown fracture involves not only enamel and dentin but the soft tissue of the pulp as well. Immediate dental referral is mandatory if the tooth is to be saved.

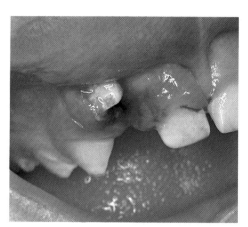

FIG. 18.49 This primary lateral incisor was traumatically intruded. Such intrusions will usually spontaneously reerupt.

CROWN FRACTURES WITH PULPAL EXPOSURE

Such fractures usually involve a significant loss of tooth structure. On physical examination, the fracture surface exhibits a pulpal exposure (Fig. 18.48). Such teeth must be treated as soon as possible with pulp capping, pulpotomy, or root canal therapy, depending on severity.

ROOT FRACTURES

Root fractures are less common in the primary dentition, and when they do occur they usually require no therapy. Root fractures of permanent teeth may occur with or without loss of crown structure, and may be asymptomatic. If a seemingly normal tooth becomes tender or exhibits increased mobility following trauma, root fracture should be suspected and radiographs obtained. Generally the prognosis is good, and treatment may include splinting the involved segment for 6 to 10 weeks, with or without root canal therapy.

DISPLACEMENT INJURIES

These injuries result in extrusion, intrusion, or lateral displacement, and are most commonly seen in the primary dentition where the combination of a short root length and a very "pliable" bony structure seem to permit displacement to occur (Fig. 18.49). They are often associated with significant discomfort, bleeding, and possible interference with mastication, occlusion, and the normal development of permanent tooth buds; therefore, immediate care is advised. Treatment may include observation with or without prophylactic antibiotic coverage, immediate correction in cases of posterior displacement due to interference with mastication, or extraction of the displaced tooth in cases of severe labial or vertical displacement. Most intruded primary teeth will reerupt within 6 to 8 weeks with antibiotic coverage, sensible oral hygiene, and an appropriate diet. In general, displaced permanent teeth should be surgically repositioned and splinted, and follow-up root canal therapy should be seriously considered.

AVULSION AND REIMPLANTATION

Avulsion is the complete displacement of a tooth from its socket, and is seen mostly in preschool and early school-aged children. Reimplantation of primary teeth is still experimental and should only be done under selective conditions. However, the prognosis is usually poor, and splinting is not easily carried out.

On the other hand, reimplantation of permanent teeth is an acceptable technique with a relatively good prognosis (Fig. 18.50). The major factors in improving prognosis are:

1. A short period between avulsion and reimplantation, preferably less than half an hour.
2. Appropriate storage of the avulsed tooth. The most desirable "media" would be the socket itself, followed by saliva and milk.
3. Appropriate irrigation of the surgical site, replacing the tooth into the socket *without* pressure, and the use of an acid-etched splint.
4. Appropriate removal of the pulp within 2 weeks as a first step in completing root canal treatment, unless the tooth was immature with incomplete root formation.
5. Removal of the splint within 2 weeks.

It is generally accepted that scraping of the root or the socket is contraindicated.

Trauma to Supporting Structures

Injuries to the bony supporting structures of the mouth may result from birth trauma, bicycle accidents, car accidents, various physical activities, child abuse, and animal bites. First, a concise history including information concerning the circumstances of the accident must be obtained. Then, a careful clinical examination is necessary to determine the extent and nature of injury, which will help the physician select the needed diagnostic tools and take the appropriate course of action. The examination should include:

1. The overlying skin and soft tissues
2. The dentition
3. The gingiva and oral mucosa
4. The facial and jaw bones
5. Dental occlusion

Tenderness on palpation, trismus, hemorrhage from the nose or the ear, deviation on opening or closing the mouth, periorbital ecchymosis or edema, subconjunctival hemorrhage or edema, diplopia, or the presence of sinus clouding on radiographs should call for a detailed evaluation of the suspected area.

FRACTURES OF THE MANDIBLE

Excluding nose fractures, the most common facial fracture in children is the mandibular fracture. These fractures seem to occur in the weakest part of the bone, in the condylar neck, or through the sites of developing tooth buds. The most impor-

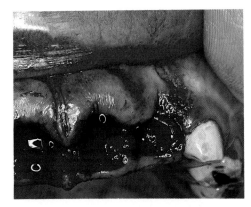

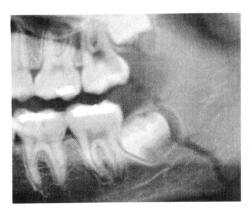

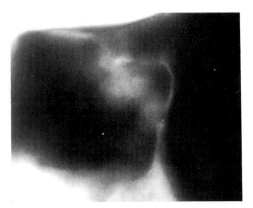

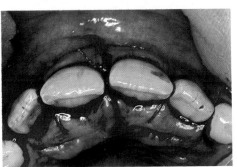

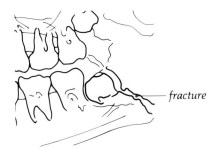

FIG. 18.51 *A panoramic radiograph reveals a nondisplaced mandibular fracture originating in the third molar tooth bud.*

fracture

FIG. 18.50 (Top) *Four permanent incisors have been avulsed.* (Bottom) *The teeth have been reimplanted successfully.*

FIG. 18.52 *Lateral radiograph (top) reveals increased opacity in the maxillary sinus, an indication that a fracture may have occurred. This may be confirmed by tomography (bottom).*

tant diagnostic clues in addition to localized tenderness include gingival tears, ecchymosis, malocclusion, limitation of movement, or deviation on opening or closing the mouth. A panoramic radiograph and a mandibular series should be ordered if there is clinical suspicion of a fracture (Fig. 18.51). If routine views are unrevealing, tomography may be called for in certain unusual, difficult, or complex cases.

Management requires careful assessment of the stability and type of erupted dentition as well as the location of the tooth buds. Nondisplaced fractures with no occlusal abnormalities may require no treatment other than a soft diet. Most displaced fractures can be treated conservatively: first, by appropriate reduction, followed by either simple intermaxillary fixation or by intraoral splints and circumferential wiring (closed reduction). Seldom is open reduction indicated. Careful placement of intraosseous holes is essential to avoid damage to the developing tooth buds.

FRACTURES OF THE MAXILLA AND THE MIDFACE
Fractures of the midface are especially uncommon in younger children and infants because of their relatively large cranial vault and the elasticity of their bones. When such fractures do occur, they are often associated with injuries to the frontal region, the orbits and overlying soft tissues, and the nose.

In 1901, LeFort divided midfacial fractures into three groups:

LeFort I, which primarily involves the maxilla
LeFort II, which primarily involves the maxilla and the nasal complex
LeFort III, which involves separation of the midface from the cranium

These fractures require a thorough and detailed examination to ensure proper care. Diagnosis can be challenging and frequently requires specialized tomography since routine views such as anteroposterior, lateral, and Towne's are often inadequate (Fig. 18.52).

Early treatment of facial injuries requires careful monitoring of vital signs, maintenance of an adequate airway, observation for progression of edema, and a careful neurologic evaluation. The need for intubation or even tracheotomy must be considered if airway difficulties arise. The next most important factor to consider is hemorrhage, which may become a critical problem in younger children. In such cases, total blood loss should be monitored, the patient typed and cross-matched, and replacement therapy initiated if necessary. Definitive treatment can be completed following stabilization and appropriate radiographic evaluation.

BIBLIOGRAPHY

Bhaskar SN: Oral lesions of infants and newborns. Dent Clin North Am 421–435, July 1966.

Christensen RE Jr: Soft tissue lesions of the head and neck. In Sanders B (ed.) Pediatric Oral and Maxillofacial Surgery. Mosby, St. Louis, 1979, pp 221–272.

Nazif MM, Ruffalo RC: The interaction between dentistry and otolaryngology. Pediatr Clin North Am 28 (4): 997–1010, 1981.

Rapp R: Dental and gingival disorders. In Bluestone CD, Stool SE (eds.) Pediatric Otolaryngology. Saunders, Philadelphia, 1983, pp 931–955.

Sanders B et al: Injuries. In Sanders B (ed.) Pediatric Oral and Maxillofacial Surgery. Mosby, St. Louis, 1979, pp 330–399.

Schuitt KE, Johnson JT: Infections of the head and neck. Pediatr Clin North Am 28 (4): 965–971, 1981.

PEDIATRIC ORTHOPEDICS

Edward N. Hanley Jr., M.D.
W. Timothy Ward, M.D.
Holly W. Davis, M.D.

Children with musculoskeletal injuries and afflictions seek help because of pain, deformity, or loss of function. Often the clinical challenge lies not so much in recognizing the impaired or injured part, which in most cases is readily accessible to inspection and examination, but in making an accurate diagnosis in order to plan and initiate appropriate treatment. Because of their rapid physical growth and the special properties of their developing bones, children often pose special problems for the clinician.

Discussion is divided into five sections: (1) musculoskeletal trauma; (2) disorders of the spine; (3) disorders of the upper extremity; (4) disorders of the lower extremity; and (5) generalized musculoskeletal disorders. Brief discussions of treatment are included because timing for orthopedic referral is so important for children.

A number of other disorders generally classified under other subspecialties, but involving the musculoskeletal system, are covered in other chapters. Bone and joint infections are discussed in Chapter 12, collagen vascular diseases in Chapter 7, nutritional deficiencies and renal disorders affecting the skeletal system in Chapters 10 and 13, and neuromuscular disorders and spinal dysraphism in Chapter 14. Additional examples of trauma are presented in Chapter 6.

There are a number of other disorders in which trauma plays a partial role. Mild trauma can serve to disclose an underlying abnormality. Some of these conditions and a few posttraumatic deformities will be discussed in subsequent sections.

MUSCULOSKELETAL TRAUMA

The normal impulsiveness and inquisitiveness of children combined with their lack of caution and love of energetic activities place them at a relatively high risk for accidental injury. The incidence of trauma is further elevated by the prevalence of child abuse (see Chapter 6). In fact, beyond infancy, trauma is the leading cause of death in children and adolescents, and is the source of significant morbidity. Musculoskeletal injuries are very common whether seen in isolation or as part of multisystem trauma. While management of life-threatening injuries to the airway, circulation, and CNS must take precedence over accompanying musculoskeletal injuries in cases of multiple trauma, it must be kept in mind that fractures can result in significant blood loss. This is particularly true of pelvic and femoral fractures. Furthermore, prompt attention must be given to assessment of the status of neurovascular structures distal to obvious fractures; failure to recognize compromise may result in permanent loss of function.

Accurate diagnosis and optimal management of pediatric orthopedic injuries also requires a clear understanding of the physiology of the growing musculoskeletal system and of the unique properties of growing bone especially. At birth only a few epiphyses have begun to ossify; the remainder are cartilaginous and, thus, are invisible radiographically. With development, other epiphyses begin to ossify, enlarge and mature in an orderly fashion, such that one can estimate a child's age from the number and configuration of ossification centers (Fig. 19.1). The epiphyseal plates (physes), being sites of cartilaginous proliferation and growth, do not begin to ossify until puberty (Fig. 19.2). When skeletal injuries involve sites where ossification has not begun or is incomplete, radiographs may appear normal or may not reflect the full extent of the injury. This necessitates greater reliance on clinical findings.

Prior to closure of the physis during puberty, the growth plate is actually weaker than nearby ligaments. As a result, injuries that occur near joints are more likely to result in physeal disruption than in ligamentous tearing (i.e., sprains and dislocations are unusual prior to puberty). When there is displacement of an epiphyseal fracture and the fragments are not anatomically reduced growth disturbances may occur. Because the epiphysis may not be ossified radiographs often may fail to reveal the injury, and for this reason children with injuries at or near joints must be examined with meticulous care in order not to miss epiphyseal fractures.

The periosteum of a child is much thicker than that of an adult, strips more easily from the bone, and rarely is disrupted completely when the underlying bone is fractured.

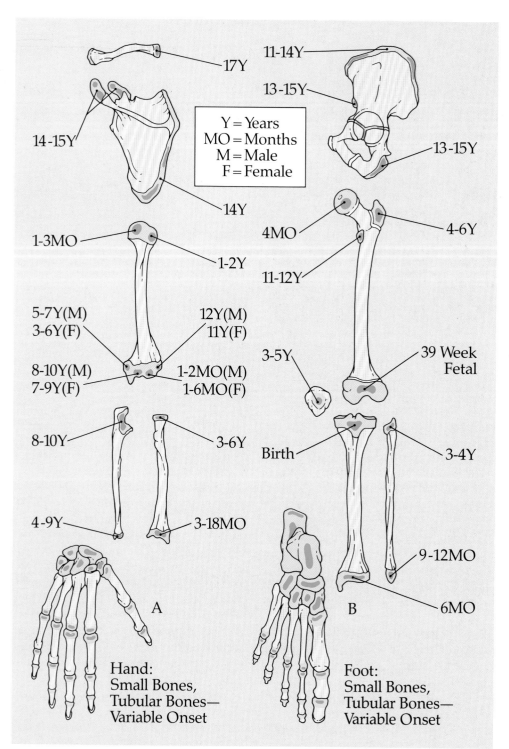

FIG. 19.1 Ages of onset of ossification. At birth only a few epiphyses have begun to ossify. The remainder are cartilaginous and therefore invisible radiographically. With development other epiphyses begin to ossify, enlarge, and mature in an orderly fashion, making it possible to estimate a child's age from the number and configuration of ossification centers. This forms the basis for the use of bone age as part of the evaluation of children with growth disorders. It is of crucial importance to bear in mind when evaluating the radiographs of injured children that fractures involving nonossified epiphyses are radiographically invisible until healing begins (see Figure 19.33).

The immature, rapidly growing bone of the child is more porous than that of the adult and has a greater capacity for plastic deformation but less ability to withstand compressive or tensile forces. Consequently, a given compressive force that would produce a comminuted fracture in an adult tends to be dissipated in part by the bending that occurs in the more flexible bone of the child. Such a force is thus more likely to result in plastic deformation or to produce an incomplete fracture, such as a torus fracture or a greenstick fracture, in a child.

Thus, fracture patterns in children often differ from those in adults. Their fractures can be considerably harder to detect clinically and radiographically, and can potentially result in long-term growth abnormalities. Children do have advantages, however, in that their actively growing bones heal with greater rapidity and have a remarkable capacity for remodeling.

Fractures

DIAGNOSIS

One of the many variables that complicate the diagnosis of the skeletally injured child is that the child, already in pain, is frightened by his recent experience and by the strangeness of the hospital or emergency room setting. Many children are too young to give a firsthand history, and the cooperation of toddlers is often limited. The parents are likely to be anxious as well. A calm empathetic manner is needed to allay their fears. Taking a thorough history prior to any attempt at physical assessment will help establish rapport with the patient and the family. This should include questions concerning the type and direction of the injuring force, the position of the involved extremity at the time of the accident, as well as the events immediately following the injury,

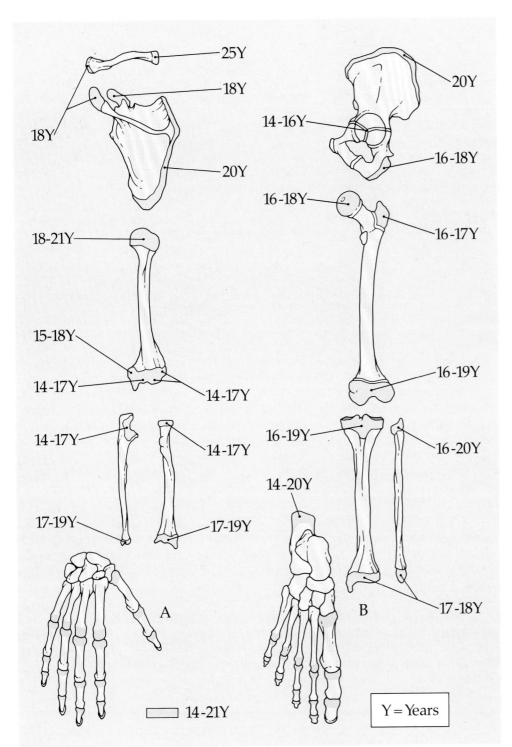

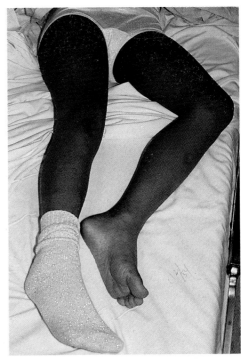

FIG. 19.3 Proximal femur fracture. Note the characteristic shortened, externally rotated position of the lower extremity following a fracture of the proximal femur. The patient was struck by a car sustaining a fracture of the femoral neck.

FIG. 19.2 Ages of physeal closure.

such as measures taken at the scene of the accident. The presence of underlying disorders and the possibility of contamination of an open wound should be determined as well. Physicians also should be alert to signs suggestive of inflicted injury or child abuse (See Chapter 6).

In cases of suspected fracture, splinting, elevation, and topical application of ice may help reduce discomfort and local swelling. Splinting is particularly important for displaced and unstable fractures as it prevents further soft tissue injuries and reduces the risk of fat embolization. When pain is severe and there are no cardiovascular or CNS con-

traindications, analgesia should be administered promptly. Contrary to the opinion of many physicians, this does not obscure physical findings. Tenderness will not be reduced significantly, swelling will remain, and patient cooperation for the examination may be considerably greater.

The first step in a physical examination is visual inspection of the injured area. The gross position of the extremity should be noted, and attention given to the presence or absence of deformity, distortion or abnormal angulation, and longitudinal shortening (Fig. 19.3). The overlying skin and soft tissues are examined for evidence of swelling, ecchy-

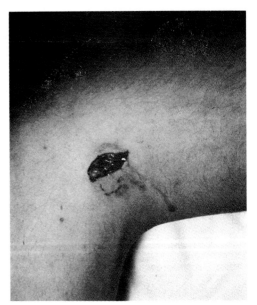

FIG. 19.4 Penetrating injury of the knee. This child was struck by a stone propelled by the blades of a power lawn mower. Though the laceration appeared to be a minor one, on movement of the knee serosanguinous fluid flowed from it suggesting penetration of the joint capsule. This was confirmed on exploration in the operating room. (Courtesy of Dr. B. Watson)

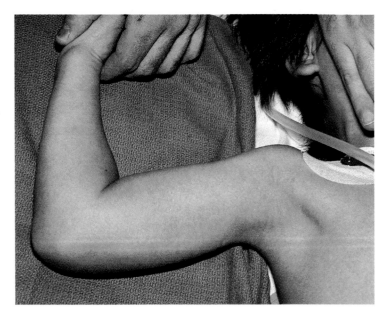

FIG. 19.5 Fracture with overlying soft tissue swelling. This child has a dislocated supracondylar fracture of the distal humerus with moderate soft tissue swelling. The degree becomes evident when the size of the elbow area is compared with the size of the patient's wrist.

moses, abrasions, punctures or lacerations. Comparison with the opposite extremity and measurement of circumference can be very helpful when findings are subtle. The location of open wounds is important in ascertaining whether an underlying fracture is open or closed and in assessing risk of joint penetration. Small puncture wounds or lacerations overlying bony structures which appear to be oozing a bloody, fatty exudate usually reflect communication with the medullary cavity of a fractured bone. Similarly punctures or tears over joints which weep serous or serosanguinous fluid, especially when drainage is increased on moving the joint, must be assumed to communicate with the joint capsule (Fig. 19.4). Probing of open wounds which have a high likelihood of communication with a fracture or a joint is contraindicated. The wound should be cleaned and covered with a sterile dressing until its extent can be determined under sterile conditions in the operating room.

Following inspection of the most obviously injured area, palpation and assessment of active and passive motion can be performed. It is crucial to remember that in examining an injured limb the entire extremity must be evaluated in order to detect less obvious associated injuries. Localized swelling and tenderness on palpation are significant findings and should alert the examiner that there is a high likelihood of an underlying fracture. Pain on motion and limitation of motion signal the need for careful scrutiny as well. Assessment of motion involves observation of spontaneous movement, attempts to get the patient to voluntarily move the involved part through its expected range, and passive movement. Particular attention should be paid to the adjacent joints both proximal and distal to avoid missing associated injuries. It can be difficult, however, to determine whether motion is limited because of pain, an associated injury, or fear and lack of cooperation.

Clinical findings vary depending on the nature of the fracture. Undisplaced growth plate fractures typically present with mild localized swelling and point tenderness at the level of the epiphysis. Since ligamentous injury is relatively uncommon in a child, the finding of such point tenderness

should be sufficient evidence to treat the injury as a fracture until proven otherwise. Often initial radiographs appear normal and the fracture is confirmed only on follow-up when repeat radiographs disclose evidence of healing. Swelling is typically mild and occasionally imperceptible in cases of torus or buckle fractures and of undisplaced transverse and spiral fractures. Careful palpation should disclose focal tenderness, however. Usually, the patient will also experience some degree of discomfort on motion in some planes or on weight-bearing, but it must be remembered that limitation of movement or function can be minimal with such incomplete fractures. In contrast, fractures that completely disrupt the bone and displaced fractures are accompanied by more prominent swelling, more diffuse tenderness, and severe pain which is markedly increased on motion (Fig. 19.5). Crepitance may be evident also on gentle palpation. In examining children with these findings manipulation must be kept to a minimum to prevent further injury.

Assessment of neurovascular function distal to the injury is essential in evaluating any child with a potential fracture. This includes checking the integrity of pulses and speed of capillary refill as well as testing sensory and motor function. Strength and sensation should be compared to the contralateral extremity. Assessment of two point discrimination is probably the best test of sensory function. Evidence of neurovascular compromise necessitates urgent, often operative, orthopedic treatment. In addition, this assessment is crucial prior to and following reduction of displaced fractures in order to determine if the procedure itself has impaired function in any way. Supracondylar fractures of the humerus, fractures of the distal femoral shaft and proximal tibia, fracture/dislocations of the elbow and knee, and severely displaced ankle fractures have a particularly high risk of associated neurovascular injury. It is also important to be aware of the fact that vascular compromise can be present in a patient who has normal distal pulses and good peripheral perfusion. This should be suspected in patients who complain of intense muscle pain that is aggravated by stretching the muscle in an area distal to a displaced fracture. Persis-

PATTERNS OF FRACTURES

Fracture Pattern	Major Feature	Radiographic Appearance
Longitudinal	Fracture line is parallel to the axis of a long bone	Fig. 19.7
Transverse	Fracture line is perpendicular to the axis of a long bone	Fig. 19.8
Oblique	Fracture line is at an angle relative to the axis of a bone	Fig. 19.9
Spiral	Fracture line take a curvilinear course around the axis of a bone	Fig. 19.10
Impacted	Bone ends are crushed together producing an indistinct fracture line	Fig. 19.11
Comminuted	Fracturing forces produce more than two separate fragments	Fig. 19.12
Bowing	Bone bends to the point of plastic deformation without fracturing	Fig. 19.13
Greenstick	Fracture is complete except for a portion of the cortex on the compression side of the fracture which is only plastically deformed	Fig. 19.14
Torus	Bone buckles and bends rather than breaking	Fig. 19.15

FIG. 19.6 Patterns of fractures.

tance of intense pain following fracture reduction should also provoke suspicion of ischemia.

In all cases of suspected extremity fractures the injured part should be properly splinted and elevated, and an ice pack should be applied while awaiting transport to the radiography suite. However, in order to obtain high-quality radiographs, obstructing splints must be removed temporarily. This presents no major problem with partial or nondisplaced fractures, but can create difficulties in patients with severe displaced fractures. To insure that manipulation is minimal in these cases, splint removal, positioning for radiographs and splint reapplication should be supervised by a physician and not done merely at the discretion of the X-ray technician.

At minimum, two radiographs taken at 90° angles are obtained, anteroposterior and lateral views being the most common. Oblique views are helpful in fully disclosing the nature and extent of many fracture patterns especially when the injury involves the ankle, elbow, hand, or foot. They can also prove useful in detecting subtle spiral fractures, and in cases in which AP and lateral views are negative, yet a fracture is strongly suspected. Radiographs should include the joints immediately proximal and distal to a fractured long bone as there may be associated bony and/or soft-tissue injuries in these areas, as well. Such associated injuries easily can be missed on clinical examination when assessment of motion is limited by pain or when patient cooperation is limited. It is also advisable to obtain comparison views of the opposite side, especially when evaluating patients with suspected physeal injuries who may have very subtle radiographic abnormalities. In some cases of displaced and/or angulated fractures, tomograms and CT scans can be useful. Particular care should be taken in interpreting pediatric radiographs because of the high incidence of subtle or even negative findings in patients with fractures. When the clinical picture strongly suggests a fracture, appropriate treatment should be initiated even if the radiograph appears normal. Reassessment in 1 to 2 weeks can then clarify the exact nature of the injury.

FRACTURE PATTERNS

Fractures should be described in terms of anatomic location, direction of the fracture line, type of fracture, and degree of displacement. When the growth plate is involved, use of the Salter-Harris classification system is recommended.

Any specific mechanism of injury results in a readily definable pattern of force application, which tends to produce a typical fracture pattern. Because of this, it is often possible to infer the likely mechanism of injury once the fracture pattern is documented radiographically. If the vector of the direct force is perpendicular to the bone, a transverse fracture is most likely to result, whereas direct force applied at any angle to the bone produces an oblique fracture pattern. Examples of situations resulting in transverse and short oblique fractures include falls in which an extremity strikes the edge of a table, counter or chair, direct blows with an object such as a stick, and karate chops. These fractures are commonly seen as a result of accidents, fights, and in the battered child syndrome. Comminuted fractures generally are the result of high velocity direct forces such as those characteristic of vehicular accidents, falls from heights, or gunshot wounds. Impacted fractures are produced by forces oriented in a direction parallel to the long axis of the bone. Application of indirect force commonly results in spiral, greenstick, or torus fractures in children. A common example of a nondisplaced spiral fracture is the "toddler's fracture" which results from a fall with a twist. Typically, the child either was running, turned, and then fell, or had gotten his foot caught and fell while twisting to extricate himself. When a child's arm or leg is forcibly pulled and twisted a similar fracture pattern may be seen. Greenstick and torus fractures of the radius and/or ulna are incurred usually by falling on an outstretched arm with the wrist in a dorsiflexed position. Vigorous repetitive shaking while holding a child by the hands or feet results in small metaphyseal chip or avulsion fractures, a major feature of the shaken baby syndrome (see Chapter 6). Figure 19.6 describes the major features of these various fracture patterns, which are illustrated in Figures 19.7 through 19.15.

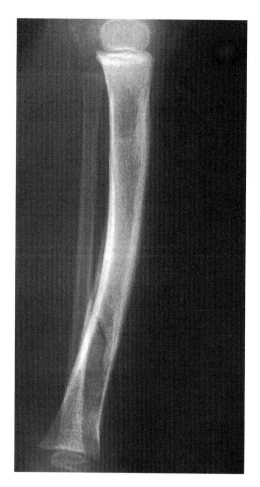

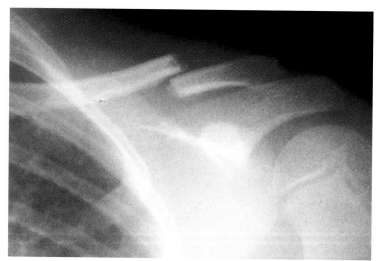

FIG. 19.8 Transverse fracture of the midportion of the clavicle. Fracture line is perpendicular to the long axis of the bone.

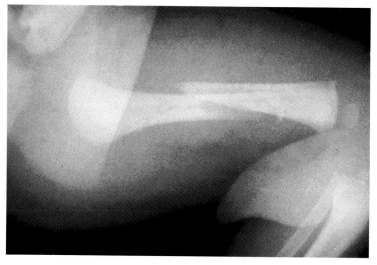

FIG. 19.9 Oblique fracture of the midportion of the femur. Fracture line is angled relative to the axis of the bone.

FIG. 19.7 Longitudinal fracture of the distal tibia still evident 4 weeks following injury in a 4-year-old boy. Slight periosteal callous formation can be seen posteriorly.

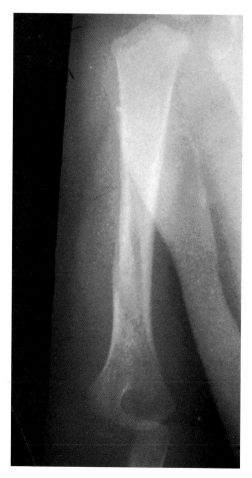

FIG. 19.10 Spiral fracture of the humerus. Fracture line takes curvilinear course around the axis of the bone.

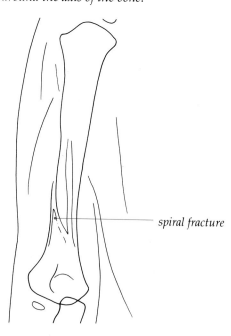

spiral fracture

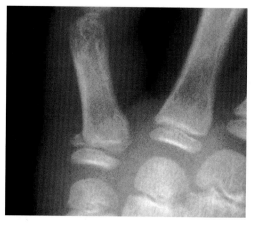

FIG. 19.11 Impacted fracture of the base of the proximal phalanx. The fracture line is indistinct and the fragments appear crushed together. The fracture does not actually involve the growth plate but is located just distal to it in the proximal metaphysis.

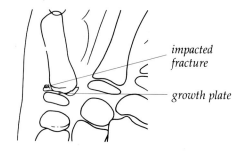

impacted fracture

growth plate

PEDIATRIC ORTHOPEDICS

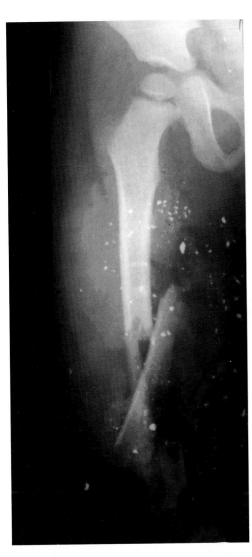

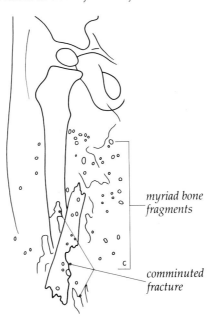

FIG. 19.12 *Comminuted fracture of the femur secondary to gunshot wound. Notice the multiple small fragments of bone present in the adjacent soft tissues.*

myriad bone fragments

comminuted fracture

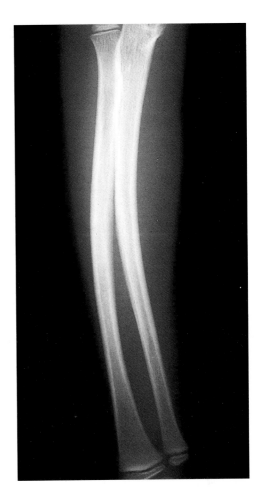

FIG. 19.13 *Bowing of the forearm bones in an 8-year-old. This type of plastic deformation can be expected to remodel with time.*

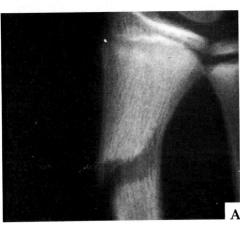

A

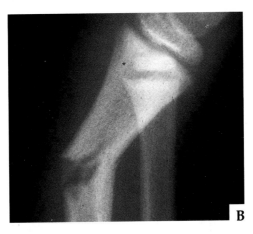

B

FIG. 19.14 *Greenstick fracture of the distal radius. In the AP view of the distal radius (A) a fracture line is seen that is complete except for a portion of the cortex on the compression side of the fracture. The lateral radiograph (B) demonstrates more clearly the disrupted and compressed cortices.*

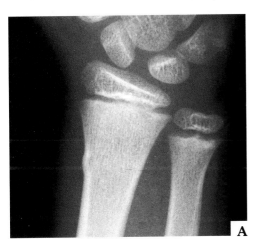

A

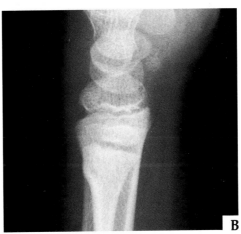

B

FIG. 19.15 *Torus fracture of the distal radius. An AP radiograph of the wrist (A) demonstrates a minor torus or buckle fracture of the radius. The lateral radiograph (B) shows the dorsal location of the deformity. This injury can be expected to completely remodel.*

Type	Site	Radiographic Appearance
Diaphyseal	Fracture involves the central shaft of a long bone	Fig. 19.17
Metaphyseal	Fracture involves the widened end of a long bone	Fig. 19.18
Epiphyseal	Fracture involves the chondro-osseous end of a long bone. Such fractures can also be classifed as Salter-Harris fractures.	Fig. 19.19
Articular	Fracture involves the cartilaginous joint surface	Fig. 19.20 (see Figs. 19.29 and 19.30)
Intercondylar	Fracture is located between the condyles of a joint. This is one variant of articular fracture and could also be subclassifed as a Salter-Harris fracture.	Fig. 19.20
Physeal	Fracture involves the growth center of long bone. These are subclassified according to the Salter-Harris system.	Fig. 19.21
Transcondylar	Fracture traverses the condyles of a joint	Fig. 19.22
Supracondylar	Fracture line is located just proximal to the condyles of a joint	Fig. 19.23
Epicondylar	Fracture involves an area juxtaposed to the condylar surface of a joint	Fig. 19.24
Subcapital	Fracture is located just below the epiphyseal head of certain bones	Fig. 19.25

FIG. 19.16 Classification of fractures by anatomic location.

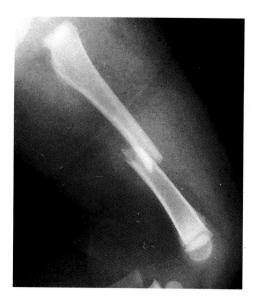

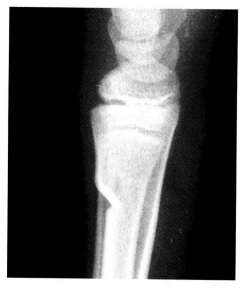

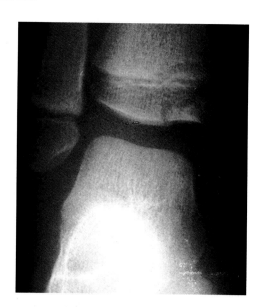

FIG. 19.17 Diaphyseal fracture. A transverse fracture line crosses the diaphyseal region of the femur. There is a moderate amount of overlap at the fracture site.

FIG. 19.18 Metaphyseal fracture. This lateral radiograph of the wrist shows a dorsal buckle fracture of the distal radial metaphysis. This fracture resulted from a fall on the outstretched arm with the wrist dorsiflexed and is a common injury in children.

FIG. 19.19 Epiphyseal fracture. A fracture involving the medial aspect of the epiphysis of the distal tibia is seen in this AP radiograph of the ankle in a 4-year-old girl. A slight stepoff is present at the articular surface. This could also be classified as a Salter-Harris type III fracture.

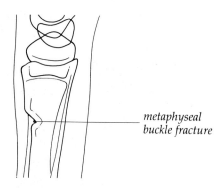

metaphyseal
buckle fracture

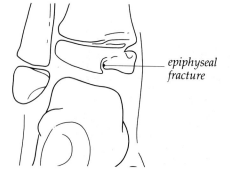

epiphyseal
fracture

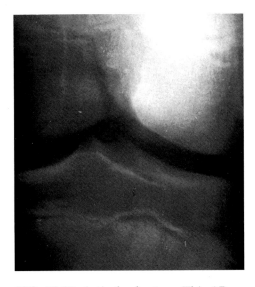

FIG. 19.20 Articular fracture. This AP radiograph of the knee demonstrates intraarticular extension of a fracture line exiting at the junction of the medial and lateral femoral condyles. The condyles are separated by only a few millimeters. This can also be termed an intercondylar fracture.

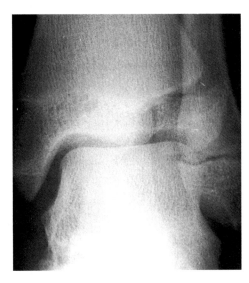

FIG. 19.21 Physeal fracture. A fracture of the lateral aspect of the epiphysis through the lateral aspect of the physeal plate is seen in this AP view of ankle of 13-year-old boy. Also called a "Tillaux" fracture, this pattern is seen in adolescents in whom the medial aspect of the distal tibial physis has closed but not the lateral aspect. Also termed a Salter-Harris type III fracture.

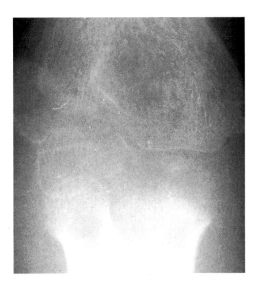

FIG. 19.22 Transcondylar fracture. This AP radiograph of the elbow reveals a fracture of the lateral condyle of the distal humerus. The condyle is displaced proximally and radially. The fragment is always larger than it appears on radiograph because of the large amount of unossified cartilage present in the distal humerus.

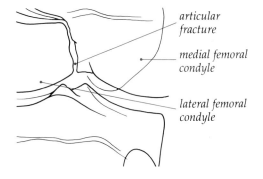

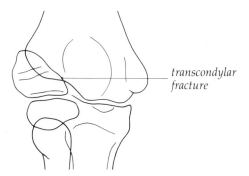

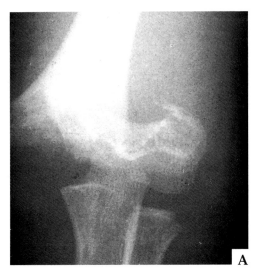

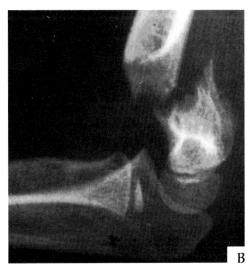

FIG. 19.23 Supracondylar fracture. These radiographs show the most common pattern of supracondylar humerus fracture seen in children. This injury commonly results from a fall on the outstretched arm with forces transmitted to the distal humerus driving the distal fragment posteriorly. The AP radiograph (A) shows the distal fragment displaced radially. In the lateral view (B), posterior displacement is evident as well.

The anatomic location of the fracture line simply refers to that portion of the bone to which the injuring force was applied. Figure 19.16 presents types of fractures classified by anatomic location. These fractures are illustrated in Figures 19.17 through 19.25. It should be noted that there is some degree of overlap in this method of categorization.

PHYSEAL FRACTURES

An estimated 15 percent of all fractures in children involve the physis. Because the adjacent epiphyseal plate is not ossified in the young child and therefore is invisible on a radiograph, the fracture may be mistaken for a minor sprain or missed altogether, only to manifest itself at a later date in

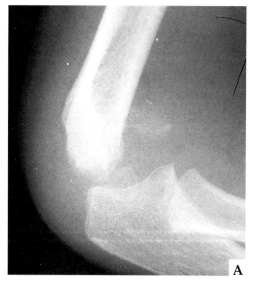

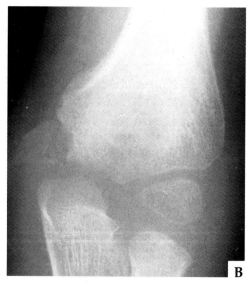

A

B

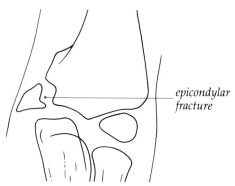

FIG. 19.24 *Epicondylar fracture. Lateral radiograph* **(A)** *reveals significant proximal migration of medial epicondyle of distal humerus. The AP view* **(B)** *shows slight medial displacement of medial epicondyle.*

epicondylar fracture

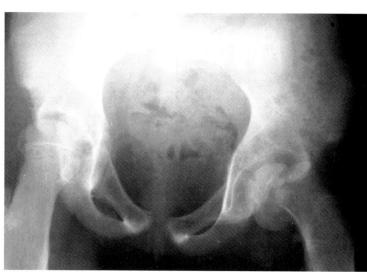

FIG. 19.25 *Subcapital fracture. This AP radiograph of the pelvis shows a displaced subcapital fracture of the right femur. This particular injury may be seen acutely due to significant trauma, or may develop slowly as a result of gradual slipping at the physeal level.*

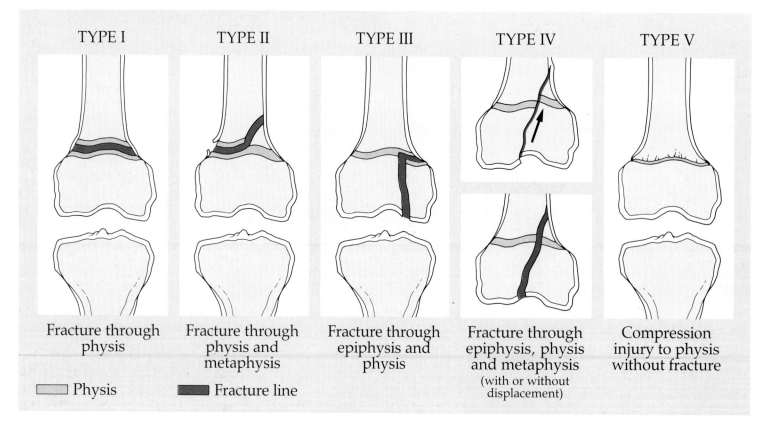

TYPE I	TYPE II	TYPE III	TYPE IV	TYPE V
Fracture through physis	Fracture through physis and metaphysis	Fracture through epiphysis and physis	Fracture through epiphysis, physis and metaphysis (with or without displacement)	Compression injury to physis without fracture

☐ Physis   ▬ Fracture line

FIG. 19.26 *Salter-Harris classification of physeal injuries.*

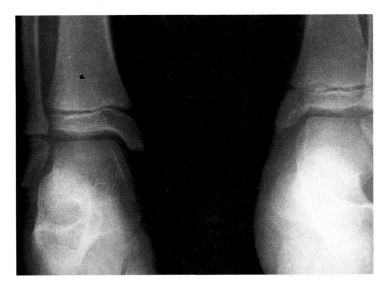

FIG. 19.27 Salter-Harris type I injury. Close inspection of the right ankle shows slight widening of the distal fibular physeal plate compared to the normal appearance of the left ankle. This patient's only clinical finding was point tenderness over the fibular growth plate.

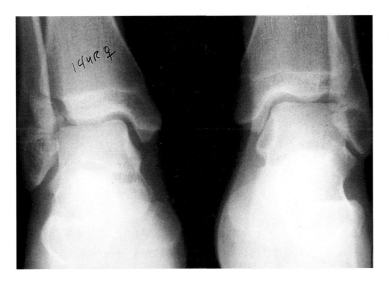

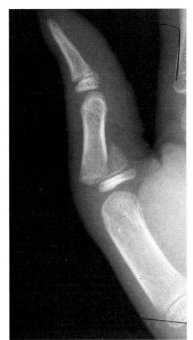

FIG. 19.28 Salter-Harris type II injury. On this lateral radiograph of the thumb the fracture is seen to involve the proximal phalanx. The fracture line runs through the physis and exits through the metaphysis on the side opposite the site of fracture initiation. A fragment consisting of the entire epiphysis with the attached metaphyseal fragment is produced.

FIG. 19.29 Salter-Harris type III injury. Comparison view of both ankles reveals a fracture involving the lateral aspect of the right distal tibial epiphysis. This configuration creates a separate fragment without any connection to the metaphysis.

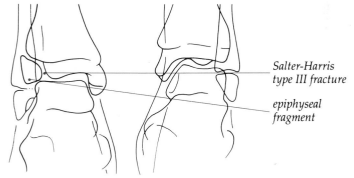

Salter-Harris type III fracture

epiphyseal fragment

slowed or failed longitudinal limb growth or in the development of an angular deformity. Even if diagnosed and properly treated, physeal injuries may still result in longitudinal or angular abnormalities. Most physeal disruptions occur through the zone of cartilage cell hypertrophy within the physeal plate and thus do not result in permanent damage to the plate. However, a small proportion of disruptions involve the resting or germinal layer of the physis and may disrupt the cells permanently, resulting in eventual deformity despite adequate reduction of the fracture fragments.

Because of their potential for long-term morbidity, great attention has been focused on the classification, diagnosis, treatment, and prognosis of physeal fractures. The Salter-Harris classification scheme is the system most commonly used to classify physeal injuries in North America (Fig. 19.26).

Salter-Harris Type I

This injury consists of a fracture running horizontally through the physis itself resulting in a variable degree of separation of the epiphysis from the metaphysis. The amount of separation depends on the degree of periosteal disruption. Radiographs are often normal, hence, the diag-

nosis frequently must be made clinically on the basis of point tenderness and mild soft tissue swelling over the site of an epiphysis (Fig. 19.27). This injury usually results from a shearing force. Prognosis is usually favorable.

Salter-Harris Type II

Also produced by shearing forces, this injury consists of a fracture line running a variable distance through the physis and exiting through the metaphysis on the side opposite the site of fracture initiation. A fragment consisting of the entire epiphysis with an attached metaphyseal fragment is thus produced (Fig. 19.28). Prognosis is generally favorable with adequate reduction.

Salter-Harris Type III

Intra-articular shearing forces can produce a fracture line running from the articular surface through the epiphysis then exiting through a portion of the physis. This creates a separate epiphyseal fragment with no connection to the metaphysis (Fig. 19.29). Prognosis may be quite poor. Accurate anatomic reduction is required to achieve the best possible outcome.

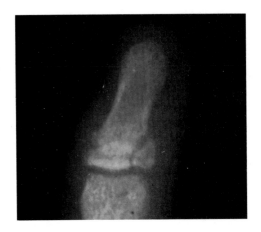

FIG. 19.30 Salter-Harris type IV injury.
This patient incurred a fracture of the distal
phalanx of the index finger. The fracture
line starts at the articular surface runs
through the epiphysis, across the physis,
and exits through the metaphysis. A single
fragment consisting of both epiphysis and
attached metaphysis is thus created.

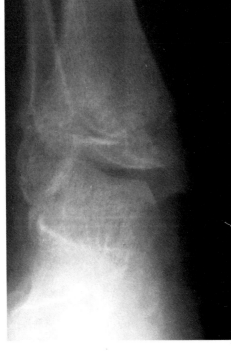

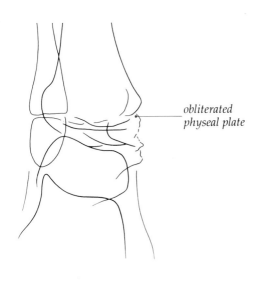

obliterated
physeal plate

metaphysis

physis

epiphyseal/
metaphyseal
fragment

epiphysis

FIG. 19.31 Salter-Harris type V injury.
This AP radiograph of the ankle taken several weeks after a crush injury sustained in
an automobile accident reveals obliteration
of the distal tibial physeal plate. As is often

the case, original radiographs taken at the
time of injury looked normal. Fracture must
be suspected on clinical grounds and the patient treated and followed accordingly.

Salter-Harris Type IV

In this type the fracture line starts at the articular surface,
runs through the physis across the epiphysis, and exits out
the metaphysis. A single fragment consisting of both epiphysis and attached metaphysis is thus created (Fig. 19.30).
Like Salter-Harris Type III, the injury results from the application of a shearing force. Prognosis may be poor despite
seemingly good anatomic restoration of the fracture fragments. Open reduction and internal fixation is virtually always necessary. Both Salter-Harris III and IV fractures also
can be classified as intra-articular fractures.

Salter-Harris Type V

This type is the product of a crushing injury to the physis
without physeal fracture or displacement. Radiographic diagnosis is virtually impossible to make at the time of injury,
hence, this fracture must be diagnosed on clinical grounds.
Distinction between a Salter-Harris I and a Salter-Harris V
fracture is often possible only when a subsequent growth
abnormality has been appreciated. Prognosis is quite poor
for normal growth (Fig. 19.31).

FRACTURE TREATMENT PRINCIPLES

The healing and remodeling capacity of the growing bones
of a child is considerably greater than that of an adult; the
younger the child the greater is this capacity for regenera-
tion. As a result, healing is rapid, necessitating a shorter
period of immobilization; nonunion is rare. Furthermore, in
planning fracture reductions, remodeling capability and the

likely addition to bone length as a result of overgrowth must
be considered. For example, in managing a toddler with a
femur fracture which is displaced in the plane of motion of
the adjacent joint, the bone ends must overlap to account
for overgrowth, and a degree of angulation can be accepted,
because this will ultimately be corrected by remodeling. The
amount of angulation and the degree of overlap of fracture
fragments that can be accepted is difficult to state in nu-
meric terms. Acceptable position is determined in part by
the child's age, the nature and position of the fracture, the
bone involved, the appearance and condition of the adjacent soft tissues, and the presence or absence of other systemic injuries. Remodeling has its limitations, however. Rotational deformities and angular deformities which are not
in the axis of adjacent joint motion are not effectively re-
modeled. Thus, these must be corrected at the time of initial
fracture reduction.

Nondisplaced fractures are simply casted or splinted. Because of the relative rarity of ligamentous injuries prior to
epiphyseal closure, patients with an appropriate clinical history and point tenderness over an epiphysis are presumed
to have a fracture and should be treated accordingly even
when radiographs are negative. Most displaced fractures
not involving the physis can be treated by closed reduction
and casting. As a general rule, open reduction and internal
fixation is usually reserved for Salter-Harris Type III and
Type IV fractures which have any degree of displacement,
for certain open fractures, and for fractures associated with
continued neurovascular compromise. Depending on time

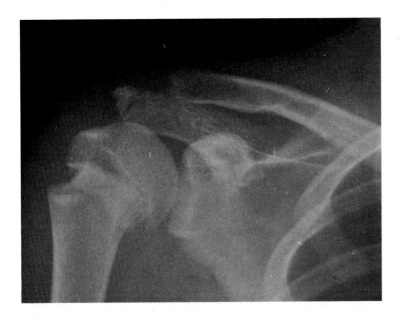

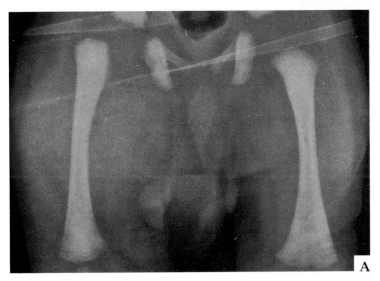

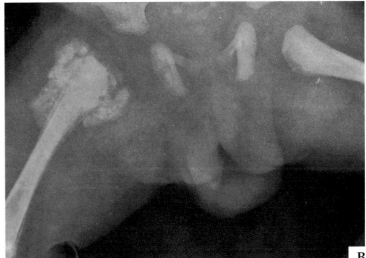

FIG. 19.32 Epiphyseal separation. Because of the elasticity and relatively greater strength of the ligaments, forces that would have resulted in dislocation in an older adolescent have instead caused epiphyseal separation and displacement of the proximal humeral epiphysis in this prepubertal child. (Courtesy of Dept. of Pediatric Radiology, Children's Hospital of Pittsburgh)

FIG. 19.33 Fracture dislocation, right hip. This young infant presented with what appeared to be a traumatic hip dislocation without an associated fracture. **A,** The right femoral head is displaced laterally and superiorly. The follow-up film taken 2 weeks later **(B)** re-

vealed vigorous callus formation around the proximal femur and periosteal new bone formation both proximally and distally, thus confirming associated fractures. (Courtesy of Dept. of Pediatric Radiology, Children's Hospital of Pittsburgh)

of presentation, degree of displacement, and severity of soft tissue swelling, reduction and/or casting may have to be deferred pending application of traction and subsidence of edema.

The importance of adequate analgesia and sedation prior to closed reduction procedures warrants emphasis. Too often reduction is performed without the benefit of analgesia and justified by the rationale that "it will only hurt for a minute." This reasoning is callous and that excruciating "minute" may seem an eternity to the child. Following reduction and/or immobilization in a cast, pain should be markedly alleviated. Persistence or recurrence of significant discomfort suggests a complication and warrants prompt reevaluation.

Care must be taken in describing the nature of the injury and its prognosis, and in explaining the rationale for proposed treatment measures to the parents. A simpler explanation in terms geared to his developmental level should be given to the child. Use of written instructions regarding home care measures, necessary parent observations, and worrisome signs that signal need for prompt reevaluation is invaluable.

Ligamentous Injuries

DISLOCATIONS

The ligaments of a child have great elasticity and are relatively strong as compared to bony structures, especially the physis (Fig. 19.32). Consequently joint dislocations and ligamentous disruptions are rather unusual in childhood; when seen, they are usually the result of severe trauma, and are commonly associated with fractures. In some instances the dislocation is obvious and the fracture subtle or even invisible radiographically (Fig. 19.33), but often the fracture is the prominent clinical finding and the dislocation less apparent. Hence, the emphasis in pediatric orthopedics is on examining the entire extremity, and including the joints proximal and distal to a suspected fracture site in radiographic examination. Failure to diagnose the full extent of injury can result in permanent morbidity. It must also be remembered that in infancy epiphyseal separations prior to ossification can simulate dislocations. For example, separation of the distal humeral epiphysis presents a radiographic picture suggesting posterior displacement of the olecranon. The

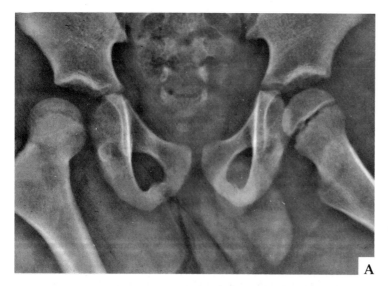

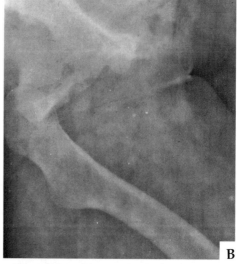

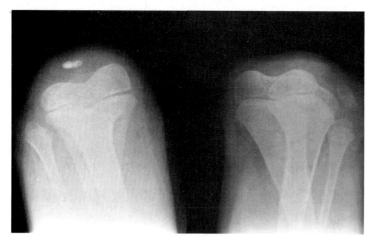

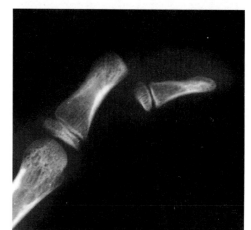

FIG. 19.36 Interphalangeal joint dislocation. The distal phalanx of the thumb is dislocated dorsally. (Courtesy of Dept. of Pediatric Radiology, Children's Hospital of Pittsburgh)

FIG. 19.35 Patellar dislocation. In this flexion view taken prior to relocation the left patella is displaced laterally and there is a marked degree of swelling. (Courtesy of Dept. of Pediatric Radiology, Children's Hospital of Pittsburgh)

most frequent sites of dislocation in childhood are the hip, the patellofemoral joint, and the interphalangeal joints.

Hip dislocations in the young are usually the result of falls. In a child under 5 years of age the softness of the acetabulum and relative ligamentous laxity enable dislocation without application of extreme force and thus there may be no associated fractures. In the older child violent force is required and dislocation is commonly accompanied by fractures of the femur and acetabulum. In most instances the femoral head dislocates posteriorly. The child presents in severe pain with the involved leg held in adduction, internally rotated and flexed (Fig. 19.34). Extension, external rotation, and abduction is the position adopted with the less common anterior dislocation. When the child also has an impressive femoral fracture, his pain may be interpreted as due to that and the positional findings missed unless the clinician specifically looks for them. Even in cases without an obvious associated fracture epiphyseal separation or avulsion of an acetabular fragment may have occurred. Prompt reduction is important both for relief of pain and to reduce the risk of secondary avascular necrosis. Post-reduction films are important as these are more likely to disclose

the fact that epiphyseal separation has occured, and will tend to show incomplete reduction if a radiolucent intra-articular fragment is present.

In patellofemoral dislocations the patella usually dislocates laterally (Fig. 19.35). This may occur as the result of shearing forces or of a hyperextension injury. Patients with ligamentous laxity appear particularly susceptible. In most instances the patella has relocated by the time the patient is seen. If not, the leg should be immediately extended and the patella pushed back into place to alleviate pain. Findings on examination include prominent swelling and hemarthrosis, tenderness along the medial patellar border and increased lateral mobility of the patella. Avulsion fractures of the lateral femoral condyle and/or medial patella are common associated injuries. Application of ice, rest, and use of a knee immobilizer for 3 weeks is recommended. Currently there is disagreement on whether operative intervention should be considered following the first episode, or deferred until a recurrence.

Dislocation of an interphalangeal joint results in an obvious deformity and is an intensely painful injury (Fig. 19.36). Avulsion fractures, volar plate fractures, and tendinous or

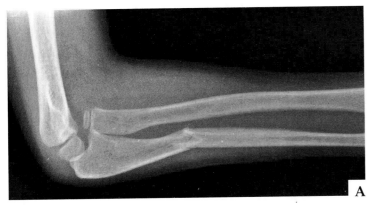

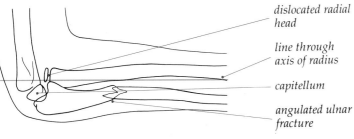

dislocated radial head

line through axis of radius

capitellum

angulated ulnar fracture

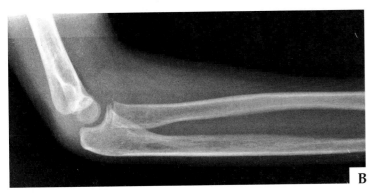

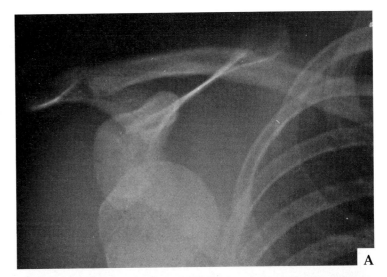

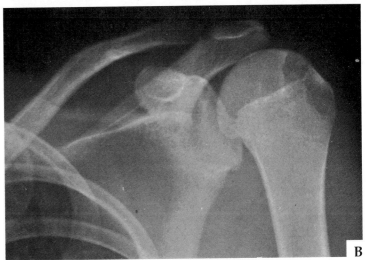

FIG. 19.37 *Monteggia fracture.* **A**, *The displaced fracture of the proximal ulna is accompanied by dislocation of the radial head. A line drawn through the long axis of the radius would intersect the distal humerus above the level of the capitellum. The comparison view of the normal arm* **(B)** *shows the normal position of the radial head. (Courtesy of Dept. of Pediatric Radiology, Children's Hospital of Pittsburgh)*

FIG. 19.38 **A**, *Anterior dislocation of the right shoulder. The humeral head is not in the glenoid fossa, but is displaced anteriorly. The normal relationship is seen in the left shoulder* **(B)**. *The injury occurred when the patient was taking a back swing for a hockey shot. The patient felt a pop and immediate onset of severe pain. Note that his epiphyses have fused. (Courtesy of Dept. of Pediatric Radiology, Children's Hospital of Pittsburgh)*

capsular injury may be associated and difficult to detect radiographically. These must be suspected if range of motion is incomplete following relocation. In some cases the associated injury makes closed reduction impossible.

Elbow dislocations are rare in the absence of an associated fracture. The fracture may be as subtle as nonossified fragment avulsed from the medial epicondyle or the ulna, or as prominent as a displaced fracture of the ulna or radius. An example of the latter is the Monteggia fracture. Here a displaced fracture of the proximal ulna is accompanied by dislocation of the radial head. A radial dislocation should be suspected if a line drawn through the long axis of the radius fails to pass through the capitellum on any view (Fig. 19.37). Less frequently, fractures of the radius are associated with dislocation of the radioulnar joint, and fractures of the olecranon may be accompanied by dislocation of the radius.

True shoulder dislocations are seen only in adolescents after epiphyseal fusion (Fig. 19.38). Separation of the proximal humeral epiphysis or major fracture dislocations are seen in younger children subjected to forces that would cause dislocation after puberty (see Fig. 19.32).

SPRAINS

A sprain is a ligamentous injury in which some degree of tearing occurs, often as a result of excessive stretching or twisting. As repeatedly emphasized in the section on fractures, sprains are relatively unusual prior to epiphyseal fusion. The growth plate, being weaker than the ligaments, tends to give before significant ligamentous tearing can develop. Thus, in children physeal fractures tend to result from forces that would produce a sprain in an older adolescent or adult. In many other instances, what appears to be a sprain is actually a small avulsion fracture. If the portion avulsed is ossified a small fragment may be detectable radiographically, but if the fragment is cartilaginous, it will be radiographically invisible. Hence, prior to epiphyseal closure, Salter-Harris fractures and avulsion fractures of the distal fibula or tibia should be strongly suspected in "sprainlike" injuries of the ankle. Similarly, injuries that rupture the

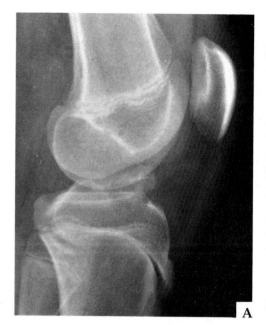
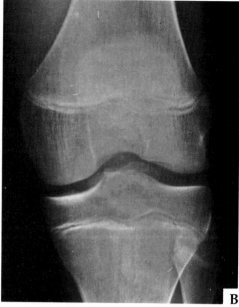
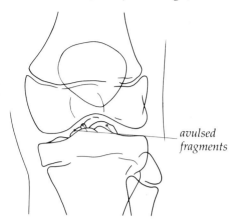

FIG. 19.39 Avulsion fracture of the left tibial spines due to soccer injury (lateral view **A**; AP view, **B**). Also present were tear in cruciate ligament and a lipohemarthrosis. (Courtesy of Dept. of Pediatric Radiology, Children's Hospital of Pittsburgh)

avulsed fragments

CLASSIFICATION OF SPRAINS

Grade of Sprain	Degree of Tearing	Clinical Findings
I	A small fraction of ligamentous fibers is disrupted	Pain on motion Local tenderness Mild swelling
II	A moderate percentage of fibers is torn	Pain on motion More diffuse tenderness Moderate swelling, may have joint effusion Mild instability
III	The ligament is completely disrupted	Severe pain on motion Marked swelling usually with joint effusion Marked tenderness Joint instability

FIG. 19.40 Classification of sprains.

cruciate ligaments of the knee in adults usually avulse the tibial spine in the child (Fig. 19.39). Following physeal closure in adolescence, sprains are seen with some frequency.

Sprains are classified in three grades according to severity (Fig. 19.40). In contrast to physeal fractures, swelling is more likely to be prominent and to occur early, and tenderness is noted over the involved ligament or ligaments, not over the epiphysis. Pain on motion is often more marked in patients with sprains than in patients with physeal fractures.

In evaluating patients with possible sprains, careful attention must be given not only to assessment of swelling, tenderness, and joint stability, but also to evaluation of adjacent bony structures and to musculotendinous function.

Rest, application of ice, use of a mild analgesic and perhaps use of an Ace wrap or taping suffice for Grade I sprains. Subjective improvement occurs in a few days. Grade II and III sprains require a longer period of immobilization. Splinting or casting for a few to several weeks is generally necessary, and Grade III sprains may necessitate operative intervention.

SUBLUXATION OF THE RADIAL HEAD (NURSEMAID'S ELBOW)

Subluxation of the radial head is the most common elbow injury in childhood and one of the most common ligamentous injuries. The mechanism is one of sudden traction applied to the extended arm. The injury is seen predominantly in children between the ages of 1 and 4 years. The typical history is one of a parent suddenly pulling the child by the arm to prevent him or her from falling or heading toward danger, or of the child, in a fit of temper attempting to pull away from the parent. After a brief initial period of crying, the child calms down, but is unable to use the affected arm which is held close to the body with elbow flexed and forearm pronated. Physical examination reveals no bony tenderness and no evidence of swelling, but on assessment of passive motion, the child resists any attempt at supination. Mild limitation of elbow flexion and extension may also be noted.

Pathologically, when the radial head is subluxed by the sudden pull on the arm, the annular ligament is torn at the

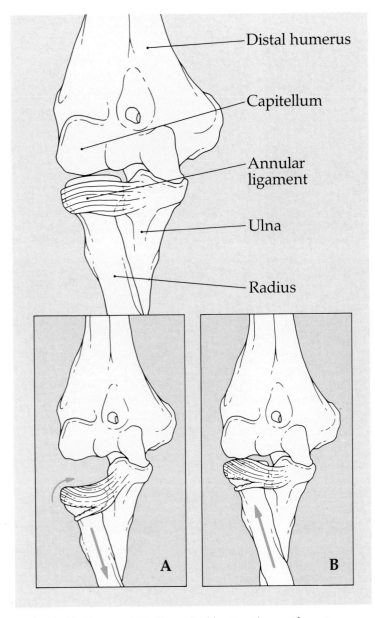

Distal humerus

Capitellum

Annular ligament

Ulna

Radius

A B

FIG. 19.41 Nursemaid's elbow. Sudden traction on the out-stretched arm pulls the radius distally causing it to slip partially through the annular ligament, and tearing it in the process (A). When traction is released, the radial head recoils trapping the proxi-mal portion of the ligament between it and the capitellum (B).

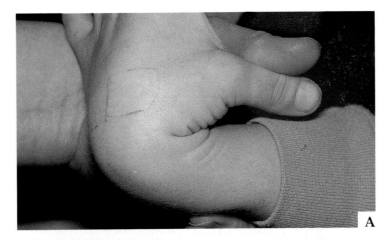

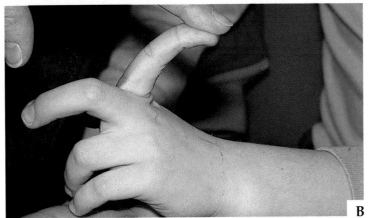

FIG. 19.42 Ligamentous laxity. This child demonstrates typical findings of joint hypermobility seen with ligamentous laxity. He is able to hyperflex the wrist on the forearm (A). He also is able to hy-perextend the distal interphalangeal joint and the metacarpopha-langeal joint (B).

site of its attachment to the radius and the radial head slips through the tear. When the traction is released and the ra-dial head recoils back, the proximal portion of the annular ligament becomes trapped between the radial head and the capitellum (Fig. 19.41). This limits motion and produces the child's pain. Radiographs are normal because the radial head is not truly subluxed.

Treatment consists of supinating the child's forearm with the elbow in a flexed position while applying pressure over the radial head. A click can be perceived as the annular liga-ment is freed from the joint. Occasionally this maneuver fails, in which case the forearm should be supinated and extended with traction applied distally while pressing down on the radial head. Pain relief is immediate and no cast is required. It is often recommended that the child wear a sling for 10 days to reduce use, and to allow the annular liga-ment to heal; compliance is difficult to assure, however.

EXTREMITY PAIN WITH LIGAMENTOUS LAXITY

Children with significant and generalized ligamentous lax-ity have hypermobile joints and are vulnerable to excessive stretching or stress on ligamentous and musculotendinous structures. They are also somewhat more susceptible to joint dislocations. The phenomenon is seen in up to 18 per-cent of girls and 6 percent of boys. Following periods of vig-orous physical activity these children often complain of ar-thralgias and/or muscular pain, and occasionally have evidence of joint swelling. Episodes tend to occur in the evening or at night, are self-limited, lasting one to several hours, and respond to rest and aspirin or acetaminophen. Many of these children have been accused of attention-get-ting behavior and hypochondriasis. Others have been passed off as having "growing pains," and some have un-dergone extensive testing for rheumatic disorders. A his-tory of greater than average activity on the preceding day and of recurrent short-lived pain usually without objective swelling, combined with findings of ligamentous laxity on examination (Fig. 19.42) should suggest this diagnosis. The rarity of joint swelling and the absence of fever and other systemic symptoms help to rule out rheumatic and collagen vascular disorders.

Once the problem is correctly diagnosed, patients can minimize discomfort by avoiding sudden increases in level of activity and by taking a mild analgesic prophylactically after a period of unusually vigorous activity. Graduated strengthening exercises may also be helpful.

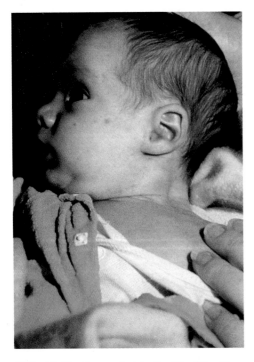

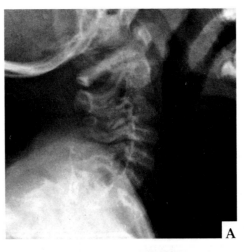

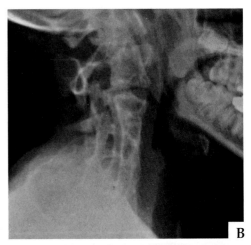

FIG. 19.43 Congenital torticollis. The "tu-mor" of congenital torticollis is seen as a swelling in the midportion of the sterno-cleidomastoid muscle. It is firm on palpa-tion, and the muscle itself is shortened. The head tilts toward the affected side and the chin rotates in the opposite direction. (Courtesy of Dr. J. Reilly)

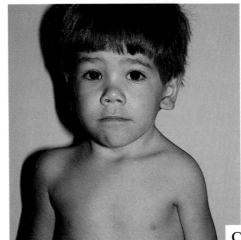

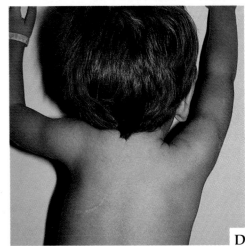

FIG. 19.44 Klippel-Feil syndrome. **A,** Mild osseous involvement is seen in this radio-graph in which there is fusion of the upper cervical segments. **B,** Severe osseous involve-ment is demonstrated in this radiograph in which C-3 to C-7 are fused and hypoplastic. **C,** The neck appears short and broad in the anterior view of this young child. **D,** In the posterior view, the hairline is low and an as-sociated Sprengel's deformity is present, the left scapula being hypoplastic and high-riding. As a result, the patient is unable to fully raise his left arm. Typical webbing is not appreciable in this child.

DISORDERS OF THE SPINE

Children with disorders of the axial skeleton most com-monly present with some type of deformity. Pain or dys-function of the associated spinal cord and nerve roots may also prompt evaluation. As these conditions often progress with growth, awareness and early recognition are impor-tant to facilitate early institution of appropriate treatment measures, and to minimize resultant morbidity.

Congenital Torticollis

Congenital torticollis or "wry neck" is a positional abnor-mality of the neck produced by fibrosis and shortening of the sternocleidomastoid muscle. It is thought to be second-ary to abnormal intrauterine positioning or birth trauma re-sulting in formation of a hematoma within the muscle belly. Usually the condition is recognized at or shortly after birth. A palpable swelling or "tumor" is often noted within the muscle. With subsequent fibrosis, the characteristic deform-ity of torticollis develops consisting of head tilt toward the affected side with rotation of the chin to the opposite side (Fig. 19.43). While the mass usually disappears in the first several weeks of life, contracture of the muscle persists and,

if untreated, may result in craniofacial disfigurement with flattening of the face on the affected side. Gentle passive stretching exercises and positioning the child's crib so that external stimuli will cause him to turn the head and neck away from the side of deformity may be beneficial. If these measures fail, surgical release of the contracted muscle may be indicated.

The differential diagnoses include Klippel-Feil syndrome, inflammatory or infectious conditions of the head, neck or nasopharanx, posterior fossa or brain stem neoplasm, trau-matic cervical spine injury, or atlantoaxial rotary sublux-ation. However, with the exception of the Klippel-Feil anomaly, the other sources tend to occur considerably later in childhood.

Klippel-Feil Syndrome

This congenital malformation of the neck is the result of a failure of segmentation in the developing cervical spine. The condition varies greatly in severity depending on the number of vertebrae that are fused (Figs. 19.44, A and B). More severely affected individuals exhibit a short broad neck with the appearance of "webbing," a low hairline, and gross restriction of motion (Figs. 19.44, C and D). The condi-

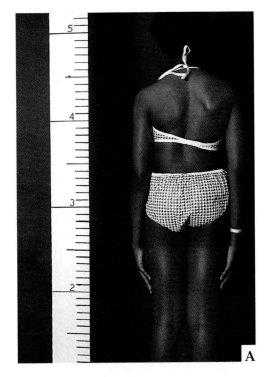

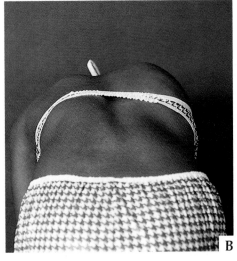

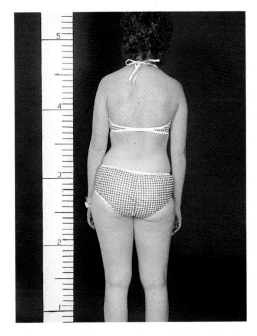

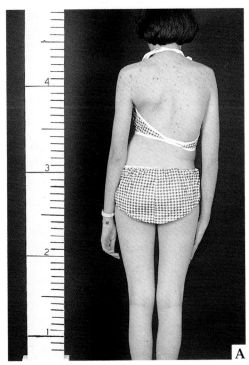

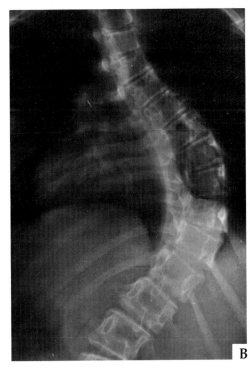

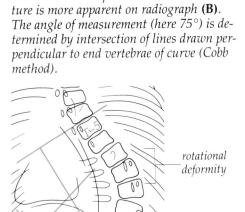

FIG. 19.45 *Moderate thoracic idiopathic adolescent scoliosis. In the upright position* **(A)**, *scapular asymmetry is easily discernible. This results from rotation of the spine and attached ribcage.* **B**, *Forward flexion reveals a mild rib hump deformity.*

FIG. 19.46 *Lumbar scoliosis. Pelvic obliquity is present, with prominence of the flank.*

FIG. 19.47 *Severe thoracic scoliosis secondary to neurofibromatosis.* **A**, *Note chest wall deformity and that patient's head is not centered over pelvis. The severe curvature is more apparent on radiograph* **(B)**. *The angle of measurement (here 75°) is determined by intersection of lines drawn perpendicular to end vertebrae of curve (Cobb method).*

rotational deformity

tion may be associated with other congenital malformations, such as Sprengel's deformity, rib deformities, scoliosis, CNS defects, and cardiac, pulmonary, and renal anomalies. Secondary neurological problems are rare, but accelerated degenerative changes may occur at mobile spinal segments adjacent to the involved vertebrae.

On occasion, range of motion exercises or bracing may be tried to improve mobility or correct deformity. Surgery, except for cosmesis or neurological dysfunction, is rarely indicated. Individuals with mild forms of the malformation may be diagnosed only as a result of radiographs taken for other reasons.

Scoliosis

Scoliosis refers to curvature of the spine in the lateral plane. By anatomic necessity, this lateral deviation is associated with vertebral rotation such that when this deformity occurs in the thoracic spine, a chest wall deformity or "rib hump" develops (Fig. 19.45). When it occurs in the lumbar spine, a prominence of the flank may be noted (Fig. 19.46). Often there is a primary structural curve with an adjacent secondary compensatory curve. The majority of cases are idiopathic and have their onset in early adolescence. Infantile (0 to 3 years) and juvenile (3 to 10 years) forms are seen, however. Scoliosis may also occur in conjunction with neuromuscular conditions (cerebral palsy, myelomeningocele, spinocerebellar degeneration, polio, spinal cord tumors, etc.); myopathic disorders (arthrogryposis or muscular dystrophy); congenital spinal anomalies; neurofibromatosis and mesenchymal disorders (Fig. 19.47); and a variety of other conditions. Apparent or "functional" scoliosis may be seen in association with limb length inequality, herniated

FIG. 19.48 *Causes of scoliosis.*

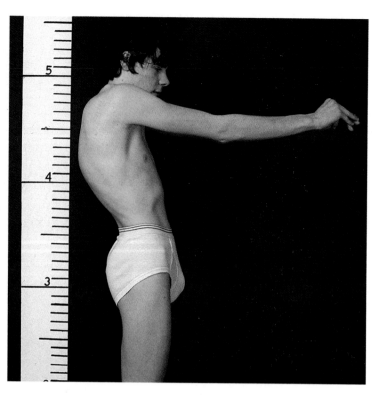

FIG. 19.49 *Moderate thoracic kyphosis secondary to Scheuermann's disease. The patient is attempting to correct the deformity, but due to its fixed nature, he cannot and must compensate for this with an increased lumbar lordosis.*

lumbar discs, inflammatory disorders, postural derangements and hysteria (Fig. 19.48). Except in curvatures resulting from inflammatory or neoplastic processes, pain is rarely a complaint.

With gross deformity the condition is readily apparent, but with minor curvatures inspection of the spine in forward flexion is required to detect scoliosis and to highlight any rotational deformity. (See Fig. 19.45B). This maneuver should be performed routinely at all well-child care visits to insure early diagnosis.

Treatment usually consists of observation for progression in mild cases, bracing to prevent progression for moderate cases, and surgical correction and arthrodesis for severe or rapidly progressing scoliosis.

Kyphosis

Kyphosis refers to curvature of the spine in the sagittal plane. As opposed to scoliosis, this condition is generally not associated with a rotational spinal deformity. It may be purely postural in nature or associated with a number of pathologic conditions. These include congenital vertebral anomalies, spinal growth disturbance (Scheuermann's disease) (Fig. 19.49), neuromuscular afflictions, skeletal dysplasias, and metabolic diseases (Figs. 19.50 A and B). Kyphosis can also develop following spinal trauma or surgery. Patients may complain of backache, aggravated by motion. The deformity is best viewed from the lateral position. Wedging of the vertebral bodies may be noted on radiographic examination (Fig. 19.50C).

Evaluation of the effects of posture and pressure over the apex facilitates therapeutic decisions. Exercises and bracing are quite effective in treating this condition in the growing spine. When the deformity is severe and fixed, surgical correction and stabilization may be indicated.

Spondylolisthesis

Spondylolisthesis is a condition characterized by the translation or forward displacement of one vertebral body over another, and is seen most commonly at the lumbosacral articulation. The problem may develop as a result of insufficiency or fatigue fractures of the pars interarticularis (isthmic), congenital dysplasia of the posterior spinal elements (dysplastic), degenerative changes of the disc and facets (degenerative), or secondary to pathologic lesions within the vertebra and its elements (pathologic). Isthmic spondylolisthesis (spondylolysis) is by far the most common type (Fig. 19.51). Patients with a congenital predisposition may show alarming degrees of slippage. The condition is often associated with pain which increases with strenuous activities and improves with rest. Some patients have symptoms of nerve root irritation. This necessitates differentiation from inflammatory and neoplastic processes, and disc herniation.

Examination often reveals loss of normal lumbar lordosis, tenderness of the involved posterior elements, paravertebral muscle spasm and secondary tightness of the hamstring muscles. A step-off deformity may be evident on palpating the spinous processes. Range of motion is often limited in extension with complaints of pain. Nerve root signs may be present. In its most severe form, spondyloptosis, the L-5 vertebral body may completely translate off of the sacrum. These patients characteristically exhibit a waddling gait, a transverse abdominal crease, flattened buttocks and flexion deformities of the hips and knees. The torso

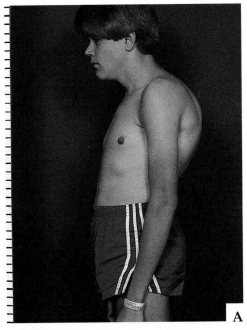

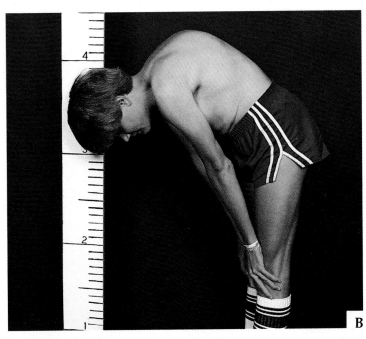

FIG. 19.50 **A**, Severe kyphosis of the thoracic spine secondary to vertebral wedging in glycogen storage disease. In order to stand upright, the patient must increase his lumbar lordosis and thrust his head forward to center it above the pelvis. **B**, The kyphotic deformity is accentuated on forward bending. **C**, Radiographically the vertebral wedging which underlies the kyphotic deformity is evident.

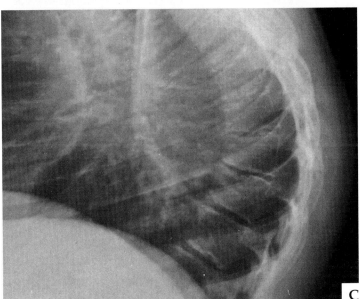

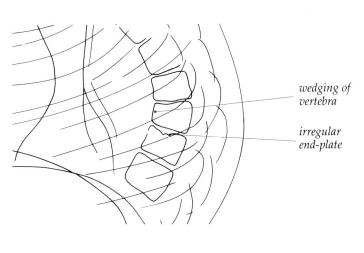

wedging of vertebra

irregular end-plate

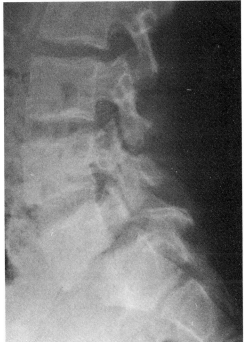

FIG. 19.51 Radiograph of moderate isthmic spondylolisthesis in a 14-year-old male. The forward slippage of L-5 on the sacrum is the result of a fatigue fracture of the pars interarticularis.

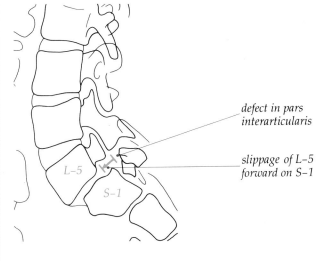

defect in pars interarticularis

slippage of L-5 forward on S-1

L-5

S-1

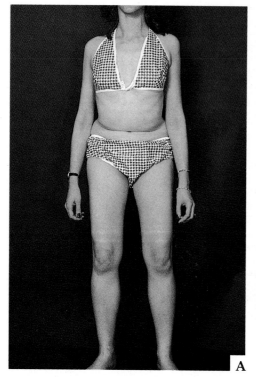

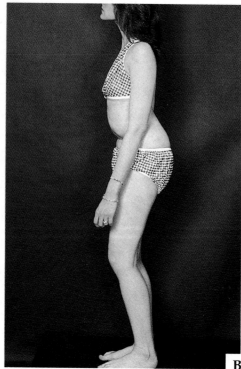

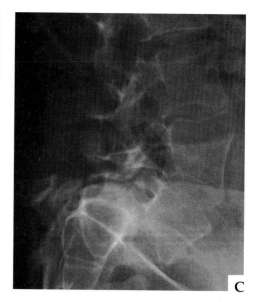

no visible
continuity
between
anterior and
posterior
elements
of spine

severe slippage
of L–5 off of S–1

vertical
orientation
of sacrum

FIG. 19.52 *Spondyloptosis in a 16-year-old female.* **A**, *A cosmetic deformity is common with this magnitude of spondylolisthesis. The torso is foreshortened and a transverse abdominal crease is present.* **B**, *In the lateral view, the torso is thrust forward, the buttocks are flattened, and there are flexion* deformities of the hips and knees. **C**, *The L-5 vertebra has completely translocated off of the sacrum due to a congenital insufficiency of the posterior elements. The lumbar spine has essentially migrated anteriorly and into the pelvis.*

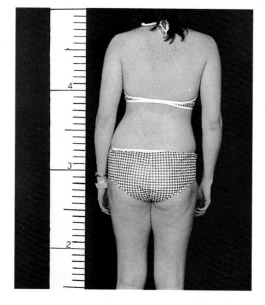

FIG. 19.53 *Discogenic scoliosis in a 16-year-old female with a herniated disc at L-4–5. The trunk is shifted away from the affected side. The normal lumbar lordosis is absent and spinal motion is severely limited.*

Herniated Intervertebral Disc

Although relatively common in adults, herniated discs occur rarely in children and are almost always limited to the lower two segments of the lumbar spine in adolescents. A history of trauma is not uncommon. Lower extremity radicular symptoms predominate. Patients often describe a peculiar "pulling" sensation in the lower extremity or liken their pain to a "toothache" in the distribution of the L-5 or S-1 nerve roots. They may complain of numbness or weakness in the involved limb. Forward flexion, sitting, coughing, or straining aggravate neural symptoms.

On examination, an antalgic scoliosis of the lumbar spine may be apparent which the patient is unable to reduce (Fig. 19.53). Inability to reverse the normal lumbar lordosis is present and symptoms may be aggravated by attempts at flexion. The straight leg raising test is often positive (radicular symptoms are reproduced when the limb is raised by the examiner) and neurological abnormalities on sensory, motor, and reflex testing may be found. Plain radiographs usually show no abnormality, but the diagnosis may be verified by a myelogram or CT scan. The differential diagnosis may include hematogenous disc space infection or vertebral osteomyelitis, spinal cord or neural element tumor, and spondylolisthesis with nerve root irritation.

Nonoperative treatment consisting of rest and anti-inflammatory agents may be successful, but if profound neurologic deficit is present or incapacitating symptoms persist, surgical disc excision may be indicated. Intradiscal chemonucleolysis, as employed for adults, is contraindicated for children.

may appear foreshortened (Figs. 19.52A and B). Characterization and grading of the process is made with radiographs. The oblique view may reveal a spondylolysis and the lateral view the degree of spondylolisthesis (Fig. 19.52C).

Treatment consists of appropriate exercises and bracing in mild to moderate cases. Patients with progressive slippage need surgical fusion, and those with neural involvement also may require nerve root decompression. In severe spondylolisthesis with cosmetic deformity, functional impairment, and neurological dysfunction, surgical reduction of the deformity may be attempted, but this is not easy, nor is it without risk to the adjacent neural structures.

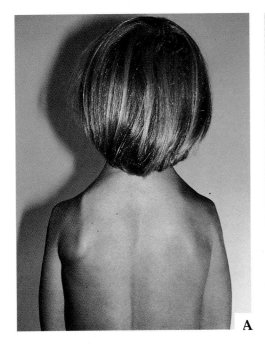
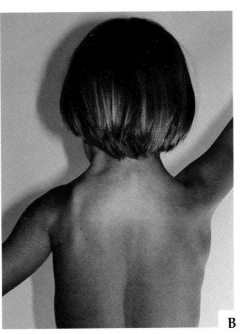
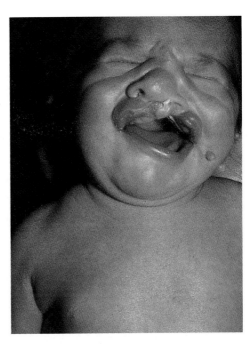

FIG. 19.54 Sprengel's deformity. The left scapula is high-riding and hypoplastic, and its vertebral border is prominent **(A)**. Shoulder motion is severely limited, particularly in abduction **(B)**. (Courtesy of Dr. D. Mears)

FIG. 19.55 Congenital pseudarthrosis of the clavicle. There is a bulbous, nontender swelling in the region of the midclavicle. The medial aspect of the clavicle is prominent. This patient has associated anomalies.

DISORDERS OF THE UPPER EXTREMITY

Because of the importance of prehensile function, disorders in any area of the upper limb can result in significant impairment of motor development during childhood. Knowledge of the normal anatomy and actions of the shoulder, arm, elbow, forearm, wrist, and hand is vital for assessment of abnormalities and institution of treatment.

Sprengel's Deformity

Sprengel's deformity is a congenital malformation characterized by an abnormally small, high-riding scapula. In the majority of cases it is unilateral. The etiology is unknown, but there appears to be a familial predisposition, and the condition may be associated with a variety of other congenital anomalies, including Klippel-Feil syndrome, and rib and vertebral malformations. The small undescended scapula may be attached to the cervical spine by a band of fibrous tissue or bone (omovertebral bone). Scoliosis and torticollis may be associated. Complaints are usually those of cosmetic deformity and limited shoulder motion on the affected side.

On examination, the scapula is noted to be hypoplastic and high-riding in association with asymmetry of the base of the neck and shoulder. Shoulder motion is usually severely limited, particularly in abduction (Fig. 19.54). Radiography confirms the abnormal size and position of the scapula.

Nonoperative treatment measures consisting of stretching and range of motion exercises may be instituted, but are rarely successful. Surgery is usually undertaken for cosmetic and functional reasons and may consist of excision of the prominent superior aspect of the scapula or release and reduction of the scapula by placing it inferiorly on the chest wall. The latter procedure is not without complication, as brachial plexus palsy may result from the maneuver.

Congenital Pseudarthrosis of the Clavicle

Congenital pseudarthrosis of the clavicle is a rare congenital disorder usually manifested by a painless, nontender bulbous deformity in the region of the midclavicle. It is thought to result from a failure of maturation of the ossification center of the clavicle. It generally involves the right side and, on occasion, may be associated with other congenital anomalies. In cleidocranial dysostosis the entire clavicle may be absent or may have an appearance similar to that of congenital pseudarthrosis.

On examination, the clavicle appears foreshortened with a prominence evident in its midportion (Fig. 19.55). Palpation reveals hypermobility of the two ends of the clavicle and crepitation. Range of motion of the shoulder is generally normal. This condition characteristically presents no functional impairment and requires no treatment. While clavicular fracture as a result of birth trauma may present a similar appearance, it is easily distinguished because of tenderness over the region of deformity.

Radial Club Hand

This condition is the result of congenital absence or hypoplasia of the radial structures of the forearm and hand. Associated muscular structures and the radial nerve are hypoplastic or absent. The anomaly is rare and affects males more frequently than females. Its characteristic clinical presentation is a small, short, bowed forearm and aplasia or

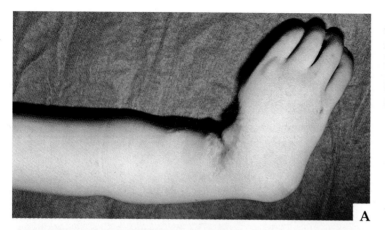

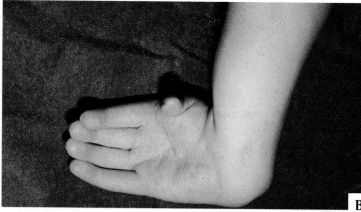

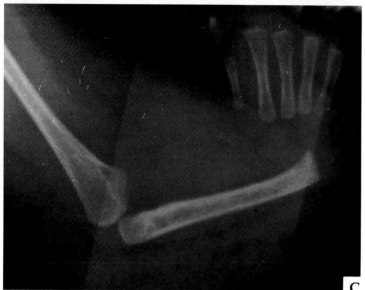

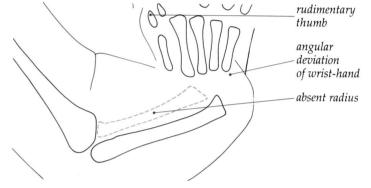

FIG. 19.56 Radial club hand deformity. **A**, The forearm is shortened with radial deviation of the hand and wrist on the ulna. **B**, There is a flexion deformity of the hand and wrist on the forearm and a hypoplastic thumb. **C**, This radiograph demonstrates absence of the radius, dislocation of the carpus, and a rudimentary thumb, all characteristic of radial club hand. (Clinical photographs courtesy of Dr. J. Imbriglia)

rudimentary thumb

angular deviation of wrist-hand

absent radius

hypoplasia of the thumb. The residual hand is deviated radially. Radiographs show absence of bones in the affected area (Fig. 19.56).

Treatment is best instituted early with passive stretching exercises and corrective casting. Surgical treatment consists of centralization of the hand on the "one bone forearm" to maximize function.

Ganglion of the Wrist

A ganglion is a benign cystic mass consisting of an accumulation of synovial fluid or gelatin in an outpouching of a tendon sheath or joint capsule. The exact etiology is unknown, but it is thought to be related to a herniation of synovial tissue with a ball valve effect. Antecendent trauma may be reported. These masses may be present over the dorsal or volar aspects of the wrist and are generally located toward the radial side (Fig. 19.57). They are occasionally seen on the dorsum of the foot or adjacent to one of the malleoli of the ankle. Their size may fluctuate with time and activity. On examination, they may be either firm or fluctuant. Transillumination is positive. While most are asymptomatic, an occasional patient may have pain and tenderness.

While treatment is unnecessary for patients who are asymptomatic, the majority desire removal for cosmetic purposes. Aspiration, injection, or rupture of these cysts often fail to permanently alleviate the problem. Surgical excision with obliteration of the base of the ganglion is the most successful treatment.

Syndactyly

Syndactyly is a relatively common congenital affliction involving failure of the digits of the hands or feet to separate. It is more common and disabling in the upper extremity. Bilateral involvement is usual and a positive family history is not uncommon. It may be associated with other congenital anomalies, particularly Apert's syndrome and Streeter's dysplasia. There is great variation in the degree of fusion. In mild cases, only the skin is joined, making reconstructive surgery simple (Fig. 19.58). In more severe cases, the nails, deeper structures and bones may be conjoined, contributing to deformity and growth abnormalities, and making reconstructive treatment more difficult.

Congenital Trigger Thumb

A congenital trigger thumb is characterized by a fixed flexion deformity of the interphalangeal joint of the thumb that may be present at birth or develop shortly thereafter (Fig. 19.59). The problem is thought to result from tightness of the tendon sheath of the flexor pollicus longus in the region of the metacarpophalangeal joint. The flexion deformity generally cannot be reduced, although in milder cases it may be passively correctable with a snapping sensation felt as the tendon passes through the stenosed pully mechanism. If passively correctable, splinting in extension occasionally will result in correction; otherwise, surgery is required.

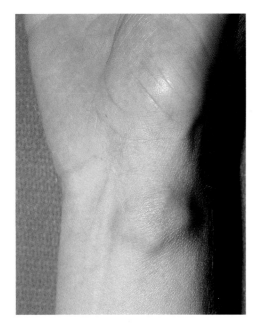

FIG. 19.57 Ganglion of the wrist. This cystic mass overlying the wrist joint and flexor tendons was asymptomatic and non-tender.

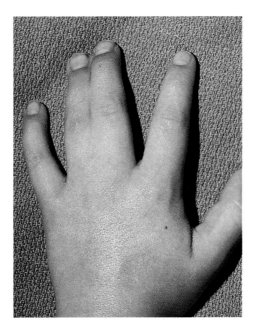

FIG. 19.58 Mild syndactyly involving soft tissues of the middle and ring fingers without bony involvement. (Courtesy of Dr. J. Imbriglia)

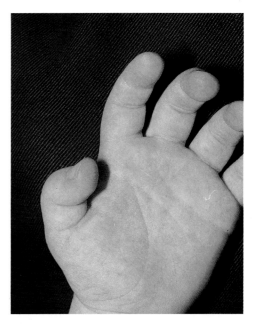

FIG. 19.59 Congenital trigger thumb. There is a fixed flexion deformity at the interphalangeal joint of the thumb due to tightness of the tendon sheath of the flexor pollicus longus. The remainder of the hand appears normal.

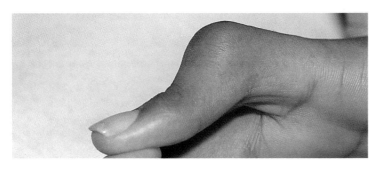

FIG. 19.60 Boutonnière deformity of the finger. There is a fixed flexion contracture of the proximal interphalangeal joint and hyperextension of the distal joint, secondary to volar migration of the lateral bands of the extensor mechanism. This is the result of unrecognized or inadequately treated injury to the extensor tendon at its insertion on the middle phalanx.

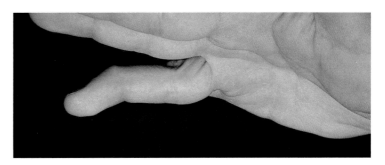

FIG. 19.61 Mallet finger with secondary "swan neck" deformity. This is the result of avulsion of the extensor tendon from its insertion at the base of the distal phalanx, which was not recognized at the time of injury. The patient demonstrates flexion deformity of the DIP joint and secondary hyperextension of the PIP joint.

Boutonnière (Buttonhole) Deformity

A boutonnière deformity of the finger is the end result of a traumatic avulsion of the central portion of the extensor tendon at its insertion on the middle phalanx of the finger which went unrecognized at the time of initial injury. The mechanism of injury is usually a blow to the tip of the finger driving it into forced flexion against resistance. A laceration over the dorsum of the finger involving the extensor tendon may produce a similar deformity if tendon involvement is not recognized and repaired at the time. Initially, there may be local tenderness over the dorsal aspect of the proximal interphalangeal (PIP) joint without deformity. With time, however, the lateral bands of the extensor mechanism migrate volarly, producing a flexion deformity of the PIP joint with a secondary extension deformity of the distal joint (Fig. 19.60). When recognized early, healing may occur with splinting of the PIP joint in extension. Later on, open surgical repair may be necessary to improve function.

Mallet Finger/Swan Neck Deformity

A mallet finger is the result of avulsion of the extensor tendon from its insertion at the base of the distal phalanx of a finger. It occurs as a result of a blow to the extended finger against resistance. The tendon alone, or a portion of the distal phalanx into which it inserts, may be involved. The clinical appearance is that of a "dropped finger" or flexion deformity of the distal interphalangeal (DIP) joint with inability to actively extend the joint. If not recognized and treated at the time of the initial injury the condition becomes chronic, and contracture of the extensor mechanism may occur with a secondary hyperextension deformity of the proximal interphalangeal joint producing a "swan neck deformity" (Fig. 19.61). Treatment consists of splinting the distal joint in an extended position, open reduction if a large fragment of bone is involved, or surgical repair in chronic cases.

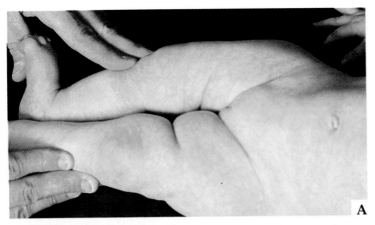

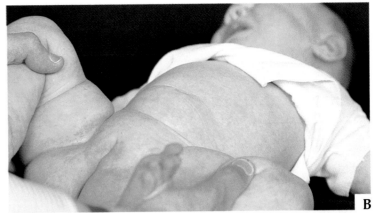

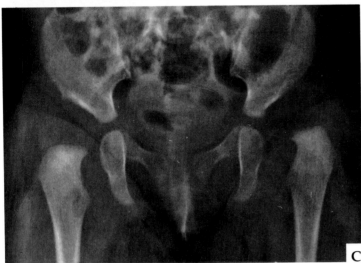

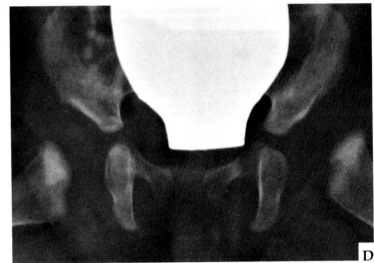

FIG. 19.62 Congenital dislocation of the hip. **A**, In cases of unilateral dislocation, the involved extremity is foreshortened and the thigh and groin creases are asymmetric. **B**, Limited abduction of the involved hip is demonstrated. This is a consistent finding in infants with a dislocated and unreducible hip. **C**, In this AP radiograph of a 3-month-old child, the proximal femur is displaced upward and lat-

erally and the acetabulum is shallow. The femoral head is not visible on the radiograph because of the delayed ossification associated with congenital hip dislocation. **D**, In the "frogleg view" the long axis of the affected left femur is directed toward a point superior and lateral to the triradiate cartilage, in contrast to that of the right, which points directly at this structure.

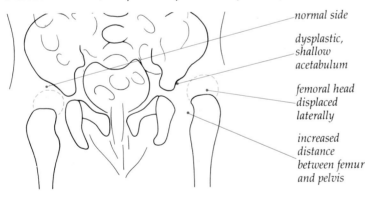

normal side

dysplastic, shallow acetabulum

femoral head displaced laterally

increased distance between femur and pelvis

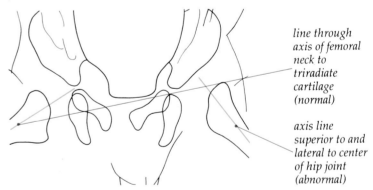

line through axis of femoral neck to triradiate cartilage (normal)

axis line superior to and lateral to center of hip joint (abnormal)

DISORDERS OF THE LOWER EXTREMITY

Normally developed and functional lower extremities permit locomotion with ease and a minimal amount of energy expenditure. Disability from a deformed, shortened, or painful lower limb can be considerable.

Many problems of the lower extremities in childhood are congenital and, if they remain unrecognized or are unsuccessfully treated, can result in life-long disability. Knowledge of the normal anatomy and function of the hip, knee, ankle, and foot is necessary to accurately recognize and treat abnormalities in this region.

Congenital Dislocation of the Hip

Congenital dislocation of the hip, or displacement of the femoral head from its normal relationship with the acetabulum, is a relatively frequent problem with an incidence of 1 to 2 per 1000 births. It is generally detectable at birth or shortly thereafter. Females are affected significantly more frequently than males and unilateral dislocation is twice as frequent as bilateral. Congenital dislocation may be divided into idiopathic and teratogenic types. Idiopathic congenital dislocation is more frequent and patients often have a positive family history. Its severity varies from subluxed, to dislocated and reducable, to dislocated and unreducable. This type of congential dislocation may be related to abnormal intrauterine positioning which impedes adequate development and stability of the hip joint complex. The relaxing effect of hormones acting on soft tissue during pregnancy may also contribute. A history of breech presentation is not uncommon and these patients often exhibit generalized ligamentous laxity. Teratogenic dislocations of the hip represent a more severe form of the disorder and are probably the result of a germ plasm defect. Associated congenital anomalies are common in infants whose dislocations are teratogenic, and there is a significant association with clubfoot deformity.

The importance of careful hip evaluation in the newborn and at early infant visits cannot be overemphasized. Early diagnosis enables prompt institution of treatment measures and results in a better outcome. An understanding of clinical signs and skill in techniques of examination is necessary.

Typically, the infant with a dislocated hip holds his leg in a position of adduction and external rotation. When unilateral, the skin folds of the thighs and buttocks are often asymmetrical and the involved lower extremity appears shorter than the opposite side (Fig. 19.62A). This foreshortening is accentuated by holding the hips and knees in 90° flexion (Galeazzi's sign). In patients with bilateral dislocations, these asymmetric findings are not present. In a truly dislocated hip, the most consistent physical finding is that of limited abduction (Fig. 19.62B). Additional diagnostic maneuvers may assist in establishing and confirming the diagnosis. In patients with reducible dislocations, Ortolani's sign is positive when a palpable clunk is felt upon abduction (relocation) of the hip. Barlow's test is positive when, with knees flexed and hips flexed to 90°, the hips are gently adducted with pressure applied on the lesser trochanter by the thumb. A palpable clunk indicating posterior dislocation is appreciated if the hip is unstable or dislocated. When the hip is dislocated and unreducible, only limitation of abduction will be apparent.

The radiographic findings of a congenital hip dislocation are characteristic. The femoral head is generally located lateral and superior to its normal position and the acetabulum may be shallow, with lateral deficiency and a characteristic high acetabular index or slope (Fig. 19.62C). Reduction of the dislocated hip is apparent when, upon abduction of the hip to 45°, a line drawn through the axis of the metaphysis of the neck crosses the triradiate cartilage (Fig. 19.62D). In idiopathic dislocation, ossification of the femoral epiphysis is delayed. Ossification is normally evident radiographically at 3 to 6 months of age, but is delayed in congenital dislocation because normal articulation forces are absent. In teratogenic hip dislocation, there may be hypoplasia of both the acetabular and femoral sides with noncongruent development of one or both of these structures. The radiographic findings early on, however, are similar to those mentioned above.

Successful correction depends on early diagnosis and institution of appropriate treatment measures. In the first 6 months of life, use of a Pavlik harness, which permits gentle motion of the hip in a flexed and abducted position, may achieve and maintain a satisfactory reduction. Between 6 and 18 months of age, gentle closed reduction and immobilization in a spica cast with or without surgical release of the contracted iliopsoas and adductor muscles is indicated. After the age of 18 months, reduction by manipulative measures is difficult owing to contractures of the associated soft tissues. In such instances, open reduction is usually indicated. In cases of teratogenic dislocation, underlying maldevelopment makes outcome less satisfactory even with optimal management.

With early recognition and appropriate treatment, a relatively normal hip with satisfactory function can be anticipated. Failure of concentric reduction or complications such as avascular necrosis of the femoral head due to overzealous attempts at closed reduction in long-standing cases, may result in a life-long disability characterized by pain and stiffness in the hip, an antalgic lurching gait, and shortening of the involved limb.

Legg-Calvé-Perthes Disease

In Legg-Calvé-Perthes disease (coxa plana) impairment of the blood supply to the developing femoral head results in avascular necrosis. Etiology is unknown. Current theories implicate traumatic disruption of the blood supply and recurrent episodes of synovitis during which increased intra-articular pressure compromises blood flow to the developing ossific nucleus. The disorder generally becomes manifest between the ages of 4 and 11 years with a higher incidence in males. Affected children often exhibit delayed skeletal maturation and are small for their age. Unilateral involvement is the rule, and if a bilateral case is suspected, some form of epiphyseal dysplasia must be ruled out. The severity of the disease varies greatly, depending on how much of the femoral head is affected. Younger children generally have milder involvement, as a larger portion of the femoral head is still cartilaginous and less dependent on vascular supply.

Onset is often insidious. The child may present with symptoms characteristic of toxic synovitis without radiographic findings. Generally, there is a flexion contracture of the involved hip with the lower extremity positioned in a slightly externally rotated position. Pain and limitation of motion are encountered on attempts at internal rotation and abduction (Figs. 19.63A and B). Trendelenburg's sign (failure to maintain a level pelvis when standing on the involved limb) is positive. Many children present with a painless limp while others complain of thigh or knee pain, fatigue on walking, or hip stiffness. Early radiographic findings may include failure of progressive development of the femoral ossific nucleus, a subchondral radiolucent fracture line (Caffey's sign), or evidence of slight subluxation. However, in very early cases, radiographs may be completely normal and a nuclear bone scan may be useful in verification of impairment of the blood supply to this region. Later on, fragmentation of the femoral ossification center may be evident with flattening of the femoral head, extrusion, and frank subluxation (Fig. 19.63C).

The disease is self-limited, typically spanning a period of 1 to 2 years. While revascularization and reconstitution of the femoral head always occurs, loss of mechanical integrity of the head with flattening and fragmentation of its surface may result in irreversible predisposition to degenerative change. Most treatment methods are based on the principle of "containment" and the maintenance of a normal relationship of the femoral head within the acetabulum so as to minimize permanent joint incongruity. In young children with minimal symptoms and radiographic findings, decreased

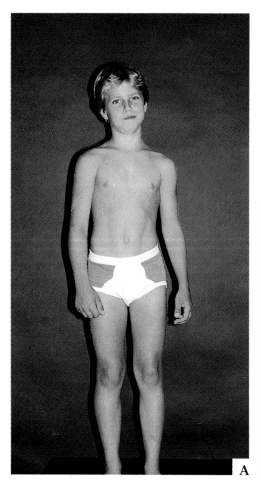

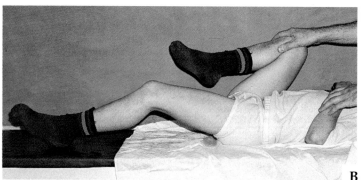

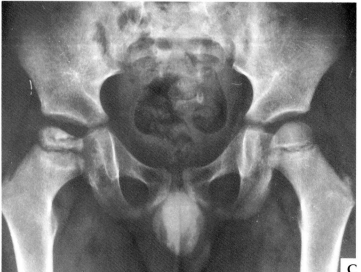

FIG. 19.63 Legg-Calvé-Perthes disease. **A,** This 7-year-old male is small for his chronologic age. The involved right extremity is slightly externally rotated and on examination a hip flexion contracture and abductor lurch gait are present. **B,** Full flexion of the opposite hip eliminates lumbar lordosis and accentuates the contracture. This is an indication of irritation of the hip joint from the disease and associated synovitis. **C,** In this AP radiograph, the right femoral epiphysis is flattened and fragmented. The proximal femur is also displaced inferiorly and laterally.

activity and close observation may be all that is necessary. Anti-inflammatory agents and traction are used during episodes of synovitis. In more severe cases, abduction casting , bracing, or operative treatment with femoral or acetabular osteotomy to reposition the femoral head deeper within the acetabulum may be employed. In cases that are recognized late or those that fail to respond to appropriate measures, permanent degenerative change is common and salvage type surgery may be necessary.

Slipped Capital Femoral Epiphysis (SCFE)

Slipped capital femoral epiphysis (SCFE) is a disorder seen early in puberty which involves displacement of the femoral head from the femoral neck through the epiphyseal plate. It is seen more frequently in males, and occurs bilaterally in approximately 25 percent of cases. Most commonly, it occurs at the onset of puberty in obese individuals with delayed sexual maturation. While etiology is unclear, it is generally thought that hormonal changes at the time of puberty may result in loss of mechanical integrity of the growth plate, and that if the epiphysis is then subjected to excessive shear stress, slippage through this area may occur. This condition differs from traumatic epiphyseal fractures because the translational displacement occurs through a different area of the growth plate. In some cases an underlying connective tissue disorder such as Marfan's syndrome or an endocrinologic problem such as hypothyroidism can be identified.

Clinical presentation is quite characteristic, although duration of symptoms varies. The patient presents with a painful limp and may or may not have a history of recent trauma. The pain may be perceived as being in the hip or in the thigh or knee. The lower extremity is held in an externally rotated position secondary to deformity at the site of physeal displacement. An antalgic and abductor lurch gait is usually apparent. A flexion contracture may be noted, and range of motion tends to be diminished in all planes, particularly internal rotation (Figs. 19.64 A and B). Slight shortening of the involved lower extremity is observed in some cases.

Radiographic findings vary in severity from a widened and radiolucent physis (preslip) to frank deformity with displacement of the femoral head on the proximal femur posteriorly and inferiorly in relation to its normal counterpart (Figs. 19.64 C and D). The degree of slippage and deformity corre-

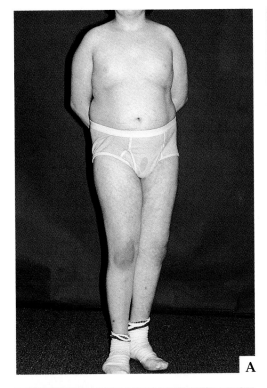

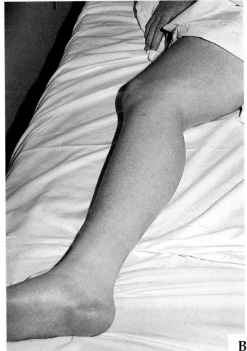

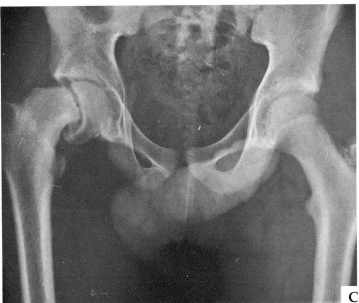

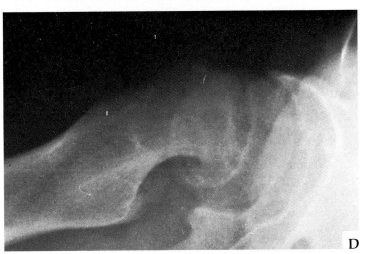

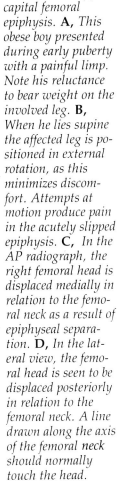

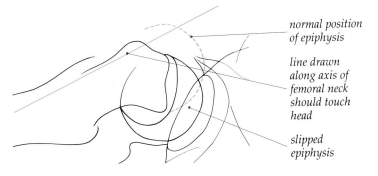

normal position of epiphysis

line drawn along axis of femoral neck should touch head

slipped epiphysis

*FIG. 19.64 Slipped capital femoral epiphysis. **A,** This obese boy presented during early puberty with a painful limp. Note his reluctance to bear weight on the involved leg. **B,** When he lies supine the affected leg is positioned in external rotation, as this minimizes discomfort. Attempts at motion produce pain in the acutely slipped epiphysis. **C,** In the AP radiograph, the right femoral head is displaced medially in relation to the femoral neck as a result of epiphyseal separation. **D,** In the lateral view, the femoral head is seen to be displaced posteriorly in relation to the femoral neck. A line drawn along the axis of the femoral neck should normally touch the head.*

lates with the extent of incongruity of the hip joint and later development of degenerative change and painful symptoms. Intervention to prevent further displacement is an important factor in preventing life-long problems, and awareness, a high index of suspicion, and early recognition are key factors in improving the prognosis.

In undisplaced or mildly displaced slips, cast immobilization or stabilization of the slip with in-situ pin fixation is indicated. In acute slipped epiphyses of moderate or severe grade, an attempt at closed reduction followed by surgical pin fixation may be indicated. When the disease is recognized late and deformity is severe, proximal femoral osteotomy may be necessary. Children with unilateral slipped epiphyses must be monitored closely for signs of involvement of the opposite limb.

Femoral Anteversion

Femoral anteversion may be viewed as a normal variation of lower extremity positioning in the developing child. In utero and at birth, the femoral neck sits in an anteverted position relative to the adult. During childhood it will remodel to a position of slight anteversion and normal alignment of the lower extremities. In certain children, however, delayed rotational correction may result in persistent intoeing. An unsightly gait, kicking of the heels, or tripping on walking or running are frequently related complaints. There may be a history of sitting on the floor with the legs out in a "reversed Tailor position". Generally the condition is bilateral, and is not associated with other musculoskeletal problems.

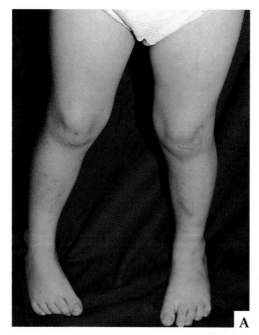

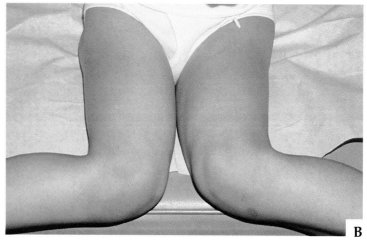

FIG. 19.65 Femoral anteversion. The condition is bilateral, and in the standing view (A), both legs appear to turn inward from the hip down. On assessment of range of motion, the degree of internal rotation of the hips is found to be greater than normal (B). (Courtesy of Dr. M. Sherlock)

A

B

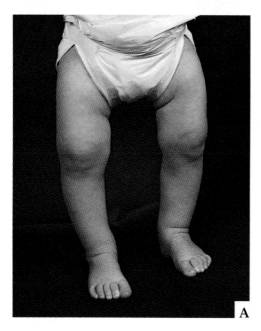

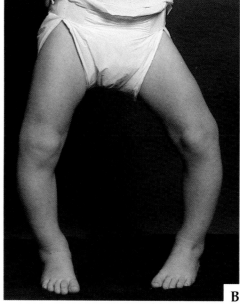

A

B

FIG. 19.66 Genu varum. The mild symmetric bowing seen in this 1-year-old male (A) represents a normal variation of lower extremity configuration in toddlers; correction occurs with growth and remodeling. The bowing is diffuse and involves the upper and lower portions of the legs. The patient (B) with severe physiologic genu varum had difficulty walking and exhibited a waddling gait. He also had associated ligamentous laxity.

On examination, the child is noted to stand with the entire lower extremities, including the knees and feet, turned inwards. An increase in internal rotation over external rotation is apparent on assessment of range of motion (Fig. 19.65). Radiographic examination is normal. No treatment is indicated other than reassurance that the condition will correct with growth and instructions to avoid sitting in the predisposing position.

Genu Varum (Physiologic Bowlegs)

Genu varum or bowlegs is a normal variation of lower extremity configuration, seen in the 1 to 3 year old age group. It is generally recognized shortly after ambulation begins and may be associated with laxity of other joints and internal tibial torsion. Examination reveals diffuse bowing of the lower extremities with an increased distance between the knees which is accentuated on standing (Fig. 19.66). Varus positioning of the heel with pronation of the feet may be noted on weight-bearing. The child may walk with a waddling gait and kick the heels on running to clear the feet from the ground

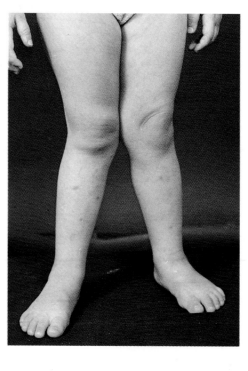

FIG. 19.67 Genu valgum. This 3½-year-old female exhibits a moderate knock-knee deformity. Ligamentous laxity and mild pes planus are associated.

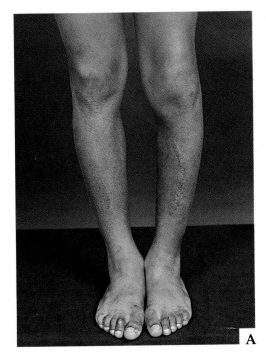
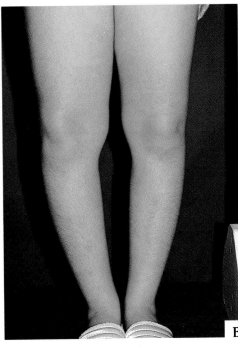
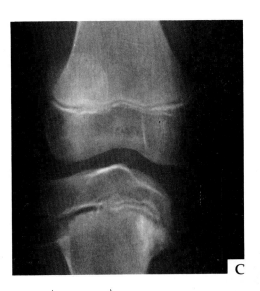
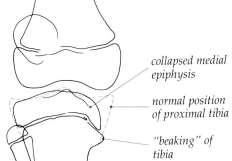

C

collapsed medial
epiphysis

normal position
of proximal tibia

"beaking" of
tibia

FIG. 19.68 Blount's disease. **A**, The patient has a unilateral angular deformity of the proximal left tibia that gives the appearance of genu varum. Both proximal tibiae are bowed in another patient **(B)**, as a result of fragmentation and loss of height of the me- dial epiphyses. In contrast to physiologic bowing, the thighs are straight. **C**, The radiograph demonstrates the typical fragmentation, loss of height, and angular deformity or beaking of the medial portion of the proximal tibia.

and avoid hitting the contralateral limb. Laxity of joint capsular structures may be noted with application of a reduction force.

Radiographs show normal osseous and physeal development and may reveal a gentle symmetrical bowing of the femur and tibia. While there may be slight beaking of the medial metaphysis of the femur and tibia adjacent to the knee joint, there is no fragmentation of the epiphysis or irregularity of the growth plate as is seen in Blount's disease. Conditions such as rickets or other metabolic abnormalities, epiphyseal dysplasia, various forms of dwarfism, or pathologic growth disturbances such as Blount's disease also must be ruled out.

Treatment is rarely indicated, as this condition corrects with growth and, in fact, a valgus deformity of the knees may be noted later, at approximately 4 to 5 years of age. Casting, bracing, and corrective shoes are unnecessary and there is no indication for surgery.

Genu Valgum (Physiologic Knock-Knees)

Genu valgum or knock-knees is a normal variation of lower extremity configuration, generally noted in children between the ages of 3 and 5 years. The phenomenon is part of the normal process of remodeling of the lower extremities during growth and development. It is more frequently seen in females and may be associated with ligamentous laxity. While standing the child is noted to have an increased distance between the feet when the medial aspects of the knees touch one another (Fig. 19.67). Not uncommonly, the child will place one knee behind the other in an attempt to get the feet together. In some cases valgus alignment of the feet and a pes planus deformity may be noted. Radiographs reveal no osseous or physeal abnormalities, but accentuation of the angular deformity of the knee is seen on weight-bearing views secondary to ligamentous laxity. One must rule out the possibility of an underlying metabolic condition such as rickets or renal disease. Treatment is generally not indicated as the condition gradually corrects with time.

Blount's Disease

Blount's disease is an isolated growth disturbance of the medial tibial epiphysis manifested as an angular varus deformity of the proximal tibia with apparent progressive genu varum. Unilateral and bilateral presentation are seen with nearly equal frequency. The etiology of this condition is unknown, although it appears to be more common in blacks. It may represent a compression injury to the medial growth plate of the proximal tibia.

On careful examination, a localized angular deformity of the proximal tibia is apparent, in contrast to the diffuse bowing of the lower extremities seen in patients with physiologic bowlegs. Generally there is no evidence of the ligamentous laxity commonly associated with physiologic bowing (Figs. 19.68A and B). Radiographs reveal fragmentation of the medial epiphysis of the tibia associated with beaking and loss of height in this region, and the characteristic angular deformity (Fig. 19.68C). Satisfactory treatment is dependent on accurate diagnosis and early recognition, as bracing or surgical osteotomy with realignment of the leg may prevent further progresson.

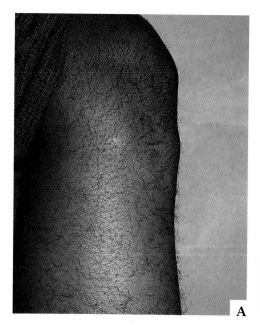
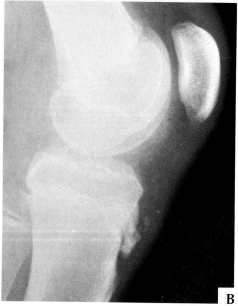
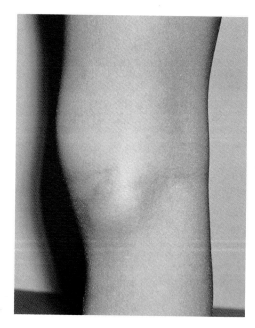

FIG. 19.69 Osgood-Schlatter disease. Localized swelling is evident in the region of the tibial tubercle **(A)**. This is generally tender on palpation. The knee is otherwise normal on examination, with the possible exception of mild limitation of flexion.

Irregularity and fragmentation of the tibial tubercle are seen in the radiograph **(B)**. In less severe cases of shorter duration, soft tissue swelling or irregularity of ossification may be the only findings.

FIG. 19.70 Popliteal (Baker's) cyst. A localized swelling appears in the region of the semimembranosus tendon. This may arise from the synovial lining of the semimembranosus bursa.

Osgood-Schlatter Disease

Osgood-Schlatter disease is a traction apophysitis of the tibial tubercle which tends to develop during the adolescent growth spurt. It occurs somewhat more frequently in males than females. It is thought that rapid differential growth between the osseous and soft tissue structures and stress on the apophysis produced by vigorous physical activity are contributing factors. Bilateral involvement is usual. Patients present with a history of gradually increasing pain and swelling in the region of the tibial tubercle. Discomfort is accentuated by vigorous physical activity, kneeling or crawling, and is relieved by rest.

On examination, a localized tender swelling is noted in the region of the tibial tubercle and patellar tendon. The knee joint is otherwise normal on examination, with the exception that some patients have findings of limitation of knee flexion with reproduction of their pain. Radiographs may reveal only soft tissue swelling in the region of the proximal tibial apophysis or irregularity of ossification of this structure (Fig. 19.69). In long-standing cases, frank fragmentation of the apophysis may be seen.

The problem, though self-limited, persists over a period of 6 to 24 months. If the condition is only occasionally bothersome and does not limit activities, treatment is unnecessary. If severe pain and a limp are present, a short period of immobilization in a splint or cast may be beneficial. Aspirin as needed and curtailing activities that produce pain is sufficient treatment for most patients. Steroid injection is contraindicated, as this may cause deterioration of the tendon and provides little in the way of long-term relief.

Popliteal (Baker's) Cyst

Popliteal cysts in childhood are encountered most commonly in children between 5 and 10 years of age and occur significantly more frequently in males than females. They are located in the posteromedial aspect of the knee joint in the region of the semimembranosus tendon and medial gastrocnemius muscle belly. The pathology is that of a fibrous tissue or synovial cyst filled with synovial-like fluid. In contrast to those seen in adults, popliteal cysts in childhood generally do not communicate with the joint capsule, but originate instead beneath the semimembranosus tendon, presumably as a result of chronic irritation. Occasionally vague pain is noted, but evaluation is usually sought because of a recently noted painless mass.

On examination, a soft, nontender, cystic mass is found in the described location (Fig. 19.70). Range of motion of the joint is normal unless the cyst is particularly large, limiting flexion. The knee is otherwise normal. Radiographs show no osseous abnormality. Popliteal cysts are benign and may resolve over time although their surgical excision is reasonable if desired.

Internal Tibial Torsion

Internal tibial torsion is a nonpathologic variation in normal development of the lower leg in children under the age of 5. It consists of a rotational deformity thought to be the result of internal molding of the foot and leg in utero. The child is usually brought for evaluation because of concern about prominent intoeing on walking and frequent tripping.

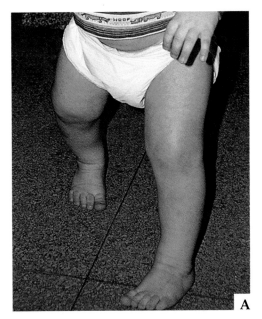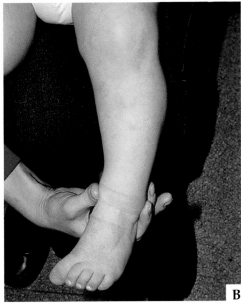

A   B

FIG. 19.71 *Internal tibial torsion.* **A**, *The hip, thigh, and knee are normally oriented and the patella faces anteriorly, but the lower leg and foot turn inward. The deformity results in prominent intoeing on walking, and may cause the child to trip frequently.* **B**, *The lateral malleolus is positioned anterior to the medial malleolus, thus shifting the ankle mortise and foot to a medially oriented position. (Courtesy of Dr. M. Sherlock)*

On examination, the hips and knees are normally aligned with the patellae facing anteriorly, and the lower legs and feet rotated inwardly. The lateral malleolus, which is normally positioned slightly posterior to the medial malleolus, may be in alignment with it or even anteriorly displaced, thus causing the ankle mortise to shift to a medially directed orientation, resulting in intoeing (Fig. 19.71). Radiographs reveal no osseous abnormalities. Treatment is seldom indicated; remodeling gradually corrects the condition as the child grows and develops. Children who have a habit of sitting on their feet on the floor may inhibit the normal remodeling process and should be instructed not to do this. Bracing and special shoes have little effect, and are not recommended.

Congenital Clubfoot

Congenital clubfoot (talipes equinovarus) is a teratogenic deformity of the foot which is readily apparent at birth. It is seen more frequently in males than females with an incidence of 1 in 1000 live births. Etiology is probably multifactorial. Proposed predisposing conditions include genetic, neural, muscular, and osseous abnormalities. There is a near equal frequency of unilateral and bilateral involvement. The deformity is characterized by three primary components: (1) the entire foot is positioned in plantar flexion (equinus); (2) the hindfoot is maintained in a position of fixed inversion (varus); and (3) the forefoot exhibits an adductus deformity often combined with supination (Figs. 19.72A, B, and C). In the newborn period the deformity may be passively correctable to some extent. With time, however, deformities become more fixed due to contracture of soft tissue structures.

The primary pathologic finding is that of a rotational deformity of the subtalor joint with the os calcis internally rotated beneath the talus producing the characteristic varus deformity of the heel and mechanically creating a block to dorsiflexion of the foot. The navicular is situated in a medially displaced position on the head or neck of the talus producing the characteristic adductus deformity of the forefoot (Figs. 19.72D and E). Contractures of the Achilles and posterior tibial tendons and medial ankle and subtalor joint capsules appear to be secondary factors that contribute to the difficulty of obtaining anatomic reduction. Congenital absence of certain tendinous structures may be found in rare instances. A small atrophic-appearing calf is frequently noted without pathologic change in its osseous or soft tissue structures. The typical congenital clubfoot deformity must be differentiated from similar deformities present in the foot secondary to neurologic imbalance from myelodysplasia, spinal cord tethering, or degenerative neurological conditions. Occasionally, tibial hemimelia with deficiency of this bone may present a similar clinical picture. The condition should not be confused with the nonteratogenic occurrence of isolated metatarsus adductus. Its association with arthrogryposis and congenital dislocation of the hips should be kept in mind.

Early treatment consists of attempts at manipulation and serial casting or cast wedging with progressive correction. When the child presents late, and/or closed treatment is unsuccessful, open reduction and surgical release of the contracted soft tissues is indicated. Generally, these measures should be undertaken before the age at which walking is expected in order to prevent the deformity from impeding the child's motor and social development.

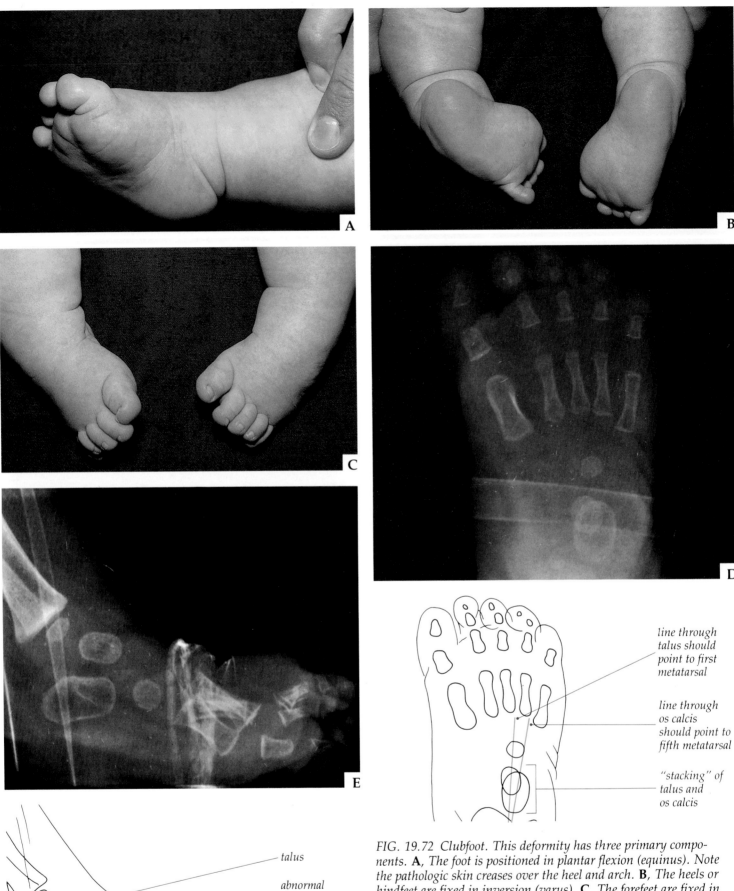

FIG. 19.72 Clubfoot. This deformity has three primary components. **A**, The foot is positioned in plantar flexion (equinus). Note the pathologic skin creases over the heel and arch. **B**, The heels or hindfeet are fixed in inversion (varus). **C**, The forefeet are fixed in an adducted and supinated position. **D**, In the AP radiographic view, the talus overlies the os calcis (stacking) and the forefoot is adducted. A line drawn through the longitudinal axis of the talus normally is in alignment with the first metatarsal, and one drawn through the axis of the os calcis normally aligns with the fifth metatarsal. **E**, The lateral radiograph shows the foot is in equinus and the axes of the talus and os calcis are nearly parallel. They normally intersect at an angle of approximately 45°.

line through talus should point to first metatarsal

line through os calcis should point to fifth metatarsal

"stacking" of talus and os calcis

talus

abnormal "parallelism" of axis lines through talus and os calcis

normal position of talus

os calcis

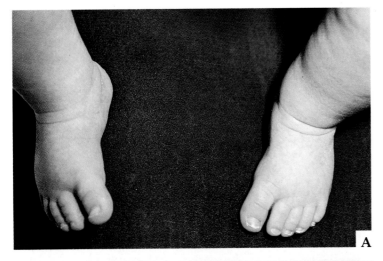

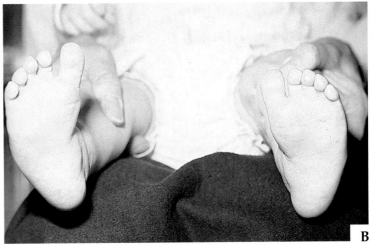

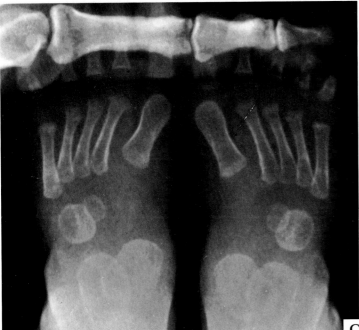

FIG. 19.73 Bilateral metatarsus adductus. **A**, In this view from above, the forefeet are seen to be deviated medially, but otherwise, the feet are normal. **B**, When viewed from the plantar aspect, rounding of the lateral border of the feet can be appreciated. **C**, In the AP radiograph note that all five metatarsals are deviated medially with respect to the remainder of the foot; otherwise, the bony structures are normal. In contrast to clubfoot deformity, the relationship of the talus and os calcis is normal.

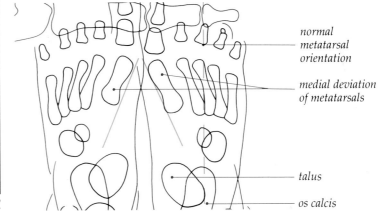

normal metatarsal orientation

medial deviation of metatarsals

talus

os calcis

Metatarsus Adductus

Metatarsus adductus (metatarsus varus) is a deformity of the forefoot in which the metatarsals are deviated medially. The condition is probably the result of intrauterine molding and is usually bilateral. Other than the deviation, there are no pathologic changes in the structures of the foot. There is a wide spectrum of severity and resultant intoeing, but otherwise, patients are asymptomatic. Clinically, it should be distinguished from the more severe and complex deformity of congenital clubfoot, as it carries a more benign prognosis.

Examination is best performed with the foot braced against a flat surface or with the patient standing. With the hindfoot and midfoot positioned straight, the forefoot assumes a medially deviated or varus position (Figs. 19.73A and B). A skin crease may be located over the medial aspect of the longitudinal arch. When mild, the deviation may be passively correctable by the physician or actively correctable by the patient. Active correction may be demonstrated by gentle stroking of the foot, stimulating the peroneal muscles to contract. In more severe cases, the deviation may be only partially correctable by these maneuvers. Some patients have an associated internal tibial torsion deformity, but the calf muscle is normal in size. Radiographs demonstrate the abnormal deviation of the metatarsals medially without other osseous abnormalities (Fig. 19.73C).

Treatment depends on the severity of the condition. In very mild cases, passive manipulation of the deformity by the mother several times a day may suffice. In moderate cases, a combination of manipulative stretching and reverse or straight-last shoes may be indicated. More severe cases which are not passively correctable and which exhibit a prominent deformity and skin crease necessitate serial manipulation and casting over a period of 6 to 8 weeks. If the deformity persists despite these measures, surgical intervention may be required. Treatment should be undertaken prior to anticipated ambulation so as to avoid impairment of the patient's motor and social development.

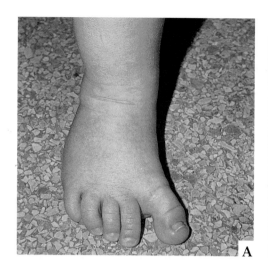
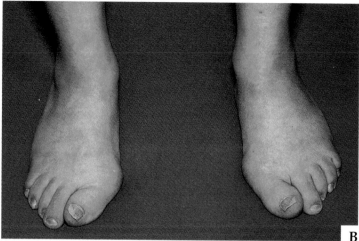

FIG. 19.74 Metatarsus primus varus. **A**, The first metatarsal and great toe are deviated medially; the forefoot is broad. The other metatarsals are normal. (Courtesy of Dr. M. Sherlock) **B**, Bilateral metatarsus primus varus with hallux valgus. The forefeet are broad and the great toes deviate laterally.

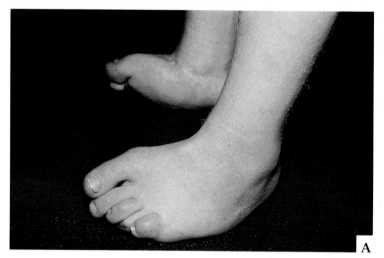
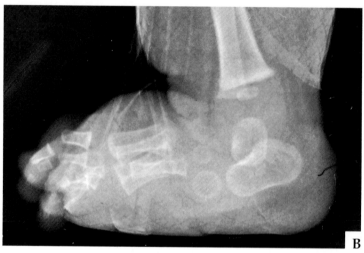

FIG. 19.75 Congenital vertical talus. The normal longitudinal arch of the foot is absent and a "rocker-bottom" type deformity is present.

The forefoot is fixed in dorsiflexion **(A)**. Note the vertical orientation of the talus in the radiograph **(B)**.

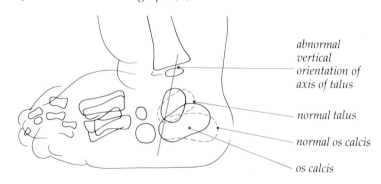

Metatarsus Primus Varus (Adductus)

Metatarsus primus varus is a congenital and often hereditary foot deformity characterized by a broad forefoot with medial deviation of the first metatarsal. It is significantly more frequent in females than males.

Examination reveals a wide forefoot with medial deviation of the first metatarsal and normal orientation of the second through fifth metatarsals. There is often an associated varus deviation of the great toe (Fig. 19.74). Over time, a secondary hallux valgus deformity and bunion may develop from the abnormal forces exerted on the great toe with weight-bearing and ambulation. The heel may seem narrow, but this is more apparent than real. Pronation of the forefoot may be present as well. Radiographs confirm the diagnosis by revealing an increased space between the first and second metatarsals and a large first intermetatarsal angle. The first ray through the tarsometatarsal joint may be medially oriented forming the basis for the deformity.

In mild cases, no treatment may be necessary. In moderate or severe cases, foot strain symptoms, bunion pain, and shoe-fitting problems may necessitate treatment. Surgical osteotomy of the medial cuneiform or first metatarsal in conjunction with bunion correction may satisfactorily correct the deformity.

Congenital Vertical Talus

Congenital vertical talus is a teratogenic anomaly of the foot noted at birth and characterized by a severe flatfoot deformity. The underlying pathology is a malorientation of the talus which assumes a more vertical position than normal. The adjacent navicular is dorsally displaced, articulating with the superior aspect of the neck of the talus and causing the forefoot to assume a dorsiflexed and valgus orientation. In effect, these deformities are the opposite of those seen in congenital clubfoot. The etiology of this condition is unknown, although it may be associated with other muscu-

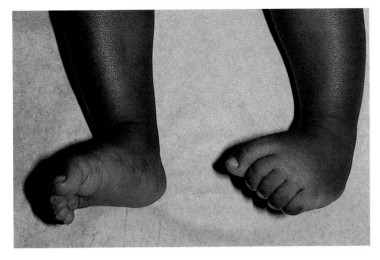

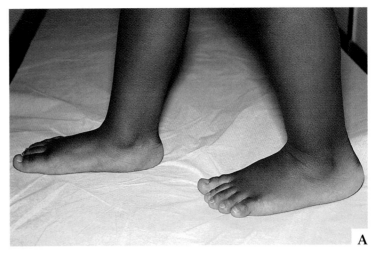

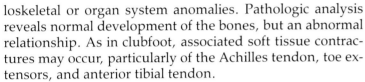

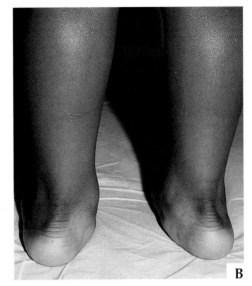

FIG. 19.76 *Calcaneovalgus foot deformity. The right foot is held in a position of eversion and dorsiflexion. This deformity is supple, and thus is passively correctable. The contralateral foot exhibits a metatarsus adductus deformity, giving the feet a "windswept" appearance.*

FIG. 19.77 *Pes planus. Laxity of the soft tissue structures of the foot results in a loss of the normal longitudinal arch and pronation or eversion of the forefoot (A). Viewed from behind (B), the characteristic eversion of the heels is appreciated more readily.*

loskeletal or organ system anomalies. Pathologic analysis reveals normal development of the bones, but an abnormal relationship. As in clubfoot, associated soft tissue contractures may occur, particularly of the Achilles tendon, toe extensors, and anterior tibial tendon.

Clinically, the deformity is recognizable as a calcaneovalgus foot with loss of the arch, or on some occasions, a rocker-bottom type foot with a prominent heel (Fig. 19.75A). The head of the talus is often palpable on the medial plantar aspect of the midfoot. The deformity is usually fixed, but passive correction may be obtainable in some instances, particularly when the talus is oriented in a less severe oblique position. Radiographs mirror the clinical appearance with a vertical orientation of the talus, calcaneous deformity of the os calcis, and valgus orientation of the forefoot (Fig. 19.75B).

Initially, attempts at manipulation and serial casting are indicated. However, if this is unsuccessful, as is often the case, surgery may be necessary.

Calcaneovalgus Foot Deformity

Physiologic calcaneovalgus is another deformity of the foot thought to result from interuterine molding. It is normally a supple deformity that is passively correctable in contrast to the rigid foot of congenital vertical talus. The condition is evident at birth and at times is associated with a contralateral metatarsus adductus deformity. There are no underlying pathologic changes in the foot and no osseous deformities other than the positional one. On examination, the foot is noted to be held in a dorsiflexed and everted position with some loss of the normal longitudinal arch (Fig. 19.76). Appreciable tightness of the anterior tibial tendon and laxity of the Achilles tendon may be noted in association with the positional deformity. Radiographs reveal no pathologic bony changes. Nonoperative treatment is usually successful and consists of serial casting to correct the deformity. Later, wearing shoes with inner heel wedges and longitudinal arch supports may help prevent recurrence and improve ambulation.

Pes Planus (Flatfeet)

Pes planus, or physiologic flatfeet, is an extremely common condition for which there is a familial predisposition. It is characterized by laxity of the soft tissues of the foot resulting in loss of the normal longitudinal arch with pronation or eversion of the forefoot and valgus or lateral orientation of the heel (Fig. 19.77). There may be secondary tightness of the Achilles tendon. The condition is generally asymptomatic in children and evaluation is sought primarily because of parental concern with the appearance of the foot and the possibility of future problems. Occasionally, affected patients report discomfort after long walks or running.

On examination, the characteristic appearance is easy to recognize and laxity of other joints, particularly the thumb, elbow, and knee may be noted. Weight-bearing radiographs reveal loss of the normal longitudinal arch without osseous abnormality. Treatment is unnecessary when the condition is asymptomatic. Corrective shoes with arch supports are of no use unless symptoms of foot strain are present.

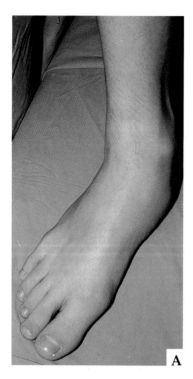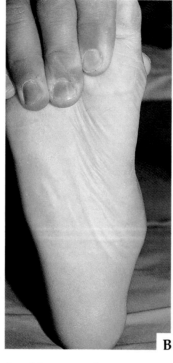

FIG. 19.78 *Accessory tarsal navicular. A bony prominence produced by formation of a separate ossification center of the tarsal navicular is present over the medial aspect of the midfoot* (A). *Patients with this problem usually have a pes planus deformity as well. In the plantar view* (B), *the bony prominence is appreciated more easily. It is covered by a painful bursa produced by chronic rubbing against the medial side of the patient's shoes.*

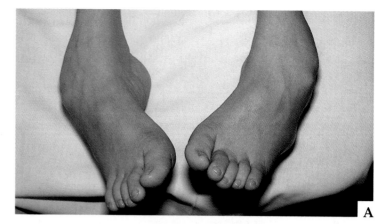

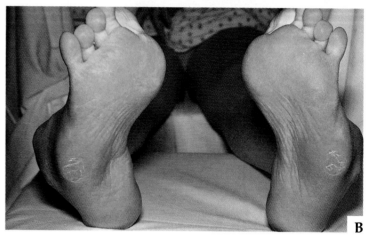

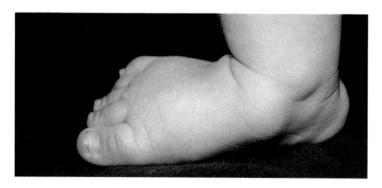

FIG. 19.79 *Ganglion of the foot. A prominent soft tissue mass is present over the medial aspect of the midfoot. This represents a ganglion of the posterior tibial tendon sheath.*

FIG. 19.80 *Bilateral cavus feet. The feet are inverted and have high arches* (A). *The deformity is often a feature of neuromuscular disorders; this case is the result of Charcot-Marie-Tooth disease. In addition to the high arches and varus (inverted) heels seen in the view of the plantar surface* (B), *the prominence of the metatarsal head region is apparent. Callosities have developed over the lateral borders of the feet as a result of abnormal weight-bearing in this region.*

Accessory Tarsal Navicular

The occurrence of an accessory tarsal navicular is the result of the formation of a separate ossification center on the medial aspect of the developing tarsal navicular at the site of insertion of the posterior tibial tendon. The condition is not uncommon and is usually associated with a pes planus deformity. Clinically, patients exhibit a bony prominence on the medial aspect of the foot that tends to rub on the shoe thus producing a painful bursa (Fig. 19.78). Radiographs reveal either a separate ossification center or bone medial to the parent navicular, or a medial projection of the navicular when fusion has occurred. Cast immobilization may be helpful in acutely painful cases. Long-term improvement can be obtained by wearing soft supportive shoes with longitudinal arches and a medial heel wedge. Recalcitrant symptoms warrant surgical intervention.

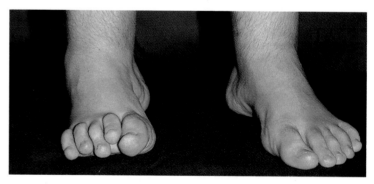

FIG. 19.81 *Unilateral claw toes. This child with a tethered spinal cord has unilateral claw toe deformities. The MP joints are held in extension while the PIP joints are fixed in flexion.*

Ganglion of the Foot

A ganglion, or synovial cyst, may occur on the foot. These benign masses are similar to those commonly seen on the wrist. They originate from outpouchings of a joint capsule or tendon sheath. Trauma may be a predisposing factor in their growth. They are most commonly seen on the dorsal or medial aspect of the foot. The mass is soft, nontender, transilluminates, and does not produce symptoms other than difficulty in fitting shoes (Fig. 19.79). If the latter occurs, surgical excision may be indicated.

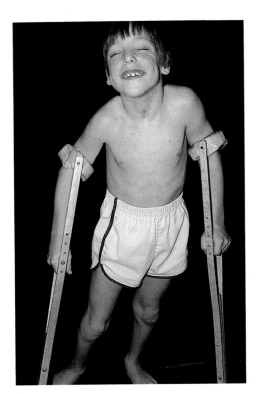

FIG. 19.82 *Cerebral palsy. Typical patient with spastic quadriplegia. Note the secondary muscle atrophy especially evident in the lower extremities. He requires crutches to ambulate, seizure medication, and a specialized educational program. His neuromuscular abnormalities are the result of a one time central nervous system insult and are not progressive.*

Cavus Foot Deformity and Claw Toes

Cavus feet and claw toes are deformities produced by muscular imbalance within the foot. Although they may occur for unknown reasons, often they are manifestations of an underlying neurological disorder such as Charcot-Marie-Tooth disease, Friedreich's ataxia, or spinal cord tethering. These conditions should be considered in each patient presenting with these deformities, particularly when the problem is unilateral. Cavus feet exhibit a high arch with a varus or inversion deformity of the heel (Fig. 19.80). Usually the metatarsal heads appear prominent on the plantar aspect of the foot. This phenomenon is accentuated by overlying callosities that develop as a result of abnormal weight-bearing. With claw toes, the metatarsophalangeal joints are held in extension with the proximal interphalangeal joints in flexion, and the distal joint in the neutral or slightly flexed position (Fig. 19.81). Callouses tend to develop over the proximal interphalangeal joints from rubbing against shoes. Neurologic examination may reveal motor weakness, most often involving the anterior tibial, toe extensor, and peroneal muscles.

Logical treatment necessitates identifying and treating the underlying pathologic condition when possible. Nonoperative measures for control of the deformities and amelioration of symptoms consist of customized shoes and use of a metatarsal bar to relieve pressure on the metatarsal heads and to correct the extension deformities at the base of the toes. However, surgical correction is often necessary.

GENERALIZED MUSCULOSKELETAL DISORDERS

A number of systemic disorders have significant musculoskeletal manifestations. Those relating to genetic, endocrine, collagen-vascular, neurologic and hematologic problems are discussed in their respective chapters. Three conditions with major musculoskeletal manifestations—cerebral palsy, osteogenesis imperfecta, and arthrogryposis—are discussed in this section.

Cerebral Palsy

The term cerebral palsy refers to a group of fixed, nonprogressive neurological syndromes resulting from static lesions of the developing central nervous system. Depending on the timing of injury, signs may be present at birth, or may become evident in infancy or early childhood. The primary cerebral insult may be intrauterine or perinatal infection; a pre or perinatal vascular accident; anoxia due to placental insufficiency, difficult delivery, or neonatal pulmonary disease; hyperbilirubinemia resulting in kernicterus; or neonatal hypoglycemia. Following the newborn period, central nervous system infections, trauma, and vascular accidents may, when severe, produce the disorder. Abnormal motor function is the most obvious result, and may take the form of a spastic neuromuscular disorder (65 percent), athetosis (25 percent), or rigidity and/or ataxic neuromuscular dysfunction (10 percent). Sensory deficits and intellectual impairment are common, and there is a significant incidence of associated seizure disorders.

Because of the number and variety of possible insulting factors, each of which has its own spectrum of severity, there is a broad range in location and extent of neural damage, and thus in degree of functional impairment. Patients with severe afflictions generally have early evidence of gross neuromuscular dysfunction. Those with milder involvement may have subtler abnormalities and may be diagnosed only after failure to achieve normal developmental and motor milestones. Patterns of involvement include affliction of one or two limbs (monoplegia or hemiplegia), of both lower extremities (diplegia), of all four extremities (quadriplegia) (Fig. 19.82), or of all limbs with poor trunk and head control (pentaplegia). Those patients with a spastic disorder exhibit flexion contractures of the involved limbs, hyperreflexia, and spasticity, while those with athetosis exhibit the characteristic movement disorder. Mixed involvement is apparent in some individuals. Neurological examination often reveals persistence of primitive reflexes.

In evaluating such patients, one must be careful to rule out a progressive neurological disorder, such as intracranial or spinal cord neoplasms, degenerative neurological conditions, or tethering of the spinal cord.

Optimal treatment necessitates a team approach. In addition to general pediatric, neurologic, and orthopedic care, these patients often need the services of a urologist, physical and speech therapists, and individualized educational programs. Family counseling is a necessity. From an orthopedic standpoint, emphasis is placed on optimizing neuromuscular function by attempting to facilitate the achievement of progressive motor milestones, including the ability to sit, stand, walk, and perform activities of daily living. Exercises, bracing and surgical procedures all have a role, and

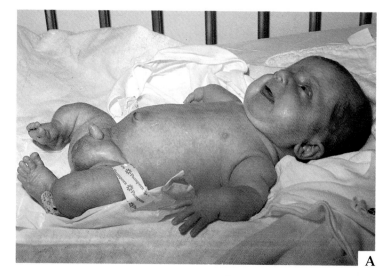

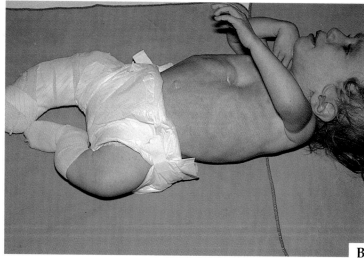

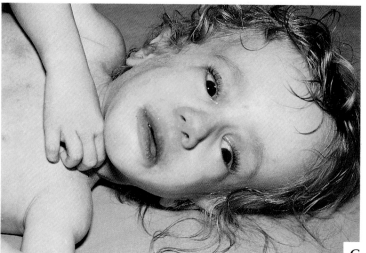

FIG. 19.83 Osteogenesis imperfecta congenita. **A**, This infant was born with multiple fractures and limb deformities. This autosomal dominant genetic disorder results in abnormal formation of collagen. Limbs are deformed, bones fracture easily, ligaments are lax, and stature is stunted. **B**, Note the extremely small stature of this 5-year-old child and the deformities of the limbs and rib cage. A recent fracture has been splinted. **C**, In this close-up, the characteristic craniofacial features are seen consisting of frontal and temporal bossing and a broad nose. In the congenita form, the sclerae are usually normal in appearance, while in the tarda form, they usually appear blue.

institution of specific measures must be timed to fit the pace of growth and development of the individual child. Encouragement and cautious optimism are important. Surgical treatment usually takes the form of soft tissue release for flexion deformities, tendon transfer to optimize functional use of the extremities, osteotomy to correct deformities, and occasionally, selective neurectomy to inhibit overactive muscle units.

Osteogenesis Imperfecta

While osteogenesis imperfecta is a disease of collagen involving all connective tissue in the body, its primary clinical manifestations involve the skeleton because of the structural demands placed on the bones. The condition is rare, and generally is transmitted as an autosomal dominant trait. Some cases are the result of new mutations, though. In its severe form (osteogenesis imperfecta congenita) the condition is apparent at birth with multiple fractures and limb deformities noted at delivery (Fig. 19.83A). Lifespan is shortened. In its less severe form (osteogenesis imperfecta tarda) fractures occur later, are fewer in number, and life expectancy may be normal with appropriate care.

The pathologic findings are those of immature collagen formation and abnormal cross-linking which may be attributed to impaired osteoblastic activity. Osteoblasts are noted to be scarce, the osteoid is disorganized and nonossified, and bony trabeculae are sparse. Clinically, patients with the congenita form have short stature, thin, frail, deformed limbs, and cranial disproportion (Figs. 19.83B and C). Ligamentous and cutaneous laxity are noted. The associated dental abnormalities are discussed in Chapter 18. Radiographs reveal thin cortises, decreased trabecular markings, and multiple limb deformities from previous fractures and structural modeling. Patients with the tarda form of the disease often exhibit blue sclera while those with the more severe form may have normal appearing sclera.

Treatment is geared towards minimizing the frequency of fractures and preventing deformities. In infancy this may mean limited handling of the child, and use of a padded carrying device. Later, bracing and surgical treatment in the form of osteotomy and internal stabilization of long bones with intermedullary rod fixation may be necessary. Maintenance of activity and the avoidance of repeated prolonged periods of immobilization aid in the prevention of disuse atrophy.

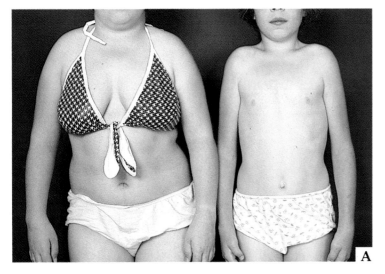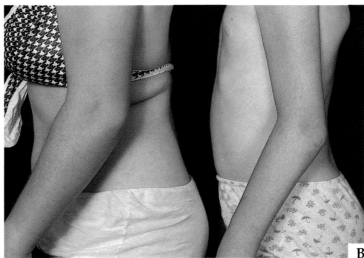

FIG. 19.84 Arthrogryposis. Two sisters with the generalized form of the disorder are shown **(A)**. Note the stiff posture and tubular appearance of the limbs. Motion of all joints is limited either due to failure in development or degeneration of muscular structures. Their stature is short. The lateral view **(B)** highlights flexion contractures of the elbows.

Arthrogryposis

Arthrogryposis is a nonprogressive muscular disorder of unknown etiology, which appears to be related either to failure of development in or degeneration of muscular structures. Neural factors have been implicated in its origin, because in some instances the spinal cord has been found to be reduced in size, with a decreased number of anterior horn cells. Generally all limbs are involved. On occasion the disease may be confined to one or a few limbs only. Primary manifestations consist of joint contractures with secondary deformities and limited motion. Deformities include clubfeet, dislocated hips, and contractures of the knees, elbows, wrists and hands (Fig. 19.84). Motion of involved joints is severely limited, but patients generally are able to compensate for this functional limitation. Radiographs show relatively normal appearing bones and joints, but fat density is noted in the areas where muscles are normally seen. On pathologic analysis, there is a striking absence of muscle tissue with strands of fat permeating the area.

Orthopedic treatment is aimed at providing optimal motor function. Range of motion exercises may maintain what motion is present, but rarely result in an increase. Surgery rarely results in improved range of motion, but is indicated to restore functional position when clubfeet and hip dislocation are part of the condition. Gradual recurrence of deformity after surgery is not uncommon, however.

BIBLIOGRAPHY

Aegerter E, Kirkpatrick JA Jr: Orthopedic Diseases, Physiology, Pathology, Radiology, 4th ed. Saunders, Philadelphia, 1975.

Edmonson AS, Crenshaw AH: Campbell's Operative Orthopedics, 6th ed. Mosby, St. Louis, 1980.

Ferguson AB Jr: Orthopedic Surgery in Infancy and Childhood, 5th ed. Williams & Wilkins, Baltimore, 1981.

Lovell WW, Winter RB: Pediatric Orthopedics. Lippincott, Philadelphia, 1978.

Moe JH, Winter RB, Bradford DS, Lonstein JE: Scoliosis and Other Spinal Deformities. Saunders, Philadelphia, 1978.

Ogden JA: Skeletal Injury in the Child. Lea & Febiger, Philadelphia, 1982.

Rang M: Children's Fractures, 2nd ed. Lippincott, Philadelphia, 1983.

Rockwood CA Jr, Wilkins KE, King RE: Fractures in Children, vol. 3. Lippincott, Philadelphia, 1984.

Salter RB: Textbook of Disorders and Injuries of the Musculoskeletal System, 2nd ed. Williams & Wilkins, Baltimore, 1983.

PEDIATRIC OTOLARYNGOLOGY

James S. Reilly, M.D.
Holly W. Davis, M.D.

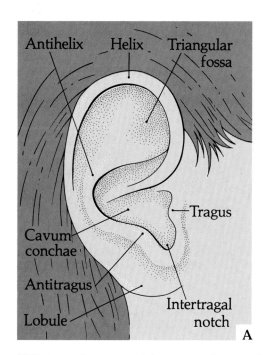

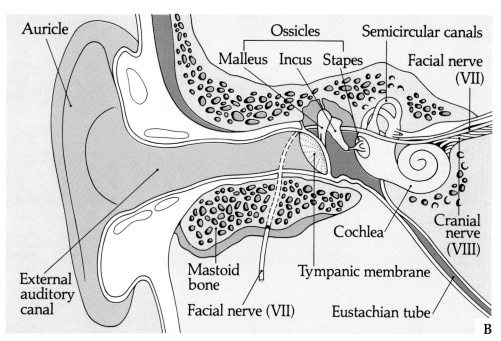

*FIG. 20.1 Anatomy of the ear. **A** A normal external ear is shown, with its various landmarks labeled. It is helpful to refer to such a diagram in assessing congenital anomalies. **B** This coronal section shows the various structures of the hearing and vestibular apparatus. The three main regions are the external ear, the middle ear, and the inner ear. The eustachian tube connects the middle ear and the pharynx and serves to vent the middle ear.*

The importance of pediatricians and family physicians having an understanding of and experience with otolaryngologic problems, and of their being skilled in techniques of examination of the head and neck region, cannot be overemphasized. A recent study revealed that over one-third of all visits to pediatricians' offices were prompted by ear symptoms. When nasal and oral symptoms are included, ear, nose, and throat pathology account for over 50 percent of all visits. With patience and proper equipment, a thorough examination can be accomplished on almost all children. Then, if the disorder fails to respond to therapy, becomes chronic or recurrent, or if an unusual problem is encountered, consultation by a pediatric otolaryngologist should be sought.

EAR DISORDERS

Ear pain (otalgia), discharge from the ear (otorrhea), and suspected hearing loss are three of the more common and specific otic symptoms for which parents seek medical attention for their children. Less specific symptoms such as pulling or tugging at the ears, fussiness, and fever are also frequently en-

The authors would like to acknowledge and thank Children's Hospital of Pittsburgh, Department of Radiology, and University of Pittsburgh, Department of Neuroradiology for providing many of the radiographs and CT scans seen in this chapter.

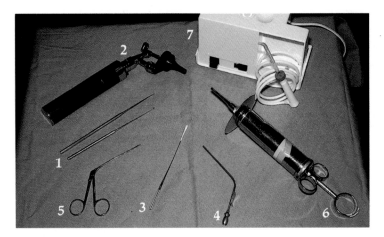

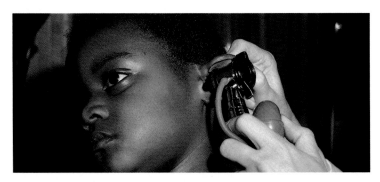

FIG. 20.2 Equipment for cleaning the external auditory canal. The curette (1) is the implement most commonly used to remove cerumen. Use of a surgical otoscope head (2) makes the process considerably easier. Additional implements include cotton wicks (3) and a suction tip (4) for removal of discharge or moist wax; alligator forceps (5) for foreign bodies; an ear syringe (6) and motorized irrigation apparatus (7) for removing firm objects or impacted cerumen. Lavage is contraindicated when there is a possible perforation of the tympanic membrane. If the motorized apparatus is used for irrigation, it must be kept on the lowest power setting to avoid traumatizing the eardrum.

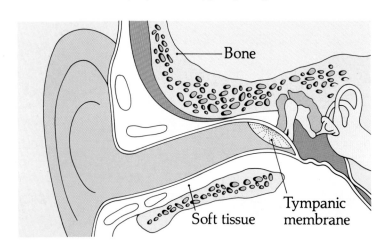

FIG. 20.3 Method of immobilization for cleaning. An assistant holds the arms and simultaneously immobilizes the child's head with the thumbs. The mother firmly holds the hips and thighs. This prevents motion by the child during cleaning of the ear canal and is also useful for otoscopy in young children.

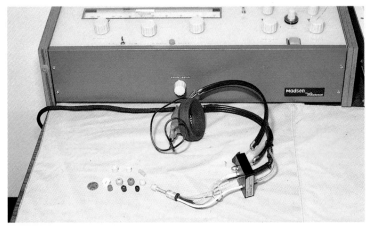

FIG. 20.4 Since the external auditory canal is usually angulated in children, lateral traction on the pinna is often required to straighten the canal and improve visualization of the tympanic membrane.

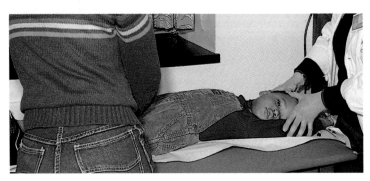

FIG. 20.5 Angulation of the tympanic membrane in infancy. The relationship between the ear canal and eardrum is different in the infant, with the drum being tilted at an angle of 130°. Greater care is required in examining the drum because of this angulation and because the landmarks are less prominent.

FIG. 20.6 Tympanometry. The apparatus and the variety of available ear tips are shown here. The tympanometer measures tympanic membrane compliance and middle ear pressure.

countered, particularly in children less than 2 years of age.

History should center on the nature and duration of symptoms, character of the clinical course, and possible antecedent treatment. Since many infections of the ear are recurrent and/or chronic, the parent should be asked about previous medical or surgical therapy (e.g., antibiotics, myringotomy, and tubes).

A brief review of the anatomy of the ear is helpful in devel-

oping a logical approach to clinical abnormalities. The ear is conveniently divided into three regions (Fig. 20.1):

1. The *external ear* includes the pinna and the external auditory canal, up to and including the tympanic membrane.
2. The *middle ear* is made up of the middle-ear space, the inner surface of the eardrum, the ossicles, and the mastoid.

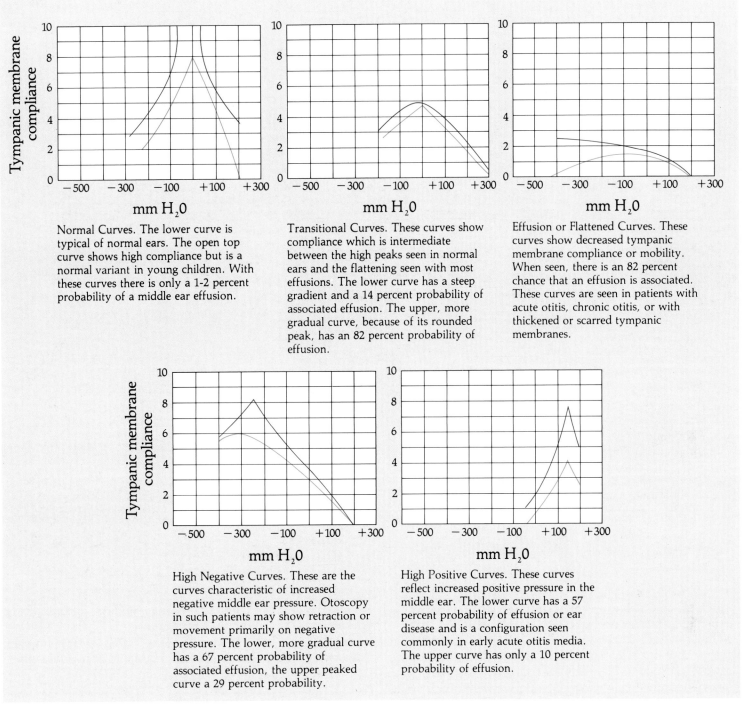

Normal Curves. The lower curve is typical of normal ears. The open top curve shows high compliance but is a normal variant in young children. With these curves there is only a 1-2 percent probability of a middle ear effusion.

Transitional Curves. These curves show compliance which is intermediate between the high peaks seen in normal ears and the flattening seen with most effusions. The lower curve has a steep gradient and a 14 percent probability of associated effusion. The upper, more gradual curve, because of its rounded peak, has an 82 percent probability of effusion.

Effusion or Flattened Curves. These curves show decreased tympanic membrane compliance or mobility. When seen, there is an 82 percent chance that an effusion is associated. These curves are seen in patients with acute otitis, chronic otitis, or with thickened or scarred tympanic membranes.

High Negative Curves. These are the curves characteristic of increased negative middle ear pressure. Otoscopy in such patients may show retraction or movement primarily on negative pressure. The lower, more gradual curve has a 67 percent probability of associated effusion, the upper peaked curve a 29 percent probability.

High Positive Curves. These curves reflect increased positive pressure in the middle ear. The lower curve has a 57 percent probability of effusion or ear disease and is a configuration seen commonly in early acute otitis media. The upper curve has only a 10 percent probability of effusion.

FIG. 20.7 Tympanometric patterns of various conditions of the middle ear are shown in this diagram. (Courtesy of Mrs. Ruth Bachman, PNP, Children's Hospital of Pittsburgh)

3. The *inner ear* comprises the cochlea (hearing), the semicircular canals (balance), and the main nerve trunks of the seventh and eighth cranial nerves.

At a minimum, examination should include inspection of the auricle, periauricular tissues, and external auditory canal, as well as visualization of the entire tympanic membrane, including assessment of its mobility in response to positive and negative pressure. This often necessitates clearing the canal of cerumen or discharge by using a curette, cotton wick, lavage, or suction (Fig. 20.2). The procedure should be done gently and attempted only after the child has been carefully immobilized to avoid trauma (Fig. 20.3). Both the patient and parent should be given a clear explanation of the procedure beforehand.

Since the external auditory canal is often slightly angulated in infants and young children, gentle lateral traction on the pinna is frequently necessary to facilitate visualization of the eardrum itself (Fig. 20.4). In infancy, the tympanic membrane also tends to be oriented at an angle (Fig. 20.5), the landmarks are less prominent, and the canal mucosa, being loosely attached, moves readily on insufflation of air, simulating a normally mobile eardrum. To avoid confusion, it is important to inspect the canal as the speculum is inserted to ensure that the transition between canal wall and tympanic membrane is visualized. When otoscopic findings are unclear or it is difficult to obtain a good air seal for pneumatic otoscopy, tympanometry can be highly useful in evaluating patients over 6 months of age (Figs. 20.6 and 20.7). The proce-

Test	External Ear			Middle and Inner Ear				
	Appearance of Tympanic Membrane (TM)	Mobility of TM	Integrity of TM	Hearing Objective	Hearing Subjective	Vestibular Semicircular Canals	Middle Ear Ossicles and Pressure	Cochlea and Internal Auditory Canal
Otoscopy	+++	++	++	–	–	–	+	–
Acoustic otoscopy	–	++	–	+	–	–	–	–
Microscopy	++++	+	+++	–	–	–	++	–
Tympanometry	–	+++	++++	–	–	–	–	–
Acoustic reflexes	–	+	+	+++	–	–	++	+
Auditory brain response	–	–	–	++++	–	–	++	+
Pure tone audiometry	–	–	–	++	+++	–	++	+
Speech audiometry	–	–	–	+++	+++	–	+	+++
Conventional polytomograms of temporal bone	+	–	–	–	–	+	++	++
CT scan with 1.5 mm section bone algorithm	+	–	–	–	–	++++	++++	++++
Calorics	–	–	–	–	–	++	–	+
Posturography	–	–	–	–	–	+	–	–
Rotational test	–	–	–	–	–	++	–	–

++++ =Excellent; +++ =very good; ++ =good; + =fair; — =no information.

FIG. 20.8 Audio/vestibular tests.

dure is not of value in young infants, because canal wall compliance influences the results.

Children with chronic effusions who complain of hearing loss (or "not listening") or with suspected congenital malformations must have their hearing evaluated—by either audiometry or brainstem-evoked potentials. Patients with vertigo and/or problems of balance and those with facial weakness or asymmetry warrant testing of hearing *and* vestibular function. These children and those suffering from malformations may require radiographic imaging in selected cases to clarify the nature of the problem. Figure 20.8 lists a variety of tests that should be considered for children with ear disorders.

Disorders of the External Ear

THE FOUR "D"s

Examination of every child's ear begins with inspection of the auricle and periauricular tissues for four very important signs: *discharge, displacement, discoloration,* and *deformity* (the four "D"s). The canal is normally smooth, and slightly angulated anteriorly. Cerumen is often present; it varies in color from yellowish-white to tan to dark brown. If cerumen obstructs the view, it must be effectively removed to achieve adequate visualization of the canal and tympanic membrane, to facilitate diagnosis. When soft and moist, it is easi-

ly removed with a curette. This may be more difficult if the cerumen is dry and flaky, and at times may require instillation of drops. In some children it solidifies, forming a firm plug which impedes sound conduction and necessitates softening and irrigation for removal.

Discharge

Discharge is a common complaint with a number of possible causes. When there is thick white discharge and erythema of the canal wall, the physician should gently pull on the pinna. If this maneuver elicits pain and the canal wall is edematous, *primary otitis externa* is the likely diagnosis (Fig. 20.9), although prolonged drainage from untreated *otitis media with perforation* may present a similar picture. When the middle ear is the source of otic discharge, the tympanic membrane will be abnormal and should have evidence of a perforation (see Fig. 20.28). The major predisposing condition to primary otitis externa is prolonged presence of excessive moisture in the ear canal which promotes bacterial or fungal overgrowth. Thus this is a common problem in swimmers. Another major source is the presence of a *foreign body* in the ear canal (see Fig. 20.19) which stimulates an intense inflammatory response and production of a foul-smelling purulent discharge. Thus, when otic drainage is encountered it must be gently cleaned away in order to assess the condition of the tympanic

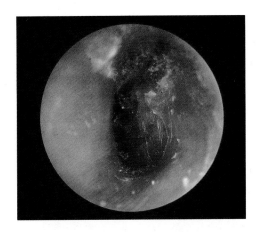

FIG. 20.9 Fungal otitis externa, shown here, is generally more chronic and recurrent than other types. The dark hyphae of **Aspergillus niger** *are visible superiorly.*

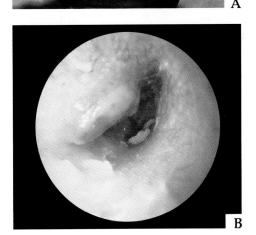

A

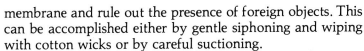

B

FIG. 20.10 Mast-oiditis. **A** *This boy's right ear is swollen, erythematous, and displaced away from his skull. Postauricular swelling is present as well. On palpation the swelling was markedly tender.* **B** *On otoscopy, the canal wall is erythematous and contains purulent drainage. The posterosuperior portion of the canal wall sags inferiorly. (**B** courtesy of Dr. Michael Hawke)*

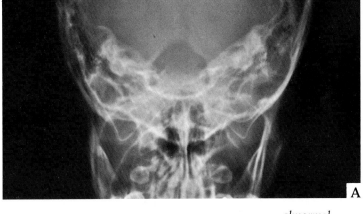

A

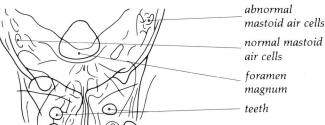

— abnormal mastoid air cells
— normal mastoid air cells
— foramen magnum
— teeth

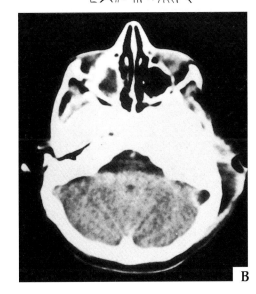

B

FIG. 20.11 Radio-graphic and CT findings in mast-oiditis. **A** *Plain radiograph shows clouding of the mastoid air cells.* **B** *CT scan clearly demonstrates edema and extent of sub-periosteal abscess.*

membrane and rule out the presence of foreign objects. This can be accomplished either by gentle siphoning and wiping with cotton wicks or by careful suctioning.

If history indicates the drainage is persistent or recurrent despite therapy, a culture should be obtained to determine both the causative organism and its sensitivity to antimicrobial agents. Treatment consists primarily of topical otic antibiotic/steroid preparations. Systemic antibiotics should be given when pain is severe, when there is evidence of otitis media, or when, despite attempts at cleaning, there is still uncertainty about an infection of the middle ear.

Displacement

Displacement of the pinna away from the skull is a worrisome sign. The most severe condition causing displacement is *mastoiditis*, resulting from extension of a middle ear infection through the mastoid air cells and out to the periosteum of the skull. In addition to displacement, important clinical signs of mastoiditis include erythema and edema of the pinna and the skin overlying the mastoid, exquisite tenderness on

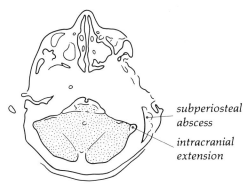

— subperiosteal abscess
— intracranial extension

palpation of the mastoid process, a sagging ear canal, purulent otorrhea, fever, and usually toxicity (Fig. 20.10). This condition is now considered unusual and is seen mainly in patients with long-standing untreated or inadequately treated otitis media. Recognition and prompt institution of parenteral antibiotic therapy are crucial, as there is significant risk of central nervous system extension. Radiographs show haziness of the mastoid air cells, and CT scanning helps delineate extent of involvement and facilitates surgical approach (Fig. 20.11). Mastoidectomy is indicated following stabilization.

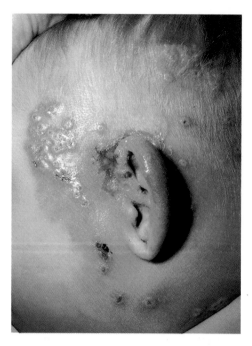

FIG. 20.12 Periauricular and auricular cellulitis. This infant had mild post-auricular seborrhea and developed varicella which rapidly became secondarily infected, producing intense erythema and edema of the auricle and periauricular tissues which were markedly tender. In this case the external canal was normal. (Courtesy of Dr. Ronald Chludzinski, Miner's Clinic, New Kensington, PA)

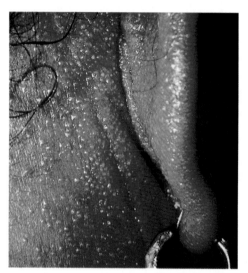

FIG. 20.13 Periauricular contact dermatitis. This young girl became sensitive to the nickel posts of her earrings and developed this contact dermatitis. The auricle and periauricular skin are erythematous and covered by a weeping, pruritic microvesicular eruption. (Courtesy of Dr. Michael Sherlock)

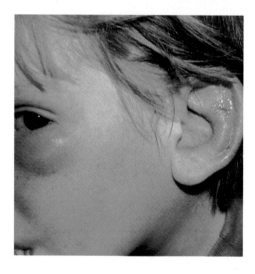

FIG. 20.14 Angioedema. This youngster presented with pruritic, nonpainful, nontender swelling of his ear and suborbital region. Close examination of the latter revealed the punctum of an insect bite. This was obscured by the crusting on his ear which he had scratched. (Courtesy of Dr. Michael Sherlock)

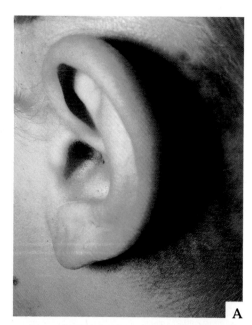

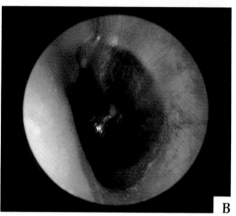

FIG. 20.15 Basilar skull fracture. **A** The presence of a basilar skull fracture involving the temporal bone is often signaled by postauricular ecchymotic discoloration, termed a Battle's sign. **B** The force of the blow may also cause tearing of the ear canal or, as shown here, middle ear hemorrhage with hemotympanum. Depending on time of examination this may appear red or blue. (**B** courtesy of Dr. Michael Hawke)

Other conditions characterized by displacement of the pinna away from the head include parotitis, primary cellulitis of periauricular tissues, and edema secondary to insect bites or contact dermatitis. *Parotitis* is differentiated by finding prominent induration and enlargement of the parotid gland anterior to the external ear, together with blunting of the angle of the mandible on palpation (see Chapter 12). *Primary cellulitis* is characterized by erythema and tenderness, but can often be distinguished clinically from mastoiditis by the presence of associated skin lesions which anteceded the inflammation (Fig. 20.12). In cases secondary to untreated external otitis or otitis media with perforation, the picture may be clinically similar, but mastoid X-rays will be normal. Localized *contact dermatitis* and *angioedema* may be erythematous but will be pruritic and nontender. The former condition is characterized by microvesicular skin changes (Fig. 20.13), while in the latter condition, a precipitating insect bite can often be identified on inspection (Fig. 20.14).

Discoloration

Discoloration is another important sign and is commonly a feature of conditions producing displacement. Erythema of the pinna is common when there is inflammation with or without infection (see Figs. 20.12–20.14). Ecchymotic discoloration may be encountered with trauma. When this overlies the mastoid area it is termed *Battle's sign* (Fig. 20.15A) and usually reflects a basilar skull fracture. In such cases, the canal wall should be checked for tears, and the tympanic membrane for perforation or a *hemotympanum* (Fig. 20.15B). In

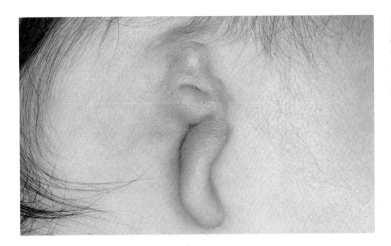

FIG. 20.16 Atresia of the external ear. In this infant, the pinna failed to develop properly and the external canal was completely stenosed. Audiometric testing revealed a 60-dB hearing loss. This isolated deformity in an otherwise normal child was the result of abnormal development of the first branchial arch. (Courtesy of Dr. Michael Hawke)

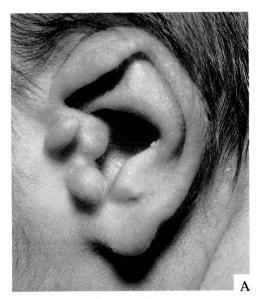

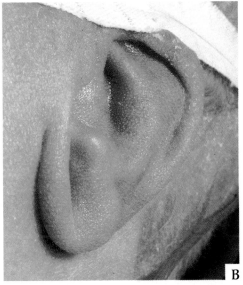

A

B

FIG. 20.17 Minor congenital auricular deformities. **A** In this infant, the superior portion of the helix is folded over obscuring the triangular fossa, the antihelix is sharply angulated, and there are three preauricular skintags. **B** This neonate with orofaciodigital and Turner syndromes has a simple helix and a redundant folded lobule. The ear is low set and posteriorly rotated, and the antitragus is anteriorly displaced. **C** This infant with Rubinstein-Taybi syndrome has an exaggeratedly elongated intertragal notch. **D** Lop ear in an otherwise normal child. The auricular cartilage is abnormally contoured, making the ear protrude forward. (**C** courtesy of Dr. Michael Sherlock)

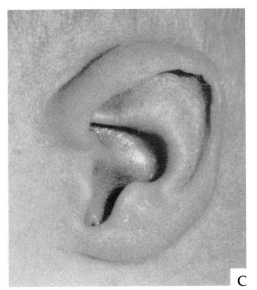

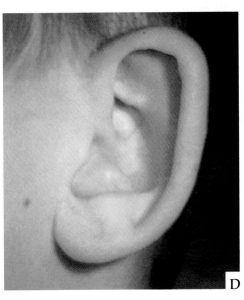

C

D

fact, these findings are generally more helpful in making the diagnosis than routine skull X-rays which are often negative.

Deformity

Deformity of the pinna is often the result of hereditary factors, but at times is produced by intrauterine positioning. When the external ear is grossly misshapen or atretic, anomalies of middle and inner ear structures are often associated, and hearing loss may be profound (Fig. 20.16). Such abnormalities warrant thorough evaluation in infancy in order to ensure early recognition and treatment of hearing loss. More frequently, deformities are minor. In some instances they may be part of a picture of multiple congenital anomalies (Fig. 20.17A–C), but in most cases they represent isolated minor malformations which are of little significance other than cosmetic (Fig. 20.17D).

Preauricular cysts constitute one of the more common congenital abnormalities. These are branchial cleft remnants lo-

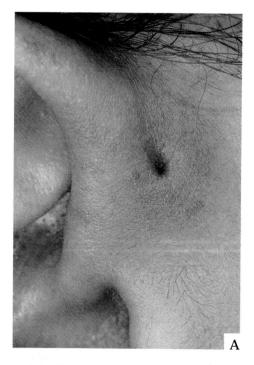

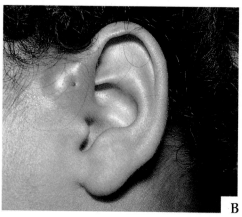

B

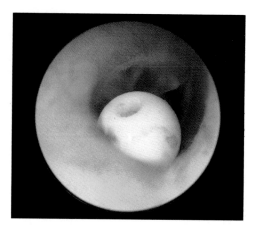

FIG. 20.18 Preauricular sinuses. **A** These branchial cleft remnants are located anterior to the pinna and have an overlying surface dimple. **B** In this child the sinus has become infected, forming an abscess. (**A** courtesy of Dr. Michael Hawke)

FIG. 20.19 Foreign body. This child had inserted a bead into her ear. Care is required in removal to prevent further trauma. (Courtesy of Dr. Michael Hawke)

A

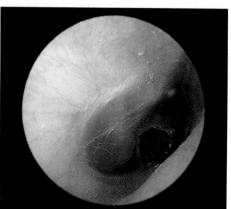

FIG. 20.20 Traumatic perforation of the tympanic membrane. This 8-year-old boy's tympanic membrane was perforated from a slap on the ear. (Courtesy of Dr. Michael Hawke)

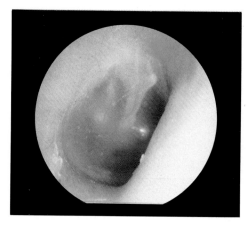

FIG. 20.21 Normal tympanic membrane. The drum is thin and translucent, and the ossicles are readily visualized. It is neutrally positioned with no evidence of either bulging or retraction. (Courtesy of Dr. Sylvdn Stool, Children's Hospital of Pittsburgh)

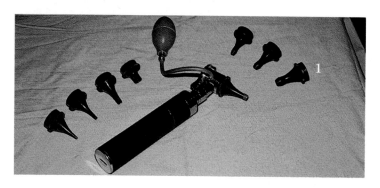

FIG. 20.22 Pneumatic otoscopy. The procedure requires proper equipment including a pneumatic otoscope head and an appropriately sized speculum to achieve a good air seal. When a seal is difficult to obtain despite proper speculum size, the head and tubing should be checked for air leaks. If none is found, application of a piece of rubber tubing to the end of the speculum (shown attached to the otoscope) or use of a soft speculum (**1**) may solve the problem.

cated anterior to the pinna with an overlying surface dimple (Fig. 20.18A). These cysts are vulnerable to infection and abscess formation (Fig. 20.18B), which necessitates incision and drainage in conjunction with antistaphylococcal antibiotics. Once infected, recurrence will be common unless the entire cyst is completely excised once inflammation has subsided.

FOREIGN OBJECTS AND SECONDARY TRAUMA

It is not unusual for children to put paper, beads, and other foreign objects into the ear canal (Fig. 20.19). In some cases small objects may be embedded in cerumen and missed on inspection. As noted earlier, if present for more than a few days, the foreign material stimulates an inflammatory response and production of a purulent discharge which is often foul-smelling and which may obscure the presence of the inciting foreign body. Removal of some objects can be accomplished by use of alligator forceps or by irrigation of the ear canal, while others—particularly spherical objects—require use of suction. Foreign objects may also be the source of painful abrasions or lacerations of the external auditory canal, or even perforation of the tympanic membrane. Insertion of pencils or sticks into the ear canal by the child and parental attempts to clean the canal with a cotton swab are the most common modes of such injury. Exposure to concussive forces such as a direct blow or an explosion can also result in perforation (Fig. 20.20). Patients with traumatic perforations must be carefully assessed for signs of injury to deeper structures. Evidence of hearing loss, vertigo, or nystagmus should prompt urgent otolaryngologic consultation.

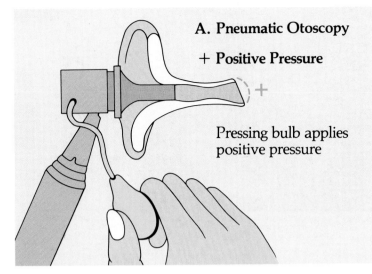

A. Pneumatic Otoscopy

+ Positive Pressure

Pressing bulb applies positive pressure

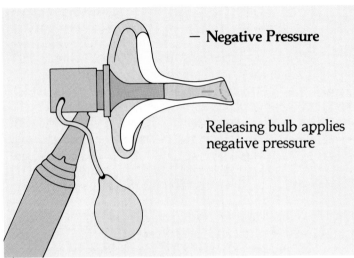

− Negative Pressure

Releasing bulb applies negative pressure

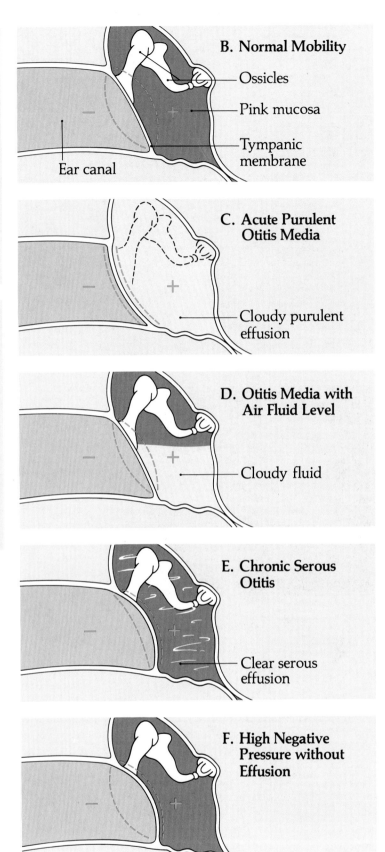

B. Normal Mobility

— Ossicles

— Pink mucosa

— Tympanic membrane

Ear canal

C. Acute Purulent Otitis Media

—Cloudy purulent effusion

D. Otitis Media with Air Fluid Level

—Cloudy fluid

E. Chronic Serous Otitis

—Clear serous effusion

F. High Negative Pressure without Effusion

FIG. 20.23 The technique and findings of pneumatic otoscopy.
A The speculum is inserted into the ear canal to form a tight
seal. The bulb is then gently and slowly pressed and then
released while the mobility of the drum is assessed. Pressing on
the bulb applies positive pressure; letting up applies negative
pressure. B With normal mobility, the drum moves inward and
then back. C In cases of acute otitis media in which the middle
ear is filled with purulent material, the drum bulges toward the
examiner and moves minimally. D In cases of acute otitis media
with an air-fluid level, mobility may be nearly normal. In some
patients, however, the drum may be retracted, indicating in-
creased negative pressure. If this is the case, mobility on positive
pressure may be reduced while movement on negative pressure
is nearly normal or only mildly decreased. This is the same
pattern as that seen commonly in children with chronic serous
otitis (E). F In cases of high negative pressure and no effusion,
application of positive pressure produces little or no movement,
but on negative pressure the drum billows back toward the
examiner.

Disorders of the Middle Ear

The normal tympanic membrane is thin, translucent, neutrally positioned, and mobile. The ossicles, particularly the
malleus, are generally visible through it (Fig. 20.21). Adequate assessment requires that the examiner note four major
characteristics of the tympanic membrane: (1) thickness, (2)
degree of translucence, (3) position relative to neutral, and

(4) mobility. Application of gentle positive and negative pressure, using the pneumatic otoscope (Fig. 20.22), produces
brisk movement of the eardrum when the ear is free of disease, and abnormal movement when fluid is present, when
the drum is thickened or scarred, or when there is an increase
in either positive or negative pressure (Fig. 20.23). An abnormality in *any one* of the four major characteristics is suggestive of middle ear pathology.

PATHOGENS OF ACUTE OTITIS MEDIA

Pathogen	%
S. pneumoniae	35.0
H. influenzae	17.0
B. catarrhalis	9.0
S. pyogenes	4.0
S. aureus	0.5
No growth	35.0
Ampicillin resistant	1.0

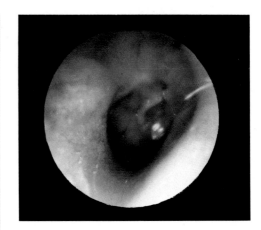

FIG. 20.26 Acute otitis media with purulent effusion. A crescent of yellow pus with bubbles in the hypotympanum. There is no erythema, and mobility was only slightly reduced. The patient was acutely febrile and had ear pain.

FIG. 20.24 Pathogens of acute otitis media. (These microorganisms have been obtained in the percentages shown from aspirates of middle ear effusions of patients seen at Children's Hospital of Pittsburgh, 1979-1980. Studies at other medical centers have yielded similar findings.)

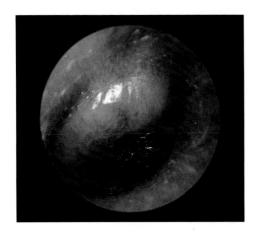

FIG. 20.25 Acute otitis media. This is the textbook picture: an erythematous, opaque, bulging tympanic membrane. The light reflex is reduced, and the landmarks are partially obscured. Mobility is markedly reduced. (Courtesy of Dr. Michael Hawke)

ACUTE OTITIS MEDIA

Acute otitis media is the term used to describe acute infection and inflammation of the middle ear. Associated inflammation and edema of the mucosa of the eustachian tube appears to play a role in the pathogenesis by impeding drainage of the middle ear fluid. (In some children anatomic or chronic physiologic abnormalities of the eustachian tube predispose to infection.) The problem is commonly seen in conjunction with an acute upper respiratory infection, and its onset is often heralded by a secondary temperature spike. The major offending organisms are bacterial respiratory pathogens. The most commonly isolated organisms and their relative frequency are listed in Figure 20.24.

In acute otitis media, the classic findings on inspection of the tympanic membrane are erythema and injection; bulging which obscures the malleus; thickening, often with a grayish-white or yellow hue reflecting a purulent effusion; and reduced mobility (Fig. 20.25). It must be remembered, however, that crying rapidly produces erythema of the eardrum, and thus erythema in the face of crying is of little value. The patient is usually febrile and, if old enough, typically complains of otalgia. However, in many cases this "textbook picture" is not seen. This is probably due in part to time of presentation, the virulence of the particular pathogen, and host factors. Accuracy in diagnosis necessitates meticulous care on otoscopy and knowledge of the various modes of presentation. Children may present with fever of a few hours duration and otalgia (or if very young with fever and irritability), yet have no abnormality on otoscopy. If reexamined the following day, many of these patients have clear evidence of acute otitis media. Other patients have erythema and bubbles or an air-fluid or air-pus level (due to venting by the eustachian tube) without bulging, and with nearly normal mobility (Fig. 20.26). In still other cases, the drum may be full and poorly mobile with cloudy fluid behind it, but minimally erythematous. In some patients the drum is retracted, moves primarily or only in response to negative pressure, and shows signs of inflammation and/or a cloudy effusion. Occasionally the signs and symptoms of otitis media may be accompanied by formation of a bullous lesion on the surface of the tympanic membrane, a condition termed *bullous myringitis* (Fig. 20.27). These children usually complain of intense pain. While this phenomenon is most commonly associated with Mycoplasma in adults, any of the usual pediatric pathogens (see Fig. 20.24) can be causative in children. Finally, acute otitis media may, by virtue of increasing middle ear pressure, result in acute perforation of the tympanic membrane. On presentation, the canal may be filled with purulent material; however, tugging on the pinna usually does not elicit pain, and erythema and edema of the canal wall are minimal or absent. Cleansing with a cotton wick will usually reveal an inflamed drum with a barely visible perforation (Fig. 20.28). Just as clinical findings vary, so do symptoms. While some patients present with severe otalgia, others may complain of sore throat, only mild ear discomfort, ear popping, or decreased hearing, yet have floridly inflamed eardrums. Fever may be absent.

In addition to treating patients with an appropriate antimicrobial agent and analgesics when needed, follow-up examination is important. This is best done 2 to 3 weeks after diagnosis, when complete resolution can be expected in over 50 percent of children. The purpose of reevaluation is to identify those patients who have persistent serous effusions and who require ongoing surveillance.

OTITIS MEDIA WITH EFFUSION ("SEROUS OTITIS MEDIA")

"Serous" effusion in the middle ear may result from an upper respiratory infection or may be the residual of a treated acute

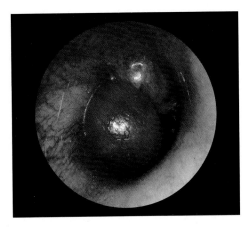

FIG. 20.27 *Acute otitis media with bullous myringitis. This patient was febrile and extremely uncomfortable. On otoscopy an erythematous bullous lesion is seen obscuring much of the tympanic membrane. This phenomenon, called bullous myringitis, is caused by the usual pathogens of childhood. The bullous lesion commonly ruptures spontaneously, providing immediate relief of pain.*

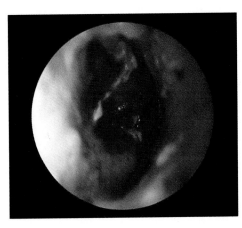

FIG. 20.28 *Acute otitis media with perforation. In this child, increased middle ear pressure with acute otitis resulted in perforation of the tympanic membrane. The drum is thickened, and the perforation is seen at 3 o'clock.*

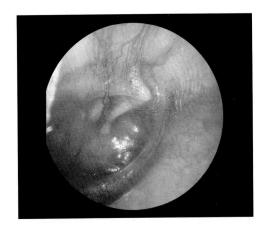

FIG. 20.29 *Serous otitis media. This patient has a chronic serous middle ear effusion. The tympanic membrane is retracted, thickened, and shiny, and has a clear yellow effusion behind it. Mobility was decreased and primarily evident on negative pressure. The child was not acutely ill but did have decreased hearing. (Courtesy of Dr. Sylvan Stool)*

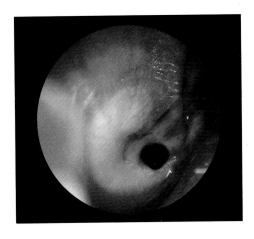

FIG. 20.30 *Sequela of chronic otitis media. The eardrum is markedly thickened, scarred in an arc from 12 to 5 o'clock, and has a large chronic perforation. (Courtesy of Dr. Sylvan Stool)*

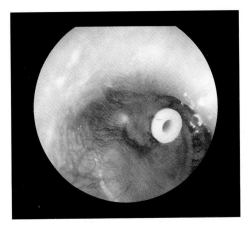

FIG. 20.31 *Tympanic membrane of patient with chronic otitis media, with tympanostomy tube in place. The tubes serve to vent the middle ear, improve hearing, and tend to reduce the frequency of infection. (Courtesy of Dr. Sylvan Stool)*

otitis. In many instances this effusion is not spontaneously cleared, but instead remains in the middle ear for weeks or months, resulting in a persistent clear gray or yellow effusion behind the eardrum (Fig. 20.29). Persistence appears due in part to eustachian tube dysfunction. Pneumatic otoscopy often reveals poor mobility of the tympanic membrane, and then primarily on negative pressure. The latter is thought to develop as a result of consumption of middle ear oxygen by mucosal cells, creating a vacuum which persists with the fluid because of failure of ventilation by the eustachian tube. Such long-standing effusions impair hearing and are subject to bacterial invasion, and thus recurrent middle ear infection. Persistence of a serous effusion for longer than 2 to 3 months is an indication for myringotomy and insertion of tubes (see Fig. 20.31) to facilitate hearing and reduce the risk of recurrent infection.

CHRONIC/RECURRENT OTITIS MEDIA
Chronic or chronic/recurrent otitis media with effusion (COME) is not an uncommon finding in young children. Patients subject to this condition appear to have significant and prolonged eustachian tube dysfunction. This "otitis-prone" state may be an apparently isolated phenomenon or can be a feature of a number of syndromes characterized by palatal dysfunction or malformation, or by facial hypoplasia or deformity. These conditions include cleft palate, Crouzon syndrome, Down syndrome, the mucopolysaccharidoses, and mucolipidoses. Chronic obstructive tonsillar and adenoidal hypertrophy may also be a predisposing condition. Chronic otitis media is associated with significant morbidity in terms of intermittent or chronic hearing impairment, intermittent discomfort, and the ill effects of recurrent infection. Over months or years, the process produces permanent myringosclerotic changes in which the tympanic membrane becomes whitened, thickened, and scarred. Chronic perforations are not uncommon (Fig. 20.30). Patients with persistent middle ear infections despite medical therapy and those with frequent recurrences appear to benefit from surgical drainage and insertion of tympanostomy tubes which vent the middle ear (Fig. 20.31). Once placed, these should be checked at intervals

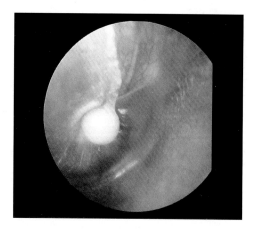

FIG. 20.32 Cholesteatoma. This mass lesion which consists of an epithelial cyst is growing within the eardrum of this child. (Courtesy of Dr. Sylvan Stool)

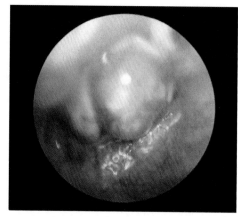

FIG. 20.33 Granuloma of the tympanic membrane. Growth of this polypoid lesion was stimulated by the inflammatory process of chronic middle ear infection. (Courtesy of Dr. Sylvan Stool)

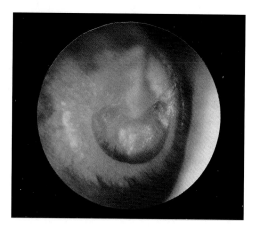

FIG. 20.34 Dimerism of the tympanic membrane. Otoscopy demonstrates a severely retracted atrophic segment of the eardrum which also has multiple white scars. The thinned portions are the result of abnormal healing of perforations, and tend to be hypermobile on otoscopy. (Courtesy of Dr. Sylvan Stool)

for presence and patency. Spontaneous extrusion generally occurs 6 to 12 months after insertion. Children with chronic perforations or tubes must protect the ear from moisture to reduce risk of contamination of the middle ear and reinfection.

OTHER MIDDLE EAR DISORDERS
A number of other disorders involving the tympanic membrane, though considerably less common than otitis media and serous otitis media, are important because of potential seriousness.

Mass Lesions Involving the Tympanic Membrane
A *cholesteatoma* appears as a pearl-like cyst of the eardrum and consists of trapped epithelial tissue which grows beneath the surface of the membrane (Fig. 20.32). While many are congenital, some are sequelae of untreated or of chronic/recurrent otitis media. If a cholesteatoma is not removed surgically, it continues to grow and results in a progressive hearing impairment.

Granulomas or polyps of the tympanic membrane (Fig. 20.33) also can occur in children with chronic middle ear infections. This tissue often bleeds easily and can be frightening to the patient, the parent, and the physician. Left untreated, polyps can enlarge to fill the canal, and by expansion can progressively damage both the drum and the ossicles. Therefore, prompt surgical removal is indicated.

Distortions of the Tympanic Membrane
Thin, dimeric portions of the eardrum may also be observed in patients with chronic middle ear disease, or may develop following extrusion of a tympanostomy tube (Fig. 20.34). These thinned areas are the result of abnormal healing of perforations and are hypermobile on pneumatic otoscopy. The important points to note on examination are whether the pocket is fully visible or partly hidden, and whether or not it is dry. If the ear canal and drum are *not* dry, then an active infection and/or cholesteatoma will be present, and aggressive therapy, including ventilation of the middle ear and excision of the pocket, may be necessary.

NASAL DISORDERS
A child's nose is most commonly examined for disturbances in external appearance, excessive drainage, or blockage of airflow and interference with breathing. Epistaxis is also frequently encountered.

Nasal Obstruction

UPPER RESPIRATORY INFECTIONS IN EARLY INFANCY
In infancy and early childhood, the nasal passages are small and easily obstructed by processes which produce mucosal edema, whether infectious, "allergic," or traumatic. In the first 1 to 3 months, infants are obligate nose breathers, and therefore can have significant respiratory distress from nasal congestion alone. Young infants with upper respiratory infections may, in addition to nasal discharge, have tachypnea and mild retractions, and often have to interrupt feeding to breathe. Instillation of saline nose drops to loosen secretions followed by nasal suctioning prior to meals and naps can provide a measure of relief. Oral decongestants are ineffective and often produce marked irritability when given to infants in the first several months of life. Fortunately, these upper respiratory infections are generally brief and clear within a few days. On occasion, the discharge persists and often becomes purulent or serosanguinous. Whether this represents an ethmoiditis (see section on Sinusitis) or simply a nasopharyngitis is unclear. However, culture of discharges persisting longer than 10 to 14 days may disclose heavy growth of a single bacterial pathogen, which when treated results in resolution of symptoms.

CONGENITAL CAUSES OF NASAL OBSTRUCTION
Congenital causes of nasal obstruction include choanal atresia, choanal stenosis, and mass lesions.

Choanal Atresia and Stenosis
Choanal atresia may be either bony (90 percent) or mem-

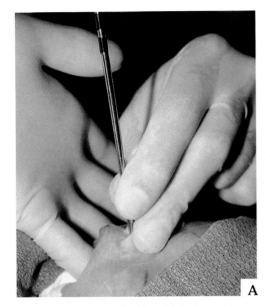
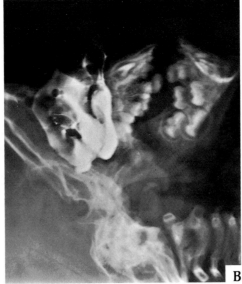
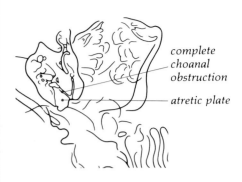

complete
choanal
obstruction

atretic plate

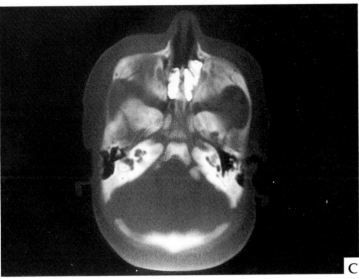

FIG. 20.35 Choanal atresia. **A** This infant manifested severe respiratory distress at delivery, with paradoxical cyanosis. Attempts to pass a urethral sound revealed bony obstruction of the choanae bilaterally. **B** A lateral radiograph, taken following instillation of radiopaque dye, reveals pooling of the dye within the nose anterior to the choane, confirming complete choanal obstruction. This was also evident on CT scan (**C**).

branous (10 percent), bilateral or unilateral. Newborns with bilateral choanal atresia manifest severe respiratory distress at delivery, with cyanosis which is relieved by crying and returns with rest (paradoxical cyanosis). The true nature of the problem can elude detection if the physician relies solely on passing soft feeding catheters through the nose to determine patency, as these can buckle or curl within the nose. The correct diagnosis is best made by using a Van Buren urethral sound or a firm plastic suction catheter (both #8 French). This is passed gently along the floor of the nose, close to the septum. If bony resistance is encountered, then the diagnosis of choanal atresia is almost certain (Fig. 20.35A). Membranous atresia, if present, can often be penetrated. Confirmation of choanal atresia is obtained by placing barium into the nose and viewing lateral and basilar X-rays (Fig. 20.35B). Immediate relief of respiratory distress may be accomplished by insertion of an oral airway (or a nipple from which the tip has been cut away) into the mouth. Definitive studies including computerized tomography can then be performed to aid in planning surgical correction (Fig. 20.35C). Infants with *unilateral choanal atresia* are usually asymptomatic at birth; however, with time they develop a persistent unilateral nasal discharge.

Choanal stenosis is also generally asymptomatic in the newborn period, but acquisition of an upper respiratory infection can result in significant respiratory compromise. When suspected, probing with a urethral sound is indicated. If this meets resistance, further evaluation is required. In most cases, symptomatic therapy using saline nose drops and nasal suctioning is sufficient to help the infants through their upper respiratory infections. With growth, the problem abates.

Congenital Mass Lesions

Congenital mass lesions are another source of nasal obstruction. These are particularly likely to become apparent during the first 2 years of life. The mode of presentation varies, some manifesting primarily by symptoms of obstruction and detected via diagnostic radiography, others being visually evident either within a nostril or seen as a subcutaneous mass located near the root of the nose. A few present with recurrent nasal infections and/or epistaxis. All such growths merit thorough clinical and radiographic evaluation, since many have intracranial connections.

An *encephalocoele* is an outpouching of brain tissue through a congenital bony defect of the skull. In some cases patients present with craniofacial deformities and a rounded

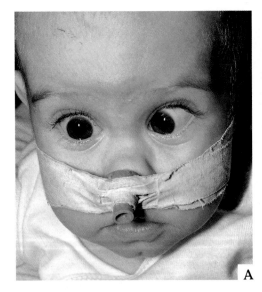
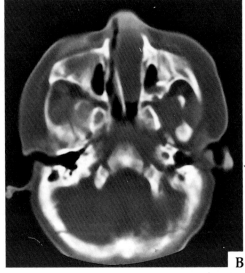
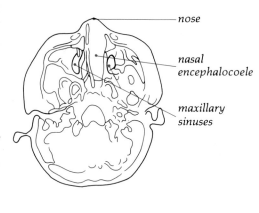

nose

nasal encephalocoele

maxillary sinuses

A   B

FIG. 20.36 Nasal encephalocoele. **A** This normal-appearing infant presented with signs of severe nasal obstruction, necessitating insertion of a nasopharyngeal airway to relieve distress. **B** A CT scan shows a large nasal mass lesion which fills one nostril and pushes the nasal septum into the other. This lesion proved to be an encephalocoele extruding through a bony defect in the skull (extrusion seen on another cut).

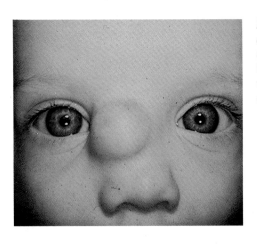

FIG. 20.37 Nasal dermoid. Note the characteristic overlying dimple from which hair may extrude.

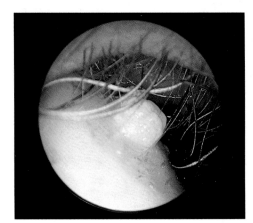

FIG. 20.38 Nasal papillomas, warty growths at the mucocutaneous junction of the nares. (Courtesy of Dr. Michael Hawke)

swelling between the eyes. In other instances the neural tissue prolapses into the nasopharynx, resulting in signs and symptoms of nasal obstruction without obvious external anomalies (Fig. 20.36A). Occasionally, a grapelike mass may be seen within the nares or (via direct nasopharynoscopy) protruding into the pharynx. The mass is usually identified by diagnostic radiography. Computerized tomography (Fig. 20.36B) is particularly helpful in delineating the extent of mass and underlying bony defect. Repair requires a collaborative effort by specialists in otolaryngology, neurosurgery, and in some cases, plastic surgery.

Nasal dermoids are embryonic cysts containing ectodermal and mesodermal tissue. They present as round, firm subcutaneous masses which are located on the dorsum of the nose close to the midline (Fig. 20.37). Examination of the overlying skin frequently reveals a small dimple, at times with extruding hair. Some of these cysts have deep extensions down to the nasal septum or through the cribriform plate into the cranium. Thorough evaluation using CT scan and perhaps standard tomograms is necessary to determine ex-

tent and plan repair. If not removed, infection is common and often results in fistula formation.

Small *skintags* are frequently seen around the nasal vestibule and should be removed to improve appearance. *Papillomas* (Fig. 20.38) are similar growths that occur on the distal nasal mucosa near the mucocutaneous junction. These should be excised both to improve appearance and confirm diagnosis; they do not cause obstructions.

ACQUIRED FORMS OF NASAL OBSTRUCTION
Adenoidal and Tonsillar Hypertrophy

The lymphoid tissue that constitutes the tonsils and adenoids is relatively small in infancy, gradually enlarges until 8 to 10 years of age, and then begins to shrink in size. In most instances this normal process of hypertrophy results in mild to moderate enlargement of these structures and does not constitute a problem. A small percentage of children, however, develop marked adenoidal and tonsillar hypertrophy, with attendant symptoms of nasal obstruction and rhinorrhea. A few even have difficulty swallowing solid foods. Re-

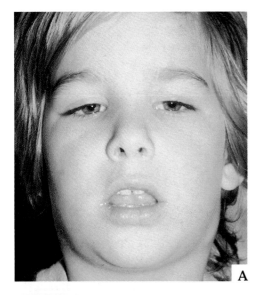

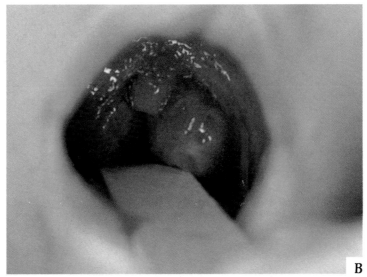

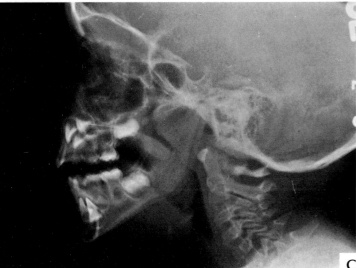

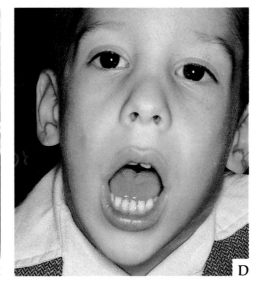

FIG. 20.39 Adenidal and tonsillar hypertrophy. **A** External appearance of a child with marked enlargement of tonsils and adenoids. He must keep his mouth open to breathe, and shows signs of fatigue as a result of sleep disturbance caused by his upper airway obstruction. **B** On examination of the pharynx, his tonsils are seen meeting at the midline. **C** A lateral neck radiograph shows a large adenoid shadow impinging on the nasal airway. **D** If obstruction is prolonged, cor pulmonale and abnormal facial growth consisting of facial elongation and widening of the nasal root may result.

current infection appears to be the most common inciting factor, although atopy may play a role in some cases. Occasionally, mononucleosis is the initiating event resulting in rapid enlargement of adenoidal and tonsillar tissues which is then slow to resolve (see section on Tonsillopharyngitis and see also Chapter 12). In most children progressive adenoidal enlargement appears to be the cumulative result of a series of upper respiratory infections. The consequent obstruction to normal flow of secretions then starts a vicious cycle, making the child even more vulnerable to recurrent bacterial infections of the ears, sinuses, and nasopharynx which further exacerbate the adenoidal and tonsillar hypertrophy.

Regardless of mode of origin, when adenoidal hypertrophy is marked, blockage of the nasal airway becomes severe and results in mouth breathing, chronic rhinorrhea, inability to blow the nose, and snoring during sleep (Fig. 20.39A). Speech has a hyponasal and muffled quality. The child holds his mouth open, has little or no airflow through the nares, and his tonsils may meet in the midline (Fig.

20.39B). A cephalometric lateral neck X-ray reveals a large adenoidal shadow impinging on the nasal airway (Fig. 20.39C). For many patients these features are seen primarily in the course of acute illness; however, a number of children have symptoms even when free of acute infection. In a minority, obstruction is so severe as to produce sleep disturbance. This is characterized by restlessness and retractions when recumbent, stertorous snoring, and sleep apnea with frequent waking. Some patients actually begin to sleep sitting up, and many manifest daytime fatigue. If the obstruction is prolonged, cor pulmonale (with signs of right ventricular hypertrophy on EKG and chest X-ray) and abnormal facial growth may result (Fig. 20.39D).

Management of patients with adenoidal hypertrophy is dependent in part upon the severity and the duration of obstruction. In milder cases of short duration, or in patients with intermittent symptoms, careful monitoring, prompt institution of antimicrobial therapy for bacterial infections, and treatment of atopy when present may bring the problem

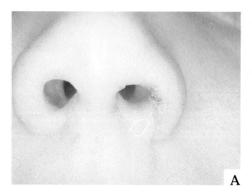

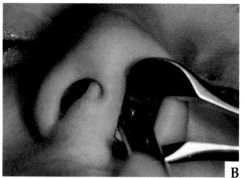

FIG. 20.40 Nasal foreign body. **A** This child presented with a unilateral, foul-smelling nasal discharge. Aspiration of the discharge revealed a red bead which was deep in the nose, necessitating removal under general anesthesia (**B**). (**A** courtesy of Dr. Michael Hawke)

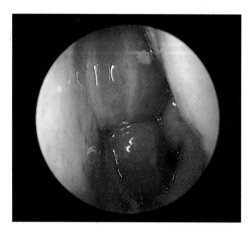

FIG. 20.41 Nasal polyp. This 2-year-old girl with cystic fibrosis was referred because of nasal obstruction and nocturnal snoring of a few months duration. A large grayish polyp was found in the left nostril.

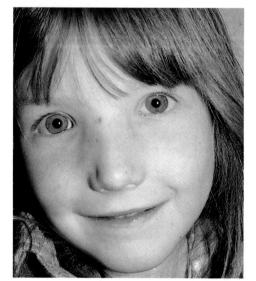

FIG. 20.42 Sequela of chronic nasal polyps. This 7-year-old girl with cystic fibrosis and recurrent nasal polyps shows secondary alteration in facial growth consisting of a broadened nasal dorsum and prominence of the malar areas. This occurred despite several resections.

under control. Children with persistent symptoms despite therapy and those with sleep disturbance or cor pulmonale warrant adenoidectomy.

Nasal Foreign Bodies

As is true of the external ear, it is not unusual for small children to put beads, paper, pieces of sponge, plastic toys, or other foreign material into their noses. Such foreign objects are irritating to the nasal mucosa and soon incite an intense inflammatory reaction with production of a thick, purulent, foul-smelling discharge that helps to hide their presence. Intermittent epistaxis may accompany the discharge. As most children below 5 years of age are unable to blow their noses and are fearful or unable to tell their parents about disapproved actions, the object is not expelled and the problem often goes unrecognized until medical attention is sought. A unilateral nasal discharge, a foul smell, or both are the typical chief complaints and should lead the clinician to suspect a foreign body immediately. Speculum examination may readily disclose the object (Fig. 20.40), but often the purulent discharge obscures the view. Even when visualization is accomplished, removal can be difficult, as children are easily frightened at the prospect of instrumentation, and their struggling can result in mucosal injury during attempts at removal. To minimize problems, topical anesthetic spray can be applied and the child restrained with a papoose board. The discharge then may be removed by swab or suction. If the object is anterior to the turbinates, removal can be attempted using suction or a right angle or Day hook for spherical objects or alligator forceps for material that can be grasped. Consultation from an otolaryngologist should be sought for removal of objects located more posteriorly or those not readily removed on initial attempts.

Nasal Polyps

Polyps are thought to be the product of recurrent infection and/or inflammation, although in a proportion of cases atopy may play a contributing role. The phenomenon is unusual in children under 10 years of age, with the exception of patients with cystic fibrosis, 25 percent of whom develop polyps, some as early as in infancy. Symptoms consist of progressive nasal obstruction, frequently with associated discharge. Recurrent sinusitis is a common complication as a result of impaired sinus drainage. Affected patients with acute infections may also have intermittent epistaxis. Involvement may be unilateral or bilateral. On examination, moist, glistening pedunculated growths are seen that may have a smooth or a grapelike appearance (Fig. 20.41). Bilateral opacification of the ethmoid and maxillary sinuses are commonly found on radiography. Polyps must be distinguished from a nasal glioma or encephalocoele which may have a similar appearance and can produce identical symptoms. These neural mass lesions are more common in infancy, but can present in older children. Therefore, computerized tomography of the nasopharynx should be considered for children under age 10 with polypoid nasal lesions without documented cystic fibrosis.

Surgical removal of the polyp is indicated to relieve nasal obstruction, reduce the risk of secondary sinusitis, and diminish the possibility of altered facial growth. The latter problem is seen in children with chronic polyps (most frequently those with cystic fibrosis) and consists of widening of the nasal dorsum and prominence of the malar areas of the face (Fig. 20.42).

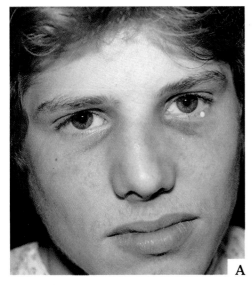 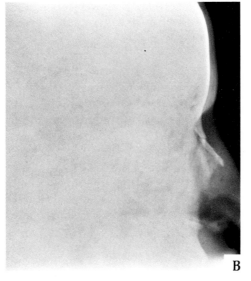 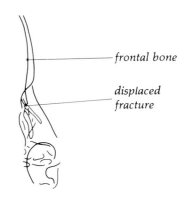

FIG. 20.43 Displaced nasal fracture. **A** This teenager was hit on the nose while playing football. On external inspection there is obvious deformity and there are ecchymoses under both eyes.

Crepitance was evident on palpation. **B** A lateral radiograph of another patient shows a displaced fracture of the proximal portion of the nasal bone.

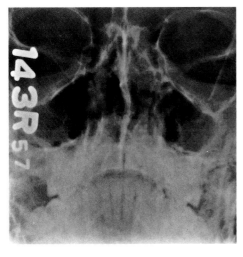

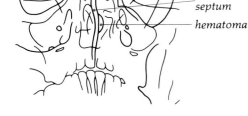

FIG. 20.44 Deviated nasal septum. This patient was punched in the nose, resulting in a leftward deviation of the cartilaginous portion of the nasal septum, clearly seen in this radiograph. The small arc of mucosal swelling along the septum proved to be a small septal hematoma. There is no visible fracture. Septal deviation requires correction to prevent deformity and relieve secondary nasal obstruction.

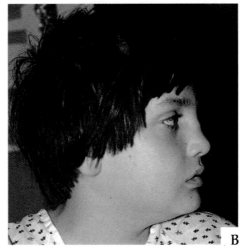

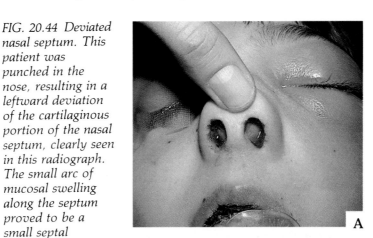

FIG. 20.45 Septal hematoma. **A** This patient incurred facial trauma resulting in multiple fractures of the nasal and orbital bones and submucosal bleeding along the nasal septum. Such septal hematomas must be drained promptly to reduce the risk of abscess formation, and to prevent cartilage necrosis which ultimately results in a saddle nose deformity (**B**).

Nasal Trauma

Blunt nasal trauma is frequently encountered in pediatrics. In the majority of instances it results only in minor swelling and mild epistaxis, which is readily controlled by application of pressure over the nares (see Chapter 2 for nasal trauma incurred during delivery). However, more severe injuries are not uncommon and have a significant potential for long-term morbidity and deformity if not identified and treated

appropriately. These include displaced nasal fractures (Fig. 20.43), which if not reduced, result in permanent deformity; septal deviation or dislocation, with or without an associated fracture (Fig. 20.44), which produces unilateral impairment of airflow; and septal hematomas (Fig. 20.45A), which if not drained promptly, cause destruction of nasal cartilage resulting in a saddle nose deformity (Fig. 20.45B). Finally, profuse bleeding which is difficult to stop or recurs readily suggests trauma to deeper structures of the face or frontal bones and warrants prompt stabilization and meticulous clinical and radiographic assessment.

In evaluating patients with nasal trauma, the nasal bridge should be inspected for swelling or deformity (the latter may not be apparent if swelling is marked), and the bony septum palpated for tenderness, crepitus, or excessive mobility. The nares should be cleared of clots and the septum assessed for position and presence of swelling suggestive of a hematoma. Examination of the oropharynx is also helpful in determining if blood is flowing posteriorly. When marked swelling, severe tenderness, deformity, crepitus, or septal deviation is found, radiographs are indicated. Septal hematomas, displaced fractures, and bleeding which fails to cease readily with direct pressure necessitate prompt consultation by an otolaryngologist.

Epistaxis

Nasal bleeding in childhood has a number of causes including trauma, infection, mucosal irritation, bleeding disorders, vascular anomalies, and hypertension. Patients with these conditions may have apparently spontaneous bleeding, or may have epistaxis triggered by minor external trauma or by forceful sneezing and blowing. Profuse bleeding which is difficult to stop is most characteristic of acute thrombocytopenia, vascular anomalies, and hypertension. Mild bleeding which is readily controlled by application of pressure is more suggestive of mucosal infection or irritation. In all cases the problem should be taken seriously and investigated carefully in order to correctly diagnose and appropriately treat the primary source of the problem. A key point to remember is that while many children pick their noses and many have nosebleeds, the two are rarely if ever related.

In approaching patients with epistaxis, the following historical points should be addressed:
1. Is the problem acute or recurrent?
2. Was external trauma, sneezing, or blowing a triggering event?
3. What is the duration of the current bleed and approximate volume of blood loss (handkerchiefs soaked, hemodynamic status, etc.)?
4. Is the bleeding unilateral or bilateral?
5. Has the patient been having symptoms suggestive of an upper respiratory infection or nasal allergy?
6. Has the child manifested other signs and symptoms of an underlying coagulopathy or of hypertension?
7. Has the patient been taking medication, especially aspirin?

Physical assessment must address the patient's general well-being in addition to careful examination of the nasopharynx. Hemodynamic status is of particular import when hemorrhage has been profuse.

After observation of the external appearance of the nares, the nose should be cleared of clots and discharge, if present. Then the septum and mucosa are inspected for possible points of hemorrhage, signs of obstruction, mass lesions, and foreign objects. The oropharynx should also be examined for posterior flow of blood, especially in cases in which no point of bleeding is evident on inspection of the nasal mucosa. Otolaryngologic consultation should be sought in cases involving profuse bleeding which does not readily cease upon application of pressure and which may require nasal packing or other surgical treatment.

INFECTION AND MUCOSAL IRRITATION

In a large number of patients with nontraumatic epistaxis, examination reveals unilateral or bilateral septal erythema and friability or excoriation (Fig. 20.46). The history given is one of intermittent bleeding, especially with sneezing or blowing the nose, or during sleep (the child's pillow is found spotted with blood). The phenomenon is commonly attributed to picking the nose in response to itching, whether due to mucosal drying or allergic rhinitis. In view of the sensitivity of the mucosa to painful stimuli, picking to the point of excoriation is rather unlikely. In many instances these lesions either are impetiginous or represent the product of the combined effects of inflammation (due to nasopharyngitis, sinusitis, or allergic rhinitis) and trauma due to forceful sneezing and blowing. Therefore, careful assessment for signs of upper respiratory infection, pharyngitis, sinusitis, and allergic rhinitis is indicated. When infection is suspected, culturing of the friable area for a predominant bacterial pathogen (especially group A beta-streptococcus or coagulase-positive staphylococcus) may prove rewarding. In patients with no history of or findings consistent with upper respiratory infection, mucosal drying may be responsible. This is seen most commonly in winter as a result of drying of the air by central heating systems. While application of topical antibiotic ointment, humidification, and antihistamines (for atopic patients) may provide some relief, oral antimicrobial therapy for bacterial pathogens, when found, is more likely to be successful.

Patients with nasal polyps who have an intercurrent infection, and children with nasal foreign bodies with secondary infection and inflammation are also highly prone to intermittent epistaxis and/or blood tinging of their nasal discharge.

BLEEDING DISORDERS

Despite application of pressure, epistaxis in patients with coagulopathies is more likely to be prolonged and carries a greater risk of significant blood loss. While many such patients have known bleeding disorders, a few may present with prolonged or recurrent nosebleeds as one of the initial manifestations of their problem. This is most typical of idiopathic thrombocytopenia, aplastic anemia, and acute leukemia. When a patient is having epistaxis due to a bleeding disorder, the personal history, family history, and/or other physical findings should point to the diagnosis (see Chapter 11), which can then be confirmed by hematologic studies (CBC and differential, platelet count, PT and PTT, and coagulation profile).

Acute management is dependent in part on the source of the coagulopathy (e.g., factor replacement or platelet transfusion), and in part on severity of bleeding. Topical application of a vasoconstrictor such as epinephrine and insertion of absorbable synthetic material that aids coagulation (Gelfoam or Surgicel) can be very helpful in patients with thrombocytopenia and an anterior point of bleeding. The risks of secondary infection with packing must be given careful consideration when treating patients undergoing immunosuppressive therapy.

VASCULAR ABNORMALITIES

In a minority of children with recurrent epistaxis, the history reveals significant bleeding which typically drains from one side of the nose. This suggests a localized vascular abnormality. The most commonly encountered problem is that of a *di-*

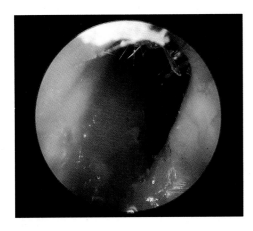

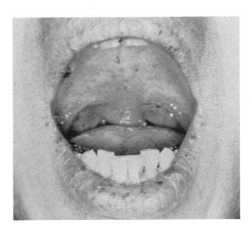

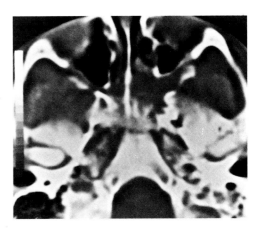

FIG. 20.46 Excoriated nasal septum. This child presented with URI and a history of intermittent epistaxis with nasal blowing and during the night. He had a purulent nasal discharge (on the lower right) and a diffusely excoriated erythematous septum. Cultures of his nose and throat grew group A beta-streptococci.

FIG. 20.47 Hereditary hemorrhagic telangiectasia. Numerous telangiectasias dot the lips and palatal mucosa of this boy who had problems with recurrent epistaxis. (Courtesy of Dr. Bernard Cohen, Children's Hospital of Pittsburgh)

FIG. 20.48 Juvenile nasopharyngeal angiofibroma. CT scan is helpful in assessing the extent of this locally invasive vascular tumor. In this cut, an enhanced mass is seen occupying the posterior portion of the nostril, deviating the septum and compressing the ipsilateral maxillary sinus.

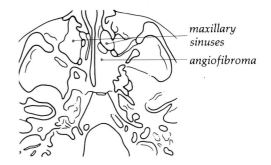

lated septal vessel or plexus, which may be a sequela of prior inflammation. This may be visible anteriorly, but can also be located high on the septum requiring nasopharyngoscopy for identification. Cauterization is generally curative. In children over 7 years of age, anterior septal lesions can be cauterized in the office with silver nitrate after application of a topical anesthetic. Younger children and many patients with posterior lesions may need general anesthesia for cauterization.

Two relatively rare vascular anomalies may also be the source of recurrent nasal bleeding: telangiectasias and angiofibromas. Patients with *hereditary hemorrhagic telangiectasias* (Osler-Weber-Rendu disease) have an autosomal-dominant disorder characterized by formation of cutaneous and mucosal telangiectatic lesions which begin to develop in childhood and gradually increase in number with age. These lesions appear as bright red, slightly raised, star-shaped plexuses of dilated small vessels which blanch on pressure (Fig. 20.47). Mucosal telangiectasias may bleed spontaneously or in response to minor trauma. Recurrent epistaxis is a common mode of presentation in childhood. Multiple telangiectasias are evident on close examination. Hematuria and/or gastrointestinal bleeding may be seen separately or in combination with epistaxis.

A *juvenile nasopharyngeal angiofibroma* is a rare vascular tumor seen predominantly in adolescent males. While benign, it is locally invasive and destructive and may involve the maxillary sinuses, palate, sphenoid sinus, and anterior portions of the skull. Its most common mode of presentation is profuse, often recurrent epistaxis. Some patients also have symptoms of nasal obstruction with secondary rhinorrhea, and a small percentage may have visual or auditory disturbances. On examination, a purplish soft-tissue mass may be seen through the nares or on nasopharyngoscopy. General radiographs, computerized tomography, and angiography may be needed to assess the extent of the tumor (Fig. 20.48). Carefully planned excision is then the treatment of choice.

HYPERTENSION

In contrast to the adult population, hypertension is an unusual source of epistaxis in childhood. However, it should be considered, especially in patients with antecedent headache and spontaneous profuse bleeding which is difficult to stop. It must be remembered that following significant blood loss, blood pressure may drop to normal limits. Patients with such a history may have previously undiagnosed coarctation of the aorta or undiagnosed chronic renal disease and should be examined with these possibilities in mind.

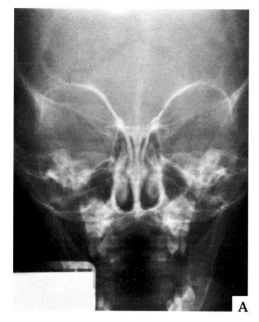 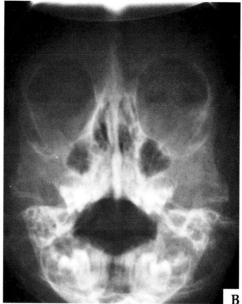 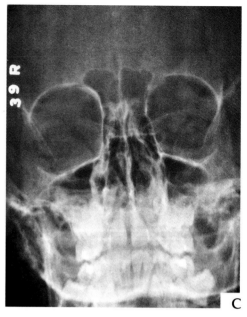

FIG. 20.49 Normal radiography of the sinuses. Radiography is currently the most helpful noninvasive tool for evaluating the paranasal sinuses. Interpretation requires appreciation of the normal pattern of development and the findings seen in health and with disease. **A** AP or Caldwell view shows clear ethmoid sinuses in an 18-month-old child. The bony margins are sharp and the sinus cavities are dark. **B** Waters view of the same child shows normal maxillary sinuses with sharply defined bony margins. The cavities appear black. **C** After age 6 or 7, the Caldwell view is taken PA. In this 8-year-old, the bony margins of both the ethmoid and frontal sinuses are sharply defined. Because the calvarium is superimposed, it can be difficult to dis-

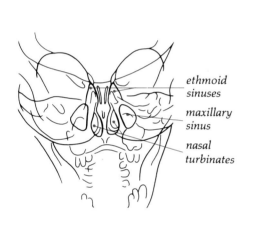 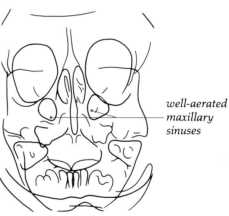 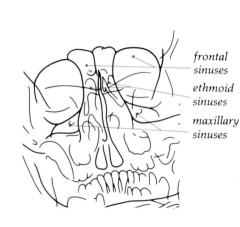

DISORDERS OF THE PARANASAL SINUSES

The paranasal sinuses are small cavities within the maxilla and bones of the skull which develop by gradual spread of pneumatized cells that evaginate from the nasal cavity. This process occurs over the course of childhood and adolescence; there is a wide range of normal in the duration of this process and in the ultimate size of the sinuses and their ostia. In infancy, the ethmoid and maxillary sinuses are partially pneumatized, but are small and not readily demonstrable on X-rays. Therefore, radiographs are of little diagnostic use until after the first year of life. The sphenoid sinus is not radiographically evident until about 5 to 6 years, and the frontal sinuses are not well developed until after 7 to 8 years of age (Fig. 20.49).

The sinuses are lined by ciliated, pseudostratified columnar epithelium which both produces and transports mucus secretions. The sphenoid and posterior ethmoids drain via the superior meatus below the superior nasal turbinate, and the maxillary, anterior ethmoid, and frontal sinuses drain into the middle meatus below the middle turbinate. Several points of clinical importance warrant emphasis. The ostia of the ethmoid sinuses are small and thus easily obstructed by mucosal edema. The ostia of the maxillary sinuses are located high on the medial wall of each sinus, placing greater demand on ciliary action for drainage. There is significant variation in the configuration of the frontal sinus ostia, ranging from wide and short to long, narrow, and tubular. Patients with the latter configuration are more vulnerable to obstruction. Finally, the roots of the maxillary teeth lie in the floor of the maxillary sinuses. Therefore, dental infections may drain into the maxillary sinus, resulting in recurrent or chronic sinusitis. The dentition should be thoroughly inspected in evaluating any child with suspected sinus infection (see Chapter 18).

Sinusitis

During the first several years of life, infection of the maxillary and/or ethmoid sinuses is more common than is general-

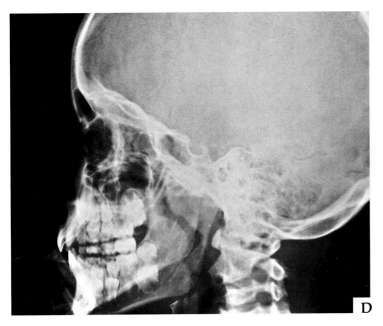

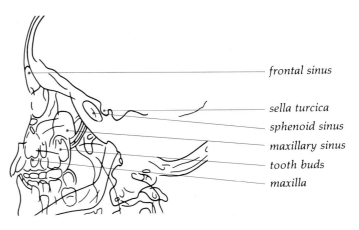

frontal sinus

sella turcica

sphenoid sinus

maxillary sinus

tooth buds

maxilla

*tinguish frontal sinus clouding on this view alone, particularly with bilateral disease. Therefore, evaluation of the frontal sinuses requires close scrutiny of both Caldwell and lateral views. **D** Lateral view of an 8-year-old child shows pneumatization of the frontal and sphenoid sinuses. Bony margins are sharply defined. The frontal sinuses appear black,*

but the sphenoid is somewhat gray because there are more overlying structures. Note how the roots of the maxillary teeth are imbedded in the floor of the maxillary sinus.

ly appreciated. Frontal sinusitis assumes importance after about 10 years of age. The probable pathogenesis is mucosal swelling and vascular congestion, whether incited by upper respiratory infection or allergic rhinitis. This results in obstruction of the sinus ostia impeding drainage of secretions, and if prolonged, sets the stage for proliferation of bacterial pathogens with resultant infection. Interference with ciliary function and increased mucus production, possibly with attendant mucus plugging, may also play a role, as do host variations in anatomy. Both bacterial and viral pathogens have been isolated from pediatric patients. The most commonly identified bacteria are *Streptococcus pneumoniae,* nontypable *Hemophilus influenzae,* and *Branhamella catarrhalis.* The viral agents include adenoviruses and parainfluenza viruses. As in adults, there is no good correlation between results of nasopharyngeal and sinus aspirate cultures.

As is true of otitis media, a number of conditions have been identified as predisposing children to sinus infections by virtue of alterations in anatomy, physiology, or both. These include midfacial anomalies or deformities, particularly when maxillary hypoplasia is part of the picture; cleft palate; nasal deformity and/or septal deviation, whether congenital or acquired; mass lesions including hypertrophied adenoids, nasal foreign bodies, polyps, or tumors; abnormalities of mucus production and/or ciliary action such as cystic fibrosis

and the immotile cilia syndrome; immunodeficiency; atopy; dental infection; and barotrauma.

In young children, sinusitis is primarily a disorder of the ethmoid and maxillary sinuses, and the clinical picture differs considerably from that of adolescents and adults. Two major modes of presentation have been described. The most common picture is one of a prolonged upper respiratory infection which has shown no sign of amelioration after 7 to 10 days. Cough and/or persistent nasal discharge (which may be of any character—thin, thick; clear, cloudy; white, yellow, or green) are the major complaints. The cough is usually loose or wet; it is prominent during the day, but may be worse on waking in the morning and/or on first going to bed at night. Patients tend to clear their throats and sniff or snort frequently. Halitosis or "fetor oris" is commonly noted by parents. In a minority of children, periorbital swelling, most noticeable on awaking, may be reported. A small percentage of patients have low-grade fever, and a few may complain of headache, facial discomfort, or sore throat.

Often physical examination is of little help in distinguishing sinusitis from rhinitis alone. Findings may include purulent nasal and postnasal discharge with erythema of the nasal mucosa and pharynx; but, as noted above, this is not uniformly seen. Halitosis may be pronounced and is strongly suggestive of sinusitis in the absence of evidence of dental

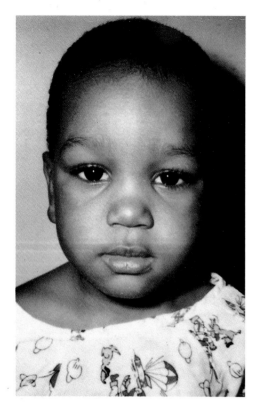

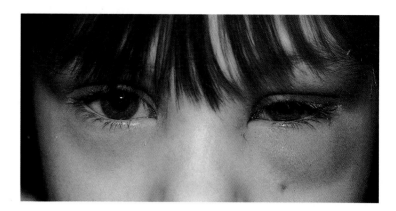

FIG. 20.50 Sympathetic periorbital swelling with sinusitis. This 2-year-old boy was seen late in the afternoon with high fever, wet cough, decreased activity, and mild infraorbital puffiness. The latter was not red, nonindurated, and nontender, and reportedly had been more marked upon awakening in the morning. He also had a scant cloudy nasal discharge. His chest X-ray was normal, but sinus films showed opacification of the maxillary sinuses.

FIG. 20.51 This child with sinusitis presented with prominent erythematous periorbital edema and signs of purulent conjunctivitis. The redness raised concerns of periorbital cellulitis, but the area was nontender and not indurated. Presence of periorbital swelling is a helpful clue in diagnosing sinusitis in children with other suggestive signs and symptoms. (Courtesy of Dr. Ellen Wald, Children's Hospital of Pittsburgh)

infection, severe pharyngitis, or nasal foreign body. Sinusitis is also probable when features of the above picture are accompanied by signs of a maxillary dental abscess (see Chapter 18). Nontender, nonindurated periorbital edema (Fig. 20.50) and/or tenderness to percussion over the sinuses are very suggestive of—but are not seen in the majority of patients with—the "prolonged URI" picture. One very strong clue is the observation of drainage of purulent material from the middle meatus following topical application of a vasoconstrictor to the nasal mucosa. It is important to recognize that the clinical spectrum is wide, that any combination of the above symptoms and signs may be seen, and that sinusitis should be suspected even if the course is relatively brief in duration, when clinical findings are strongly suggestive.

A less frequent mode of presentation in young children is one of an acute upper respiratory infection that is unusually severe, characterized by high fever and copious purulent nasal discharge. Facial discomfort and periorbital swelling (nontender, nonindurated, and most marked on awaking) are not uncommon with this picture. The edematous area may be normal in color or mildly erythematous. (If erythema is intense or the area is indurated or tender, periorbital cellulitis should be suspected.) This phenomenon is thought to be the result of impairment of venous blood flow caused by increased pressure within the infected sinuses. Some of these patients will also have conjunctival erythema and discharge (Fig. 20.51). Occasionally, a child with sinusitis will present with the typical findings of sympathetic edema but without high fever or the prolonged URI picture.

Older children and adolescents with acute maxillary and/or ethmoid sinusitis may present with either of the above symptom pictures, but are more likely to complain specifically of headache and/or facial pain. The headache may be perceived as frontal, temporal, or even retroauricular. Facial discomfort can be described as malar pain, or a sense of pressure or fullness. Occasionally, patients may complain that their teeth hurt (in the absence of dental pathology). When the frontal sinuses are involved, frontal or supraorbital headache is prominent, often perceived as dull or pulsating. The sphenoid sinus is rarely a site of isolated sinus infection, but is often involved in pansinusitis, in which case occipital and postauricular pain may be reported in addition to other sites of discomfort. Not infrequently the headache is intermittent; or when constant, varies in severity. This variability appears related to degree of drainage. Patients reporting copious "postnasal drip" tend to have less pain. Others may have periods of headache alternating with relief which is associated with an increase in volume of nasal and postnasal discharge. Discomfort and congestion are often most marked on waking, probably as a result of recumbency and failure during sleep to actively promote flow of drainage by snorting (creating a vacuum) and blowing. As as result, secretions collect, pressure increases, and mucus plugging of the ostia may occur. Some patients also report aggravation of pain with head movement, particularly with bending down and then straightening up. Swallowed discharge often produces significant abdominal discomfort as well. Cough is often a feature but tends to be less prominent than in younger children. Physical findings may include purulent (often blood-streaked) nasal and postnasal discharge with erythema of the nasal mucosa and halitosis. Tenderness on sinus percussion is more common, and transillumination is more likely to be absent or impaired. As with younger children the clinical spectrum is wide and highly variable.

The usefulness of diagnostic methods in evaluating suspected sinusitis is still under study. Radiography does appear to be the most helpful noninvasive tool in children over 1 year of age. (In infancy, if sinusitis occurs at all, the diagnosis must be made on grounds of prolonged nasal discharge and possibly results of nasopharyngeal cultures.) Findings of complete opacification, mucosal thickening greater than 4 mm, or an air-fluid level (Fig. 20.52) have a strong association with positive findings on sinus aspiration. However, the wide range of variability in development and configuration of the sinuses can make interpretation difficult. Ultrasono-

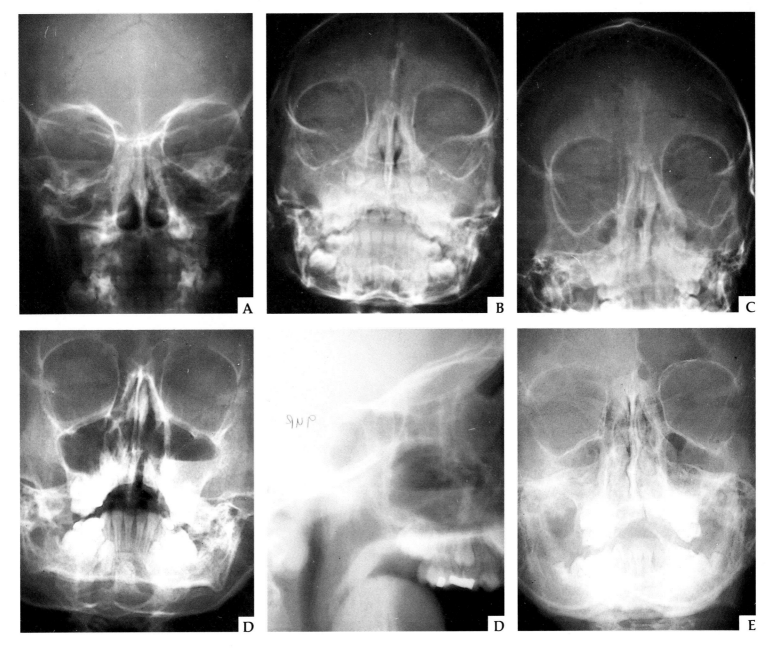

FIG. 20.52 Radiographic findings of sinusitis. **A** In this Caldwell view, the right ethmoid is clouded, and the bony margins are less distinct than on the left. **B** In this Waters view, complete opacification of both maxillary sinuses is evident. The bony margins are visible but faint. **C** This child has significant mucosal thickening of the maxillary sinuses. Thickening of greater than 4 mm has a strong association with positive culture on sinus aspirate. **D** An air-fluid level can be seen in the left maxillary sinus on both Waters (left) and lateral (right) views. **E** Differential opacification of the right frontal sinus is evident in this child who presented with fever and headache. (**D** courtesy of Dr. J. Ledesma-Medina, Children's Hospital of Pittsburgh; **E** courtesy of Dr. C. D. Bluestone, Children's Hospital of Pittsburgh)

graphic examinations have been useful, but as yet the procedure continues to have a significant rate of false-negative and indeterminate readings. Transillumination has not been adequately studied in children, but is of value in adolescents and adults. Needle aspiration of the sinuses is conclusive but invasive, and not without risk. It is, however, justified in patients with very severe symptoms, patients with CNS or orbital extension, those not responding to treatment, and children who are immunocompromised or immunosuppressed.

Therapy consists of *at least* a 10- to 14-day course of an antimicrobial agent suitable to the likely spectrum of orga-nisms, analgesia as needed for discomfort, and perhaps an oral antihistamine in patients known to have allergic rhinitis.

COMPLICATIONS OF SINUSITIS
Infectious sinusitis is important not only because of the discomfort it causes, but also because there is a significant risk of extension of infection and secondary complications. This risk stems from several anatomic factors. First, the sinuses surround the orbits superiorly, medially, and inferiorly. The bony plates that make up their walls are very thin and porous, and their suture lines are open in childhood. This is especially true of the lamina papyracea which separate the

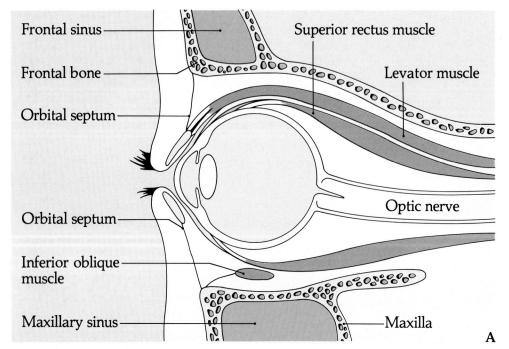

Frontal sinus

Frontal bone

Orbital septum

Orbital septum

Inferior oblique
muscle

Maxillary sinus

Superior rectus muscle

Levator muscle

Optic nerve

Maxilla

A

FIG. 20.53 The anatomy of the orbit. **A** *Sagittal section shows the relationship of the orbit to the maxillary and frontal sinuses, and the position of the orbital septum within the eyelid. The latter structure appears to serve as an anatomic barrier, helping to prevent the spread of infection from periorbital tissues into the orbit.* **B** *In this horizontal section, the close relationship of the orbit to the ethmoid sinuses is apparent.*

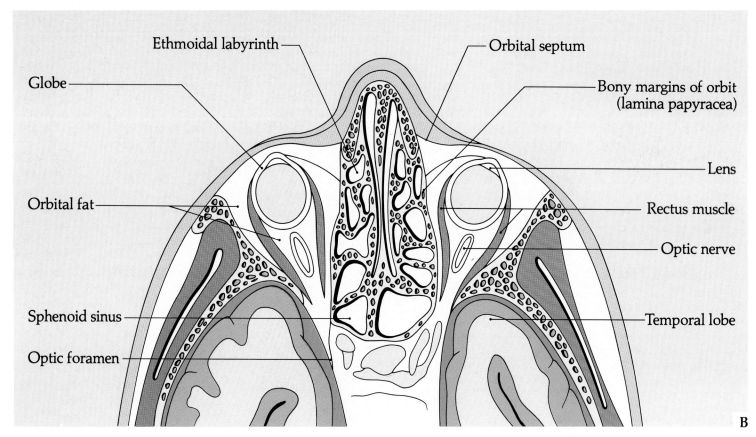

Ethmoidal labyrinth

Orbital septum

Globe

Bony margins of orbit
(lamina papyracea)

Lens

Orbital fat

Rectus muscle

Optic nerve

Sphenoid sinus

Temporal lobe

Optic foramen

B

ethmoid air cells from the orbits (Fig. 20.53). Increase in sinus pressure as a result of ostial blockage and fluid collection can cause separation of portions of these bony septa and can compromise their blood supply with resultant necrosis, thus promoting extension of infection. Facial vascular anatomy also contributes to the spread of infection. The veins of the face, nose, and sinuses drain in part into the orbit, then into the ophthalmic venous system which is in direct continuity with the cavernous sinus. The ophthalmic veins are valveless and thus may present less of a defense against spread of infec-

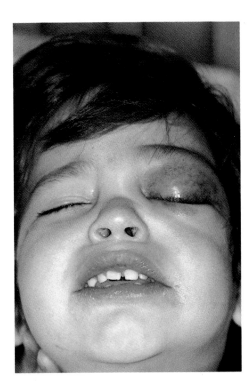

FIG. 20.54 Periorbital cellulitis. Intense erythema and edema of the lids are evident. The swollen tissues were indurated and very tender on palpation. Ocular motion was normal. (Courtesy of Dr. Ellen Wald, Children's Hospital of Pittsburgh)

tion. The orbit is also devoid of lymphatics, a fact that helps explain the ease of periorbital edema collection when there is increased sinus pressure. The relative looseness of the subcutaneous tissues of the face augments this and may also aid in spread of infection. As a result of these factors, direct extension of infection through bony walls into the orbits—outward through the frontal bone or inward into the cranium—and hematogenous spread of infection are the major complications seen. Fortunately, improved recognition of sinus infection and early use of antimicrobial therapy, whether before or early in the course of recognized extension, have reduced the frequency and severity of these disorders.

Periorbital Cellulitis

This condition is the mildest of the complications of infectious sinusitis. The cellulitis is confined to tissues outside the orbit, with spread blocked in part by the orbital septum (see Fig. 20.53A). When sinusitis is the underlying condition, the ethmoids and/or maxillary sinuses are the structures primarily affected. Patients typically are under 4 or 5 years of age and have an antecedent history of upper respiratory infection (with or without conjunctivitis), otitis, or one consistent with sinusitis. Occasionally, a dental abscess with secondary maxillary sinusitis is the predisposing problem (see Chapter 18). This is superseded by the sudden appearance of lid and periorbital swelling. In contrast to the uncomplicated sympathetic edema seen in some patients with sinusitis, the swelling in these children is usually unilateral, definitely erythematous, and is indurated and tender (Fig. 20.54). Conjunctival injection and discharge may also be seen. In many patients a secondary increase in temperature accompanies the onset of swelling, but while most appear uncomfortable, toxicity is unusual.

The course of periorbital cellulitis resulting from extension of sinus infection is milder and is characterized by much slower progression than is true of cases believed due to hematogenous spread. In the latter there is sudden onset of high fever (often following a mild URI) accompanied by the appearance of erythematous, indurated, and tender periorbital swelling which progresses with striking rapidity and is accompanied by signs of systemic toxicity. The majority of these patients are under a year of age or only slightly older, and bacteremia with *H. Influenzae* type B or *S. pneumoniae* is usual.

About 50 percent of periorbital cellulitis cases have neither sinusitis nor bacteremia as a predisposing condition. Rather, these patients appear to suffer from extension of facial infection to periorbital tissues. They tend to have a history either of antecedent trauma to the orbit or nearby facial structures (often with a break in the skin), or a history of nearby skin infection (impetigo, a pustule, a chalazion, or an infected dermatitis or insect bite). They subsequently experience a temperature spike and evolution of periorbital and eyelid edema, but this is often less abrupt than in patients with underlying sinusitis. This group is somewhat older, generally over 5 years of age. *S. aureus* and group A beta-hemolytic streptococci are the predominant offending organisms.

A number of cultures are often done in an attempt to isolate the causative pathogen. Needle aspiration of the leading edge of the cellulitis has perhaps the highest yield, but requires caution and is perhaps best avoided when the inflamed area does not extend beyond the orbital rim. Culture of adjacent skin wounds, when present, also is commonly positive. Nasopharyngeal and conjunctival drainage reveals the offending organism in about one-half to two-thirds of cases, respectively. Blood cultures are positive in about one-third of patients overall, with the highest incidence found in cases due to hematogenous spread. Sinus X-rays show opacification in over two-thirds of patients without antecedent trauma or skin lesions, and in about 40 to 50 percent of patients with such a history. Ethmoid opacification is the predominant finding. Radiographic interpretation can be difficult, however, as overlying edema may give a false impression of clouding. In addition, X-rays are relatively useless in most cases of hematogenous origin as the patients are typically under 1 year of age.

Because of the severity and potential for further extension and hematogenous spread, aggressive intravenous antimicrobial therapy is urgently required. This necessitates empiric selection of agents to cover likely pathogens, pending culture results. Patients also require close monitoring for signs of complications.

Orbital Cellulitis

In this condition, infection has extended into the orbit itself, and may take the form of undifferentiated cellulitis or can evolve to result in a subperiosteal or orbital abscess. Patients tend to have a history similar to those with periorbital cellulitis, but are generally more ill, toxic and lethargic. As with periorbital cellulitis, extension may be from an infected sinus or a nearby facial infection, although sinusitis probably accounts for a larger percentage. Causative organisms are the same. Patients old enough to be articulate describe intense deep retroorbital pain aggravated by ocular movement. Edema and erythema of the lid and periorbital tissues are so marked that it is often impossible to open the eye with-

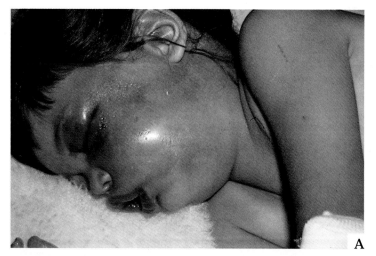

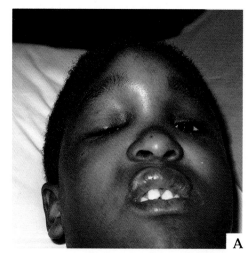

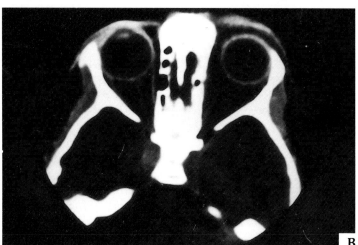

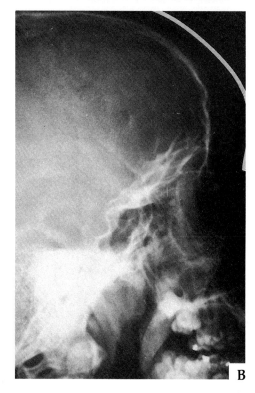

FIG. 20.55 Orbital cellulitis. **A** This preschool child presented with fever, severe toxicity, and marked lethargy. The entire left side of his face was erythematous, indurated, and exquisitely tender. Retraction of his lids revealed mild proptosis, conjunctival inflammation with chemosis and purulent discharge, and decreased range of motion of the globe. **B** CT scan demonstrates preseptal swelling, mild proptosis, and lateral displacement of the globe. There is no evidence of periosteal abscess formation. (**A** courtesy of Dr. Michael Sherlock; **B** courtesy of Dr. Joseph Horton, Dept. of Neuroradiology, University of Pittsburgh)

FIG. 20.56 Pott's puffy tumor. **A** This patient presented with fever, headache, and an erythematous swelling over the forehead which had a doughy consistency and was exquisitely tender. **B** A lateral radiograph shows frontal sinus clouding, irregularity of the frontal bone, and marked soft-tissue swelling which is highlighted by a wire placed over the forehead and scalp. (Courtesy of Dr. Kenneth Grandfast, National Children's Medical Center)

out use of lid retractors (Fig. 20.55A). Tenderness is exquisite. If the lid can be retracted, proptosis, conjunctival inflammation with chemosis and purulent discharge, decreased extraocular motion, and loss of visual acuity may be found.

Aggressive intravenous antimicrobial therapy and close monitoring for evolution and central nervous system complications are vital in management of orbital cellulitis. Computerized tomography is proving exceptionally useful for determining extent and location of orbital involvement, and for following the evolution of the process (Fig. 20.55B). Findings are also highly useful in planning surgical intervention when needed for drainage. Optimal management necessitates a team approach involving pediatrics, otolaryngology, ophthalmology, and at times neurosurgery.

Local complications of orbital cellulitis include abscess formation, optic neuritis, retinal vein thrombosis, and panophthalmitis. Central nervous system complications may result from direct extension or spread of septic thrombophlebitis. Meningitis, epidural and subdural abscesses, and cavernous sinus thrombosis have been described. All are characterized by marked toxicity and alteration in level of consciousness. Meningeal signs are seen with meningitis, but may be absent with abscesses. The latter may or may not produce focal neurologic signs. Cavernous sinus thrombosis is heralded by sudden, bilateral, pulsating proptosis in association with increased toxicity and obtundation.

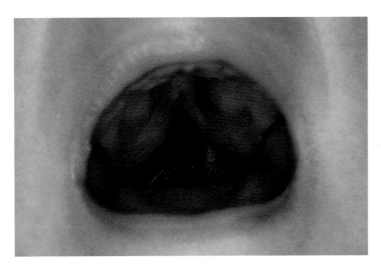

FIG. 20.57 *Cleft palate. This child has a midline cleft of the soft palate. The hard palate, alveolar ridge, and lip are spared. (Courtesy of Barbara Elster, RN, PNP, Cleft Palate Center, Pittsburgh)*

Pott's Puffy Tumor

Frontal sinusitis, which assumes importance after 8 to 10 years of age, is potentially dangerous as well, particularly when neglected or inadequately treated. Bony erosion is the major mechanism of extension. Posterior erosion can result in formation of an epidural or brain abscess. Less frequently, erosion occurs anteriorly resulting in formation of a subperiosteal abscess of the frontal bone, *Pott's puffy tumor.* This is seen as an erythematous frontal swelling which has a doughy feeling and is exquisitely tender (Fig. 20.56). Affected patients are toxic, febrile, and acutely uncomfortable. A CT scan should be obtained to evaluate the extent of the abscess and identify other sites of spread prior to surgical drainage.

Atopic Sinus Disorders

ALLERGIC SINUSITIS WITH POSTNASAL DISCHARGE

Patients with allergic rhinitis appear to be more susceptible to infectious sinusitis than nonatopic individuals, probably as a result of mucosal swelling in response to exposure to allergens, and perhaps as a result of alterations in ciliary action. They can also present with symptoms mimicking sinusitis in the absence of infection, and this can be a source of confusion. Two major clinical pictures are seen. In the first, nasal congestion, nighttime cough, and morning throat clearing are prominent. Some may complain of morning nausea, and a few may have morning emesis containing large amounts of clear mucus. Fever is absent, and in contrast to infectious sinusitis, nasal discharge is never purulent, there is no halitosis, and daytime cough is not prominent. Patients may complain of itching of the nose and eyes, and some have frequent sneezing. On examination, the nasal mucosa is edematous but does not appear inflamed. Discharge, if present, is clear. Patients also tend to have the typical allergic facies (see Chapter 4) with Dennies lines, allergic shiners, and cobblestoning of the conjunctivae. Environmental control and antihistamines provide symptomatic relief for most of these children.

VACUUM HEADACHE

The second potentially confusing clinical picture is that of the allergic sinus headache or vacuum headache. In this condition, older atopic individuals complain of intense facial or frontal headache, without fever or other evidence of infection. This is seen during periods in which they are having exacerbation of allergic symptoms or following swimming in chlorinated pools. The phenomenon appears to be due to acute blockage of sinus ostia by mucosal edema, with subsequent creation of a vacuum within the sinus as a result of consumption of oxygen by mucosal cells. The resultant negative pressure pulls the mucosa away from the walls of the sinus, producing the pain. In these patients the nasal mucosa will tend to be pale and swollen, but without discharge. Sinuses may be tender to percussion, but will be clear radiographically. Symptoms respond promptly to application of a topical vasoconstrictor and warm compresses over the face. Improvement is maintained by antihistamines.

OROPHARYNGEAL DISORDERS

Adequate examination of the pharynx is highly important in pediatrics because of the frequency of pharyngeal infections. The procedure can be challenging at times, however. The small size of the mouth and difficulty of depressing the tongue in infancy, lack of cooperativeness in toddlers, and fear of gagging with use of the tongue blade in older children can impede efforts. These problems can be minimized by a few simple techniques. Infants and young children, when placed supine with the head hyperextended on the neck, tend to open their mouths spontaneously, enabling visualization of the anterior oral cavity and facilitating insertion of a tongue blade to depress the tongue and inspect the posterior palate and pharynx. When examining older children, asking them to open their mouths as wide as possible and pant "like a puppy dog" or say "ha ha" usually results in lowering of the posterior portion of the tongue, revealing posterior palatal and pharyngeal structures. Having presented conditions involving the lips, mucosa, and dentition in Chapter 18, this section will concentrate on palatal and pharyngeal problems.

Palatal Disorders

Palatal malformations range widely in severity and can have significant impact on feeding, swallowing, and speech. In addition, by altering normal nasal and oropharyngeal physiology, they place affected patients at increased risk for chronic recurrent ear and sinus infections.

CLEFT PALATE

Palatal clefts are among the most severe abnormalities encountered. They stem from a failure of fusion during the second month of gestation and have an incidence of about 1 in every 2000 to 2500 births. They are usually but not always associated with a cleft lip. The defect is often isolated in an otherwise normal child. In many cases there is a positive family history for the anomaly. A number of teratogens have also been linked to the malformation. In a small percentage of cases the cleft palate is one of multiple congenital anomalies in the context of a major genetic syndrome.

The extent of the cleft varies: some involve only the soft palate (Fig. 20.57), others extend through the hard palate but spare the alveolar ridge and still others are complete (Fig.

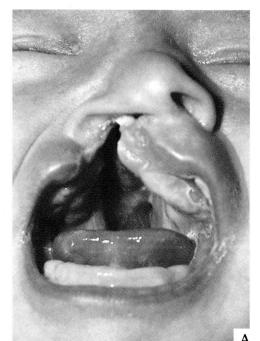 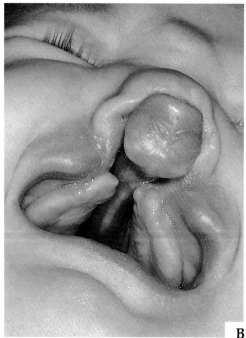

FIG. 20.58 Cleft palate. Complete clefts of the palate, alveolar ridge, and lip may be unilateral (A) or bilateral (B). (A courtesy of Dr. Michael Sherlock; B courtesy of Dr. William Garrett)

20.58). The defect may be unilateral or bilateral. The four major types of congenital cleft palate are:

Type I: Soft palate only

Type II: Unilateral cleft of soft and hard palate

Type III: Unilateral cleft of soft and hard palate extending through the alveolar ridge

Type IV: Bilateral cleft of soft and hard palate extending through the alveolar ridge

This anomaly creates a number of problems beyond the obvious cosmetic deformity. In infancy it prevents the child from creating an effective seal when nursing and hampers feeding. In addition, formula tends to reflux into the nasopharynx with resultant choking. This necessitates patience in feeding and careful training of parents in feeding techniques to facilitate nursing and prevent failure to thrive. Eustachian tube function is uniformly abnormal, and prior to repair, all patients have chronic middle ear effusions which are frequently infected. Even following repair, recurrent middle ear disease (characterized by negative pressure and effusions) remains a problem. Hearing loss, with its potential for hampering language acquisition, ultimately occurs in over 50 percent of patients. Despite corrective surgery, palatal function is never totally normal, and many patients continue to have hypernasal speech and difficulties in articulation, necesssitating long-term speech therapy. Secondary dental and orthodontic problems are routine as well.

The multitude of problems and the need for frequent medical visits and multiple operations, in combination with the oft-associated cosmetic deformity, can have significant psychological impact on both child and family. Optimal management necessitates a multidisciplinary team, preferably coordinated by a primary care physician who is aware of the patient's individual needs and those of his or her family. Timing of corrective surgery remains somewhat controversial. Cleft lips are repaired at about 3 months, but scheduling of palatal repair must be individualized depending on the size and extent of the cleft. Defects of the soft palate are generally repaired at about 8 months, and the hard palate is either closed surgically or by use of a prosthetic plate. Most patients also require early myringotomy with insertion of tubes to help in managing the chronic middle ear disease. Tonsillectomy and adenoidectomy are contraindicated because of adverse effects on palatal function.

Another disorder of clinical importance, *submucous cleft of the palate,* is often missed in infancy. The condition is characterized by a U-shaped notch, palpable in the midline, at the juncture of the hard and soft portions of the palate (Fig. 20.59A). There may also be palpable midline thinning of the soft palate. The anomaly results from a failure of the tensor veli palatini muscle to insert properly in the midline. Some children have an associated double or notched uvula which, when present, serves as a clue to the existence of the palatal abnormality (Fig. 20.59B). The latter may be an isolated anomaly, however. While not subject to the feeding difficulties seen in children with overt clefts, children with submucous clefts do have similar problems with eustachian tube dysfunction and recurrent middle ear disease. Speech is often mildly hypernasal. Recognition is particularly important when considering tonsillectomy and adenoidectomy for recurrent tonsillitis and otitis, as surgical removal of the adenoids in these children can result in severe speech and swallowing dysfunction, and thus may be contraindicated.

HIGH-ARCHED PALATE

This minor anomaly is a common clinical finding (Fig. 20.60). While usually an isolated variant of palatal configuration, it is occasionally seen in association with congenital syndromes. Long-term orotracheal intubation of premature infants is now creating an iatrogenic form of the problem. While generally insignificant clinically, the high arch can be associated with increased frequency of ear and sinus infections, and with hyponasal speech when it is severe.

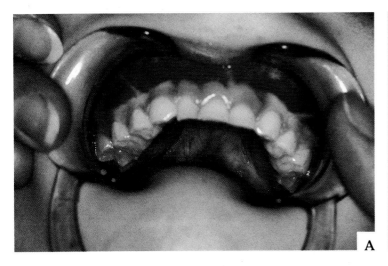

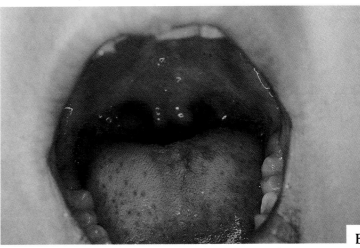

FIG. 20.59 Submucous cleft of the palate. **A** This boy shows failure of normal midline fusion of the palatal muscles, resulting in midline thinning of the soft palate. Palpation confirms the area of weakness. A U-shaped notch can also be felt in the midline at the junction of the hard and soft palate. **B** This child was found to have a notched or bifid uvula on pharyngeal examination. This may serve as a clue to the presence of a submucous palatal cleft, or it may be an isolated anomaly.

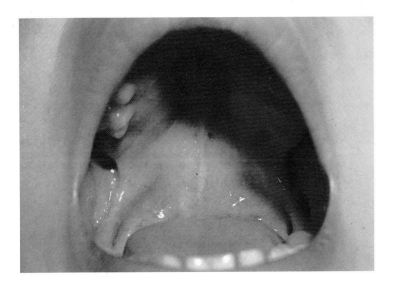

FIG. 20.60 High-arched palate. This is a common minor anomaly, usually isolated, but occasionally associated with genetic syndromes.

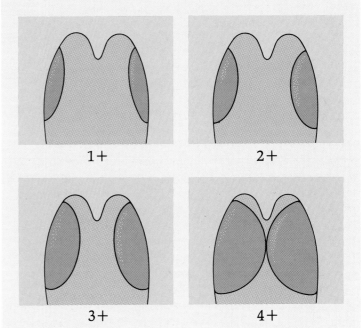

FIG. 20.61 Grading of tonsillar size, for use in children with acute tonsillopharyngitis and those with chronic tonsillar enlargement. This grading system is particularly useful in the serial examinations of the patient. (Adapted from Feinstein and Levitt: Role of tonsils. New Engl J Med 282:285, 1970)

Tonsillar Disorders

TONSILLOPHARYNGITIS

As noted earlier in the section, Acquired Forms of Nasal Obstruction, the tonsils and adenoids are quite small in infancy, gradually enlarge over the first 8 to 10 years of life, then start to regress in size. In evaluating the tonsils, particularly during the course of an acute infection but also when following patients for chronic enlargement, it is helpful to use a standardized grading system of size, as shown in Figure 20.61. Inspection of the palate is also important in assessing patients with tonsillopharyngitis, as lesions characteristic of particular pathogens are often present on the soft palate and tonsillar pillars (see Fig. 20.62B and Chapter 12).

The tonsils appear to serve as a first line of immunologic defense against respiratory pathogens and are frequently infected by both viral and bacterial agents. The most commonly identified organisms are group A beta-hemolytic streptococci, adenoviruses, coxsackieviruses, and Epstein-Barr (EB) virus. There is a wide range of severity in symptoms and signs, regardless of the pathogenic organism. Sore throat is the major symptom and may be mild, moderate, or severe. When severe it is typically associated with dysphagia. Erythema is the most common physical finding and var-

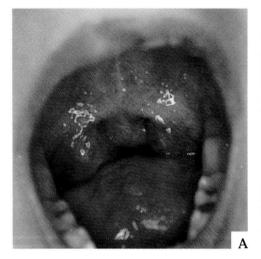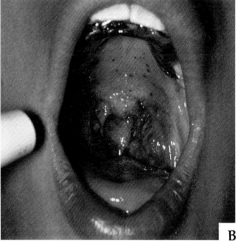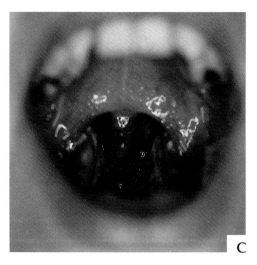

FIG. 20.62 Tonsillopharyngitis. This common syndrome has a number of causative pathogens and a wide spectrum of severity. **A** The diffuse tonsillar and pharyngeal erythema seen here is a nonspecific finding that can be produced by a variety of pathogens. **B** This intense erythema seen in association with acute tonsillar enlargement and palatal petechiae is highly suggestive of group A beta-streptococcal infection, though other pathogens can produce these findings. **C** This picture of exudative tonsillitis is most commonly seen with either group A streptococcal or EB virus infection. (**B** courtesy of Dr. Michael Sherlock)

ies from slightly to intensely red (Fig. 20.62A). Additional findings may include cervical adenopathy, acute tonsillar enlargement, and formation of exudates over the tonsillar surfaces. In a small percentage of cases the findings are highly suggestive of a given pathogen. Patients with fever; headache; bright red, enlarged tonsils (with or without exudate); palatal petechiae (Fig. 20.62B); tender and enlarged anterior cervical nodes; and perhaps abdominal pain are highly likely to have streptococcal infection. Patients with marked malaise, fever, exudative tonsillitis, generalized adenopathy, and splenomegaly are probably suffering from EB virus mononucleosis (Fig. 20.62C and Chapter 12). Those with conjunctivitis, nonexudative tonsillar inflammation, and cervical adenopathy may have adenovirus. Presence of yellow ulcerations with red halos on the tonsillar pillars is highly suggestive of coxsackievirus infection whether or not other oral, palmar, or plantar lesions are present. Unfortunately, the majority of patients with tonsillopharyngitis do not present with such clear-cut clinical syndromes. Patients with streptococcal infection may have only minimal erythema; in its early stages, mononucleosis may consist of fever, malaise, and nonexudative pharyngitis without other signs; and while streptococci and EB virus are the most common sources of exudative tonsillitis and palatal petechiae, other pathogens can produce these findings as well.

Because of the variability in the clinical picture and the importance of identifying and treating group A beta-streptococcal infection to prevent both pyogenic (such as cervical adenitis, peritonsillar and retropharyngeal abscesses) and nonpyogenic (rheumatic fever) complications, a screening throat culture is advisable for patients presenting with signs and symptoms of tonsillopharyngitis. In obtaining this culture both tonsils and the posterior pharyngeal wall should be swabbed to maximize the chance of obtaining the organism. In the first 3 years of life, when streptococcal infection is suspected, it is helpful to obtain a nasopharyngeal (NP) culture as well. For reasons as yet unclear, the NP culture will often be positive while the throat culture is negative in this age group.

Treatment is symptomatic for all forms of tonsillopharyngitis except that due to group A beta-streptococci, which requires a 10-day course of penicillin or erythromycin. Follow-up is also important. As noted earlier, the tonsillitis of mononucleosis may appear mild early in the course of the illness, yet tonsillar inflammation and enlargement may progress over a few to several days to produce severe dysphagia and even airway obstruction. Thus, mothers should be instructed to notify the physician if such signs develop. Follow-up is also important in monitoring for other complications and for frequent recurrences.

RECURRENT TONSILLITIS

Frequent recurrences of tonsillitis despite antibiotic therapy, when indicated, must be handled on an individual basis. In some cases, frequent recurrences of streptococcal infection can be traced to another family member or members. When they are treated along with the patient, the cycle of recurrences often ends. In other instances, frequent recurrent tonsillar infections have no traceable source within the family and are significantly debilitating. In children with six or more episodes per year, tonsillectomy does have a favorable outcome in reducing both frequency and severity of sore throats.

UVULITIS

Uvulitis is characterized by inflammation and edema of the uvula. Affected patients commonly complain of a sense of "something in their throat," or a gagging sensation. The phenomenon has been reported in association with pharyngitis due to the group A beta-hemolytic streptococcus, in which cases the uvula was bright red and often hemorrhagic. We

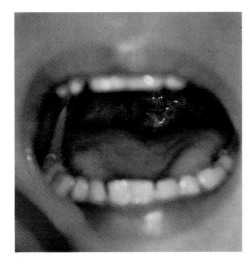

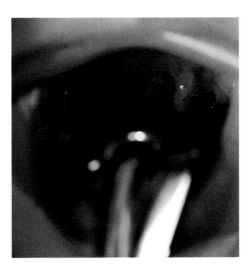

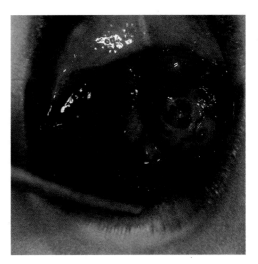

FIG. 20.63 Uvulitis. The uvula appears markedly erythematous and edematous.

FIG. 20.64 Peritonsillar abscess. This photograph, taken in the operating room, shows an intensely inflamed soft palatal mass that obscures the tonsil and bulges forward and toward the midline, deviating the uvula.

FIG. 20.65 Tonsillar lymphoma. This adolescent presented with painless dysphagia and on examination was found to have marked unilateral tonsillar enlargement. The asymmetry and degree of enlargement prompted tonsillectomy. Pathologic examination confirmed a tonsillar lymphoma.

have also noted the condition in association with mononucleosis, both in the presence of and in the absence of exudative tonsillitis (Fig. 20.63). Uvulitis has also been reported in a patient with concurrent epiglottitis. In this case the child was anxious, toxic, had high fever, and was drooling, a more severe clinical picture than that seen with streptococcal or EB virus infection. Culture of the uvular surface grew *Hemophilus influenzae*, type B.

PERITONSILLAR ABSCESS

A peritonsillar abscess is actually an abscess which not only surrounds the tonsil but also extends onto the soft palate. Patients are usually school age or older and typically have a history of an antecedent sore throat a week or two earlier. This either was not cultured or treated, or the patient took an incomplete course of antimicrobial therapy (suggesting this as a pyogenic complication of untreated or undertreated bacterial pharyngitis). The patient may subsequently improve, then experiences sudden onset of high fever and severe throat pain worse on one side. The pain usually radiates to the ipsilateral ear and is associated with marked dysphagia, such that the patient spits out his saliva to avoid swallowing. On examination the child often appears toxic and has obvious enlargement of the ipsilateral tonsillar node, which is exquisitely tender. Many patients have torticollis, tilting the head toward the involved side to minimize pressure of the sternocleidomastoid over the inflamed node. Speech is thick and muffled, and trismus is often noted as a result of sympathetic inflammation of the adjacent pterygoid muscles. If visualization of the pharynx is possible (despite the trismus), a bright red, smooth mass is seen in the supratonsillar area projecting forward and medially, obscuring the tonsil, and deviating the uvula to the opposite side (Fig. 20.64). Group A beta-streptococci and *Staphylococcus aureus* are the most common pathogens. Patients with mononucleosis,

concurrently infected with group A strep and treated with steroids, have been reported to be at risk for a rapidly evolving peritonsillar abscess as well.

If the abscess has matured and become fluctuant, operative drainage is needed in addition to parenteral antibiotic therapy to prevent spontaneous rupture and secondary aspiration. When fluctuance is not present and the patient is in a cellulitic stage, management consists of intravenous antimicrobial therapy and serial reexamination. Because of the risks of rupture, prompt otolaryngologic consultation is suggested from the outset.

TONSILLAR LYMPHOMA

The vast majority of children, whether well or acutely ill with tonsillitis, have tonsils that are symmetrical in size. When a child is found to have an asymmetrically enlarged tonsil without evidence of infection, the possibility of a lymphoma should be considered (Fig. 20.65). Thorough history of recent health, and meticulous regional and general examination are in order. Particular attention should be paid to cervical and other nodes, and to the size and consistency of abdominal viscera. Hematologic studies may be helpful as well. In the absence of other evidence, a brief period of observation may be justified. If other findings are suggestive, or enlargement continues during observation, excisional biopsy is indicated.

Penetrating Oropharyngeal Trauma

Penetrating oral injuries are fairly frequent in childhood and are usually the result of falling with a stick, pencil, or lollipop in the mouth, or of the child fooling around with such an object and inadvertently stabbing himself. Gunshot wounds and external stab wounds are unusual sources in the pediatric population, but begin to increase in incidence in adolescents.

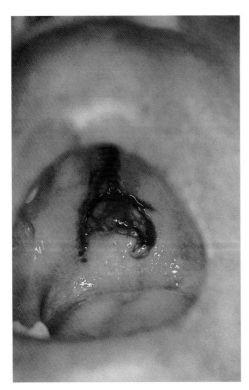

FIG. 20.66 Palatal laceration. This large, complex laceration resulted when this boy fell with a piece of metal tubing in the mouth. A flap of palatal tissue has retracted away from the tears. Surgical approximation was required.

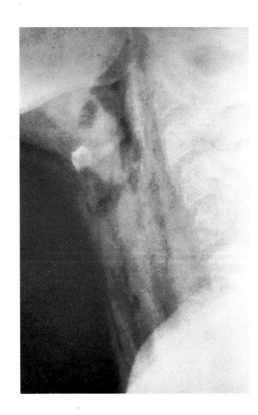

FIG. 20.67 Retropharyngeal air dissection. This lateral neck radiograph of a child with a puncture wound of the posterior pharyngeal wall reveals extensive air dissection through the retropharyngeal soft tissues. Subcutaneous air has tracked anteriorly as well.

CLINICAL FEATURES OF ACUTE UPPER AIRWAY DISORDERS

	Supraglottic Disorders	Subglottic Disorders
Stridor	Quiet and wet	Loud
Voice alteration	Muffled	Hoarse
Dysphagia	+	−
Postural preference*	+	−
Barky cough	−	+ especially with croup
Fever	+	+ usually in croup
Toxicity	+	−
Trismus	+ usually in peritonsillar abscess	−
Facial edema	−	+ usually with angioedema

*Epiglottitis—patient characteristically sits bolt upright, with neck extended and head held forward; retropharyngeal abscess—child often adopts opisthotonic posture; peritonsillar abscess—patient may tilt head toward affected side.

FIG. 20.68 Clinical features of acute upper airway disorders. (From Davis et al, 1981)

The majority of intraoral injuries involve the palate and consist of simple lacerations. Many of these heal spontaneously and require no repair. Large lacerations producing mucosal flaps must be sutured (Fig. 20.66). Prophylactic penicillin is also indicated, because of the high risk of secondary infection.

Penetration of the posterior pharyngeal wall may result in a number of complications. Therefore, these patients merit careful clinical evaluation of the oropharynx and neck, and neck radiographs should be obtained. When the child has presented promptly with a simple tear and no evidence of secondary problems, he can usually be followed closely at home on penicillin prophylaxis. Findings indicative of complications and certain high-risk lesions necessitate more conservative management.

Whenever an object penetrates the pharyngeal wall, it introduces oral flora into the retropharyngeal soft tissues, setting the stage for development of infection and abscess formation (see section on Retropharyngeal Abscess). This complication is seen predominantly in patients who failed to seek care immediately following the injury and who thus were not placed on antimicrobial prophylaxis. However, it can develop even in treated patients. Symptoms generally begin a few to several days following the initial trauma. Fever, pain, dysphagia, and signs of airway compromise predominate (see Fig. 20.70).

In a number of patients with posterior pharyngeal tears, penetration results in dissection of air through the retropharyngeal soft tissues (Fig. 20.67). Such children may complain of throat and neck pain. Subcutaneous emphysema may be noted clinically. Occasionally, signs of airway compromise develop with this complication. Therefore, hospitalization for observation is advisable when this sequela is encountered.

When penetration involves posterolateral structures (e.g., the tear is located near the tonsil or tonsillar pillar), the possi-

	Mild	Moderate	Severe
Color	Normal	Normal	Pale, dusky or cyanotic
Retractions	Absent to mild	Moderate	Severe and generalized with use of accessory muscles
Air entry	Mild ↓	Moderate ↓	Severe ↓
State of consciousness	Normal or restless when disturbed	Anxious, restless when undisturbed	Lethargic, depressed

FIG. 20.69 Estimation of severity of respiratory distress. (From Davis et al, 1981)

bility of vascular injury must be considered. Deep penetration in this area can puncture or nick the internal carotid artery or nearby vessels, resulting in hemorrhage or more commonly in gradual hematoma formation. Clues to vascular injury are lateral pharyngeal or peritonsillar swelling and fullness and/or tenderness on palpation of the neck on the side of the wound. X-rays should confirm soft-tissue swelling. Patients with peritonsillar tears generally should be admitted for observation even in the absence of these signs. Those with findings suggestive of vascular involvement warrant angiography.

UPPER AIRWAY OBSTRUCTION

Acute Upper Airway Obstruction

Few conditions in pediatrics are as emergent and potentially life-threatening as those causing acute upper airway obstruction. In these conditions expeditious assessment and appropriate stabilization are often lifesaving. In contrast, underestimation of severity of distress, overzealous attempts at examination or invasive procedures, and efforts by the unskilled to intervene may have catastrophic results.

The major causes are severe tonsillitis with adenoidal enlargement (see section on Tonsillar Disorders), retropharyngeal abscess, epiglottitis, croup or laryngotracheobronchitis, foreign body aspiration, and angioedema (see Chapter 4 for obstruction due to angioedema). All are characterized by stridor and retractions that are primarily suprasternal and subcostal (unless distress becomes severe and retractions generalize), and mild to moderate increases in heart rate and respiratory rate. For purposes of assessment we have found it helpful to classify the disorders into two categories—supraglottic and subglottic—based on major signs and symptoms listed in Figure 20.68.

The key to appropriate management is a brief history detailing the course and associated symptoms, followed by rapid assessment of clinical signs to determine the approximate level of involvement and degree of respiratory distress (Fig. 20.69). This can be done for the most part by visual inspection, without ever touching the patient. It is particularly important to avoid upsetting a child with upper airway obstruction who shows signs of fatigue, cyanosis, or meets any of the other criteria for severe distress. Such disturbances

can only serve to worsen distress and may precipitate complete obstruction. Therefore, when a child has signs of moderately severe or severe obstruction, his parents should be allowed to remain with him, positional preference (if present) should be honored, and oral examination, venipuncture, IVs, and X-rays should be deferred until the airway is secure. Once assessment is done, the most skilled personnel available are assembled to stabilize the airway. This procedure is best accomplished under controlled conditions in the operating room.

RETROPHARYNGEAL ABSCESS

A retropharyngeal abscess usually involves one of the retropharyngeal lymph nodes which run in chains through the retropharyngeal tissues on either side of the midline. Since these nodes tend to atrophy after 4 years of age, the disorder is seen primarily in children under 3 or 4 years. The major causative organisms are group A beta-streptococci, although *Staphylococcus aureus* is found in some cases. The child generally has a history of an acute febrile upper respiratory infection or pharyngitis beginning several days earlier, which may have improved transiently. Suddenly his condition worsens with development of high spiking fever, toxicity, anorexia, drooling, and dyspnea. On examination the patient is restless and irritable and tends to lie with his head hyperextended, simulating opisthotonus. Quiet gurgling stridor is heard. If respiratory distress is not severe, the pharynx can be examined and a firey red asymmetrical swelling of the posterior pharyngeal wall may be observed (Fig. 20.70A). Even with direct examination, this can be difficult to appreciate at times. A portable lateral neck X-ray (with a physician in attendance) taken on inspiration will show marked widening of the prevertebral tissues (Fig. 20.70B), which normally are no wider than the width of a vertebral body. When diagnosed, prompt otolaryngologic consultation should be sought to determine if the mass is fluctuant, necessitating surgical drainage, or is in an early cellulitic phase requiring serial reexamination. A CT scan can be helpful in this regard (Fig. 20.70C). High-dose intravenous antimicrobial therapy is needed whether or not drainage is necessary.

As noted earlier, a retropharyngeal abscess may occasionally form in an older child following a puncture wound of the posterior pharyngeal wall. Signs of infection develop acutely a few days later. Oral flora are found on culture.

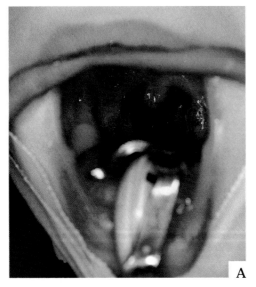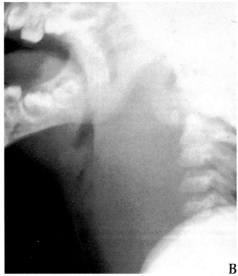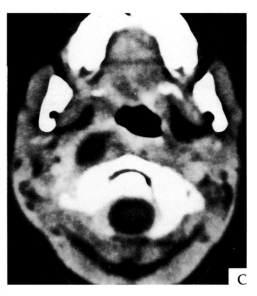

A   B   C

*FIG. 20.70 Retropharyngeal abscess. This young child presented with high fever, drooling, quiet stridor, and an opisthotonic postural preference. **A** Pharyngeal examination, in the operating room, reveals an intensely erythematous unilateral swelling of the posterior pharyngeal wall. **B** A lateral neck radiograph shows prominent prevertebral swelling displacing the trachea forward. **C** On CT scan a thick-walled abscess cavity is evident in the retropharyngeal space. The highly vascular wall enhanced with contrast injection.*

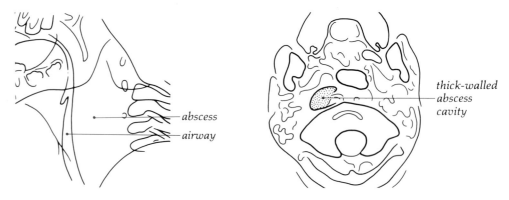

PARAPHARYNGEAL ABSCESS

Lateral neck space abscesses can also occur in infants and young children. Most are toxic with high spiking fevers. The history and clinical picture are nearly identical to that of children with retropharyngeal abscess. However, these patients will have torticollis, bending toward the affected side, and examination of the neck reveals diffuse anterolateral swelling which is exquisitely tender. Oral inspection may show medial displacement of the tonsil or lateral pharyngeal wall. A CT scan is essential to confirm the diagnosis. Prompt drainage is important to prevent extension into the mediastinum.

EPIGLOTTITIS

Epiglottitis is an infection caused by *Hemophilus influenzae* type B which is characterized by marked inflammation and edema of the pharynx, epiglottis, aryepiglottic folds, and ventricular bands. The peak age range is 2 to 7 years, but infants and older children may be affected. Onset is sudden and progression rapid, most patients being brought to medical attention within 12 hours of the first appearance of symptoms. Generally the child was entirely well until several hours prior to presentation, when he abruptly spiked a high fever. This was rapidly followed by severe throat pain with dysphagia and drooling, and soon thereafter by dyspnea and anxiety. On examination the child is usually toxic, anxious, and remarkably still, sitting bolt upright with neck extended and head held forward (unless obstruction is very mild or fatigue has supervened) (Fig. 20.71A–C). Quiet gurgling, stridor, and drooling are evident along with dyspnea and retractions. If the child will talk, which is unusual, his voice is muffled. This clinical picture is so typical that when seen, the best course of action following initial assessment is prompt airway stabilization, usually intubation under controlled conditions by experienced personnel in the operating room. At this time the epiglottis will be found to be markedly swollen and erythematous (Fig. 20.71). Following airway stabilization, cultures can be obtained and intravenous antimicrobial therapy initiated.

On occasion children present with a similar history but milder symptoms and signs. In these cases presentation is either very early, or the child is older than average. Respiratory distress is minimal, and visualization of the pharynx can be attempted (without use of a tongue blade) if the child will voluntarily open his mouth. In some instances a swollen epiglottis is seen projecting above the tongue. Where the history suggests epiglottitis but clinical findings are mild and the diagnosis is not confirmed by attempted noninvasive visualization, a portable lateral neck X-ray (done in the emergency room with physician in attendance) can be useful. It may reveal epiglottic enlargement (Fig. 20.72) or merely swelling of

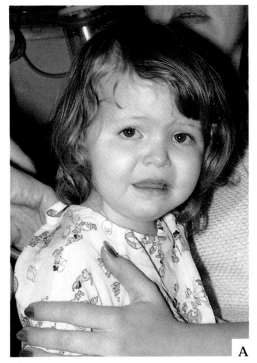

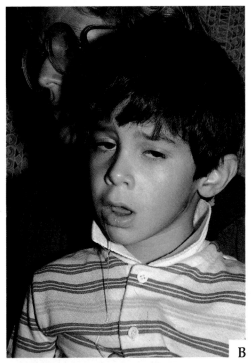

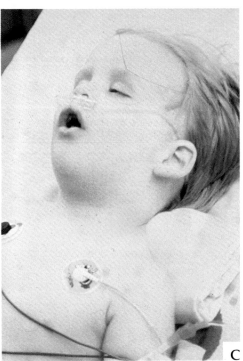

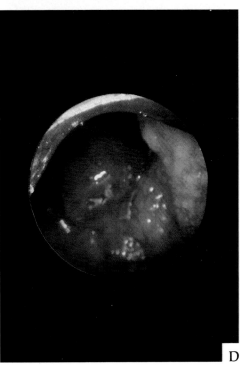

FIG. 20.71 Epiglottitis. **A—C** These three patients with acute epiglottitis demonstrate the varying degrees of distress that may be seen depending on age and time of presentation. **A** This 3-year-old seen a few hours after onset of symptoms was anxious and still, but had no positional preference or drooling. **B** This 5-year-old who had been symptomatic for several hours holds his neck extended head-forward, is mouth-breathing, drooling, and shows signs of tiring. **C** This 2-year-old was in severe distress and was too exhausted to hold his head up. **D** In the operating room the epiglottis can be visualized and appears intensely red and swollen.

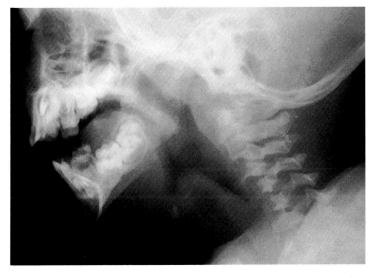

FIG. 20.72 Mild epiglottitis/supraglottitis. This lateral neck radiograph demonstrates mild epiglottic swelling and thickening of the aryepiglottic folds.

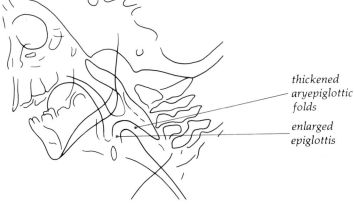

thickened
aryepiglottic
folds

enlarged
epiglottis

CROUP SCORING SYSTEM

	0	1	2	3
Stridor	None	Mild	Moderate at rest	Severe, on inspiration and expiration, or none with markedly decreased air entry
Retraction	None	Mild	Moderate	Severe, marked use of accessory muscles
Air entry	Normal	Mild decrease	Moderate decrease	Marked decrease
Color	Normal	Normal (0 score)	Normal (0 score)	Dusky or cyanotic
Level of consciousness	Normal	Restless when disturbed	Anxious, agitated; restless when undisturbed	Lethargic, depressed

FIG. 20.73 Croup scoring system. (Modified from Taussig et al: Treatment of laryngotracheobronchitis (croup): Use of intermittent positive pressure breathing and racemic epinephrine. Am J Dis Child 129:790, 1975)

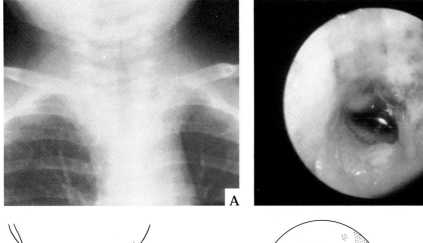

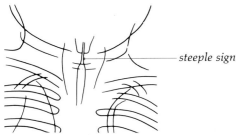
steeple sign

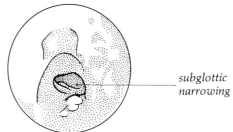
subglottic narrowing

FIG. 20.74 Croup. **A** This radiograph reveals a long area of narrowing extending well below the normally narrowed area at the level of the vocal cords. The finding is often termed the "steeple sign." **B** In this patient direct visualization revealed subglottic narrowing that was so severe, only tracheostomy would enable establishment of an adequate airway.

the aryepiglottic folds and ventricular bands: *supraglottitis.* If either is found, the diagnosis is confirmed. Intubation is generally advisable in the former instance despite mild symptoms, but close observation on intravenous antibiotic therapy (covering for *H. influenzae*) may suffice when supraglottitis is the only finding.

CROUP OR LARYNGOTRACHEOBRONCHITIS
This acute respiratory illness is characterized by inflammation and edema of the pharynx and upper airways with maximal narrowing in the immediate subglottic region. There is probably a component of laryngospasm as well. The vast majority of cases are caused by viral pathogens, with parainfluenza, respiratory syncitial virus, adenoviruses, influenza viruses, and Echoviruses the agents most commonly identified. The peak season is between October and April in the northern hemisphere. The disorder affects children between the ages of 3 months and 3 years primarily. This is probably because their airway is narrower, and its mucosa is both more vascular and more loosely attached than in older children, enabling greater ease of edema collection. Older children can be affected, however.

Typically the child has had symptoms of a mild upper respiratory infection with rhinorrhea, cough, low-grade fever, and perhaps a sore throat for 1 to 5 days prior to developing symptoms of croup. The change is generally sudden and usually occurs at night. The child awakens with fever, loud inspiratory or inspiratory and expiratory stridor, a loud "barky" or "seal-like" cough, and hoarseness. The severity of symptoms and the course vary widely and are highly unpredictable. Duration averages 3 days but can be as brief as 1 day or as long as a week. Most patients have a waxing and waning course with symptoms more severe at night, but it is impossible to predict which night will be the worst. Some pa-

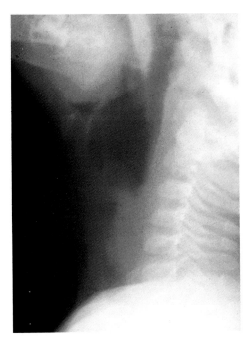

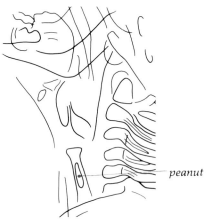

peanut

FIG. 20.75 Foreign body aspiration into the trachea. In this child who presented with a croup-like picture consisting of loud stridor, cough, and severe respiratory distress, a history of a choking spell while eating peanuts was obtained. His lateral neck radiograph reveals an ovoid foreign object lodged in the subglottic area. An intact peanut was removed at bronchoscopy.

Management is dependent largely on severity of distress when seen, and on clinical response to mist therapy. Most patients have mild disease, improve considerably on mist alone, and can be managed at home with humidification. Parents must, however, be instructed to watch for signs of increasing distress which would warrant return to the hospital. Aerosolized racemic epinephrine has been proven to be effective in reducing airway obstruction due to croup. It is particularly useful for children with moderate obstruction who do not show marked improvement on mist alone, and can provide significant relief for children with severe distress. This agent, though effective, is short-acting and rebound tends to occur. Thus, patients requiring racemic epinephrine should generally be admitted for further observation. The effectiveness of steroids is as yet unproved. While numerous studies have been done, some suggesting their efficacy, design flaws make it impossible to draw firm conclusions. Patients with severe distress who do not improve dramatically following treatment with racemic epinephrine and patients who steadily worsen in the hospital warrant airway stabilization, either via intubation or tracheostomy under controlled conditions. The choice of procedure remains controversial and is perhaps best made in accordance with the skills of personnel and facilities available at the individual institution. In some instances narrowing is so severe as to necessitate tracheostomy (Fig. 20.74B). Attempts at emergency tracheostomy are fraught with hazard and should be avoided at all costs.

BACTERIAL TRACHEITIS

In a small percentage of cases, children presenting with a croup-like picture are atypically toxic, markedly febrile, and have rapidly progressive airway obstruction necessitating urgent intubation and frequent suctioning. Bronchoscopy prior to airway stabilization reveals severe inflammation and edema, and a purulent subglottic exudate which contains large numbers of bacteria. Most of these patients appear to have a history of viral croup with sudden worsening. It is thus thought that the disorder may represent secondary bacterial infection. However, there is still some question that this disorder may represent an unusually virulent form of viral laryngotracheobronchitis.

FOREIGN BODY ASPIRATION

This problem is seen for the most part in older infants and toddlers. The story is usually one of a sudden choking episode while eating material that their immature dentition is ill equipped to chew. Such foods include nuts, seeds, raw vegetables such as carrots and celery, and hot dogs. Occasionally the episode occurs when the child is chewing on a small object, a toy or a detachable portion of a toy. If the object lodges in the larynx, asphyxiation results unless the Heimlich maneuver or backslaps are performed promptly. In the majority of cases the foreign material clears the larynx and lodges in the trachea or a bronchus. Following the choking spell, there is a silent period of a few to several hours, after which the child develops cough and either stridor (lodged in trachea) or wheezing (lodged in a bronchus), and respiratory distress. In this acute phase when the object is situated in a bronchus, wheezing may be unilateral and associated with decreased breath sounds. Later, diffuse wheezing may be heard simulating asthma or bronchiolitis. Lateral neck radiography occasionally reveals objects lodged in the upper airway (Fig. 20.75). Chest fluoroscopy may show differential

tients remain relatively mild throughout their course, while others progress either slowly or rapidly to severe distress. Airway drying, probably in part as a result of mouth breathing necessitated by nasal congestion, appears to aggravate the cough and possibly the element of laryngospasm.

Physical findings are highly variable depending on degree of distress at the time of presentation. Most affected children are moderately febrile but not toxic, and have a loud barky cough and loud inspiratory stridor, with suprasternal and subcostal retractions, and a mild decrease in air entry. A small percentage of patients with more extensive airway inflammation may have wheezing on auscultation. Many have improved substantially as a result of exposure to cool night air during the trip to the ER. Some have restlessness or agitation reflecting hypoxia, and a few have severe distress. In these more severely affected patients, stridor may be both inspiratory and expiratory with generalized retractions. If impairment of air flow is extreme, fatigue supervenes, stridor abates, and retractions diminish. This must not be mistaken for clinical improvement. A clinical scoring system which helps in grading severity of distress is presented in Figure 20.73. In mild to moderate cases, the pharynx can be visualized and reveals only mild erythema. Oral examination should be deferred in severe cases until the airway is secure. Radiography can be helpful in demonstrating subglottic narrowing—the "steeple sign" (Fig. 20.74A).

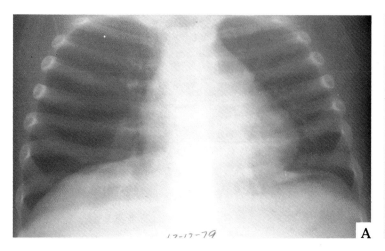 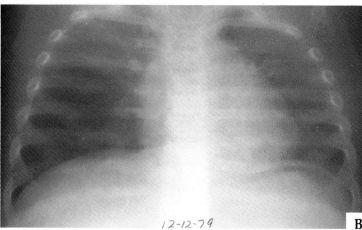

FIG. 20.76 Foreign body aspiration into a bronchus. This 14-month-old presented with a persistent cough about 12 hours after choking on a piece of walnut. He had decreased breath sounds and wheezing on the right side. **A** An inspiratory chest X-ray suggests hyperinflation of the right lung. **B** The expiratory film shows a decrease in volume of the left lung and right upper lobe but no change in volume of the right lower and middle lobes. Fluoroscopy revealed mediastinal shift to the left on expiration and decreased movement of the right diaphram. At bronchoscopy a walnut fragment was removed from the mid-segment of the right mainstem bronchus. (Courtesy of Dr. J. L. Medina, Children's Hospital of Pittsburgh)

lung inflation and deflation if aspiration is recent and the foreign material is located in a bronchus (Fig. 20.76). When suspicion is raised, endoscopic examination of the airway is indicated.

Unfortunately, in up to 50 percent of cases the aspiration episode is not reported, either because the parent does not relate it to the child's symptoms or did not witness the choking spell. For this reason this diagnosis should be considered and specific questions asked regarding possible aspiration whenever a young child presents with acute onset of cough and stridor or a first episode of wheezing.

Chronic Upper Airway Obstruction

SUBGLOTTIC STENOSIS

This is a disorder in which the subglottic region of the trachea is unusually narrow in the absence of infection. In some instances the stenosis is the result of abnormal cricoid development and is therefore congenital. In other cases narrowing is the long-term result of injury and scarring from prior intubation. Regardless of source, these children tend to develop stridor and respiratory distress with every upper respiratory infection. A few are identified by virtue of having an atypically prolonged episode of croup. Some also have stridor with crying, even when well. Neck X-rays present a similar appearance to that seen with croup. The problem generally improves with growth, but a few of these children develop such severe distress with colds that tracheostomy is required.

JUVENILE LARYNGEAL PAPILLOMATOSIS

This is a condition in which multiple benign papillomas develop and grow on the vocal cords. In a few patients they may extend to involve the pharyngeal walls or tracheal mucosa. They are apparently of viral origin, and there is some evidence of transmission during delivery to children born to mothers with condyloma accuminata. The main symptom is hoarseness, but stridor may develop in children with large lesions or tracheal extension. Radiographs are usually normal. The diagnosis should be considered in patients with chronic hoarseness and in those with atypically prolonged croup. At laryngoscopy, irregular warty masses are seen (Fig. 20.77). Biopsy is required to confirm the diagnosis. Excision can be attempted using forceps or a laser, but is often followed by regrowth. Tracheostomy should be avoided if at all possible, as this often promotes seeding further down the tracheobronchial tree.

ESOPHAGEAL FOREIGN BODIES

Ingestion of foreign objects is relatively common in older infants and toddlers, who are prone to putting almost anything they can pick up into their mouths. Coins, small toys, and pieces of toys are the objects most frequently found. Most traverse the esophagus, stomach, and intestines without incident and are of little concern. When the object carries a risk of toxicity such as a lead pellet or a battery, endoscopic removal is required. A small percentage of swallowed foreign bodies become lodged in the esophagus, being too large to pass through to the stomach. With mild obstruction the child may refuse solid foods; with moderate obstruction liquids will often be refused as well, or the child may appear to choke with drinking. When the lumen is completely obstructed, the child may present with drooling. If the object is particularly large it may compress the trachea as well, producing signs of upper airway obstruction. Because of the young age of most of these patients, it is difficult to determine if pain is associated.

While in many cases there is a clear history of ingestion, in a significant percentage the ingestion was not witnessed. A high level of suspicion is often required to make the diagnosis, and the possibility of an esophageal foreign body should be considered in evaluating any young child for a sudden change in eating pattern. Plain radiographs will detect metallic and other radiopaque objects (Fig. 20.78). Most objects are plastic, however, and require barium swallow or in some cases endoscopy for detection. Delays in diagnosis can result in stricture formation or, more rarely, in esophageal perforation with secondary mediastinitis, and/or large vessel hemorrhage.

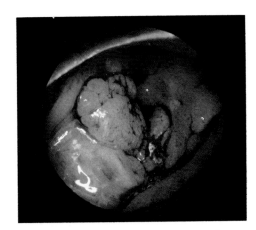

FIG. 20.77 Laryngeal papillomas. Multiple smooth warty growths are seen nearly occluding the larynx in this child who had a history of chronic hoarseness.

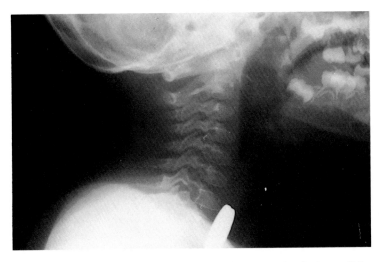

FIG. 20.78 Esophageal foreign body. A history of refusing solid foods following a choking spell prompted radiographic examination. AP radiograph showed what appeared to be a quarter lodged in the esophagus, but this lateral view reveals two coins superimposed.

NOTE

Neck disorders including adenitis, congenital cysts, vascular and lymphatic masses and tumors are commonly managed by otolaryngologists. Limitations of space have required us to be selective in presenting disorders in this chapter. The reader is referred to Chapter 12 for a discussion of cervical adenitis, and to Chapter 15 for a description of mass lesions.

BIBLIOGRAPHY

Bluestone CD, Stool SE (eds): Pediatric Otolaryngology. Saunders, Philadelphia, 1983

Bluestone CD: Recent advances in the pathogenesis, diagnosis, and management of otitis media. Pediatr Clin N Amer 28:727–755, 1981.

Bowen A'D, Ledesma-Medina J, Fujioka M, et al.: Radiologic imaging in otorhinolaryngology. Pediatr Clin N Amer 28:905–939, 1981.

Davis HW, Gartner JC, Galvis AG, et al.: Acute upper airway obstruction: Croup and epiglottitis. Pediatr Clin N Amer 28:859–880, 1981.

Gellady AM, Shulman ST, Ayoub EM: Periorbital and orbital cellulitis in children. Pediatrics 61:272–277, 1978.

McGuirt WF (ed): Pediatric Otolaryngology Case Studies. Medical Examination Publishing Company, Garden City, New York, 1980.

Wald ER: Acute sinusitis in children. Pediatr Inf Dis 2:61–68, 1983.

Wald ER, Milmoe GJ, Bowen A'D, et al.: Acute maxillary sinusitis in children. N Engl J Med 304:749–754, 1981.

INDEX

Facies
in allergic rhinitis, 4.3–4.4, **4.4–4.9**
in Cushing syndrome, 9.9, **9.15**
in DiGeorge syndrome, 4.18, **4.38**
in Down syndrome, **1.14**
in failure to thrive in infancy, 6.12, **6.24**
in hyper-IgE syndrome, 4.19, **4.43**
in large-for-gestational age infant of diabetic mother, **2.15**
in Potter syndrome, 13.4, **13.12**
in scleroderma, 7.12, **7.28**
in trisomy 13, **1.21**
in Williams syndrome, 5.4, **5.9**
Factor VIII deficiency, 11.21
Factor IX deficiency, 11.21
Failure to thrive in infancy, 6.12, 6.13, **6.24**
Fallot tetralogy, 5.6–5.7, **5.17–5.19**
Fanconi syndrome, 11.20, **11.63**, 13.11
Farsightedness, 17.2, **17.3**
Fasciitis, necrotizing, 12.28–12.29, **12.48**
Fascioscapulohumeral dystrophy, clinical features of, **14.30**
Fat necrosis from forceps trauma, 2.7, **2.20**
Fecalith, appendiceal, 10.8, **10.19**, 15.23, **15.65**
Felty syndrome, 7.4
Female genitalia, normal, 16.1–16.2, **16.1–16.3**
Female karyotype, normal, 1.1
Feminization, testicular, 9.12
Femoral hernia, 15.30, **15.87**
Femur, disorders of. *See* Hip
Fencer position in asymmetric tonic neck reflex, 3.1, **3.2**
in cerebral palsy, 3.7
Fibroplasia, retrolental, 17.18–17.19, **17.74**
Fibrosis
cystic, 4.12, 10.11, **10.27–10.29**. *See also* Cystic fibrosis
hepatic, congenital, 10.13, **10.36–10.37**
Fifth disease, 12.6, **12.12**
Fissure-in-ano, 15.20, **15.56**
Fistula
branchial arch, 15.2, 15.4, **15.10**
rectourethral, 15.18, **15.54**
rectovaginal, 15.18, **15.53**, 16.13
tracheoesophageal, 15.10, **15.31–15.32**
urachal, 15.27
vesicovaginal, 16.13
Fitz-Hugh-Curtis syndrome, 16.23–16.24
Flatfeet, 19.37, **19.77**
Fluorescence under Wood's light, 8.3
Folate deficiency, megaloblastic anemia in, 11.7, 11.8
Follicles
conjunctival, 17.11, **17.37**
hair, 8.1, **8.1**
Follicle-stimulating hormone, 9.1
feedback regulation of, 9.1, **9.2**

Folliculitis, 12.21, **12.33**
staphylococcal, differential diagnosis, 8.4
vulvar, 16.16
Foot
accessory tarsal navicular, 19.38, **19.78**
calcaneovalgus deformity, 19.37, **19.76**
cavus deformity, 19.39, **19.80**
in Charcot-Marie-Tooth disease, 14.14
claw toes, 19.39, **19.81**
clubbing of toes in heart disease, 5.2, **5.4**
clubfoot, **1.13**, 19.33, **19.72**
creases in sole, 2.2, **2.6**
digital anomalies, 2.8–2.9, **2.25–2.26**
ganglion of, 19.38, **19.79**
metatarsus adductus, 19.35, **19.73**
metatarsus primus varus, 19.36, **19.74**
pes planus, 19.37, **19.77**
toe spacing in Down syndrome, **1.14**
in trisomy 13, **1.21**
in trisomy 18, **1.22**
in Turner syndrome, **1.23**
vertical talus, congenital, 19.36–19.37, **19.75**
warts, plantar, 8.20, **8.75**
Foramen of Morgagni, hernia through, 15.8, **15.27**
Forceps delivery, trauma from, 2.7
Foreign bodies
aspiration of, 4.12, 20.37–20.38, **20.75–20.76**
ear, 20.4–20.5, 20.8, **20.19**
esophageal, 20.38, **20.78**
nasal, 20.16, **20.40**
vaginal, 16.13
Forscheimer spots in rubella, 12.3, **12.5**
Fractures, 19.2–19.13
as abusive injuries, 6.5–6.6, **6.15**
analgesia in, 19.3, 19.13
articular, 19.12, **19.16**, 19.20, **19.29**, **19.30**
avulsion, tibial, 19.16, **19.39**
bowing, **19.6**, **19.14**
classification by anatomic location, **19.16–19.25**, **19.29–19.30**
comminuted, 19.5, **19.6**, **19.12**
diagnosis, 19.2–19.5
diaphyseal, **19.16**, **19.17**
dislocations with, 19.13–19.15, **19.33**
epicondylar, **19.16**, **19.24**
epiphyseal, 19.9–19.13, **19.16**, **19.19**
greenstick, 19.5, **19.6**, **19.14**
impacted, 19.5, **19.6**, **19.11**
intercondylar, **19.16**, **19.20**
longitudinal, **19.6**, **19.7**
metaphyseal, **19.16**, **19.18**
Monteggia, 19.15, **19.37**
nasal, 20.17–20.18, **20.43–20.45**

oblique, 19.5, **19.6**, **19.9**
in osteogenesis imperfecta, 19.40, **19.83**
patterns of, 19.5, **19.6**
physeal, 19.9–19.13, **19.16**, **19.21**
position of extremity in, 19.3, **19.3**
radiography in, 19.5, **19.7–19.15**
Salter-Harris, 19.11–19.12
type I, 19.11, **19.27**
type II, 19.11, **19.28**
type III, 19.11, **19.19**, **19.21**, **19.29**
type IV, 19.12, **19.30**
type V, 19.12, **19.31**
spiral, 19.5, **19.6**, **19.10**
subcapital, **19.16**, **19.25**
supracondylar, **19.16**, **19.23**
swelling in, 19.4, **19.5**
Tillaux, **19.21**
torus, 19.5, **19.6**, **19.15**
transcondylar, **19.16**, **19.22**
transverse, 19.5, **19.6**, **19.8**
treatment principles, 19.12–19.13
Francisella tularensis, adenitis from, 12.36
Frenula, oral, abnormalities of, 18.4, **18.13–18.15**
Friedreich ataxia, cardiovascular findings in, **5.10**
Frontal sinus, 20.20, **20.49**
sinusitis, 20.21, 20.22
Pott's puffy tumor in, 20.27, **20.56**
Fungal infections
cutaneous, 8.18–8.19, **8.66–8.69**
ear, 20.4
hair, 8.3, **8.4**
Wood's light in, 8.3
nails, 8.26
oral, 18.10, **18.42**
scalp abscess, 12.26
Funnel chest, 15.5, **15.16**
Furuncle, 12.24, **12.40**

Gait in cerebral palsy, 3.8
Galeazzi's sign in dislocation of hip, 19.27
Gallstones, 15.23, **15.66**
Galgion
foot, 19.38, **19.79**
wrist, 19.24, **19.57**
Gangrene
in necrotizing fasciitis, 12.28–12.29
testicular, from torsion, 15.31
Gardner syndrome, 10.8, 15.22
Gardnerella vaginalis infection, 16.20–16.21, **16.21**, **16.38**
Gastroenterology, 10.6–10.13
abdominal pain, 10.8
colon. *See* Colon
constipation, 10.8
cystic fibrosis, 10.11, **10.27–10.29**
diarrhea, 10.8–10.10
disorders in scleroderma, 7.12
esophagus. *See* Esophagus
hemorrhage, 10.8
liver disease, 10.11–10.13, **10.30–10.36**